Also available from the
American Academy of Pediat...

Caring for Your Baby and Young Child: Birth to Age ...

Heading Home With Your Newborn: From Bi... Reality

Mommy Calls: Dr. Tanya Answers Parents' Top 101 Questions
About Babies and Toddlers

The Wonder Years: Helping Your Baby and Young Child Successfully Negotiate
the Major Developmental Milestones

Raising Twins: From Pregnancy to Preschool

Your Baby's First Year *(English and Spanish)*

New Mother's Guide to Breastfeeding *(English and Spanish)*

Food Fights: Winning the Nutritional Challenges of Parenthood Armed With Insight,
Humor, and a Bottle of Ketchup

A Parent's Guide to Childhood Obesity: A Road Map to Health

Guide to Your Child's Nutrition

ADHD: A Complete and Authoritative Guide

Waking Up Dry: A Guide to Help Children Overcome Bedwetting

A Parent's Guide to Building Resilience in Children and Teens:
Giving Your Child Roots and Wings

Sports Success Rx! Your Child's Prescription for the Best Experience

Less Stress, More Success: A New Approach to Guiding Your Teen
Through College Admissions and Beyond

Mental Health, Naturally: The Family Guide to Holistic Care
for Healthy Minds and Bodies

Caring for Your School-Age Child: Ages 5 to 12

Caring for Your Teenager

Guide to Your Child's Allergies and Asthma

Guide to Toilet Training *(English and Spanish)*

For more information, visit www.aap.org/bookstore.

Newborn Intensive Care

What Every Parent Needs to Know

3rd Edition

Jeanette Zaichkin, RN, MN, NNP-BC

Editor in Chief

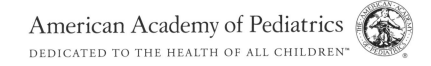

American Academy of Pediatrics

DEDICATED TO THE HEALTH OF ALL CHILDREN™

American Academy of Pediatrics Department of Marketing and Publications

Maureen DeRosa, MPA
Director, Department of Marketing and Publications

Mark Grimes
Director, Division of Product Development

Eileen Glasstetter, MS
Manager, Product Development

Carrie Peters
Editorial Assistant, Product Development

Sandi King, MS
Director, Division of Publishing and Production Services

Linda Diamond
Manager, Art Direction and Production

Kate Larson
Manager, Editorial Services

Shannan Martin
Print Production Specialist

Jill Ferguson
Director, Division of Marketing

Linda Smessaert
Manager, Clinical and Professional Publications Marketing

Bob Herling
Director, Division of Sales

Cover photography by Gigi O'Dea, memoryportraitsbygigi.com. Used by permission.

Library of Congress Control Number: 2009906425

ISBN: 978-1-58110-307-6
MA0451

The recommendations in this publication do not indicate an exclusive course of treatment or serve as a standard of medical care. Variations, taking into account individual circumstances, may be appropriate.

Products are mentioned for informational purposes only. Inclusion in this publication does not imply endorsement by the American Academy of Pediatrics.

The publishers have made every effort to trace the copyright holders for borrowed material. If they have inadvertently overlooked any, they will be pleased to make the necessary arrangements at the first opportunity.

9-216/Rep0513

Contributors

Julie M. R. Arafeh, RN, MSN
Obstetric Simulation Specialist
Center for Advanced Pediatric
    and Perinatal Education
Lucile Packard Children's Hospital
Stanford University
Palo Alto, CA
1: Expecting the Unexpected

Debbie Fraser Askin, MN, RNC-NIC
Associate Professor, Centre for Nursing
    and Health Studies
Athabasca University
Athabasca, Alberta, Canada
Neonatal Nurse Practitioner, NICU
St Boniface General Hospital
Winnipeg, Manitoba, Canada
*8: Mother-Baby Factors: Effects on
    Newborn Health*
Appendix B: Medications and Your Baby

J. Craig Jackson, MD, MHA, FAAP
NICU Medical Director, Seattle
    Children's Hospital
Professor of Pediatrics, University
    of Washington
Seattle, WA
10: Major Medical Problems

Patricia Jason, RN, BSN, CCRN
Neonatal Intensive Care Transport Nurse
Seattle Children's Hospital
Seattle, WA
2: A Different Beginning

Terrie Lockridge, MSN, RNC-NIC
Staff Nurse–Neonatal Intensive Care Unit
Swedish Medical Center
Seattle, WA
6: Parenting in the NICU

**Diane B. Longobucco, RNC-NIC, MSN,
APRN, NNP-BC**
Clinical Nurse Specialist
Maternal/Child Services
Saint Francis Hospital and Medical Center
Hartford, CT
11: Neonatal Surgery

David J. Loren, MD, FAAP
Division of Neonatology
University of Washington
Department of Pediatrics
Seattle Children's Hospital
Seattle, WA
3: NICU Players: Working With the Team

Brenda Lykins, RNC-NIC, BSN
Neonatal Outreach Coordinator
MultiCare Regional Perinatal Outreach
    Program
Tacoma, WA
4: Getting Acquainted

Denise Maguire, PhD, RN-BC, CNL
Assistant Professor
Interim Assistant Dean of Academics,
    Masters Program
Director, CNL Concentration
University of South Florida
Tampa, FL
13: When a Perfect Baby Is No More

Lori A. Markham, MSN, MBA, NNP-BC, CCRN
Program Manager, Neonatal Nurse Practitioners
Clinical Manager, Neonatal Transport Team
Seattle Children's Hospital
Seattle, WA
10: Major Medical Problems

Cindy C. Martin, MSN, RN, IBCLC, CKC
Lactation Consultant, Neonatal Intensive Care Unit Level III
Sarasota Memorial Hospital
Sarasota, FL
5: Feeding Your Baby

Karin Menghini, RN, MSN, NNP-BC
Neonatal Nurse Practitioner
St Joseph Mercy Hospital
Ann Arbor, MI
14: One Step Closer to Home: The Intermediate Care Experience
15: Homeward Bound

Katie Stiver, MSW, LICSW
Neonatal Intensive Care Unit Social Worker
Seattle Children's Hospital
Seattle, WA
7: Organizing Your Finances

Ellen Tappero, DNP, RN, NNP-BC
Director, Neonatal Nurse Practitioner Programs
Neonatology Associates, Ltd
Phoenix, AZ
12: Diagnostic and Therapeutic Techniques: Progress and Promise

Lauren Thorngate, PhD(c), RN, CCRN
Clinical Nurse Specialist, NICU
University of Washington Medical Center
Seattle, WA
6: Parenting in the NICU

Gary M. Weiner, MD, FAAP
Clinical Associate Professor
St Joseph Mercy Hospital
Ann Arbor, MI
Wayne State University
Detroit, MI
9: Problems Associated With Premature Birth

Jeanette Zaichkin, RN, MN, NNP-BC
Neonatal Outreach Coordinator
Seattle Children's Hospital
Seattle, WA
1: Expecting the Unexpected
2: A Different Beginning
5: Feeding Your Baby
Appendix C: Car Safety Seats

TrezMarie T. Zotkiewicz, RNC-NIC, MN, APRN
Maternal-Child Clinical Nurse Specialist
Child Developmental Consultant
New Orleans, LA
16: Home at Last
17: Looking Ahead

Reviewers

Robert M. Arensman, MD, FAAP

Keleen H. Arnold, LOTR

Henry H. Bernstein, DO, FAAP

Joseph Anthony Bocchini Jr, MD, FAAP

Michael Thomas Brady, MD, FAAP

Carrie Lynn Byington, MD, FAAP

Dennis R. Durbin, MD, MSCE, FAAP

Jaime Fernandez, MD, FAAP

Mary P. Glode, MD, FAAP

Jay P. Goldsmith, MD, FAAP

Karen D. Hendricks-Muñoz, MD, FAAP

Mark L. Hudak, MD, FAAP

Bonnie Kozial

Susan Landers, MD, FAAP

Karen Emmerman Mazner

H. Cody Meissner, MD, FAAP

Suhas M. Nafday, MD, FAAP

Sheri L. Nemerofsky, MD, FAAP

Angel Rios, MD, FAAP

Dedication

To parents of babies who require newborn intensive care.

Find strength in knowledge. Face challenges with teamwork.

Celebrate each step forward.

Table of Contents

Table of Contents

Foreword

The birth of a baby is one of the most rewarding, exhausting, exciting, beautiful, personal, and emotionally charged events of a lifetime. When everything proceeds perfectly, it is also one of the most joyous and satisfying experiences. But when everything does not go well—when labor is complicated or the baby is born prematurely or with a congenital malformation or an illness of one sort or another—different emotions take over. If your baby is now in an intensive care nursery, you may be feeling anxiety, confusion, sadness, guilt, anger, and even grief over the loss of the normal, healthy birth experience you had envisioned. But your primary focus is likely obtaining as much information as you can about this new situation.

You probably have a multitude of questions—for which you want concrete, simple answers. You want to know what will come next, whether your baby is suffering, and what is being done to alleviate his or her pain. But most of all, you want to know the implications and eventual outcome of your child's condition, both over the next few days and for your child's lifetime. All too frequently the answers to many of these questions are not immediately available. Despite our tremendous progress in both the science and the art of neonatology over the past 2 to 3 decades, we can seldom predict the outcome of most neonatal conditions for an individual baby until we have had the benefit of some time to watch those conditions—and the complications associated with them—evolve. But we do know a great deal about your baby's medical condition, what may come next, and what can be done to decrease pain and suffering. In fact, the amount of information is so voluminous, it is unlikely that you will be able to absorb it all during the many discussions you will have with the doctors and nurses caring for your baby. This book will help you prepare for those discussions and know what questions to ask. It will also serve to reinforce, review, and clarify the information you receive from those who are helping your baby.

Neonatal intensive care has evolved from a single physician and a single bedside nurse caring for a baby to one or more complex teams of physicians, nurses, and allied personnel working together to apply their combined expertise to deliver optimum care to your baby. Although this team approach compounds the knowledge and skills available to help your child, it can also sometimes cause confusion, particularly when you receive information about the same subject from multiple sources in different forms and from different perspectives. Remember that you are also a critical member of this team and your questions, opinions, and recommendations should be highly valuable and respected by the other members.

This book can help you make sense of your baby's complicated situation. Most of all, it can help you feel more in control, and it can show you how you can participate in the team effort to make your baby well. Although there is a considerable amount of science associated with neonatal intensive care, there is also a certain degree of art—and often several different styles of practice. Multiple possible therapies can be applied in several different ways for almost every condition. I came to know Jeanette Zaichkin through our mutual service on a committee that was organized to set national standards for neonatal resuscitation, where addressing multiple options and different styles consumed many of the discussions. It became evident during those discussions that Ms Zaichkin has a tremendous fund of knowledge and a real knack for representing multiple viewpoints—and this book, with its information coordinated from multiple authors, confirms that assessment. As you read this book, you will frequently find several possible therapies presented for a single condition. The therapies your baby is receiving are likely included, but you may also find it helpful to be knowledgeable of the other options for use in future discussions with your baby's physicians and nurses.

Ms Zaichkin and her colleagues have done a superb job of addressing complex problems and making them understandable to people with little or no medical training. And yet they have not oversimplified. Although the chapters may not have been written specifically for your baby, you will likely find that they explain the care being delivered to your baby in your neonatal intensive care unit and offer strategies for becoming a valuable partner in your baby's health care. This is a wonderful book; one I think you will find very helpful as you negotiate this emotionally challenging time in your and your baby's life.

John Kattwinkel, MD, FAAP
Charles Fuller Professor of Neonatology
University of Virginia
Charlottesville, VA

Acknowledgments

I am pleased to announce that the third edition of *Newborn Intensive Care: What Every Parent Needs to Know* starts a new life as a publication of the American Academy of Pediatrics (AAP). This edition is not only revised and updated by authors who are experts in the field of neonatology, but is now supported by the education, national policy, and research efforts of the AAP.

This third edition is a major accomplishment from a dedicated group of physicians, nurse practitioners, neonatal nurses, social workers, and neonatal intensive care unit (NICU) parents who were supported by the AAP publications team of content reviewers, copy editors, designers, and project staff.

Thanks to my family for their understanding and support during this intensive project. Thanks to the authors of this book for contributing their valuable time, writing talent, and professional expertise.

Thanks to Charles and Suzanne Rait of NICU Ink Book Publishers for accepting the original proposal for this book and for guiding me through the first 2 editions. Most important, thank you for your valuable and enduring friendship.

Thanks to the AAP team.
Mark Grimes, Director, Division of Product Development, for his support of this project and his willingness to explore acquisition of this book for publication.

Eileen Glasstetter, Manager, Division of Product Development, who kept everyone on track and on time, encouraged and supported me at every turn, and guided our project to completion on a very aggressive timeline.

Wendy Marie Simon, Director, Division of Life Support Programs, who has always believed in the value of this book for NICU parents and introduced it to colleagues at the AAP. Thank you for being my friend and Destiny Person.

Thank you to the many people who contributed to the photographs and artwork for this book. Your pictures are worth a thousand words.

Gigi O'Dea of Memory Portraits by Gigi, Sarasota, FL, for contributing her amazing photographs of NICU babies and their families, including the 3 photos for our cover.

Heidi Nakamura, University of Washington Medical Center NICU.

Lauren Thorngate, University of Washington Medical Center NICU, who facilitated the acquisition of numerous photographs and parent permissions.

Acknowledgments

Lori Markham, Seattle Children's Hospital, for taking photos at Providence Regional Medical Center, Everett, WA.

Maureen Goins, Providence Sacred Heart Medical Center & Children's Hospital, Spokane, WA.

Julie Arafeh, Lucile Packard Children's Hospital at Stanford University.

Shelly Vaziri Flais, MD, FAAP, for the photos on pages 488 and 555.

David W. Ehlert, medical illustrator, University of Washington, who created the gastroschisis series on page 332.

Jordan Hartman, Pacific Lutheran University, Tacoma, WA.

Linda Diamond, for the layout and design of this book.

Kenneth Gow, MD, Seattle Children's Hospital, for the photos on page 331.

I wish to thank my fellow colleagues who contributed to this book in so many ways.

Seattle Children's Hospital
Nate Brown
Shauna Carrette
Vicki Cronin
Denise Dubuque
Kenneth Gow
Stephanie Hillman
Meg Larkin
Wendy Nicon
Cathie Rea
Paige Richardson
Jennifer Seymour
Mirtha Vaca-Wilkens
Lani Wolfe

University of Washington Medical Center
Catherine Cordner
Heidi Nakamura
Lauren Thorngate

Airlift Northwest, Seattle
Frare Davis Photography
Kim Lambert
Mardie Rhodes
Nan Walker

A special thanks to the hospital staff, the babies, and their families from all over the United States who allowed us to share their NICU experiences through photos for this third edition.

The Bugbee family

The Burns family

The Clark Denny family

The families of Gigi O'Dea photographs

The Feldpausch family

The Garka family

The Hendler family

The Kellington family

The Lindsay family

The Mera family

The McDonald family

The Parent family

The Walters family

The Reynolds family

The Zaichkin family

Thank you to the health care professionals whose unique contributions are much appreciated.

Marcy Mallouf, Lucile Packard Children's Hospital at Stanford University

Kimberly Radtke, Manager, Breastfeeding Coalition of Washington

Kathryn E. Barnard, Professor Emeritus, Family and Child Nursing, University of Washington

Kathleen Southerton, State University of New York

Liz Carr and David McBride, Washington State Department of Health

We wish to acknowledge the chapter authors of the first 2 editions of this book. Their excellent work provided the foundation on which this third edition was created.

Debbie Fraser Askin

Susan Tucker Blackburn

Ann Flandermeyer

Kathleen A. Green

Sharon Gregory

Susan M. Kearns

Carole Kenner

Denise Merrill

Margaret M. Naber

Kathleen M. Pompa

Ellen P. Tappero

Patricia Thornburg

Ginna Wall

TrezMarie T. Zotkiewicz

Introduction

Having a baby is a miraculous accomplishment. But your baby is not perfect, which seems unfair and shatters any illusions of a traditional beginning. At first, most parents of sick and premature babies don't know how to feel and are often torn between joy and sadness. For almost every parent in the neonatal intensive care unit (NICU), though, one desire remains consistently strong—and that is to be recognized as the baby's parent. In other words, NICU parents need to be included in the care of their own special babies. The authors of this book invite you to become an important member of your baby's health care team. We believe that parents can and should play an active role in their baby's care. This book was written for parents who wish to learn about their baby's illness, how to overcome the barriers to NICU parenting, and how to prepare for and nurture their NICU graduate at home.

Some of the information in this book may seem frightening at first, but knowledge is empowering. When you understand your baby's illness and treatments, you will gain confidence and be able to communicate effectively with your baby's caregivers. You can then form the working partnership with the medical and nursing staff that is essential for your sense of control and for mutual problem-solving.

Neonatal intensive care is a huge subject, and your baby will certainly not have every problem in this book. Because your NICU experience is unique, this book cannot answer every question or prepare you for every situation. Read through the table of contents to find the sections that interest you most—and know that what interests you will change as your baby progresses through hospitalization. We hope that this information answers many of your questions, and we encourage you to ask your NICU team about what you do not understand. We hope you will feel better informed and prepared to celebrate the achievements—and manage the crises—that are an inevitable part of every family's life.

It would be unrealistic to expect a carefree journey through the NICU. Intensive care is stressful by nature and overwhelming at times. Reading this book and learning about what happens in the NICU will help you gain confidence and feel more relaxed. You will meet some incredible people to help you through the experience. You will meet other parents whose support will give you strength. You will meet health care professionals who have devoted their careers to helping babies like yours. You will discover that the NICU offers a unique blend of technology and compassion that encourages healing and growth not only for babies, but also for parents.

This is probably not the experience you had hoped or planned for, but the NICU offers opportunities you otherwise would have missed. Right from the beginning, you can learn how to communicate effectively with health care professionals and how to use community resources. You will learn to value what is unique and special about your baby and what is most important for your baby's future. And when your baby's hospital stay is over, you will probably realize that your NICU experience has made you stronger, smarter, and more aware of what is most important in your life.

We want you to have a positive NICU experience. Even though your baby has had a difficult start, it is an amazing beginning just the same. Use this book to guide you through your experience, and remember that your baby's nurses and physicians are your most important sources of information. As your baby grows, you will continue to learn things about your child from teachers, coaches, health care professionals, and all of the people who influence your child's life.

Learning how to be a good parent never ends. We hope you get a good start here—and enjoy learning about your very special baby.

Jeanette Zaichkin, RN, MN, NNP-BC

We know that you would prefer to read "he" if your baby is a boy and "she" if your baby is a girl. It is difficult to communicate with the distraction of "his/her" and "he/she," however. Therefore, the baby's gender in this book alternates by chapter. Likewise, we know that both men and women are nurses; however, we refer to nurses as "she."

Chapter 1
Expecting the Unexpected

"As soon as he saw the Big Boots,

Pooh knew that an Adventure was going to happen,

and he brushed the honey off his nose

with the back of his paw, and

spruced himself up as well as he could,

so as to look Ready for Anything."

Jeanette Zaichkin, RN, MN, NNP-BC
Julie M. R. Arafeh, RN, MSN

Giving birth is an adventure unmatched by few other life experiences. Most parents anticipate the big event with a mixture of excitement and apprehension, yet few are truly prepared for complications that may result in a sick newborn.

No one chooses a complicated pregnancy or an experience in the neonatal intensive care unit (NICU). Finding out that pregnancy, labor, and birthing your baby may pose risks to your health or that your unborn baby may be at risk for health problems can be frightening and changes your life in more ways than you can imagine. Understanding the basics of birthing "at risk" may help you cope with the inevitable anxiety that accompanies a different beginning.

If you are reading this chapter before giving birth, you have the opportunity to learn about some aspects of high-risk delivery and participate in the plan. If you have already given birth, things may have happened quickly. This chapter will help you understand parts of your birth experience that are still unclear.

Where Will You Give Birth?

Your baby's quality of life may depend on decisions made before his birth. By working with your team of doctors, nurses, and other health care professionals in making these decisions, you are acting as a responsible parent even before your baby is born. Your team's first recommendation may concern the hospital where your baby will be born.

Levels of Care

Your hospital's designated level of maternal and neonatal care (also called *perinatal care)* may affect where you give birth or where your baby receives special care. Although every hospital is equipped to handle emergencies, including newborn resuscitation, many community hospitals prefer to transport pregnant women who are at risk or whose babies may be at risk to a nearby medical center where staff is experienced at managing complicated pregnancies and sick newborns.

In 1976 the March of Dimes categorized hospital obstetric and newborn services as Level I, II, or III, depending on the availability of resources and the complexity of the patients served. This was especially important in the 1970s and 1980s because neonatology was a developing medical specialty and not every hospital was equipped to care for sick and premature babies. Categorizing perinatal services into Levels I, II, or III helped ensure that the highest-risk patients were sent to the Level III units where experienced teams had state-of-the-art resources to best care for mothers and babies with complex health issues. At that time, most NICUs were located in university medical centers.

Most maternal and neonatal care units continue to describe their level of care by using a numerical classification, with a higher number indicating more comprehensive services than a lower number. Now most cities have at least one hospital that provides neonatal intensive care, and many communities have several hospitals that provide Level II and Level III obstetric and nursery services. Several different levels of care may be provided in different areas of the same hospital.

The American Academy of Pediatrics (AAP) has proposed these uniform definitions for neonatal levels of care.

- A hospital that provides Level I (basic) nursery services is designed to care for healthy term babies. The Level I nursery may stabilize and care for babies at 35 to 37 weeks' gestation if they have no complex problems. Babies born at less than 35 weeks' gestation are transferred to a facility that can provide the appropriate level of care. It is important that hospitals in this category have a system for quickly identifying high-risk patients and transferring them to a facility that provides specialty or subspecialty care.

- A Level II (specialty) service is equipped to care not only for healthy newborns, but also for some types of high-risk newborns. A Level II nursery cares for babies who are more than 32 weeks' gestation and weigh more than 1,500 grams (3 pounds, 5 ounces). This level of nursery cares for moderately ill newborns, preterm babies whose problems are expected to resolve quickly, and sick newborns who have been stabilized pending transport to a Level III NICU. Level II nurseries also care for babies convalescing from neonatal intensive care. Because this category covers a huge range of possibilities, the AAP has divided Level II into Level IIA and Level IIB. A Level IIB differs from a Level IIA in that it has the capability to care for babies who need mechanical ventilation (respirator) for a day or less or continuous positive airway pressure (CPAP), a form of support for babies with breathing problems. See Chapters 2 and 12 for more information about mechanical ventilation.

- A Level III (subspecialty) service offers comprehensive care for all newborns. Often located in a regional medical center, this type of facility is equipped to provide neonatal intensive care. The AAP designates 3 categories for Level III nurseries. Level IIIA cares for infants born at more than 28 weeks' gestation and weighing more than 1,000 grams (about 2 pounds, 3 ounces). This nursery cares for typical premature babies and has resources to perform minor surgical procedures. Level IIIB provides care for babies born at less than 28 weeks' gestation and weighing less than 1,000 grams. The Level IIIB NICU offers different types of ventilators, a full range of pediatric specialty services, and the ability to perform major surgery. The Level IIIC NICU provides the highest category of care and is equipped to manage patients with the most complex health issues, including those who need extracorporeal membrane oxygenation (cardiac or lung bypass) and surgical repair of complex birth defects. Level III nurseries offer state-of-the-art equipment and teams of highly trained specialists in medicine, nursing, and other related health care fields.

Interpretation and application of these definitions vary widely across the United States. In some states, regulations govern how many Level II and Level III NICUs may exist and where they can be built; other states offer no such regulation or enforcement. You may even hear about a Level IV designation, which means the hospital has determined that its NICU has even higher capabilities than the Level IIIC defined by the AAP.

The most important aspect of your community hospital may be its staff's expert ability to determine where both you and your baby will have the best outcome. If the perinatal team at your community hospital determines that your labor or your baby's birth may become complicated, its best recommendation may be that you be transported to a hospital that offers a higher level of care before your baby is born.

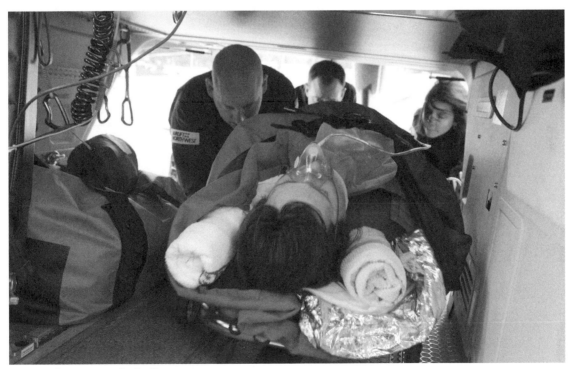

Maternal transport by helicopter.
This expectant mother prepares for transport by helicopter. The transport team provides expert care, reassurance, and a safe trip.

Courtesy of Frare Davis Photography, Airlift Northwest, Seattle, WA.

Maternal Transport

Even if your health care professional anticipates an uncomplicated labor, maternal transport may be recommended so that your newborn will have the advantage of immediate admission into a NICU if he is born with complications. If you give birth in a community hospital that does not provide neonatal intensive care, your newborn faces the possibility of transport, which is stressful for the baby and may separate you and your baby.

Maternal transport is not possible if you are so seriously ill that transport would further endanger your health or safety, or if labor has progressed to the point where birth could happen during transport. In these cases, it is safer to give birth at the community hospital and stabilize your newborn for transport.

Methods of maternal transport depend on the seriousness of your condition and how close you are to the medical center. Some medical centers send their specially trained perinatal transport team to the community hospital; that team accompanies you as you travel by ambulance, helicopter, or other aircraft. Other community hospitals use a local ambulance company for transport, sending members of their own labor and delivery staff with you to ensure your safe arrival at and admission to the medical center. Not often, but in certain non-emergent situations, a family member or friend may drive you to a higher-level perinatal facility.

Even though transport may be in your or your baby's best medical interest, it comes with a personal price. When you change hospitals, you usually lose the services of your own physician or midwife and your chosen pediatrician. You may be far from home, without the support of family and friends. In addition, maternal transport may mean making long-term arrangements for the care of your household and other children in your absence.

Your partner or support person may worry about your health and safety and the uncertain health of your unborn baby. Witnessing the flurry of activity that accompanies transport and sensing the urgency of the situation, your partner may feel all the responsibility for holding things together.

During this stressful time, partners need to communicate honestly with each other. Lend each other support, and be together if possible when information is given. Stress makes it difficult to hear everything that health care providers tell you. Partners may be able to clarify the facts for one another.

Your labor and delivery nurse at the community hospital or a member of the transport team should provide your partner or support person with directions to the medical center and to its perinatal unit. Your case manager or the hospital social worker should be able to tell your partner about inexpensive lodging and parking discounts at or near the medical center. They can also provide other important information to help navigate an unfamiliar hospital system.

The transport process can be frightening for parents. Not only is it an unanticipated new experience, but you can no longer deny the reality of your complications. If you are able, tell your health care team what you are feeling, and ask questions about what will happen next. The members of your perinatal team realize that you are apprehensive and will make every attempt to keep you informed and as comfortable as possible.

"Our health insurance let us choose the hospital where our baby would be born. We chose the one with the nicest interior decorating. Our priorities changed when we had an emergency cesarean. Thank goodness there was also an expert staff that saved my baby's life."

Your Care Providers

The personnel attending your labor and your infant's birth will depend on your circumstances. When you become sick or your labor becomes complicated, many interventions become necessary. People and machines may fill the room until you wonder if anyone remembers you are in the bed.

Following are descriptions of the care providers you may encounter during labor. Chapter 3 is devoted to helping you understand the roles of the many people involved in caring for your baby in the NICU and how best to communicate with them.

Your Labor Nurse

Most women establish firm bonds with the nurse who guides and supports them through labor and birth. Your labor nurse will be your primary source of information, your advocate, and your link to the many people involved in your care. Your nurse's expertise will become obvious as she manages and coordinates everything necessary to ensure a safe labor and birth. But just as important as technical skills are abilities to promote the natural processes of birth and to help keep you and your partner involved in the overall plan of care.

Physicians

If your labor becomes complicated, your family physician or midwife may call specialists to assist. An obstetrician is a physician who specializes in women's health care issues. A perinatologist is an expert in high-risk maternal and fetal medical care. In large medical centers, most women with high-risk pregnancies also meet with a neonatologist. A neonatologist is an expert who works with perinatologists to advise on newborn care.

In a teaching hospital, fellows, residents, and interns may also be involved in your care. Participation by health care professionals at different stages of their learning is an important part of the team approach in large medical centers. Large centers may also include physician extenders or physician assistants as team members in your care. Because they often do very detailed histories and examinations, your care may be enhanced by their participation. However, if you find all of this attention overwhelming, you may ask your labor nurse to help you limit the number of students and interns involved in your labor and birth.

Your obstetrician may administer pain control if needed. Some facilities use the services of anesthesiologists, physicians trained to administer medications that reduce pain and/or cause unconsciousness. Nurses with advanced practice education, called *certified registered nurse anesthetists,* can also administer anesthesia in collaboration with an anesthesiologist. If you have questions about pain control during labor, be sure to ask your nurse or doctor or someone from the anesthesia department.

Other Hospital Personnel

In addition to your labor nurse and physician, other specialized hospital staff may participate in your care. Laboratory personnel will draw your blood, a sonographer may

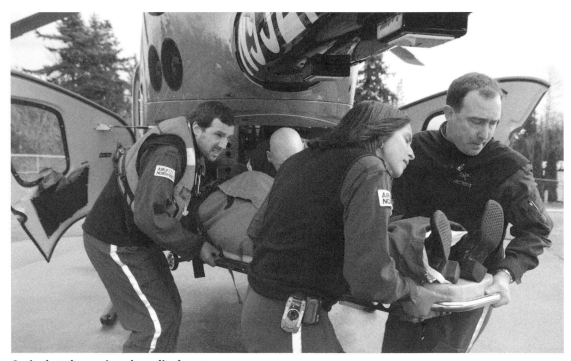

Arrival at the regional medical center.
The expertise of the transport team ensures a safe arrival and a smooth transition to new caregivers.

Courtesy of Frare Davis Photography, Airlift Northwest, Seattle, WA.

conduct your ultrasound, and a social worker may meet with you to discuss available resources and your personal needs. Each member of the hospital team supports an important aspect of your care.

What to Expect From the Team

In general, you should expect courteous and respectful treatment at all times. All members of your health care team should introduce themselves by name and title before examining you or asking questions about your history. Even in an emergency, team members should protect your privacy by closing hallway doors and using privacy screens during caregiving.

Most hospital care providers make an effort to ask you the same questions only once or twice; however, sometimes repetition is unavoidable and even important. You may feel that a multitude of caregivers whom you have never before met and who never seem to talk to one another are asking you the same questions. It may help to realize that different members of the health care team look for specific sorts of information within your answers so that they can make the best possible nursing and medical decisions for you and your baby. Communication will probably not be easy for you at this difficult time. You may relate to some members of your health care team better than others. But do keep in mind that you and your partner are also important members of the team, and your input is valuable. Mutual respect among all members of the team is the key to success. If possible, communicate your needs to your physician and labor nurse and ask them to act as your advocate.

You will likely have many questions about your plan of care. However, if you are in a new hospital surrounded by a new health care team, you and your partner may have difficulty remembering all of your questions. It may help to write down your questions. Some questions you may have for your team are listed below.

- How long will I need to be in the hospital?
- What activities can I do while I am in the hospital? Can I get out of bed to use the bathroom and shower?
- Will I be able to eat and drink as usual while I am here?
- What signs and symptoms should I look for and report to the team?
- Why might an emergency birth be necessary in my situation?
- If an emergency birth is necessary, what can I expect? How can I assist the team? Will my partner be able to stay with me?
- What can I do to keep my baby and myself as healthy as possible?

When you are nervous, it is normal to forget what you are told and not hear all of the information you are given. Write down the answers to your questions. Discuss any areas of uncertainty with your team so you can contribute to the plan of care and be better able to cooperate if emergency action must be taken. If you have more questions or have forgotten the answers, you may always ask questions again. The health care team wants you to be as comfortable as possible in this situation.

Interventions

When your labor becomes complex or if your health care team anticipates problems with your baby, you can expect basic interventions to ensure the best possible outcome. Your health care team is committed to providing you with as satisfying a birth experience as possible. If complications develop, however, your safety and that of your baby become the biggest priority. The goal is for you and your baby to be as healthy as possible at the time of delivery. Following are explanations of some of the equipment that may be used to accomplish that goal.

Intravenous Line

Your physician may limit your intake of food and beverages shortly before you give birth. This is to prevent vomiting and potential aspiration (inhalation of fluid into the lungs) if cesarean birth becomes necessary. To provide a route for fluids and medications, an intravenous (IV) line will be inserted into a vein somewhere on your hand or arm. The IV line may be "capped off" and reconnected to the tubing only when a constant infusion of fluid or medication is necessary. Having this cap, called a *heparin* or *saline lock,* is less cumbersome than being continuously "hooked up" to IV tubing. You can anticipate the heparin or saline cap will be flushed with a small amount of solution 3 to 4 times a day to ensure the cap remains open and ready to use in the vein if a constant infusion is needed.

Electronic Fetal Monitoring

Fetal heart rate monitors were introduced to hospitals in the late 1960s. It was hoped that fetal monitoring could identify fetal distress in time for health care providers to perform emergency procedures—and thus eliminate newborn brain damage and death. Research and experience have since shown that fetal monitoring has limitations and cannot achieve this result for several reasons. Changing conditions within the uterus or fetus can affect fetal well-being at any time during pregnancy, not just in the hospital or during labor and birth. Furthermore, years of experience with fetal monitoring have demonstrated that fetal heart rate abnormalities (such as intermittent slowing of the baby's heart rate) are common in labor, can be interpreted in various ways, and do not always result in an unhealthy newborn.

Your obstetrician, labor nurse, and perinatal team are aware of the abilities and limitations of electronic fetal monitoring (EFM). They use EFM to track your baby's heart rate and monitor maternal uterine contractions. Electronic fetal monitoring also helps the nurse evaluate the adequacy of uterine contractions and the progress of labor. Although fetal monitoring can detect complications that require evaluation, your perinatal team uses EFM as only one tool for assessing how well you and your baby are progressing through labor and birth.

The fetal heart rate monitor gives a digital readout of the baby's heart rate, and in some systems, 2 wave-like patterns showing both the baby's heart rate and your contractions are printed on a strip of graph paper. In state-of-the-art systems, the nurse and physician use a computer or video system to review your data rather than analyzing output on graph paper. The recent advances in computer technology also allow the team to see the monitor at a central location, as well as in your hospital room. Technology allows some hospitals to communicate your EFM tracing via modem to obstetric experts in other institutions for consultation.

Two different types of EFM are available. External fetal monitoring uses 2 elastic belts fastened around the mother's abdomen. One belt holds an ultrasound transducer

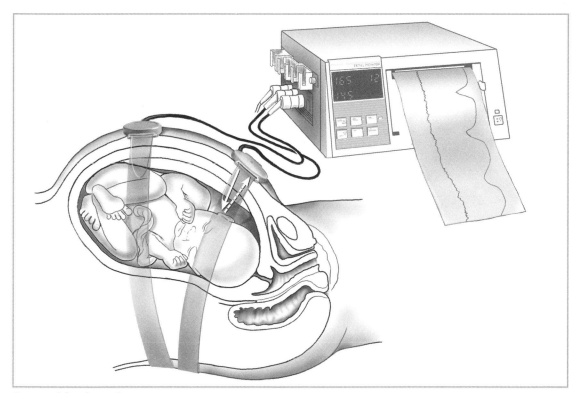

External fetal monitor.
The external fetal monitor uses 2 belts across the mother's abdomen. One belt holds a tocotransducer that senses the abdominal pressure changes of uterine contractions. The other belt holds an ultrasound transducer that detects fetal heart sounds.

From: American College of Obstetricians and Gynecologists. Your Pregnancy and Birth. *4th ed. Washington, DC: ACOG; 2005. Reprinted by permission.*

(Doppler) and detects your baby's heart beat. The second belt holds a disc called a *tocotransducer* that senses pressure changes on the abdomen. The tocotransducer records the frequency and duration of uterine contractions, but the intensity of the contractions cannot be accurately recorded using external fetal monitoring. Internal fetal monitoring allows precise measurement of the strength of uterine contractions and provides a continuous tracing of your baby's heart rate in situations when the ultrasound transducer is unable to do so.

An internal fetal monitor involves 2 pieces of monitoring equipment. The first piece is the internal scalp electrode that measures your baby's heart rate. An internal electrode looks like a spiral wire. Your nurse or doctor guides the electrode up through the birth

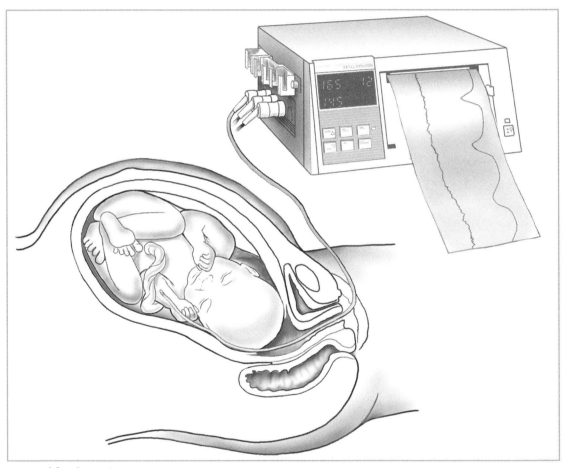

Internal fetal monitor.
The internal fetal monitor uses a fetal scalp electrode and an internal pressure catheter. The internal monitor provides more accurate information about your contractions and fetal heart rate than the external fetal monitor.

From: American College of Obstetricians and Gynecologists. Your Pregnancy and Birth. *4th ed. Washington, DC: ACOG; 2005. Reprinted by permission.*

canal and through the cervix (the opening to the uterus) and attaches it to your baby. The tip of the electrode slides just under the surface of the baby's skin nearest to the mother's cervical opening (usually the baby's head or bottom, depending on the baby's position). Care is taken to avoid your baby's face or genitals. Your baby's electrode wire leads back out of the birth canal, attaches to a small plate wrapped around or taped to the mother's thigh, and connects to the fetal monitor by a cord. The wire is removed from the baby at birth. The second part of the internal fetal monitoring system is called an *internal uterine pressure catheter (IUPC)*. This pressure-sensing catheter is guided up through the birth canal and through the cervix and is placed inside the uterus. The IUPC accurately records the frequency, duration, and strength of the mother's contractions.

In order to use internal monitoring, your membranes must be ruptured (your water must be broken) and your cervix must be dilated enough that the 2 parts of the monitoring equipment can be placed into the uterus. Internal fetal monitoring is not used as often as external fetal monitoring but is valuable if external fetal monitoring is not providing an adequate digital readout. Internal fetal monitoring is more invasive and carries more risk than external fetal monitoring but is necessary and worthwhile if your physician requires more comprehensive information to help ensure a safe labor and birth.

Oxygen

An unborn baby depends on his mother for oxygen and nutrition. Oxygen supply to the baby decreases during every uterine contraction. A healthy baby tolerates this normal part of labor without problems. The baby may receive an unusually low oxygen supply during contractions, however, if the placenta is not functioning at its best or if a maternal medical condition (such as high blood pressure or heart disease) is present and reduces oxygen circulation in the mother's body. Your baby's oxygen supply may also be insufficient if maternal contractions come too close together or if the baby's umbilical cord becomes temporarily squeezed during contractions. In any of these cases, your doctor or nurse may request that you wear an oxygen mask to help the baby receive extra oxygen during labor.

Corticosteroids

If there is a strong chance that your baby will be born between 24 and 34 weeks' gestation and within the next 7 days, you will most likely be given injections of corticosteroids (often referred to as *steroids*). Depending on the type of steroid given, you will receive either 2 injections 24 hours apart or 4 injections 12 hours apart in your hip or other muscular area, such as your thigh.

Steroids help your baby's lungs mature. Steroids work best about 48 hours after the first administration and continue to work for about 7 days. The goal is to decrease the incidence and severity of respiratory distress syndrome and bleeding in the brain—both serious complications of premature birth (see Chapter 9). This single course of steroid therapy given to the mother does not adversely affect growth or development of the child. Steroid therapy is a proven emergency intervention that can make a positive difference in the health of your child.

"My family made me call the doctor about the back pain I was having but I didn't think I was in labor. My doctor said I was in labor and should be transferred to another hospital because the baby was too early. Things happened really fast after that, and Amy was born the next day. At first it was scary to be away from home but I'm glad my doctor sent me where my baby had everything she needed right away."

Labor and Birth Management

Once you are declared "at risk," technology and intervention replace your anticipated birth experience in the homelike atmosphere of your community hospital. The mood is more serious, the medical personnel are more numerous, and your anxiety is understandably higher. Most parents feel powerless in this situation. It is true that many factors are no longer within your control. But understanding the reasons behind the decisions medical personnel are making and how those decisions affect you and your baby will help you cope with this experience.

A Difficult Question: Will My Baby Live?

"Will my baby live?" is the most common question asked by parents who are surprised by an unexpected high-risk birth. This is a difficult question, and the answer depends on your situation.

If time allows before you give birth, your health care provider and your baby's medical provider will speak with you about what to expect when your baby is born. As your baby's parent, you are expected to help make health care decisions in your baby's best interests. Depending on your situation, you may be asked for input about choices and decisions that affect your baby's care at birth. If birth is imminent or has become an emergency, it may be difficult to get all of the information you need and have the time to think about your choices. This makes clear and ongoing communication with the resuscitation team most important, so you can be kept updated on your baby's condition. A baby of more than 25 weeks' gestation who has no other complications besides prematurity has a good chance of survival. In most cases, every additional week of pregnancy improves the baby's chances. Most NICU graduates, especially those born at 28 weeks' gestation and more, grow into healthy children and adults.

If your baby is less than 25 weeks' gestation, your health care providers will talk with you about your baby's chances for survival and use statistics to give a prognosis about problems that may develop later, such as vision and hearing problems and learning disabilities. You may be asked if you prefer a full resuscitation or if you prefer no resuscitation and want instead to hold your baby immediately after birth for comfort only (no intensive care interventions).You may prefer something in between an all-or-nothing approach, such as asking the team to begin resuscitation by providing oxygen and initial breathing assistance and then, depending on how the baby responds and the advice of the medical provider, deciding to proceed with more complex resuscitation or stop and provide comfort only. It is important to know that resuscitation can be followed by withdrawing support; however, it is not in the best interests of the baby to make a decision to provide comfort care only and then change the plan and initiate resuscitation many minutes after the baby is born. A baby who survives a delayed resuscitation is at risk of serious disability.

Your baby's health care provider cannot make any promises about what will happen at the delivery. If the baby's condition at birth is different than expected, the plan may change. In this case, the neonatal resuscitation team will keep you informed about your baby's condition and may ask for your input in decision-making. Sometimes resuscitation and stabilization give the neonatal medical team additional time to gather more information about the best course of action, which also gives you time to ask questions and participate in the plan of care after your baby's birth.

Talking with the baby's team and asking questions will give you vital information about your baby. Discussing this information with your partner or others you trust will help you and your health care team make the best decisions for your baby and your family.

Negotiating

If you have reached the point in your pregnancy when you have planned your labor and birth experience but then find that you are at risk, you may be able to keep part of your plan. When your physician recommends cesarean birth, for example, ask if you may play the music you planned for labor in the operating room. If you have an internal fetal monitor in place and can no longer walk around the room, ask if you may sit in the rocking chair next to the bed. Having some control over your care may reduce the intensity of your feelings of loss for the "perfect" labor and birth and may help them resolve more quickly.

Vaginal Birth or Cesarean Birth?

The members of the health care team want your birth experience to be meaningful even under difficult circumstances. Their overall goals are to ensure a safe labor and to deliver your baby to the neonatal team in the best possible condition. This can be a special challenge when the forces of labor and birth present potential hazards for you and your baby.

When spontaneous vaginal birth is deemed safe for you and your baby, this is the option of choice. Because it is a "normal" birth experience, some women find a vaginal birth more emotionally satisfying. More important, a vaginal birth eliminates the risks of operative and postoperative complications and shortens your hospital stay and recovery period.

An obstetric condition that causes concern about the baby's well-being—such as fetal distress, acute maternal bleeding, or serious maternal illness—usually makes cesarean birth the choice for the best possible outcome. Other common reasons for cesarean birth include a previous cesarean, failure to progress in labor, and breech presentation (the baby is positioned to deliver the buttocks or feet first instead of headfirst). The experience and training your health care professionals have in this type of medical and nursing care will guide their clinical judgment. The information they give you is based on careful consideration of the risks and benefits of each birthing method.

Current research does not suggest that all preterm infants should be delivered by cesarean birth. A cesarean birth may be performed for very low birth weight infants demonstrating fetal stress, breech presentation, or intrauterine growth restriction; when labor fails to progress; or for maternal conditions such as high blood pressure (hypertension) or serious bleeding. If the mother is not in labor but maternal or fetal well-being necessitates immediate delivery, cesarean birth may be indicated to avoid a long induction of labor that the preterm or sick fetus might not tolerate.

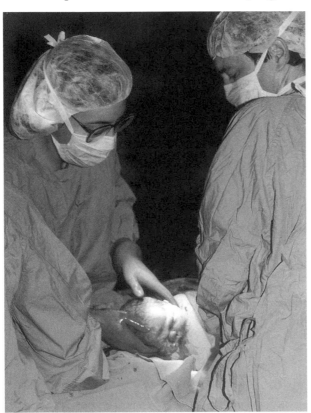

Cesarean birth.
This baby was positioned head down in the uterus. The obstetrician first guides the baby's head through the abdominal incision, then delivers the rest of the baby's body.

If you are in preterm labor and are giving birth vaginally, you may discover that labor and birth progress quickly once things begin to happen. Even though a vaginal birth is a natural process, an unusually fast birth (called a *precipitous birth*) can be frightening. Mothers who birth precipitously often feel out of control and as if they missed the whole thing. Because caregivers and equipment must move quickly, a precipitous birth often feels like an emergency. Your obstetric care provider and labor nurse, who are your advocates and primary information source during labor, will support you through the urgency of the birth. Afterward, ask them to help you review what happened, validate what you remember, and clarify details that are important to you.

Special Interventions During Labor and Birth

Induction of Labor

Under special circumstances, your labor may be induced. This means that uterine contractions are deliberately stimulated before labor begins on its own. The goal is vaginal birth.

Labor is induced when a specific obstetric or medical problem is present. Labor would not be induced for a woman whose labor should be delayed or who has a high chance of needing cesarean birth (for example, for twins or more babies, because of placental problems, or if the baby is positioned differently than head down). Induction may be indicated for a variety of conditions that complicate a pregnancy—as a response to gestational hypertension (explained in Chapter 8), some types of diabetes, or risk of infection because of prematurely ruptured membranes (the "bag of water" breaks before labor begins). Labor may also be induced for an "overdue" baby or for a sick or compromised fetus whose chances of a healthy outcome would be improved with immediate neonatal intensive care.

For labor induction, a drug called *oxytocin* (Pitocin) is given through an IV line to stimulate uterine contractions. Sometimes a prostaglandin preparation is used before oxytocin to soften, or "ripen," the cervix.

Your nurse closely monitors your condition during labor induction. Your vital signs (temperature, pulse, respirations, and blood pressure) are checked frequently. Electronic fetal monitoring is used to assess your baby's well-being and your contraction pattern. Your nurse will provide encouragement and keep you informed of your progress.

Labor Augmentation

Augmentation is used when labor has already begun but is not progressing satisfactorily or has stopped altogether. *Labor augmentation* refers to methods used to promote more effective uterine contractions. Successful labor augmentation reduces the incidence of cesarean birth and also reduces the risk of infection sometimes seen with prolonged labor.

As in labor induction, oxytocin can be used to augment labor. Expert and supportive nursing care can be expected during labor augmentation. Your nurse will take your vital signs frequently and use EFM to assess fetal well-being and your contraction pattern. Another method of augmentation uses a procedure called *artificial rupture of the fetal membranes (AROM)*, or *amniotomy*. This means that your doctor or midwife "breaks" your bag of water to stimulate contractions. Often AROM brings the baby's head down onto the cervix. A combination of effective uterine contractions and pressure on the cervix helps dilate the cervix and allows the baby to be born.

Episiotomy

You may wonder if your vaginal birth will include an episiotomy (a surgical incision to enlarge your vaginal opening). The purpose of an episiotomy is to allow easy passage of your baby's head in the final moments of birth. Although an episiotomy used to be a common procedure, it is less so now.

An episiotomy may be considered if your physician or midwife is concerned about your baby's heart rate at the time of birth or if there is difficulty delivering the baby's shoulders. However, every birth is unique, and your care provider will make a decision about an episiotomy based on your individual circumstances.

Vacuum Extraction

Sometimes a laboring woman is unable to push her baby out of the birth canal without assistance. In some cases, vacuum extraction may be used to shorten the time the woman must push before the baby is born. In this method, a soft suction cup is applied to the top

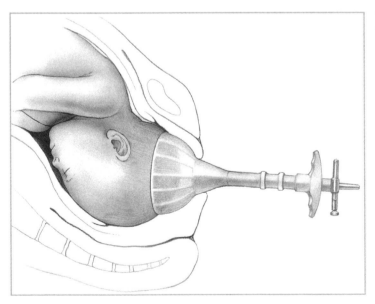

Vacuum extractor.
The suction cup of the vacuum extractor is applied to the top of the baby's head. Working with the mother's contractions, the physician uses traction to deliver the baby's head.

From: American College of Obstetricians and Gynecologists. Your Pregnancy and Birth. 4th ed. Washington, DC: ACOG; 2005. Reprinted by permission.

of the baby's head, and firm suction is applied. Working with the mother's contractions, the physician gently applies traction and delivers the baby's head. The vacuum extractor usually leaves a soft, temporary swelling on the baby's head, which resolves in the first week of life. In general, vacuum extraction is not used on a baby of less than 34 weeks' gestation.

Indications for vacuum extraction include maternal exhaustion, reduced ability or urge to push as a result of anesthesia, or a maternal medical condition (cardiac or circulatory disease) requiring that the mother receive assistance in the pushing stage. Vacuum extraction should be used only for specific obstetric indications. If steady progress is not being made toward delivery when a vacuum extractor is used, your doctor will abandon attempts to deliver the infant with this type of assistance.

Forceps

Forceps are curved metal tongs used to shorten the pushing stage of labor and to deliver the baby's head. Forceps delivery may be considered when the baby's head is low in the birth canal. This type of assistance may be indicated for fetal distress, when the mother's power or urge to push has decreased as a result of anesthesia or exhaustion, or when a maternal medical condition (such as cardiac or circulatory disease) requires that the mother receive assistance in the pushing stage. Just as in vacuum-assisted delivery, your doctor will stop this procedure if any unexpected difficulty occurs.

It used to be thought that forceps delivery would protect the preterm infant's fragile head from the pressures of a long pushing stage during childbirth. Subsequent research did not support this practice, and forceps are now used during preterm birth for the same reasons for which they would be used in a term birth.

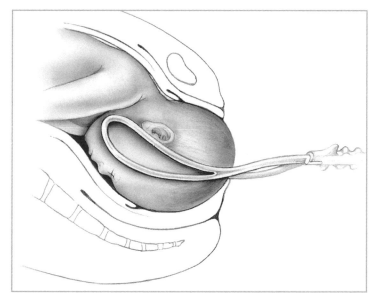

Forceps delivery.
Forceps are used to shorten the pushing stage of labor. Unlike the vacuum extractor, forceps can be used to accomplish a fast birth if the mother or baby experiences distress late in this stage of labor.

From: American College of Obstetricians and Gynecologists. Your Pregnancy and Birth. *4th ed. Washington, DC: ACOG; 2005. Reprinted by permission.*

Pain Management During Labor and Birth

Medications and anesthesia affect not only the mother, but the unborn baby as well. Your physician, labor nurse, and anesthesiologist or nurse anesthetist will work with you and assess your needs while bearing in mind the goal of delivering your baby in good condition.

Every labor situation is different, and no one method of pain relief is superior under all conditions. Pain medication and anesthesia will depend on the many factors that contribute to the complexity of your labor and birth. Ask your physician or labor nurse what aspects of your health may influence decisions regarding pain medication and anesthesia.

If you have the opportunity, tell your labor nurse your plans for pain management. If you plan to have an unmedicated birth, she will work with you to accomplish this goal. If you change your mind and decide to use pain medication, you should feel equally supported in this decision. Sometimes your pain management plan will not be in the best interests of your baby. In this situation, you and your health care team will make a plan to ensure that you are as comfortable as possible and your newborn is as vigorous as possible at birth.

If your labor or birth becomes complicated and medical intervention makes medication or anesthesia necessary, your nurse will explain why and what you should expect next. When you work as a team, you can maintain a sense of control and trust your nurse's assessment of your needs.

Labor Management Without Medication

Walking, if permitted, usually helps a woman cope with the early stages of labor. Sitting in a rocking chair; changing positions in bed; and using massage, visual imagery, or breathing techniques help many women cope as labor intensifies. Your labor nurse or midwife may offer more suggestions for managing discomfort.

Fear can intensify pain. For this reason, it is important to ask about anything that worries you. Education about the labor process and what to expect during labor and birth can help allay many fears and the accompanying discomfort.

A supportive partner is so important during childbirth. This person may not only respond to your requests for physical comfort through touching or providing a cool washcloth, but also provide security just by being there and sharing this experience with you. Keep communication open, and tell your partner what you expect of him or her during labor and birth. A plan may make things easier if your situation becomes complicated.

Analgesia

Medication that relieves pain or decreases awareness of pain is called *analgesia*. Examples of medications used for labor analgesia include meperidine hydrochloride (Demerol), butorphanol tartrate (Stadol), and fentanyl (Sublimaze). Their use during labor may be limited, however, because of the unpredictable speed of the labor and the inability of the sick or preterm baby to handle the medication. These drugs cross the placenta and are metabolized more slowly by the fetus than by the mother. Babies born with maternal pain-relief narcotics in their system may experience respiratory depression (decreased breathing effort) that may take hours to resolve. Respiratory depression caused by maternal medication further challenges the uncertain ability of immature or sick babies to breathe on their own.

Anesthesia

Anesthesia refers to a method of pain control that involves partial or total loss of sensation in the affected area. Anesthesia may or may not include loss of consciousness. The 2 major types of anesthesia are regional (including epidural and spinal) and general.

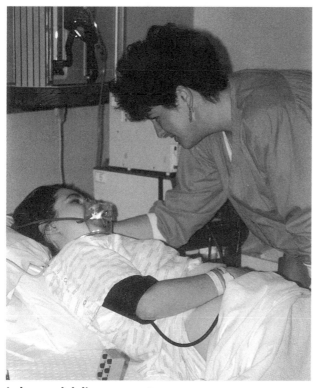

Labor and delivery expert.
Your labor nurse provides expertise and support during this very important event in your life.

Regional anesthesia is used for moderate to severe pain or when cesarean birth is a possibility. During labor, your anesthesiologist or nurse anesthetist may administer an epidural or spinal block, types of regional anesthesia that block pain sensation from the navel to the mid-thigh. An epidural block is used for labor pain and can also be used for cesarean birth. The medication is injected through a catheter into the space outside the covering of the spinal cord. Unlike an epidural block, a spinal block is injected with a needle through the covering of the spinal cord. A spinal block can be administered more quickly than an epidural block and is also used for cesarean birth.

Epidural and spinal anesthesias do not cause drowsiness or loss of consciousness in the mother and allow her to be awake during vaginal or cesarean birth. Regional anesthesia carries fewer risks to mother and baby than general anesthesia and does not cause respiratory depression of the baby at birth.

Emergency cesarean birth may require the use of general anesthesia, which means the patient is unconscious ("asleep") during surgery. This type of anesthesia is administered to the patient in the operating room through inhaled medication and/or IV medication. Although this type of anesthesia can be an important lifesaving tool, it carries risks for the mother and her fetus and prevents the mother from seeing her newborn in the first moments of life. It is not often used for childbirth.

Remembering What's Important

As pregnancy progresses, parents-to-be usually focus most of their energy and attention on labor and birth because giving birth is the biggest and most immediate challenge. Much of your prenatal education may have focused on "planning" the birth and even on such topics as how to avoid cesarean delivery. Especially for first-time parents, imagining actually caring for the infant can be more difficult than thinking about the very real task of giving birth.

When you face a complicated labor and birth, the plan of care may change rapidly depending on the status of you or your baby. Some lifesaving actions may need to occur very quickly, and you will likely feel a loss of control over the decision-making process. When the birth is over, you may feel that you "didn't do it right." It might help to know that most birth complications are not caused by anything parents do or fail to do, and most are unforeseen. If there is time before your birth, you can discuss with your health care team what will happen if an emergency birth is necessary. Most health care professionals will try to explain what is happening during an emergency so you can assist them as much as possible. Even so, feelings of disappointment may occur and often take time to resolve. In the meantime, remember that the most important goal for you and your health care team is for you and your baby to be as healthy as possible.

Keep in mind that the most important part of parenting is not vaginal versus cesarean birth or pain medication versus a non-medicated birth. Much more important is the quality of parenting you bring to your baby after birth and the values you teach that will influence your child's entire life.

Chapter 2
A Different Beginning

"But the more Tigger put his nose into this
and his paw into that, the more things
he found which Tiggers didn't like.
And when he had found everything
in the cupboard, and couldn't eat any of it,
he said to Kanga, 'What happens now?' "

Jeanette Zaichkin, RN, MN, NNP-BC
Patricia Jason, RN, BSN, CCRN

The moment of birth is usually a triumphant celebration. Not only have you made it through labor and birth, you've welcomed into your family a new little person who carries your dreams for the future.

When things don't go as expected, you face a more stressful beginning than most parents. You and your partner need to deal with the feelings of loss that accompany the birth of a sick or premature baby. For most parents, the neonatal intensive care unit (NICU) is a new world of medical vocabulary and technology that may, at first, seem foreign, cold, and hostile.

Sometimes parents know in advance that their baby's birth may be difficult or that their newborn may need the special care of a NICU. This chapter will help you prepare for these events. It explains what you can expect and should ease your anxiety about the sights and sounds surrounding the birth and your baby's NICU admission. If your baby has already been admitted to the NICU, this chapter will explain what you may have seen or heard in the delivery room and will acquaint you with the NICU environment.

What Can Happen at Birth

Infrequently, a baby is born sick without warning. Most of the time, though, the obstetric and neonatal team of doctors, nurses, and other trained personnel anticipate problems and are ready to deal with them. At every birth, members of the neonatal team work together to assess the baby's condition. Caregivers are ready to help the newborn breathe and achieve or maintain the pulse and blood pressure necessary for life.

Every birthing area is equipped to resuscitate (revive) a sick baby. Resuscitation may take place in the delivery room or in a room near the birthing area. In any case, the birth of a sick newborn brings inevitable tension into the birthing area. Equipment is checked and checked again. A physician or a nurse practitioner usually leads the neonatal resuscitation team. You may hear the team leader assigning duties and checking your baby's condition with your health care provider.

Resuscitation Equipment

Every delivery room contains equipment that the neonatal team may use to resuscitate your baby if necessary. Following are descriptions of the items found in most birthing areas.

Radiant Warmer

A radiant warmer is a type of bed that consists of a mattress, usually on a mobile cart, with a heat source overhead. The mattress area is used for resuscitation and immediate stabilization of the baby after birth, while the overhead heater helps to keep the baby warm. If your baby is placed on a radiant warmer, the staff will tell you that your newborn is "on a warmer."

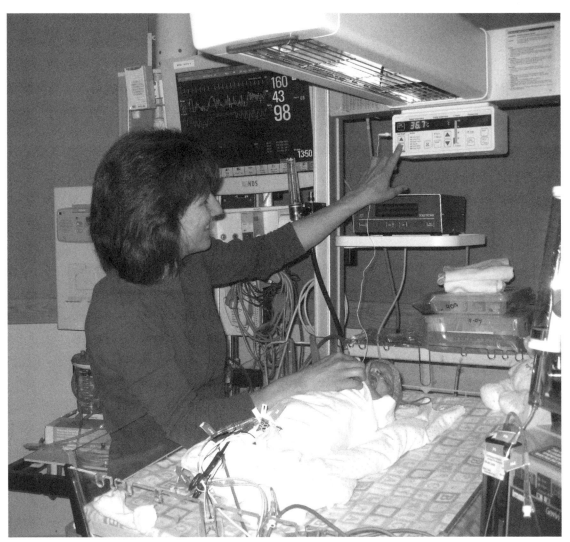

Radiant warmer.
The radiant warmer provides a mattress for the baby to lie on and overhead heat for warmth.

Courtesy of Seattle Children's Hospital.

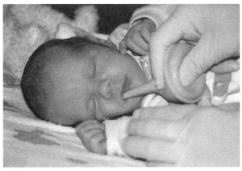

Bulb syringe.
The bulb syringe uses gentle suction to remove fluid from the baby's nose or mouth.

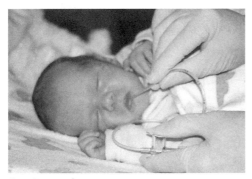

Suction catheter.
The suction catheter is attached to a wall or portable unit that uses a vacuum system to generate a preset amount of suction to clear secretions from the baby's nose, mouth, throat, or stomach.

Suction

Babies are often born with mucus and fluid in the mouth, nose, and throat. Suction may be needed to clear those areas and to prevent choking.

The most basic suction tool is called a *bulb syringe*. The caregiver first squeezes all of the air out of the bulb, then gently places the pointed end in the baby's nose or mouth. When the caregiver releases her grip on the bulb, mucus and fluid are drawn into the bulb syringe, clearing the baby's breathing passages, or airway.

Wall suction is another method for clearing a baby's airway. A mechanical suction apparatus is built into the wall or radiant warmer and a suction setup hangs on it. A thin tube (called a *suction catheter*) is passed into the baby's nose, mouth, throat, and perhaps stomach. Then the fluid is "vacuumed" out at a preset, safe suction pressure.

Oxygen

The oxygen we breathe (called *room air*) contains about 21% oxygen. If your baby requires extra oxygen at birth, you may hear the NICU team say, "The baby needs some Os" (pronounced "ohs") or "The baby needs O2" (the molecular term, pronounced "oh-two"). A concentration of 100% oxygen comes either from a portable tank on or near the radiant warmer or directly from pipes built into the wall. When the oxygen valve is open, oxygen flows through a length of flexible tubing to your baby's location on the radiant warmer. Many delivery room settings use an oxygen blender, which is a machine that mixes 100% oxygen that comes from the portable tank or pipes in the wall with room air. This enables the team to use any concentration of oxygen depending on your baby's needs, from room air (21%) to 100% oxygen.

For decades health care providers in the United States agreed that newborns who require breathing assistance should receive 100% oxygen. Emerging research, though still inconclusive, now seems to indicate that room air resuscitation may be just as successful as resuscitation using supplemental oxygen. There is concern that too much oxygen may be toxic to body tissues, especially for very preterm babies. During resuscitation, your baby's response to oxygen may be monitored using pulse oximetry (see page 40). The goal is to use the lowest oxygen concentration necessary to adequately supply the neonatal brain, vital organs, and body tissues with oxygen. It is still unknown what the oxygen target levels should be and how these levels differ for term babies and preterm babies. Recommendations for how much oxygen to use during resuscitation are still developing. At this point, each hospital has its own protocol for starting the resuscitation with any concentration of oxygen, including room air; however, the recommendation is to increase the oxygen concentration if the baby does not respond well to resuscitation efforts within a few minutes after birth.

All babies are blue at birth. Healthy babies may take as long as 5 to 10 minutes to become pink, and parents should not be concerned if the baby is vigorous but slightly blue in the first few minutes after birth. If your baby is breathing and has a good heart rate but does not turn pink after a few minutes, a stream of oxygen will be aimed toward her nose and mouth. This is called *free-flow oxygen* and provides oxygen-enriched air for your baby to breathe. Free-flow oxygen is given by blowing oxygen from tubing toward her mouth and nose, placing an oxygen mask on the baby's face, or allowing oxygen to flow through the face mask or open-end tubing of a resuscitation bag.

Breathing Assistance

When your baby does not breathe on her own, or is not yet strong enough to breathe effectively, breathing assistance called *positive pressure ventilation* is required. A resuscitation bag is commonly used to ventilate (breathe for) a baby who needs this type of assistance. A resuscitation bag, also called a *bag and mask,* connects to a tank or wall source of oxygen and consists of a small pouch that fills with oxygen and a soft mask that fits over the baby's nose and mouth. A member of the resuscitation team places the face mask firmly over the baby's nose and mouth and provides positive pressure ventilation by squeezing the bag, thereby delivering "breaths" into the baby's lungs. The person

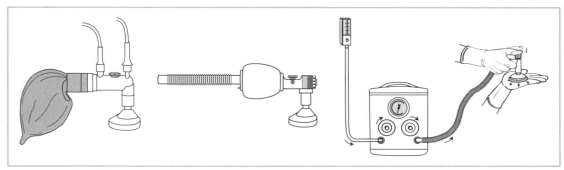

Devices used to deliver positive pressure ventilation.
Resuscitation bags are pictured on the left and in the center. A T-piece resuscitator is pictured on the right.

From: American Academy of Pediatrics, American Heart Association. Textbook of Neonatal Resuscitation. 5th ed. Kattwinkel J, ed. Elk Grove Village, IL: American Academy of Pediatrics; 2006:3-34.

who is using the resuscitation bag controls the size (pressure) of the breath by how hard the bag is squeezed and the rate of breathing by how often the bag is squeezed. This type of positive pressure ventilation is called *bag and mask ventilation* or *bagging the baby.*

The T-piece resuscitator may also be used in the delivery room or nursery to assist your baby's breathing. The T-piece resuscitator is a mechanical device that delivers blended oxygen in a "breath" given at a preset pressure that ensures the same-sized breath is delivered each time. The T-piece can be connected to a face mask and would be used instead of the resuscitation bag described above. The T-piece can also be connected to an endotracheal tube (see below) and deliver breaths much like a respirator (ventilator).

Endotracheal Tube

If your baby is very premature, very ill, or requires more than a few minutes of positive pressure ventilation, an endotracheal (ET) tube may be inserted. This thin plastic tube is placed deep into the baby's throat, directly into the trachea (windpipe). It is then connected either to the resuscitation bag, T-piece resuscitator, or a ventilator. Placement of an ET tube is called *intubation.* Because the ET tube is positioned between your baby's vocal cords, your baby will not be able to make crying noises while the tube is in place.

An ET tube provides a direct route to your baby's lungs and is the most effective means for delivering positive pressure ventilation to help your baby breathe. The ET tube can also be used for delivering emergency medication into the baby's lungs. When a

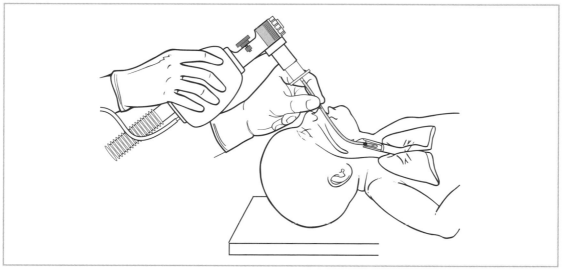

Endotracheal tube.
The endotracheal tube is positioned in the baby's trachea (windpipe) between the vocal cords.
A baby with an endotracheal tube is intubated and requires mechanical assistance to breathe.
When the endotracheal tube is removed, the baby is extubated.

*From: American Academy of Pediatrics, American Heart Association. Textbook of Neonatal Resuscitation.
5th ed. Kattwinkel J, ed. Elk Grove Village, IL: American Academy of Pediatrics; 2006:5-21.*

resuscitation bag is attached to the ET tube and the caregiver squeezes breaths from the bag into your baby's lungs, the baby is being hand-bagged. When a ventilator is connected to the ET tube, the baby is being mechanically ventilated.

Laryngeal Mask Airway

Relatively new to delivery room resuscitation, the laryngeal mask airway (LMA) looks like a tiny inflatable raft connected to a tube. The LMA slides easily into the baby's throat, covers the baby's esophagus (food pipe), and holds open the trachea (windpipe). The LMA works much like an ET tube to provide direct access for delivering breaths into the baby's lungs. The LMA is usually used as a "rescue airway" when intubation with an ET tube is difficult or not possible. Unlike the ET tube, the LMA is too large to fit newborns weighing less than about 1,500 grams (3 pounds, 5 ounces) and cannot be used to deliver medication into the lungs. If the newborn needs assisted ventilation after resuscitation, the LMA is usually replaced with an ET tube if possible, or a surgically placed airway if necessary.

Emergency Medications

In rare cases, a baby is born so seriously ill that fluid and medication must be administered to save her life in the delivery room. Various medications are available to stimulate the heart, increase blood pressure, and correct chemical imbalances in the baby's blood. Some medication can be administered through the ET tube, but most must be injected directly into the baby's bloodstream or work more effectively when given by this route. The umbilical cord provides a large and easily accessible vein through which emergency medications can be given during birth resuscitation (see page 33 to learn about umbilical lines).

Resuscitation Activities

The steps taken to resuscitate a newborn depend on the infant's condition at birth and on the baby's special needs. A full-term baby who is pink and crying but has internal organs exposed on her abdomen (gastroschisis), for example, will require interventions different from those needed by a preterm infant who has difficulty taking that first breath. Although babies require resuscitation because of various problems, the following concerns are typical in most infant resuscitations.

Initial Steps

When your baby is born, the delivering physician or midwife will suction her mouth and nose and clamp the umbilical cord. The baby is immediately placed under the warmer, and her head is positioned in "sniffing" position (nose pointed to the ceiling) to open her airway. Then her mouth and nose are cleared of fluids with the bulb syringe. Most babies are quickly wiped dry to prevent chilling; however, preterm babies may be covered with a clear plastic sheet from the neck down and wear a soft cloth hat to help prevent heat loss.

Breathing

Breathing supplies oxygen and maintains the heart rate. It may seem like forever before you hear your baby's first cry, but most babies make some crying efforts in the first minute after birth. The neonatal team may provide tactile stimulation (gentle rubbing of the baby's back and flicking of the feet) to encourage breathing. If your baby does not breathe in a few moments, is too weak to breathe regularly, or has a heart rate (pulse) of less than 100 beats per minute, a resuscitation bag or T-piece resuscitator will be used to provide positive pressure ventilation.

Ventilation (breathing) is the most important aspect of neonatal resuscitation. Most babies respond quickly to effective positive pressure ventilation with a heart rate that rises to over 100 beats per minute. Positive pressure ventilation will continue until your baby's heart rate is over 100 beats per minute and she is breathing on her own.

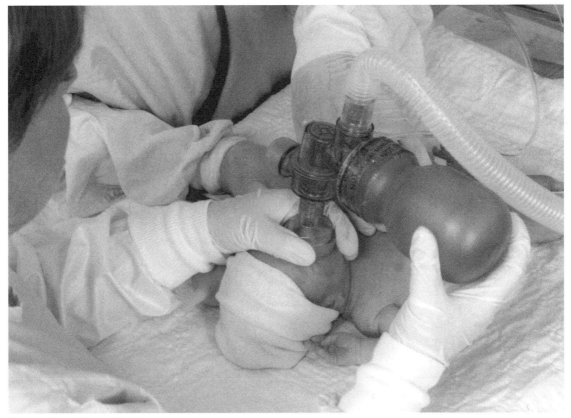

Bag and mask ventilation.
The caregiver places the resuscitation bag firmly over the baby's nose and mouth and pumps air/oxygen into her lungs. Positive pressure ventilation is necessary when the baby is not breathing on her own or when her heart rate is less than 100 beats per minute.

From: American Academy of Pediatrics, American Heart Association. Textbook of Neonatal Resuscitation. *5th ed. Kattwinkel J, ed. Elk Grove Village, IL: American Academy of Pediatrics; 2006.*

When a baby is bagged, some of the oxygen also goes down the baby's esophagus (food pipe) and collects in the stomach. If the baby's stomach is allowed to fill with air, it will push up on the diaphragm, leaving less room for the baby's lungs to inflate. Just as you have trouble taking a deep breath after eating a big meal, air in your baby's stomach will keep her from breathing effectively. Therefore, if your baby needs more than several minutes of bagging or if her stomach looks bloated, her stomach will be suctioned with a tube that goes through her mouth into her stomach. This not only removes the air, but also cleans out any fluid that the baby could vomit and aspirate (breathe into the windpipe and lungs). Then, with a suction tube functioning as an air vent, bagging can continue.

After a few breaths from the bag, most babies perk up and begin to breathe on their own. Your baby may need free-flow oxygen to keep her oxygen levels normal while she gets used to breathing on her own.

Heart Rate

A baby's heart rate is normally 120 to 160 beats per minute. Many preterm babies and those experiencing complications at birth will be born with a heart rate less than 100 beats per minute, but most respond quickly to effective positive pressure ventilation. If your baby's heart rate stays dangerously low (less than 60 beats per minute) despite good positive pressure ventilation, a member of the neonatal team will begin chest compressions

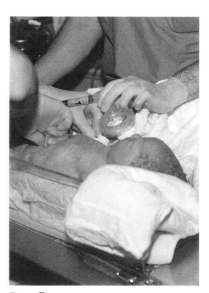

Free-flow oxygen.
A baby who is breathing but stays blue receives a steady stream of oxygen-rich air from oxygen tubing or from the resuscitation bag. This newly delivered infant receives free-flow oxygen while another caregiver monitors the baby's pulse through the umbilical cord.

(pushing on your baby's chest to artificially pump your baby's heart). At this point, the situation is considered very serious, and a member of the neonatal team will prepare to intubate your baby and/or give lifesaving medication.

Endotracheal Intubation

If the baby does not begin to breathe well on her own after a minute or two of positive pressure ventilation or if her heart rate remains less than 100 beats per minute, she will probably be intubated. Intubation, placing an ET tube in the baby's trachea (windpipe), is sometimes performed even before a baby receives positive pressure ventilation. Babies at risk for meconium aspiration (explained in Chapter 10) are usually intubated and suctioned immediately. Extremely premature babies and babies who are expected to be in very serious condition at birth may be intubated as soon as possible because this is the most effective method of ventilation. The ET tube also gives the neonatal team immediate access for administration of surfactant (see Chapter 9) or emergency medication during resuscitation.

Umbilical Catheter Placement

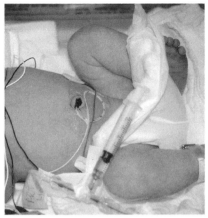

Umbilical catheter.
An umbilical catheter may be placed in one or more of the large blood vessels where the umbilical cord was connected to the placenta. When the umbilical catheter is placed in an artery, it is called an *umbilical arterial catheter*. When it is placed in the vein, it is called an *umbilical venous catheter*.

When a baby's umbilical cord is cut, a portion of the white, jellylike cord remains attached to the baby's abdomen. The umbilical cord contains 3 important blood vessels: 2 small arteries and 1 large vein. These vessels provided blood flow to and from the placenta (the "afterbirth") and provided oxygen and nutrients to the baby before birth. For a while after delivery, it is possible to thread a thin tube (called a *catheter)* into these vessels directly into the baby's bloodstream. If lifesaving medication or fluids are needed during resuscitation in the delivery room, a catheter can be threaded into the umbilical vein for this purpose and is called an *umbilical venous catheter (UVC)*. The UVC is generally used only temporarily to allow medications and/or intravenous (IV) fluids to be "pushed" (given quickly and directly) into the baby's bloodstream. If no longer necessary, it may be removed before your baby is transferred to the nursery. See page 42 for information about the umbilical arterial catheter (UAC).

Apgar Score

At 1 minute of age, again at 5 minutes, and every 5 minutes during resuscitation, your baby is assessed and given a number score to reflect her general condition. This scoring system was created by a physician, Dr Virginia Apgar, in the 1950s and is named after her. Apgar scores do not indicate what needs to be done during resuscitation; instead, they give the neonatal team an indication of your baby's overall condition and your baby's response to resuscitative efforts. The Apgar score does not accurately reflect the

Apgar Scoring

Sign	0	1	2
Heart Rate	Absent	<100	>100
Breathing	Absent	Weak	Strong cry
Color	Blue	Body pink; arms and legs blue	Pink
Tone	Limp	Some flexion	Well flexed
Reflexes	None	Grimace	Cough or sneeze

From: Apgar V. A proposal for a new method of evaluation of the newborn infant. *Anesth Analg:* 1953;32:260. Reprinted by permission.

Expanded Apgar Score

Gestational age: _____ weeks

Sign	0	1	2	1 min	5 min	10 min	15 min	20 min
Color	Blue or pale	Acrocyanotic	Completely pink					
Heart Rate	Absent	Less than 100/min	Greater than 100/min					
Reflex Irritability	No response	Grimace	Cry or active withdrawal					
Muscle Tone	Limp	Some flexion	Active motion					
Respiration	Absent	Weak cry, hypoventilation	Good, crying					
			Total					

Resuscitation

	1	5	10	15	20
Minutes					
Oxygen					
PPV/NCPAP					
ETT					
Chest compressions					
Epinephrine					

Comments

From: The Apgar Score. ACOG Committee Opinion No. 333. American College of Obstetricians and Gynecologists. *Obstet Gynecol.* 2006;107(5):1209–1212.

baby's future. A low score indicates that the baby had a difficult time making the transition necessary for adequate breathing and circulation at birth, but a high Apgar score does not predict high intelligence.

To determine your baby's Apgar score, her health care team assesses 5 categories: heart rate, breathing, color, tone, and reflexes. Babies are assigned a score of 0, 1, or 2 in each category, with 0 indicating very depressed responses and 2 indicating very active responses. The final Apgar score is the total of the 5 numbers. When the baby receives assistance at birth, an expanded Apgar score may be used (see Expanded Apgar Score chart on page 34) to document what kind of assistance the baby was receiving when the score was assigned in each category.

Few babies receive a perfect score of 10 because a baby's hands and feet usually remain blue for a while. A baby with a score of 7 to 10 is considered a "normal" newborn. An Apgar score of 4 to 6 indicates a moderately depressed newborn, and an Apgar score of 0 to 3 reflects a severely depressed newborn. Keep in mind, however, that very premature babies receive lower Apgar scores than full-term infants simply because they are immature and unable to respond with loud crying and because they do not have strong muscle tone.

Transfer to the Nursery

"The nurse asked if I had any questions. I looked at all those plugs and cords and the only question I could think of was, 'What happens if the power goes out?'"

Babies are usually transported to the nursery when they are breathing (either on their own or with positive pressure ventilation in progress), their heart rate is acceptable, and special problems have been stabilized. Depending on your baby's condition and established hospital procedures, she may be taken to the NICU or special care nursery on a radiant warmer or transferred in an incubator.

NICU Sights and Sounds

Each neonatal intensive care nursery has its own routines, but most share certain common priorities during infant stabilization. Following are explanations of the initial activities and basic equipment used during NICU admission. Chapters 9, 10, and 12 cover medical problems and the equipment used to treat them.

The Admission Process

When your baby enters the NICU, many things happen at once. You and your family probably will not be allowed into the NICU during this busy time. This is not to exclude or keep information from you, but rather to give the nurses, respiratory care practitioners, and medical providers time and space to stabilize your baby, begin diagnostic tests if necessary, and plan her immediate care.

Priorities in the first hour include making sure your baby is reaching normal oxygen levels, breathing well on her own or with assistance, maintaining an adequate heart rate and blood pressure, sustaining a normal blood sugar level, and reaching an appropriate body temperature. Soon after birth, routine admission procedures are completed. A hospital identification bracelet is placed on your baby. Your baby receives an injection of vitamin K to prevent potential bleeding difficulties and antibiotic ointment is placed in her eyes to prevent possible infection. Additional routine procedures, such as weighing, measuring, and footprinting, may be delayed until life-threatening conditions have been stabilized.

Becoming Part of the Team

The NICU team is very busy during your baby's first hours in the nursery. On the other hand, you are waiting and worrying, and that makes minutes seem like hours. Tell the NICU team member at the front desk where you will be, and ask to be called at the first break in the action. Check back with the NICU at least every 30 minutes. You should expect some kind of update in the first 90 minutes.

Most NICU nurses and physicians are good at keeping parents informed. They will probably tell you more than you can understand at first, so don't worry if things seem unclear. Once you see your baby, you will begin to understand her problems, learn what the staff is doing to help, and begin to participate as partners in her care.

The experience of becoming a NICU parent is different for everyone. These first hours may seem unreal; in fact, parents often describe their first day or two in the NICU as "foggy and dreamlike." You may feel helpless and wonder how you will ever be able to participate in your baby's care, especially if the baby is transported to another hospital. But there is something very important mothers can do to participate in their baby's care: provide breast milk for feedings when your baby is ready. Breast milk is by far the best and safest nutrition for your baby, and only a mother can provide it. Even if you and your partner had not planned on breastfeeding, consider it now because this is an important part of your baby's care and has long-term implications for her future health. Providing breast milk is a vital way in which you can contribute to the health care of your baby. See Chapter 5 for more information about the indisputable benefits of breast milk for NICU babies.

"We told the family we were pregnant on Sunday. I wore my first maternity outfit on Tuesday. On Thursday, I had a crash C-section, and my daughter weighs 675 grams. We missed the entire pregnancy."

Basic NICU Tests

At the same time the nurse is making sure your baby is stabilizing, other members of the neonatal team are preparing to process x-rays, blood, and urine to monitor your baby's progress.

X-rays

X-rays are an important diagnostic tool in the NICU. Although your baby is exposed to a certain amount of radiation with every x-ray, the amount is carefully controlled in relation to your baby's size and weight. Unnecessary x-rays are avoided. If the baby's genital area is in the primary x-ray beam, it is shielded with a lead cover.

Blood Gases

A blood gas is a small amount of your baby's blood used to analyze the levels of oxygen, carbon dioxide, and other chemical components that help the practitioner assess breathing status. Results are used to determine what kind of breathing assistance is needed, and may also help assess heart function and shock. At first, as your baby's condition changes moment to moment, frequent blood gases may be necessary so that adjustments can be made to the concentration of oxygen or to the rate and pressure of breaths coming from the ventilator. A small sample of blood for a blood gas can be taken from your baby's artery (an *arterial blood gas* or *ABG),* from your baby's vein (a venous blood gas or VBG), or by pricking your baby's heel (a capillary blood gas or CBG).

Obtaining an ABG requires arterial blood, which is obtained by inserting a needle into one of the baby's arteries (usually in the wrist or ankle, where a pulse is felt) or by simply withdrawing blood through the UAC. The piercing of the baby's artery in the wrist or ankle with a needle requires special training and considerable skill. Using the UAC to draw a blood gas does not involve a needle stick because the catheter is already positioned in a major artery.

Arterial blood best indicates the oxygen available to the tissues, whereas capillary and venous blood has already been "used" by the body and is on the way back to the heart and lungs for a fresh oxygen supply. Therefore, an ABG provides the most precise measurement of oxygen in the blood and would be the first choice for the most accurate assessment of the baby's oxygen status.

When a baby needs a blood gas but does not have a UAC, the baby's caregiver can choose to do a CBG or a VBG instead of obtaining an ABG. Oxygen analysis is just one component of the blood gas. With the exception of the oxygen value, all 3 blood gas techniques are fairly comparable for measuring the components needed for blood gas analysis.

Additional Blood Tests

Many other blood tests (also called *lab work* or *blood work)* can be done, depending on the information desired. A complete blood count (CBC) and blood culture may be collected to detect infection. A hematocrit and hemoglobin assess red blood cells and your baby's ability to carry oxygen to her body tissues, and electrolytes ("lytes") determine the balance of basic body chemicals.

A baby that needs resuscitation is at high risk for abnormal blood sugar levels. A common blood test to screen your baby's blood sugar (glucose) is done right at the baby's bedside. A tiny drop of blood is placed on a chemically treated test stick. An approximation of the baby's blood glucose is displayed by a number value on a glucose meter. The result on the glucose test strip gives the nurse a close estimation of your baby's actual blood glucose. If the test strip indicates a blood sugar outside the normal range, the nurse will draw blood for a laboratory test so she will have a precise measurement of your baby's blood sugar.

A more sophisticated apparatus may be used to reveal the actual diagnostic result instead of giving an approximate value. A few drops of blood are placed into an electronic cartridge and within 2 minutes the blood glucose result is available. If the test result indicates a blood sugar outside the normal range, the nurse will report that to your baby's physician or neonatal nurse practitioner so that steps can be taken to normalize the blood glucose level.

Urine Tests

Kidneys are very sensitive to changes in the body. The amount of your baby's urine and what is in it can tell the NICU team much about your baby's general condition and progress after birth. Hospital laboratory technicians or the NICU nurse can do simple urine screening by placing a few drops of urine on a chemically treated dipstick. The urine dipstick reveals color values for things such as acidity, sugar, protein, and blood.

If more than a few drops of urine are needed for laboratory testing, a specially designed plastic bag may be taped over your baby's vaginal area or penis and scrotum. When the baby urinates, the urine collects in the bag. This type of urine collection is called a *clean catch.*

If infection is a concern, urine may be sent to the laboratory for a "culture and sensitivity" test. This means the urine is tested for bacteria. If any are found, further tests will be done to help medical personnel determine the best antibiotic to use against the bacteria. This urine can be obtained in several ways. A clean catch urine comes from the urine collection bag. Collecting urine in this way can be difficult and the urine is often contaminated by stool. A catheterized urine sample is obtained by inserting a small sterile tube into the baby's bladder and withdrawing the urine. This type of urine collection is called a *straight cath* or an *in-and-out cath* because the catheter is removed after the urine is obtained. A suprapubic tap (bladder tap) is thought by many to be the preferred method of obtaining urine for culture and sensitivity. This procedure is performed by inserting a needle through the baby's lower abdomen and piercing the baby's bladder. The urine is then drawn up into a syringe and sent to the laboratory for analysis.

If your baby is very sick, the nurse may insert a urinary catheter into your baby's bladder and leave it in place. This is called an *indwelling catheter*. The catheter drains the baby's urine into a bag or syringe, where it is accurately measured and collected for testing.

Many babies in the NICU are said to be on "strict intake and output," more commonly called "strict I & O." An accurate record is kept of all fluids that go into the baby (such as IV fluids, blood products, and oral fluid) and all fluids that come out (such as urine, stool, blood, and so on). The baby's fluid intake is carefully calculated and administered, usually for each 24-hour period. The baby's output is measured by weighing each diaper before and after the baby has wet or soiled it. The difference between the before and after weight of the diaper is calculated and measured as fluid output. Chapter 9 gives more information about your baby's kidneys.

Typical NICU Equipment

Just as the delivery area is set up with basic equipment for birth, the NICU is equipped with machinery to stabilize a sick baby. Each baby's condition determines the types of technological support she receives, but the following equipment is used during many NICU admissions.

Radiant Warmer/Incubator

In the NICU, your baby will be placed on a radiant warmer or in an incubator (isolette) to stabilize her temperature. Some incubators are designed with round portholes through which you and the NICU team can touch the baby. Others are opened by pushing up the front covering or raising the entire incubator cover. Even though the models differ, the priority of every radiant warmer and incubator is warmth; a baby can lose body heat quickly, and many body processes depend on maintenance of a normal temperature.

Every radiant warmer and incubator is equipped with a thermostat apparatus. An incubator can use this mechanism or may maintain a constant preset temperature. The thermostat works by measuring the baby's skin temperature through a probe taped to your baby's body. When your baby's skin has warmed to the preset high temperature, the heat turns down; when the infant's skin temperature cools, the heat turns back up.

Cardiorespiratory Monitor

Most NICU babies are placed on a cardiorespiratory monitor, a device that tracks the heart rate and the rate of breathing. Three adhesive patches (leads) are placed on the baby's chest and attached by cable to the monitor. The monitor picks up the electrical activity of your baby's heart, transmits the information onto a screen, and digitally displays it as a number. The monitor also detects your baby's chest movement and displays it as respirations (breaths) per minute. The cardiorespiratory monitor is used to detect a heart rate or a respiratory rate that becomes too fast or too slow.

Pulse Oximetry

Pulse oximetry is often used to immediately assess how well a baby is using the oxygen available to her. Although pulse oximetry does not indicate the exact amount of oxygen in the blood, a reading above or below the accepted target range alerts the nurse that the baby's oxygen level may not be acceptable. The baby's caregiver may intervene by increasing or decreasing the amount of supplemental oxygen (discussed in the next section) and/or by ordering a blood gas to determine the baby's exact respiratory status.

The pulse oximetry sensor is attached to your baby's hand or foot. It uses a light sensor to read the amount of oxygen attached to the hemoglobin molecules in the blood. Your baby's nurse can tell you about what saturation range is acceptable for your baby. Frequently the baby's saturation will be temporarily outside of the targeted range and the nurse or respiratory therapist will take steps to bring the saturation back to the desired values.

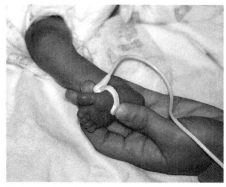 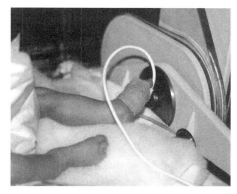

Pulse oximeter.
The pulse oximeter sensor is positioned around the baby's foot or hand and then secured with a type of wrapping, such as this stretchy bandage.

Blood Pressure Monitor

Your baby's blood pressure may be taken in much the same way as your own. A small blood pressure cuff is wrapped around your baby's arm or leg and automatically inflates at preset time intervals to display the blood pressure reading. Your baby's blood pressure may also be continuously measured through an umbilical arterial or peripheral artery catheter inserted in the arm or leg (see page 42) and displayed on the cardiorespiratory monitor screen.

Intravenous Line

Few babies are allowed to eat during their first hours in the NICU, and very sick or preterm babies may not take food by mouth for many days. An IV line may be placed to provide your baby with fluids, glucose, necessary body chemicals (such as sodium and potassium), and medications. Your baby's IV may be placed in her hand or lower arm, foot or lower leg, or scalp.

This IV line (also called a *peripheral line)* is positioned in a tiny vein very near the surface of the skin. Because a baby's veins are so small, the IV can shift or move out of place, allowing the IV fluid to leak out of the vein and into the surrounding tissue. This is called an *infiltrated IV line.* If an IV line becomes infiltrated, it must be discontinued (taken out) and restarted (placed again) at another site. Because IV placement can be stressful for your baby, the nurse safeguards the IV line so that it functions at one site for as long as possible. Even under the best circumstances, a peripheral IV line may last less than a day or two.

Peripherally Inserted Central Catheter

Another kind of IV line is called a *peripherally inserted central catheter,* or *PICC* ("pick"), *line* or *central line.* A PICC line is used when your baby needs an IV for longer than a few days. It is inserted into the arm or leg and threaded into a larger blood vessel deep

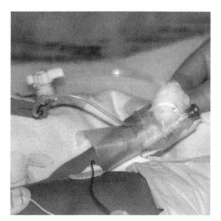

Intravenous line and monitor leads.
This IV line is placed in the baby's hand. The nurse may also place the IV line in the baby's scalp or foot. The round, adhesive patches on the baby's chest are called *monitor leads,* or *electrodes,* and attach to the cardiorespiratory monitor.

inside the body. This long, thin flexible tube is used to give medicines, fluids, nutrients, or blood products over a long period, usually several weeks or more.

Umbilical Arterial Catheter

Remember the 2 arteries and the vein in your baby's umbilical cord? An arterial line, called an *umbilical arterial catheter (UAC),* may be threaded deep into a major blood vessel (the aorta) through 1 of the 2 arteries. A UAC is necessary if your baby has significant problems that require frequent blood testing and continuous blood pressure measurement. Because the UAC feeds into a major blood vessel, the baby can receive fluids and medications through it, and most blood for laboratory testing can be drawn from it.

If your baby has an umbilical arterial line, it will be connected to a transducer so that your baby's blood pressure can be displayed on the cardiac monitor. The normal range for a baby's blood pressure is much lower than an adult's and depends on gestational age, size, activity level, and condition. If you are concerned, ask your baby's nurse what range would be considered appropriate for your baby.

Transcutaneous Monitor

A transcutaneous monitor (TCM) is a noninvasive system for monitoring oxygen and carbon dioxide levels in the bloodstream. The TCM does not substitute for blood gas sampling; it is a useful tool that helps assess your baby's status. The TCM sensor attaches to your baby's skin and warms the area under the probe. Oxygen diffuses from the skin capillaries to the probe, and a numerical value for the amount of oxygen in the blood is electronically calculated. Respirator settings and oxygen levels can then be changed without frequent blood gases being drawn. Because of the warmth of the probe, the TCM may leave a temporary red circle on your baby's skin.

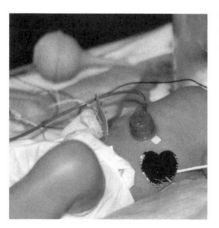

Transcutaneous monitor.
The round probe of the transcutaneous monitor sits on top of the baby's skin and monitors the oxygen and carbon dioxide levels in her blood. The warmth of this probe leaves a temporary red spot on the baby's skin. A shiny foil heart secures the thermostat of the radiant warmer to the baby's skin.

Basic Information About Oxygen

Because of prematurity or illness, your newborn may need to breathe air with a higher concentration of oxygen than is available in room air. This extra oxygen is called *supplemental oxygen.* The concentration of oxygen delivered to your baby is expressed as a percentage. The air we breathe every day contains about 21% oxygen; supplemental oxygen is any amount exceeding 21% up to 100%. Supplemental oxygen, unless it is being used for a short period or set at a very low flow, is warmed and humidified. It can be delivered in several different ways.

Oxygen in a Hood or Tent

For babies breathing independently and efficiently, supplemental oxygen can be supplied inside an oxyhood (a plastic box or hood placed over the baby's head) or, for larger infants, inside an oxygen tent (a plastic apparatus placed around the baby's upper body). If the baby is temporarily removed from the oxyhood or oxygen tent (for example, to be weighed or held for a short time), the tubing delivering the oxygen can be disconnected from the hood or tent and held in front of the baby's face.

Oxygen in an Incubator

For babies requiring low levels of supplemental oxygen (usually less than about 25%), some nurseries pipe the prescribed amount directly into the incubator. This method lets parents and caregivers see and care for the baby without interference from an oxyhood. Opening the incubator to care for the baby can allow the supplemental oxygen to escape and can dilute the oxygen level in the incubator with room air, but most babies receiving such low levels of supplemental oxygen are not affected by these temporary fluctuations.

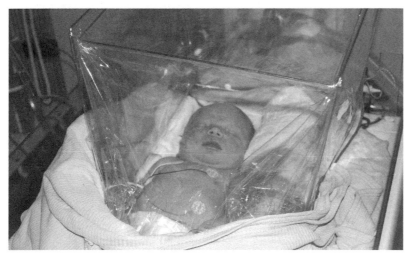

Oxygen tent.
This plastic tent fits over the baby's head and encloses warm, humidified, oxygen-enriched air for the baby to breathe.

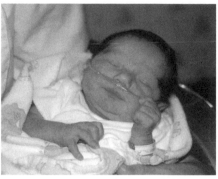

Nasal cannula.
Oxygen is delivered to this baby through a nasal cannula, a flexible hollow tube with openings, or "prongs," that fit just below the baby's nostrils.

Oxygen Cannula

An oxygen cannula is used to deliver supplemental oxygen to babies who require extra oxygen but are breathing well on their own. A cannula is a soft plastic tube that is placed under the baby's nose and encircles the baby's head; oxygen is delivered through openings ("prongs") in the tubing. Your baby may sleep with the oxygen cannula in place or in an oxygen tent placed inside the crib. An oxygen cannula is convenient for feeding, physical therapy, bathing, and other activities that are difficult to accomplish when the baby is inside a tent or oxygen hood.

Continuous Positive Airway Pressure

Continuous positive airway pressure (CPAP, pronounced "SEE-pap") is a method of assisted ventilation. With CPAP, your baby breathes on her own, but a machine keeps a steady supply of air/oxygen under pressure pushing into her lungs. This helps keep the tiny air sacs in the lungs from collapsing after each breath, reducing the effort that the baby must use to breathe. Continuous positive airway pressure can be delivered through the baby's nose (in which case some of the pressurized air can escape through the baby's mouth and/or down into her stomach), or the baby may be intubated so that the pressurized air is delivered directly into her lungs. The CPAP device in the nose can be attached to a ventilator, which delivers breaths to the baby several times each minute. (Chapter 9 provides more information about CPAP.)

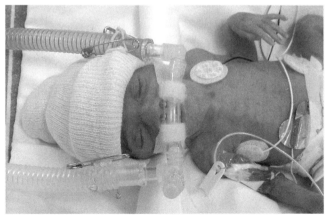

CPAP.
This baby is breathing on her own while receiving oxygen under steady pressure through her nose. CPAP makes it easier for the baby to breathe and prevents the small air sacs of the lungs from collapsing after each breath. A different CPAP device is found on page 227.

Courtesy of Deborah E. Campbell, MD, FAAP.

Mechanical Ventilation

A ventilator (also called a *respirator*) is a mechanical breathing machine that delivers a controlled mixture of air and oxygen, in a preset pressure for each breath, and at a certain number of breaths per minute (rate). The "stiffer" a baby's lungs, the higher the pressure must be to move the air/oxygen through the air sacs and into the bloodstream. Very sick babies require a high level of oxygen (up to 100%), a high pressure, and a high rate. (See Chapter 12 for an additional discussion about high-frequency ventilators.)

The ventilator is attached to your baby's ET tube. In some NICU settings, the respiratory therapist will use a capnography cable attached to your baby's ET tube to continuously monitor carbon dioxide levels in each exhaled breath. These continuous readings help your baby's care team as they adjust the amount of ventilator support. Your baby can take breaths on her own while on the ventilator unless the baby has been given medicine to suppress spontaneous breathing. As your baby weans (needs less assistance) from the ventilator, caregivers reduce the amount of pressure supplied with each breath and the number of breaths per minute.

When your baby is doing most of her own breathing, the ET tube is removed (a process called *extubation*); supplemental oxygen, which is usually required at first, is delivered by oxyhood, CPAP, or nasal cannula.

Your baby can accidentally become extubated because of her own movement or because the tape or stabilizer holding the ET tube in place slips slightly. Some babies will show obvious signs of distress, such as a dropping heart rate or a color change from pink to blue, when accidentally extubated. Other babies tolerate extubation quite well for a while and may even begin to cry. A cry from your baby indicates that the ET tube has slipped out from between her vocal cords and that she is extubated. Depending on her condition, a baby who accidentally extubates may be given a trial period to see if she can breathe effectively without the ventilator. If she tires or shows signs of increasing distress, or if her blood gases reveal low levels of oxygen and/or high levels of carbon dioxide, CPAP or mechanical ventilation will be restarted.

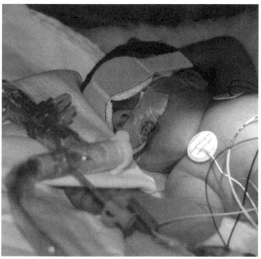

Intubated baby attached to mechanical ventilator tubing.
This endotracheal tube is secured to the baby's mouth and attached to the tubing of the ventilator. The ventilator tubing attaches to the ventilator itself, which stands on the floor near the baby's bed.

Newborn Transport

If your baby is born in a community hospital but requires additional specialized care, neonatal transport to an NICU is a possibility. Many nurseries can manage babies whose care requires oxygen by hood or cannula, and some can care for babies with umbilical arterial lines. If your baby needs a ventilator or surgery, or if the neonatal team predicts that your baby's care will become complex, your baby will be transported to a NICU, also referred to in many regions as a Level III neonatal facility. For more information about the different levels of newborn care in hospitals, see Chapter 1, page 4.

How the Transport Process Works

Your baby's physician or nurse practitioner will arrange the transport. Depending on the condition of your baby and the distance of your community hospital from the regional center, your baby may be transported by ambulance, helicopter, or aircraft.

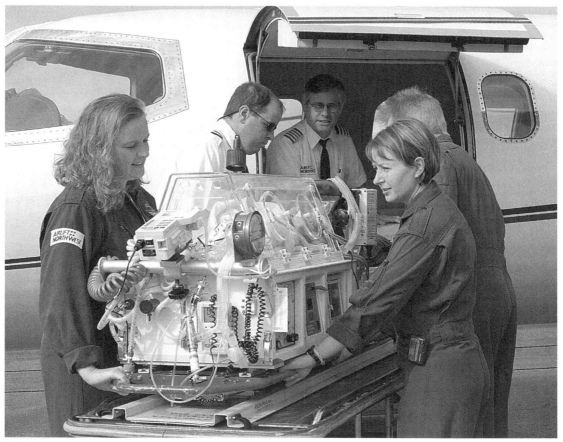

Newborn transport.
Your baby can be transported by ambulance, helicopter, or aircraft. The transport team provides critical care en route and will call you with a progress report on arrival to the NICU.

Courtesy of Frare Davis Photography, Airlift Northwest, Seattle, WA.

Some community hospitals will provide a transport team of their own to take your baby to the medical center where the NICU is located. It is more common for the medical center to send a specially trained neonatal transport team to assess your baby, stabilize her for the trip, and continue intensive care therapies en route to the NICU. Your baby will be inside a transport incubator, which is designed to provide warmth while allowing immediate access for any care she may need during transport to the regional center.

Immediately before your baby leaves the hospital, the transport team will bring her to visit with you, if possible. The transport team or nursery nurses will photograph your baby for you, and if time and circumstance allow, footprint your baby.

Saying good-bye to your baby is difficult at best. If you are still recovering from surgical anesthesia, you may not even remember seeing your baby before transport. Ask your partner or nurse to recount the events for you afterward if necessary. Even if your baby is not critically ill, separation is frightening and increases your stress. The transport team will leave you information about the NICU: their phone number, address, and directions to the receiving hospital.

Staying in Touch

The transport team should telephone you after arrival at the NICU and update you on your baby's condition. If you do not understand what you are told, ask your nurse to talk to your baby's NICU nurse and explain the situation in words you can understand. Be sure you have the NICU phone number and know how to call the NICU from your hospital room so that you can check on your baby's status whenever you wish.

If the NICU is far from the hospital in which your baby was born, you and your partner may be faced with the additional challenge of figuring out how to be in 2 places at once. Long-distance transport is especially difficult if you have other children at home who need your attention.

Ask your hospital discharge planner or social worker to help you find inexpensive lodging near your baby, and try to spend some time with your baby as soon as possible. If you must return home right away, figure out a system for staying in touch with the NICU. Your baby's nurse may set up a time to call you every day and tell you about your baby's progress, and you will be given the phone number to call whenever you wish. Some NICUs will send or e-mail you a photograph and short note "from your baby" each week. Ask your baby's nurse about the possibility of your baby returning to a hospital near your home for convalescence after she no longer needs intensive care. Being a "commuter parent" is not an ideal situation. The NICU should work with you to keep you informed and involved in your baby's progress.

Sorting It Out

To process and understand the birthing experience, every new parent, especially the mother, feels the need to tell and retell the story of the labor and birth. This recounting of events is especially important for parents of a sick newborn. When your baby's birth becomes a crisis, the whole experience takes on a dreamlike quality, making it hard for you to know what actually happened. Until the experience becomes real to you, coping with the challenges of NICU parenting will be difficult.

Fathers and other family members should participate in discussions of the birth events. Each person will have a different perception of what happened and feel varying levels of responsibility and powerlessness. Mothers of NICU babies may feel a sense of loss and failure. Fathers may feel torn in all directions in trying to meet the needs of other children, parents and in-laws, a sick newborn, and their partner. Nurses can be a great help as you search for answers to your questions and sort out your feelings. Once you begin to understand what happened and can place the events in order, you can begin to move ahead. This will not happen all at once or at the same time for everyone. Allow yourself time for personal recovery and take advantage of supportive people who will listen to your story. You will also discover that NICU parents share many feelings. Your ability to cope will grow over time as you learn about the resources available and gain the strength to move forward.

Chapter 3
NICU Players: Working With the Team

"Would you mind coming with me,
Piglet, in case they turn out to be Hostile Animals?"
—Winnie-the-Pooh

David J. Loren, MD, FAAP

Congratulations on your expanding family! Welcome to your new land, the neonatal intensive care unit (NICU). The NICU is a complicated environment populated by a cadre of people speaking a language you couldn't imagine in your most bizarre dreams.

The NICU can feel intimidating and you may feel overwhelmed with lights, alarms, and smells. Many parents feel frightened just seeing their baby, sometimes so small and hidden by equipment. Your time here is a journey, paved with the preservation of dignity and built on layers of trust.

For some babies, the NICU is a place to finish pregnancy. For others, it's a place to receive specialized care to overcome a problem. In many ways, the NICU tries to fulfill what you were doing in pregnancy, providing a nurturing place for your baby's growth and development.

The NICU is a relatively modern invention, yet its roots extend deep into medical history. The world's first maternity hospital (the ancestor of what we now know as a NICU) opened in 1752 in London at Queen Charlotte's Hospital. Neonatal intensive care units now exist in hospitals around the world in a wide array of practice settings. Some are large (able to care for 80 babies or more) while others are quite small (caring for 6–10 babies). Found in rural settings and urban centers, affiliated with academic institutions or private hospitals, NICUs come in many shapes, sizes, and designs. (See Chapter 1 to learn more about levels of care.) Despite this variation, most NICUs have in common a highly specialized team that provides care for its infants. Who are all of these people, and what are they doing for your baby? Who can best answer your questions? How can you build relationships with these people to stay informed and participate in your baby's care? Who will help you develop your own parenting skills? And who can provide support for you and your emotions?

Your Baby's Team

A small universe, including you, provides care for your baby. Various professionals make up the NICU team in each hospital, and may include different mixtures of neonatal nurse practitioners, neonatal physician assistants, and a variety of physicians, including residents, fellows, neonatologists, and hospitalists. These team members may work in 24-hour shifts or in daytime and nighttime shifts over several weeks. You will come to know many of these team members during your baby's stay in the NICU. While the following descriptions of team members are in discrete groups, each is equally important and all work cooperatively in providing care for your baby. You may meet some of these people after your baby has been admitted to the NICU, at your baby's delivery, or before your baby is even born. Each NICU may have some, or all, of the following individuals.

Nursing Team

Although many people think all nurses do the same things, nothing could be further from the truth. All nurses do have knowledge that provides the foundation for nursing practice (achieved through either an associate's or bachelor's degree), but most also choose an area of specialty and acquire additional skills and expertise specific to that area. In addition, a nurse may hold an advanced master's or doctorate degree.

Registered Nurse

The person who provides the moment to moment care for your baby (besides you!) is your baby's bedside nurse, usually a registered nurse (RN). A neonatal nurse is an RN

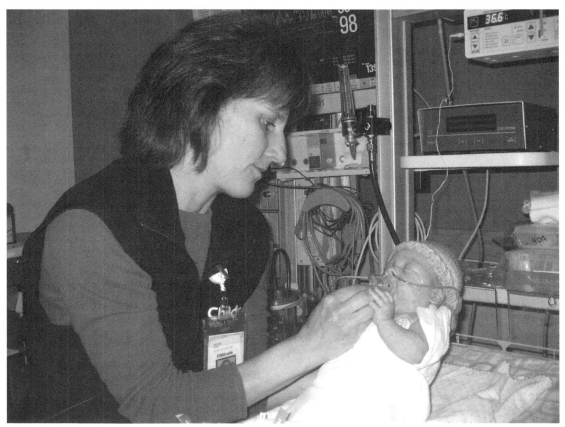

The NICU nurse.
Your baby's nurse is at the bedside more than any other professional. She is your baby's caregiver and advocate, as well as your primary source of information.

Courtesy of Seattle Children's Hospital.

who is highly educated to provide nursing care for infants and their families. The nurse caring for your baby learned NICU clinical skills through an extensive orientation program and clinical preceptorship in the NICU. You may see an RN with the designation "RNC-NIC," which means the nurse has also passed a national specialty examination in neonatal intensive care nursing.

This person may be assigned to care for just your baby or for up to 3 additional babies. The staffing assignment is determined by the skills of your nurse and how much support your baby requires at that time.

Nurses work collaboratively with physicians and other members of the health care team; they are not assistants. Nurses function independently, and their specific roles vary depending on the setting. An RN may supervise a team of other professionals and assistants who help care for patients.

Neonatal nurses are at your baby's bedside 24 hours a day. They assess your baby's current condition and progress, carry out the physician's orders, and notify the physician team (physician, neonatal nurse practitioner [NNP], or neonatal physician assistant) of any changes in your baby's status. The RN may make recommendations to the physician or the team based on his or her assessment of your baby. The RN also plans and implements all nursing care, such as bathing, feeding, positioning, administering prescribed medications, and managing intravenous (IV) and arterial lines. In addition, RNs are very involved in parent education and discharge planning.

The nursing team is supported and led by a charge nurse who oversees the nursing operation for each nursing shift. Behind the scenes, you will often find a NICU nurse manager who provides nursing supervision and leadership for the whole unit and all of the nursing staff.

Clinical Nurse Specialist

A clinical nurse specialist (CNS) (or clinical nurse educator) helps advance the practice of the nursing team. A CNS is an RN with an advanced degree who acts as an expert and resource person for nursing staff. Clinical nurse specialists are involved in many different areas on the unit, including staff education, nursing research, quality improvement, consultation, direct patient care, and program development. Together with the medical team and the nursing staff, the CNS assists the NICU team with your baby's care by making specific recommendations and offering new ideas or techniques to ensure the best possible plan of care.

Licensed Practical Nurse/Licensed Vocational Nurse

A licensed practical nurse (LPN) or licensed vocational nurse (LVN) has graduated from a state-approved technical school or community college and must pass a national written examination. The LPN/LVN provides basic bedside care and works under the direction of an RN.

Medical Team

Your baby may have more medical professionals than you have encountered in your entire lifetime. In every NICU, a member of the medical team is present in the NICU 24 hours a day, and a neonatologist is always on-call for that unit.

Neonatologist

A neonatologist is a physician who specializes in the diagnosis and treatment of sick newborns. Neonatologists have 3 years of specialized training, specifically to treat newborns, beyond that required for general pediatricians. The neonatologist is usually the most knowledgeable member of the team treating your newborn and directs the medical care of your baby. The lead physician in most NICUs is a neonatologist and, in the hierarchy of the medical team, is referred to as the attending physician.

The neonatologist's availability varies from NICU to NICU. In some units, care is directed by a team of neonatologists. That team then shares the responsibility for providing care on a 24-hour basis with a different member of the team being responsible for your baby's care each day. In other facilities, especially in large centers that are also accredited for training the next generation of neonatologists or pediatricians, the neonatologist may be present in the unit for only a portion of each day (and will usually be present during patient rounds). During rounds (see Rhythms and Schedules on page 60), members of the health care team discuss and review your baby's current condition and determine a medical plan of care. The neonatologist makes recommendations to ensure that the NICU team provides the best care for your infant based on a daily plan. If unexpected problems arise, the neonatologist is available to the health care team 24 hours a day.

The neonatologist is responsible for overseeing the medical decisions regarding your baby. The attending neonatologist may also supervise other physicians, some of whom are in varying levels of their professional training, including residents, and fellows. In many large centers the medical team is supported by clinical directors or chiefs of the NICU who may not have direct care of your child at all times but who work with the entire team of neonatologists as well as the nurse managers to oversee the general operations of the whole unit.

Neonatal Nurse Practitioner

An NNP or advanced registered nurse practitioner (ARNP), also called an *advanced practice registered nurse,* or *APRN,* is an RN who has completed advanced education and training in the care and treatment of newborns and their families. In most institutions, a nurse practitioner must have a master's degree in nursing. Working in collaboration with a neonatologist or attending physician, the NNP is an expert in neonatal resuscitation;

examines, diagnoses, and designs a care plan for your baby; and serves as an education resource for all members of the NICU team. The NNP may also perform procedures such as intubation, central line placement, chest tube insertion, and lumbar puncture. In most US states, NNPs (and ARNPs or APRNs) may prescribe medications.

Neonatal Physician Assistant

A neonatal physician assistant (NPA) is a specialist who has earned a certificate or degree from an accredited school and passed a state licensing examination. An NPA has the same general background as other physician assistants, but has completed education and training in the care and treatment of infants and their families. The NPA works under the supervision of a neonatologist or attending physician. An NPA performs delivery room resuscitation and has been trained to assess, diagnose, and design a care plan for your baby. The NPA may also perform procedures such as intubation, central line placement, chest tube insertion, and lumbar puncture and may serve as an education resource for members of the NICU team. An NPA may prescribe medications in most US states.

Hospitalist

A pediatric hospitalist is a physician who has completed a pediatric residency and has developed specific skills and interest in caring for infants and children who require inpatient hospital care. Some hospitalists choose to spend part or all of their time working in a NICU. Hospitalists work under the supervision of a neonatologist and are capable of performing many of the procedures and care for babies in the NICU.

Resident

A resident is a physician who has graduated from medical school and is enrolled in a hospital-based program of specialized training called a *residency program.* Residency programs vary according to specialty (pediatrics, obstetrics, surgery, and so on) and in the amount of time required to complete the training. Pediatric residencies usually take 3 years to complete. A resident can be in his or her first year of training or a physician in the second or third year of the program. You may also hear a resident called an R-1, R-2, or R-3 (denoting a first-, second- or third-year resident) or PGY-1, PGY-2 or PGY-3 (for postgraduate year 1, 2, or 3) or PL-1, PL-2, or PL-3 (for post-licensure year 1, 2, or 3). Most residents in the NICU are enrolled in pediatric residencies, but residents from other specialties, such as family practice, anesthesia, or obstetrics, may be involved as well.

Residents are usually very visible on the unit. They are closely involved with your baby's daily care as members of the medical team. Residents assess your infant daily, then plan and revise the medical care. Residents perform many NICU procedures, such as intubation, placement of IV and arterial lines, lumbar puncture, and chest tube insertion

Resident teams may be composed of members in varying years of their residency training; often senior residents will help supervise junior residents.

Neonatal Fellow

A neonatal fellow is a physician who has completed medical school as well as a pediatric residency and is currently training to become a neonatologist. The fellow works closely with the attending neonatologist and may be more visible on the unit than the neonatologist. Responsibilities of a fellow vary widely. In some units, a fellow may be there all day overseeing the daily plans for each baby in the NICU and at delivery room resuscitations. In other units, the fellow makes rounds in the mornings and provides consultation for residents, NNPs, and NPAs during the rest of the day or night.

Pediatrician

A pediatrician is a physician who has completed a pediatric residency and who provides medical care for children from birth to 18 years (sometimes up to 21 years). In some hospitals, pediatricians with interest in the care of babies with special needs may provide care for babies in the NICU. Other pediatricians may not have special training in NICU care and may therefore refer your baby to a neonatologist. After your baby is discharged from the NICU, your pediatrician commonly becomes your baby's primary care provider. Depending on the needs of your baby, a family practitioner may also be your baby's primary care provider.

Other Medical Personnel

Your baby's medical team may call on other specialists to assist them in providing care for your baby. These consultants may be present in your hospital, available on an intermittent basis, or by telephone.

- Cardiothoracic surgeon: specializes in performing surgery on the heart
- Pediatric cardiologist: specializes in diagnosis and treatment of heart problems (nonsurgical)
- Pediatric gastroenterologist: specializes in treatment of stomach and intestinal problems (nonsurgical)
- Geneticist: studies birth defects and their causes
- Pediatric hematologist: specializes in diagnosis and treatment of blood problems
- Pediatric nephrologist: specializes in the diagnosis and treatment of kidney problems
- Pediatric neurologist: specializes in diagnosis and treatment of the nervous system
- Neurosurgeon: specializes in surgery of the brain and nervous system
- Pediatric surgeon: specializes in performing general surgery for newborns and children
- Otolaryngologist: specializes in ear, nose, and throat surgery

- Pediatric pulmonologist: specializes in diagnosis and treatment of certain lung conditions
- Urologist: specializes in surgery of the urinary tract

Support Team

"My husband has never been comfortable asking for directions or help of any kind. But even he has to admit that the support staff who guided us through our NICU stay were necessary and important for a good experience."

It takes a village to raise a child, and in the NICU, a "village" supports the medical team, nursing team, and your baby. Again, each NICU may have some or all of these team members, and not every baby will require the services of every one of these team members.

Respiratory Therapist

If your baby needs help breathing, a respiratory therapist, also known as a *respiratory care practitioner,* will help manage the appropriate equipment and associated monitoring devices. Some respiratory therapists are trained in endotracheal intubation and may also draw blood to obtain a blood gas from your baby.

Nutritionist

The nutritional aspects of your baby's care may be supported by a pediatric or neonatal nutritionist who will help optimize your baby's growth and development and may recommend specific additives for your baby's breast milk or formula.

Lactation Specialist

Breastfeeding support may be provided by lactation specialists, or by lactation nurses or doctors who have specialized training within your NICU. The lactation specialist manages complex problems of breastfeeding mothers and babies.

Infant Developmental Specialist

Infant development specialists are individuals with training who work with the NICU team to assess your baby's development. These services may be provided by a variety of people, all ensuring that your baby's environment in the NICU and after discharge is optimal for his or her development.

Pediatric/Family Clinical Psychologist

Clinical psychologists may also be available in your NICU to help the team provide support to you. These specialists focus on supporting parents as they develop relationships with their infants and with the NICU staff.

Social Worker

A social worker in the NICU will help coordinate a myriad of services including your own support structure, financial and insurance arrangements, and even housing and transportation needs.

Parent Educator

Your unit may also have a parent educator, usually a nurse, who provides information and instruction for NICU families. This education is usually offered in a group setting, such as through scheduled classes.

Pharmacist

A pharmacist with specific training in neonatal drugs and doses helps ensure the safety of medications and IV nutrition used to treat your baby.

Therapists

Occupational, physical, and speech therapists all have special skills to help foster your baby's neurologic and physical development. These therapists may help with establishing a nipple-feeding program for your baby and may also recommend a range of exercises and stretches for your baby.

Case Manager/Discharge Planner

Some NICUs use the services of a case manager or discharge planner who may follow your baby's hospital course and ensures that orderly progress is being made toward discharge. Either of these people may also help arrange for your baby's transfer to a NICU closer to home.

Medical Students/Nursing Students

If your baby's NICU is part of an academic medical center, medical students and nursing students may also be present in the unit. These students are not yet physicians or RNs but have typically completed all of their core medical or nursing training. Medical and nursing students are closely supervised while working in the NICU.

Chaplain

Your NICU may also have a chaplain or spiritual representative from a specific religion. If one is not present in the NICU, you can often request a member of your religious affiliation to visit the NICU. The chaplain's role is not to convince you to believe or practice religion in any particular way, but rather to help you use any spiritual resources comfortable for you.

Research Investigators

Many NICUs participate in research projects to improve the quality of care for babies or to better understand and treat the diseases of newborns. To help facilitate these research projects, your NICU may have one or more clinical investigators (nurses and/or physicians) present who can discuss whether your baby might be eligible to participate in one of these research projects. Rest assured that your choice to participate or not participate in any research will not change the quality of your baby's care or the devotion of the team in providing that care.

Parent-to-Parent Providers

Your NICU may have a team of parents, some of whom are still in the unit and others of whom have gone home with their babies, who serve as a resource to newer parents in the NICU. These "veteran" parent groups do not provide any care for your baby; rather, they help provide care for you. Referred to as *family* or *parent support groups, parent-to-parent providers,* or *peer advocates,* these parents have "been there" and know the details specific to your unit. Your unit may also participate in the March of Dimes NICU Family Support Program. Whatever the name of these parents in your NICU, they can provide a listening ear, validate your experiences, provide suggestions on who can best answer your questions, and remind you that you are not "in this" alone.

Unit Clerk

When you enter the NICU, you are greeted by the unit clerk who handles the flow of people, paper, and information into and out of the NICU. This person may be identified by other titles, such as unit secretary, patient services coordinator, or health unit coordinator.

Financial Counselor

Your hospital's financial counselor can answer questions concerning your hospital bill, help you submit your bill to the appropriate agencies for payment, and set up a payment plan if you are responsible for any portion of the bill (see Chapter 7).

Simulation Center Staff

Your NICU or hospital may have a simulation center where both care team members and parents can undergo simulated experiences with mannequin babies to improve care and learn necessary skills for taking care of the baby after discharge. You may learn specialized care techniques for your baby in one of these simulation centers or simply have a chance to practice CPR or rescue breathing as part of routine first aid training. If your NICU has a simulation center, you may meet a simulation center coordinator or coach sometime during your baby's hospitalization.

Still More People

Other personnel in the NICU may include laboratory technicians (trained to obtain blood samples); x-ray technicians; ultrasound technicians; patient care associates who help keep bedside supplies stocked; and others, including housekeepers. Sometimes staff members are cross-trained; in addition to their specialty role, they can help perform unit duties such as taking routine vital signs, administering uncomplicated feedings, and transporting patients to different areas of the hospital. Whether providing direct care or mopping the floor, all hospital personnel provide vital services for your baby's care.

Rhythms and Schedules

Parents soon discover what seems to be a never-ending abundance of new faces at their baby's bedside. Even after you have sorted through all of these faces and know who does what, members of the team sometimes do not seem to be available when you want them. Communication of your needs is important at these times. Just a few people cannot possibly meet your baby's care needs 24 hours a day, 7 days a week. Hospital staffing and scheduling is a complicated exercise requiring constant adjustments to meet each unit's needs.

Physicians, Neonatal Nurse Practitioners, and Neonatal Physician Assistants

Personnel scheduling is designed to achieve around-the-clock medical and nursing care for patients. No 2 units solve scheduling needs in the same way. In some units, physicians, NNPs, and NPAs work 24-hour shifts once every 3 or 4 days. In many academic institutions, residents are present in the NICU Monday through Friday during the day and stay overnight on a structured schedule. Therefore, if you visit or have questions during the night, evening, or weekend, you may find yourself speaking with a medical team member you have not seen before.

Physician "rotation" is another area of confusion for parents. When physicians are in residency, they are in training within their specialty. During this time, they must learn everything there is to learn about their specialized population and its accompanying problems. To achieve the necessary training, they rotate (change assignments) through many different patient care areas. This means that about every 4 weeks a new resident may be assigned to care for your baby. Physician rotation may also occur for attending and fellow staff so that the attending and fellow can provide care at other centers or take days off.

Other physicians involved in your baby's care may also schedule rotations. To provide consistent care for your baby, however, physicians rarely rotate all at the same time. It is possible—in fact, highly likely—that in an academically affiliated institution, you may meet new physicians every 1 to 4 weeks. It's understandable that you would be confused or wonder who is caring for your baby.

Nurses

Nurses in the NICU work a variety of shifts, depending on the hospital's system of care delivery. Nurses may be scheduled for 4-, 8-, 10-, or 12-hour shifts and may work just 1 day or several days in a row. Many NICUs use a system called *primary nursing* to allow nurses to develop familiarity with specific patients (called *patient continuity)*. Each infant is assigned a primary nurse from the NICU staff for each shift. The primary nurses from all of the shifts make up the primary nursing team.

Primary nurses work closely with the medical team to plan, implement, and make recommendations for your baby's care. If a primary nurse is not on duty, an associate nurse or another member of the care team may be assigned. The associate nurse communicates closely with your baby's primary nurses to provide consistency for you and your baby, allowing a small number of nurses to become familiar with you and with your baby's individual needs.

Order Among Chaos: Information, Decision-making, and Negotiation

Being a parent in the NICU can be a very complicated experience. You are learning how to be a parent in an unfamiliar environment and among people you do not know. You want to help your baby, and you want to be included in what happens to your baby. You have become a member of a team. What follows is a collection of tools to help you guide the rest of the team to fulfill your hopes and dreams and to help your baby recover.

Day-to-Day Activities

As you'll quickly notice, the size and diversity of the team dedicated to caring for your baby is rather impressive. How do all of these people coordinate their ideas and plans? The most common and time-honored tradition to accomplish team communication is by a process called *rounds*. The exact origin of the term *rounds* is still debated by many medical historians, although its first use occurs well before the last century. The process of medical management—reviewing the previous day's events with the team of nurses, NNPs, NPAs, nutritionists, and others involved in your baby's care and formulating plans for the next day or more—is appropriately called *multidisciplinary care team rounds*. Many NICUs welcome parents to rounds; others ask that parents not be present at the bedside during that time to protect every family's privacy. Whether you participate in rounds or not, the language and complexity of information discussed with you may seem incomprehensible. With time, you will become an expert in your baby's preferences and patterns. Sharing your observations of your baby with the care team during and after rounds and participating in making decisions help the team provide the best care possible for your baby.

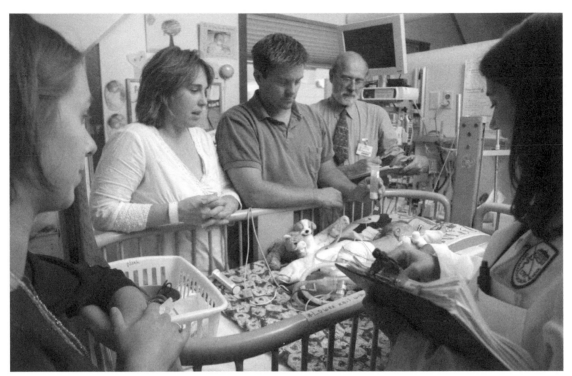

Family-centered care.
These parents are participating in rounds. Sharing with the team your observations about your baby is very important to providing the best care possible for your baby.

Courtesy of George A. Little, MD, FAAP.

Becoming a Partner, Becoming an Expert

You are a crucial part of your baby's care team, and an ally in ensuring the quality and safety of your baby's care. With your baby's admission to the NICU, you enter a partnership with the people in your unit. You enter this partnership likely frightened, somewhat unwilling, and almost certainly exhausted. Just as your baby is arising out of a challenging experience (birth), you too are emerging out of a crisis (NICU admission). Your willingness to trust your baby's care team may start haltingly, and probably somewhat blindly.

As is true in all human relationships, you will likely feel a stronger bond with some members of the medical team than you will with others. With time, you will become familiar with the people caring for your baby, and your trust and confidence will grow. Your questions are very important; for example, even asking if someone washed their hands before touching your baby allows you to participate in providing safe care.

The trust between you and your baby's health care team is built on communication. Open, direct, and honest communication is essential for family survival in the NICU. When this is lacking, parents often feel lost, frustrated, and further isolated from their baby. Now that we have explored the structure of your baby's care team and the complexities of their system, you are probably wondering how to best open the lines of communication with your baby's health care team so that you can ask the questions you need to have answered and understand the answers.

Because of the many professionals involved in your baby's care, you may feel lost in the maze. Who will update you on your baby's progress? What questions should you ask? Who will answer your questions? How can you understand and remember what you are told? There are as many solutions to these questions as there are parents asking them.

Family-Centered Care

In 2001 the Institute of Medicine published a report titled *Crossing the Quality Chasm: A New Health System for the 21st Century*. The authors issued a call for improvement in our health care systems to achieve

- Respect for patients' values, preferences, and expressed needs
- Coordination and integration of care across boundaries of the system
- Information, communication, and education that people need and want
- A guarantee of physical comfort, emotional support, and the involvement of family and friends

In 2003 the American Academy of Pediatrics issued a policy statement supporting family-centered care and reaffirmed this policy in 2007. This policy states "…family-centered care is based on the understanding that the family is the child's primary source of strength and support." Further, this approach to care recognizes that the perspectives and information provided by families, children, and young adults are important in clinical decision-making.

Participate in the Care of Your Baby

During your first days in the NICU, you may feel like unwilling passengers on a ride you never planned to take. You will notice the nurses providing all of the care for your baby, operating complicated pumps, providing medications, changing diapers, tucking in blankets, and so much more. Many parents wonder how they can "be" a parent at times like these when they aren't doing the "things" that parents usually do for their babies. As you become more familiar with your baby's care and preferences, you too will begin to provide these routine care needs. Changing your baby's diaper, taking a temperature, tucking in blankets, changing clothes, and giving a bath are all skills you will learn; let your nurse know when you are ready to begin learning how to provide these care needs. Some parents fear that asking to participate in the care of their baby will "get in the way" of the nurse. Remember that you are your baby's parent. Your baby will go home with you, not the nurses. Rest assured that most nurses are eager to help you become "the expert" in your baby's care. Sometimes participation is simply "being there." Ask about your baby's schedule, particularly about when feedings are provided, and when your baby is more awake.

Some NICUs welcome parents' presence during procedures (IV starts, placement of peripherally inserted central catheters, intubation). If you wish to be present during a procedure, please let your baby's nurse or other care team member know. If you stay in your baby's room during a procedure, you may be asked to wear a mask or hair cover to help prevent infection. If you begin to feel faint, nauseous, or emotional, let a member of the NICU team know right away so that you can get support immediately.

If your NICU is in an academic institution and you are asked to step out during complex procedures, it is most likely because the health care provider (a resident, for example) is still learning the procedure, asking questions, and possibly requesting help from the supervising physician or neonatal nurse practitioner. In some cases, the procedure is more likely to be successful if the health care provider is not under parent observation. A provider's comfort level with a parent's presence during procedures varies among providers; therefore, it is all right to ask the provider if you may stay. If you make it clear that you will step out at the provider's request, you may be more successful with making that person comfortable with your presence.

Learn About Common Terms, Phrases, and Problems

Simply having greater familiarity with the words and concepts you hear in rounds and around the NICU will help you feel more a part of what is happening. Knowledge really is power. The more informed you are, the better you will understand what is happening to your baby. Reading this book will help. Talking with other parents who have gone through a NICU experience may help (here is where the "veteran" parents can be remarkably helpful). If you like detailed information, ask your baby's nurse or physician for written materials that explain what is happening to your baby. Many NICUs have a guidebook for their parents that describes common procedures and roles of individuals in that unit. Some NICUs have a parent resource center within the unit with books and even computers for parents to research electronic resources. See Appendix D for guidance when using the Internet for information. Keep in mind that anyone can post information and ideas on the Internet; not all of it is accurate or even truthful. Ask for Web site recommendations from a parent educator, a family resource center specialist, or a member of your baby's care team. Your NICU may also have a specialized parent support and training program to help familiarize you with your baby's anticipated NICU experience. The more you understand, the more effective an advocate you can be for your baby.

Become Familiar With the Members of Your Baby's Care Team

"For new parents, the NICU experience is like being dumped into one of those complicated coffee drinks. The staff members blend smoothly and work well together. But new parents just bob around on top, feeling conspicuous and vulnerable, like puffs of whipped cream."

You are one of the most important members of your baby's care team. Your observations of your baby are very important to the team's understanding of how your baby is doing. Don't hesitate to ask your baby's nurse or other care team members how you can become more involved in the day-to-day events of your baby. Many NICUs invite parents to join and participate in rounds. And since you will eventually have your baby at home, sharing with the team your observations of what your baby enjoys and dislikes is very important to providing the best care possible for your baby.

Because of staff rotations, parents often have difficulty identifying members of their baby's team. Until you become familiar with the system, introduce yourself every time you see a new face, and never feel shy about asking a team member to identify their role on the care team. It is your right to know who is caring for your baby.

The team members working directly with your baby are the most informed and up to date about your baby's progress and plan of care. Your baby's nurse will often be the most familiar with the care plan and often can answer most of your questions in language that you can understand. The nurse spends the most time at your baby's bedside and is usually the staff member most available to you for questions and discussion. It's usually best to direct your questions to the nurse on your primary care nursing team most familiar with your baby or to the physician, NNP, or NPA directly managing your baby's care.

Different team members will have different approaches and may use different language to describe the same thing. Don't be surprised if you hear different explanations from different team members. Some parents have found that sitting down and talking with several team members at once (nursing team, medical team, social worker) can help clarify any misunderstandings that have developed from these differing explanations. (See Request a Care Conference on page 69.)

Your team members will change, both daily and over the weeks or even months. Ask your nurse or other team members how frequently team members change and how they share information with each other. The more you know about the methods of communication in your NICU, the easier it will be for you to get your questions answered and participate in your baby's care.

"I was so relieved the neonatologist asked me that question during rounds. I wanted to make sure she knew what happened to my baby the night before because it made a difference to Brian's care plan that day."

Be Clear About How Much You Want to Know

"How are things going today?" may seem like a straightforward question to you, but NICU staff may have difficulty knowing how much and what kind of information you expect in response. Some parents want specific clinical information, such as laboratory results and ventilator settings. Other parents prefer more general information, such as how well their baby slept or whether their baby is tolerating feedings.

Tell your baby's care providers about the type of information you expect to receive and when you want to know it. Give them an example. Do you want to be called immediately with abnormal (sometimes called *critical*) test results, or can you be informed of them when you visit? Do you want to be informed only of unusual test results, or do you want to know every test result? Be honest with the NICU staff. Don't expect your baby's caregivers to read your mind. Your preferences for information will likely change over time. Just tell your baby's care team what you want to know and when.

Tactics to Open Conversations

Sometimes parents in the NICU begin to feel that they are not getting all of the answers they want and need. If you feel that members of your baby's care team are not hearing your concerns or welcoming your suggestions, you may need to help guide them toward understanding your questions better. Prefacing your questions or ideas with dialogue openers can help you reach your goals. These openers reflect a "we're in this together" approach rather than ones that may be perceived as demanding or confrontational. Here are some examples.

Barriers	Openers
"I want you to…"	"Would you think about…?"
	Or "Can you share with me the pros and cons of…"
"Why can't you…?"	"What if we tried…?"
"The experts say…"	"I read about…. Do you think that might work?"
	Or "Can you help me understand why this choice was made?"
"No one told me about…"	"I'm not familiar with that, can you tell me more about…..?"

Parents who use basic negotiation and diplomacy skills when communicating with the NICU team can experience a greater sense of success in establishing a satisfying partnership. That partnership is important as you all strive to achieve the same goal—to help your baby become well. In a strong partnership, your ideas and concerns will receive the attention they deserve.

Ask for Clarification

Because professionals are comfortable with the topics they address often and the medical terminology they use among themselves, it is easy for them to forget that the NICU experience is an entirely new one for most parents and other family members. If you do not understand an explanation or cannot follow a discussion, do not be afraid to ask that terms be defined or that the explanation be repeated. You'll be surprised how quickly you'll pick up even a few common terms of NICU jargon, even though it may sound like a foreign language at first.

Keep Asking Questions

It is important to feel comfortable and satisfied with the answers you receive to your questions. If you are not satisfied with what you are being told or do not understand it, take your question to someone with more expertise. If your baby's nurse or other care provider is not giving you the information you need, ask to speak with a more senior physician, NNP, or NPA. Do not be afraid of offending members of the team because you are "going over their heads." Remember, this is your baby. You have a right to information from the most knowledgeable person available.

Keep in mind, however, that you may not get the answer you desire. Some questions have no clear answers. In other cases, too many variable factors exist to permit a specific answer. At other times, parents may be looking for an unrealistic answer to their question.

Lack of a conclusive answer can be frustrating. You may feel as if information is being kept from you, even though this is probably not the case. Acknowledging your frustration to the members of the health care team may help you deal with that feeling. Chances are that team members are also frustrated when they cannot give a conclusive answer.

Some parents find that reading the medical chart is a helpful way to understand what is happening and what the care team is thinking about their baby. You are entitled to read your baby's chart; the notes may be on paper in a physical chart book near your baby's bedside or electronically stored in a computer. Many care teams create a periodic summary of a baby's progress. This summary, often called an *interim summary,* can also be a helpful resource to you to better understand what is happening to your baby and what you might expect in the coming days or weeks. To keep communication open, inform your baby's nurse or medical care provider that you wish to read your baby's chart. Some units ask that you read the chart with a NICU team member present who can clarify information and immediately answer your questions.

An emerging practice in some pediatric hospitals and hospitals with NICUs is a place for parents to record their observations and questions as part for their baby's chart. Called *parent charting,* it is another method for you to communicate your concerns and desires with your baby's care team.

Make Appointments With People You Want to See

As you have noticed, there are both many schedules and no schedule in the NICU. Even if you have been told that the neonatologist is usually in the unit at a certain time, do not plan to "catch" the physician for a lengthy discussion during patient rounds. A more effective approach is to schedule an appointment to discuss your baby's progress. This gives the professionals involved time to review and organize the most up-to-date information regarding your baby's care. A scheduled appointment also increases your chances for uninterrupted time to discuss your questions and concerns and will most likely include more team members at the meeting.

When the Unexpected Happens

It is important to know the difference between the terms complication, adverse event, and error.

- A *medical complication* is an unwelcome but not unexpected problem that arises during the course of illness or recovery. Before your baby was born, you may have been counseled about some of the common complications that can occur when a baby is in the NICU.
- An *adverse event* is an injury caused by medical management rather than by your baby's underlying problems. An adverse event may be something as simple as a bruise from an IV or can be more serious, such as an infection resulting from the presence of a central line. Hospitals and NICU teams strive to prevent adverse events through a variety of quality assurance programs.
- An *error* is the failure of a planned action to be completed as intended. When something happens that was not expected or planned, it may have been caused by an error. Even the most skilled care team can make a mistake when providing care for a baby.

You can help prevent errors in the NICU, or call attention to an error before the consequences become more serious. If you see something that doesn't seem right, tell your baby's nurse or anyone else on the care team right away. Your baby's care team will first make sure that your baby is safe and that any problems are being properly managed. Once your baby's safety is ensured, you will want to learn more about what happened, why, and what will be done to prevent a similar error from occurring again. Members of your care team may want to apologize to you, and other representatives of the hospital may want to meet with you to provide additional support. When the unexpected happens, your trust may be impaired; your confidence may be shaken. Your team will want to repair the damage an error can cause in their relationship with you.

When Conflicts Arise

The word *intensive* in *intensive care unit* sometimes refers to the emotions felt by parents and other care team members. While your baby's care team members work in this environment, you are a temporary member and may be under significant emotional, physical, and/or financial stress. You may have expectations that are not being met, you may have responded to someone in a manner you did not plan, or you may have heard disturbing news about your baby.

If you are feeling angry, try to ask yourself if it is at a specific person or a situation in the unit. Discuss your feelings and experiences with someone on the care team whom you trust. For example, the NICU charge nurse or nurse manager may be a valuable resource to you if you need to discuss concerns regarding your interactions with your baby's nursing team. Likewise, you may want to speak with the attending neonatologist to discuss interactions with your baby's medical team. One of the "veteran" parents in the NICU may be trained to help you, or the NICU social worker can help find a solution to your conflict and help you plan how to resolve the cause of your anger.

Request a Care Conference

"I was lost at first—so many people and too much information. The care conference helped me organize my thoughts and understand much of what was happening to my baby. I could breathe again."

Even if you do not have specific questions about your baby's health or plan of care, it's often helpful to meet with members of the health care team periodically for updates. Your baby's care team may schedule a conference—commonly called a *care conference*—for you or you may request one yourself. These meetings help familiarize you with team members you may not see daily. Most of the time, meetings with your baby's care team members are informal and at your baby's bedside. A formalized care conference gives you the opportunity to ask questions of multiple team members at once, get updates on any significant changes in your baby's plan of care, and learn what progress the members of the team are hoping to see from your baby. You can ask one of the team members (most often your NICU social worker) to take notes during the meeting. Some parents find that writing down notes from the meeting or recording the conversation gives them the chance to review the meeting later, when they can be alone and not in the social pressure of a group discussion.

How frequently you meet with the team depends on your baby's medical problems. You may meet once a day if your baby is very unstable or once every few weeks if your baby has chronic problems. Usually the members of the health care team most closely involved with your baby (for example, the neonatologist, NNP, NPA, and primary nurse) attend these meetings. Depending on your baby's condition, other personnel also may be asked to attend. You may discover that you do not need to meet with the entire team and that 1 or 2 key people can provide you with the information you need. Remember that these meetings are for your benefit and can be customized to meet your needs.

Ask About Your Baby's Care Plan

Your baby is of course unique to you; however, the problems your baby experiences may be common in the NICU. Many NICUs have developed care plans, care maps, or clinical pathways to help provide consistently high-quality care to babies with specific medical problems. A general clinical pathway shows the expected progression of an illness or problem over a specific period. Clinical pathways reflect general expectations concerning a particular diagnosis; they do not incorporate your baby's individual characteristics. By

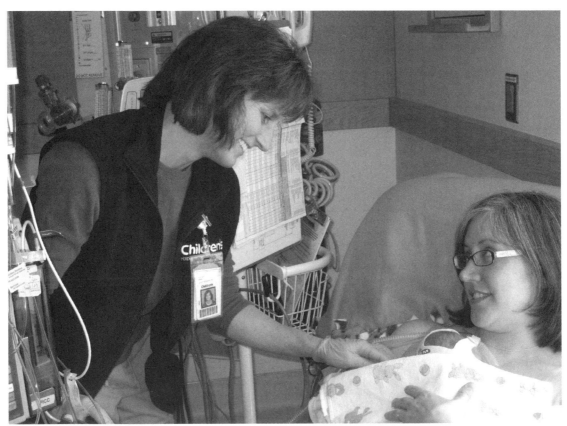

Vital communication.
The health care professionals in the NICU use every opportunity to teach you about your baby's special needs. This nurse answers the mother's questions and points out the baby's special characteristics.

Courtesy of Seattle Children's Hospital.

understanding your baby's clinical pathway, you may better understand daily routines and be able to recognize milestones in your baby's NICU experience.

The care plan guides how and when things are done. The care plan often describes how your baby's care team will respond to your baby (everything from when and how to begin or increase feedings to when your baby is ready to leave the incubator) and usually is customized to meet your baby's particular medical needs. Depending on the level of information you want, knowing about something as simple as your baby's feeding plan may be enough. Parents desiring more detailed information can ask more complex questions, such as "What is the plan for weaning my baby off of the ventilator? What is the plan for dealing with my baby's heart murmur?"

It is also important to realize that care plans change. Care plans must be flexible; they depend on your baby's response to treatments and to your baby's overall condition. Ask frequently for an update on the care plan. If the plan has changed, ask why: "What about my baby has changed to cause this change in care?" If the care plan has not changed, do not be afraid to ask about that either: "Why hasn't the plan changed despite the fact that my baby hasn't [or has] gotten better?" You are not challenging anyone's expertise or knowledge. You are merely asking for clarification.

Some parents notice that all team members may not be familiar with a baby's unique care plan elements. One strategy to help communicate your baby's specific needs is to post the relevant part of your baby's care plan at the bedside or on the wall of your baby's room.

As your baby requires less and less support from the NICU team, you may wonder what plans need to be arranged for you to go home. For some families, the path to going home is very straightforward and requires no special planning. For others, especially for babies with complicated medical needs, the path to home will demand careful consideration. In these circumstances, discharge preparation may be made much clearer by designing a specific care plan that coordinates all elements of discharge preparation, a kind of "road map" to discharge. Chapters 15 and 16 discuss preparation for discharge in more detail.

Ask "What If" Questions

All too often, parents do not ask the "What if?" questions and then become frustrated because the questions have not been addressed. "What if this drug doesn't work?" "What if we decide against surgery?" "What if this treatment doesn't work?" Asking "What if?" questions can make you better informed about the treatment, procedure, or medication in question. Keep in mind that at times a definitive answer doesn't exist. While the knowledge and expertise to care for babies keeps improving, there are times when a decision must be made by carefully weighing the risks and benefits and then choosing what simply feels like the best answer to you and the NICU team at that time.

Keep a Journal

Initially, you may feel too exhausted and overwhelmed to keep a journal, but try to make the effort as soon as you are able. You will be bombarded with an enormous amount of information as soon as you step into the NICU. Writing things down can help you keep your thoughts organized. Keep a record of who you spoke with and what was discussed. As you review your journal later, many of the things you jotted down may seem clearer.

Building Memories, Sharing Stories

"All the feedback we've received from our baby's team has made us feel confident as parents."

Sharing your baby with friends and family is an important part of becoming a parent. However, you may be inundated with calls from everyone who cares about you and wants to hear news of your baby. Your family members and friends need to know that the NICU will not release any information about your baby in order to comply with privacy laws and protect your confidentiality. Some parents find that asking one particular friend or relative to serve as a family spokesperson can help maintain your own privacy and protect you from the exhaustion of repeatedly telling your baby's story.

Many NICUs have cameras available for parents to take pictures of their baby. Often, your baby's nurse will take pictures for you so you can see what your baby is doing when you are not in the NICU. These pictures can be tremendously comforting for parents who live in a city far away from their baby's NICU. You can also share your baby's story and pictures on the Internet. CaringBridge.org is one of the most well-known sponsors of this service.

Write Down Questions as You Think of Them

Families often have many questions regarding their baby, but when the opportunity arises to ask those questions no one can remember what they were. To avoid this problem, write down your questions as they occur to you. Keep your list in your purse or wallet so that you'll have it handy when the next opportunity arises to ask your questions. You can use the same piece of paper to record the answers to your questions. When you get home, tape the piece of paper in your journal for future reference.

Take Care of Yourself

The NICU environment can be very stressful. You will encounter many unfamiliar experiences and a lot of information. You'll have a much more difficult time processing that information if you are exhausted, hungry, or sick. Try to nap during the day, or at least sit down in a quiet area and put your feet up. Try to eat regular meals or, if that is too difficult, eat frequent, healthy snacks. Allow family and friends to help out by cooking meals for you, cleaning your house, or sometimes caring for your other children. Often these people want to help but don't know how.

Because the NICU is so demanding, everyone needs an occasional break. Give yourself permission to take a day off from being with your baby and do something for yourself. It may be difficult for you to skip a daily visit, but you may find that the rest and relaxation you enjoy make the next time in the NICU even more worthwhile.

Give Yourself Some Time

"After my time in the NICU, I feel good about my baby and about us as parents."

Following your first NICU visit, you may feel overwhelmed by the environment and hopelessly outnumbered by the staff. In time, you will be able to identify the people who are caring for your baby and know what they do. With patience, you will develop effective relationships with them. These are the first important steps toward active involvement in your baby's care.

Each NICU is a village, with its own customs, language, codes of behavior, and "native" habits. Becoming part of this new community occurs at a time of significant stress when your whole world is turned upside down. Seek counsel from other parents in the NICU, and remember that some of the members of your baby's care team may have had their own children in a NICU. Give yourself some time to adjust to this difficult place, and remember that your NICU team wants you to be an informed, participating partner in your baby's care.

I would like to thank F. Sessions Cole, MD; Kim Detjen, MSW; and Joan Smith, ARPN, for their thoughtful contributions and reflections.

Chapter 4
Getting Acquainted

"Piglet was so excited at the idea of being Useful
that he forgot to be frightened any more...."

Brenda Lykins, RNC-NIC, BSN

Getting acquainted with your baby begins during pregnancy and continues at birth. However, because your baby was ill or premature, you and your partner may have seen your baby only briefly before she was taken to the nursery.

Your first time to the nursery may have brought mixed feelings of excitement and jubilation accompanied by a sense of fear and loss. You may wonder how you will ever understand what has happened, and worry if you will be able to help care for your baby. In this chapter, we will discuss your first experiences in the neonatal intensive care unit (NICU), the importance of taking care of yourself, and common feelings and reactions of NICU parents. Then we will discuss your infant's unique capabilities, behavioral states, and cues. These are important as you learn to care for and interact with your ill or premature baby. Remember, you are your baby's parents, and the foundation of your baby's NICU care team.

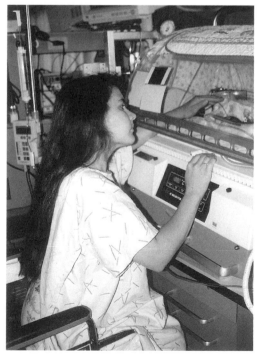

First visit.
Your first visit to the NICU can be overwhelming. Take advantage of a quiet moment to touch and talk to your new baby.

Your First Time to the NICU

Depending on your baby's condition at birth, she may have been taken immediately to the NICU, without you getting as much as a glimpse of this new member of your family. If you experienced a high-risk birth or emergency cesarean section, you may have had general anesthesia and the father of the baby or your support person may not have been able to attend the birth. Both of you may feel that you missed the birth experience. You may see your new baby for the first time in the NICU. You will likely feel a strong desire to see and hold your baby, and you probably will have many questions: How did this happen? Will I feel like her mother or father? Will my baby survive? Your first experiences in the NICU lay the groundwork for future encounters. The next section includes recommendations for taking care of yourself and learning what to expect in the NICU.

Take Care of Yourself

The birth process is amazing—and exhausting for parents, especially following pregnancy and birth complications. If possible, try to rest before you see your baby in the nursery. Writing down any questions you may have before you rest may help you relax. It is not uncommon for parents to feel energized after delivery, so watch your energy, and carefully pace yourselves.

If labor was long, you and your partner may not have eaten anything for some time. If you are able, eat something before you visit the NICU. It is normal to have no appetite when feeling stressed; however, hypoglycemia (low blood sugar) can lead to nausea, which can cut your visit short. Small, frequent healthy snacks and plenty of fluids may help, and can also help build a mother's milk supply.

The hospital environment is unpleasant for some people. The sights, sounds, and smells of the NICU, along with the stress of having an ill or premature baby, may cause you to feel faint or nauseous. Most parents find that these feelings disappear as they grow more familiar with the NICU.

Try to use the bathroom before you visit. Women who have just given birth need to urinate frequently, and the parent bathroom may be outside of the NICU.

Get Updated

If your partner or support person has already been to the NICU, talk together about the experience. Ask your partner what you can expect to see and how your baby is doing. If this is the first time to the NICU for both of you, or if your baby's condition is changing from moment to moment, ask to speak with the NICU nurse before you go. Knowing ahead of time what to expect may help you feel more comfortable.

Getting to the NICU

If you have just given birth, you will likely get to the NICU by stretcher or wheelchair. A wheelchair provides a place to sit and rest, and you can save your energy to spend special time with your new baby.

Take a Companion With You

If your partner or support person cannot be with you on your first trip to the NICU, ask your nurse to accompany you. You may remember little of what you are told about your baby this time. If someone else is with you, you will later be able to discuss details with that person.

Focus on Your Baby

All of the equipment in the NICU, such as machines, tubes, and wires, can be overwhelming. Take time to ask questions about any of this equipment, but especially take time to get acquainted with your new baby. Even at your first meeting, your baby will recognize your voice and know you are her parent. Let the staff know your baby's name. Notice her eye color, the silky touch of her hair, and her unique hands and feet. This is exciting information for you to share with others in your family. You may also want to ask for a picture of your baby to take with you. Many NICUs have cameras that provide immediate pictures to take back to your room.

What to Expect

You may not understand everything about your baby's plan of care at first. The first contact is just one step in the process of becoming acquainted with your baby and her health care team. On each subsequent meeting, you will become more familiar with your baby and more knowledgeable about your baby's condition and the technology being used to help her. Feel free to ask questions while you're at the bedside, or call after you leave. The nurses and staff caring for your baby are there to answer any questions you have, and can also provide you with other helpful resources.

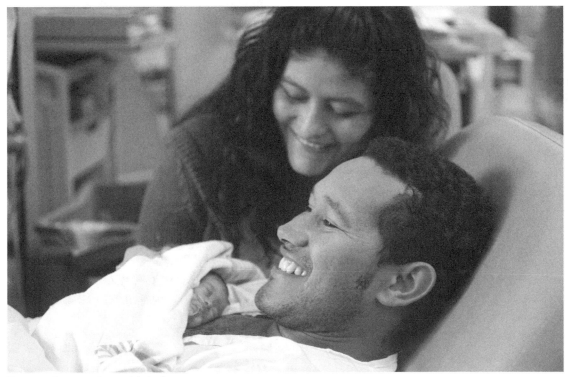

Parents interacting with baby.
Getting acquainted with your baby takes time. This father is now comfortable enough with the NICU environment to enjoy skin-to-skin care with his baby.

Courtesy of University of Washington Medical Center, Seattle, WA.

Common Parent Reactions to the NICU

The NICU is a wealth of sensory input. You may be overwhelmed by the amount of equipment. Many of these machines have unique operating noises and alarms that may frighten you or make you feel something is not right with your baby. (Chapter 2 explains equipment.) The NICU staff are specially trained to interpret and respond to any concerning alarms and explain what they mean. As you spend more time in the NICU, you too will begin to distinguish among various alarm sounds.

Depending on the time of day, the unit may be a flurry of activity. More people tend to be in the NICU during the day because this is when most physicians, nurse practitioners, and physician assistants make rounds (visit each patient) and most diagnostic testing is performed. Many different health care providers involved in your baby's care will introduce themselves to you. Don't worry about remembering their names or what they do. The staff understand that you are taking in a lot of new information and will continue to introduce themselves as you get to know each other and develop your NICU partnership. (Chapter 3 explains the roles of various NICU personnel.)

Parents report a range of reactions and emotions following their first moments in the NICU. How you feel may depend on whether you were expecting your infant to need NICU care after birth, your baby's condition, your own condition, and if you have had any past NICU experience.

Fear

Fear is a normal reaction to the unknown. Most parents have little previous experience with sick newborns; many are uncomfortable in the NICU environment and concerned about their baby. They may also fear the possibility of serious illness, disability, or even death. They may even begin to question their own abilities to take care of this ill or premature baby.

Some parents also fear their friends' and relatives' responses to the birth. Mothers sometimes fear their partner will blame them for a complicated birth and fear the loss of the relationship. Often mothers feel that their mother or their partner's mother is judging them as responsible for the baby's problems. It helps to know that most pregnancy and birth complications are not anyone's "fault" and many NICU admissions are unforeseen. Fears and misgivings usually decrease over time, but most NICU parents feel apprehensive in the early part of their NICU stay.

Anger

Anger is also a common reaction to the initial NICU experience. Many parents feel angry at the hospital staff—both the labor and delivery staff and the NICU staff. You may feel angry that your birth experience did not go as expected, or you may be angry at your inability to control events in the NICU ("They just don't know what they're doing."), at your family and friends ("They just don't understand."), and even your partner ("How can he go to work and just forget about the baby?"). You may even be angry at yourself ("Why couldn't I carry this baby to term?" or "What did I do/not do to make this happen to my baby?"). As uncomfortable as it may be, you may also feel angry at your baby ("Why couldn't you have waited for just a few more weeks?").

Most parents of NICU babies feel some anger, and they express it in different ways. Some are openly angry, demanding, and looking to blame others. Some want to retreat or run and keep their anger hidden inside. It may be difficult to acknowledge any anger, especially if that anger is directed toward your baby or partner.

To cope with anger, begin by acknowledging it to yourself, your partner, and those around you. Realize that anger is a normal, expected emotion common to most NICU parents. By discussing your feelings with NICU staff, you may begin to understand why you feel this way. Are you upset with someone in particular, or is the situation itself the problem? By discussing your feelings, you can begin to make a plan to address the problems you want to confront or things you want to try to change.

Anger requires a tremendous amount of energy. As NICU parents, you will spend a great amount of energy just getting through each day—getting to and from the hospital, absorbing the vast amounts of information you receive, spending time with your baby, caring for yourself and your household, and coping with the common emotional ups and downs of having an ill or premature baby. Dealing with your anger can give you more energy to care for yourself and your baby.

Guilt

"It took us a long time to resolve our guilt. We asked the 'what if' and 'why us' questions for months. But we did nothing wrong. We had good prenatal care. What happened to us was nobody's fault."

Most parents express feelings of guilt after the birth of a sick or premature baby. You may ask yourself, "What did I do to cause this?" or "What could I have done to prevent this?" And nearly every parent unnecessarily laments, "If only I hadn't…." Mothers, especially, examine their lives since the day they became pregnant—wondering if they could have changed the outcome by making different decisions or if their circumstances had been different.

For most babies in the NICU, the reasons they were born sick or premature are not known. If necessary, let go of guilty feelings, which will give you more energy to care for yourself and your new baby. It is also important to try and share these feelings with the NICU team. Often the NICU team can provide answers and comfort.

Loss

Throughout your pregnancy, you probably had an image of your baby. For most parents, this picture was that of a healthy full-term infant. Seeing your premature or ill baby for the first time may lead to feelings of loss for what you had expected. Most mothers of term infants report that they are glad their pregnancy is over; however, mothers of premature babies often mourn the end of their pregnancy. Mothers of premature babies frequently find that they miss feeling the baby inside of them and did not feel ready to give birth. Neonatal intensive care unit mothers may also feel jealous of women who are still pregnant, or of mothers who have given birth to healthy term babies.

If your birth didn't happen as you planned, you and your partner may also mourn the loss of that planned birth experience. Many couples today plan who will attend the birth, how the environment will look, how they will manage the labor process, and how much medical intervention they desire. Some write detailed birth plans to convey their desires to their care providers. Unfortunately, your preterm or complicated birth may have required an abrupt, unplanned change to your experience.

You may also feel the loss of your parenting role. Throughout pregnancy, you envisioned yourself as a parent. You pictured yourself and your partner playing with and caring for your baby. Now you must spend time with your baby in a foreign environment, touch your baby through an incubator porthole, and wait for someone else to tell you when it's appropriate for you to hold or feed your baby. Letting go of what has been lost is an important part of your transition to parenthood. Now you must develop a new dream of your growing family and different goals for marking progress. These new goals may be quite different (such as weaning off of oxygen or breastfeeding for the first time), and parents cannot set these new goals until they let go of the old dream of a healthy full-term infant.

It may take time to get over these feelings of loss. Many revisit these feelings frequently—sometimes for years—often around the time of their baby's birth. Again, this is a normal reaction for many NICU families. As with anger, it often helps to discuss and acknowledge these feelings of loss. You may find it helpful to talk with other parents who have had a baby in the NICU. Your NICU team can help you identify possible support in your area.

Powerlessness

You find yourself in a strange environment, surrounded by high-tech equipment and a multitude of people caring for your baby. You want to comfort your baby, but you may not know what to do. These feelings of powerlessness are common in the NICU.

Begin by understanding that most NICU parents feel powerless, and acknowledge those feelings: "I feel like I can't do anything for my baby." If you are not yet comfortable with your baby's nurses, you might begin by making observations and asking questions: "My baby looks uncomfortable. What can I do to help her?" or "My baby's lips are dry. What can I use to moisten them?" As you become more comfortable with the NICU environment and have experience touching and interacting with your baby, feelings of confidence will begin to replace your initial feelings of powerlessness.

Discuss your feelings with your baby's nursing staff. They can often suggest unique ways for you to communicate with the NICU team and participate in your baby's care. For example, providing breast milk for your baby is an important contribution to your baby's care. Even if you had planned to formula feed later, you may want to consider breastfeeding now. Breast milk is especially important for sick or premature infants because it provides ideal nutrition and other benefits that help your baby heal and grow (see Chapter 5).

Feeling "On Display"

Unlike most hospital rooms for children and adults, several NICU babies and their parents may share space in the same large room. Many parents say that this exposure makes them feel like "fish in a tank" during their early experiences in the NICU. You may feel that others are watching your every move, and this loss of privacy can be stressful. The staff in the NICU are observing you to help you learn to care for your baby. They have special training with premature and ill infants and can observe the baby for signs of stress that you may not yet understand. In addition, other NICU parents may be watching you to identify you with your baby and to compare your circumstances to theirs. This socialization is part of the getting-to-know-you process in the NICU. The more familiar you become with the environment, the more comfortable you will be with the NICU staff, the routines, and your ability to care for your baby. Your care and presence are known by your baby and are vital to your baby's growth and healing.

Learning the NICU Routine

Every NICU has an orientation program for parents. Ask about your NICU orientation, and seek out the information you need to understand your baby's care. You may find the sample orientation and learning checklists helpful as you begin to learn what you need to know.

Orientation Checklist for NICU Parents

General Information for Parents

Nursery telephone number

Visiting policy for parents, siblings, grandparents

Location of cafeteria, restrooms, public telephone, family waiting area

Hand washing policy

Infant security policy

Safekeeping place for purses, coats, briefcases, and so on, while visiting in nursery

Breast pump use; milk pumping and storing policies

Feeding schedules; how to communicate wish to perform bathing, feeding, other baby care

How to arrange consistent daily call from nursery to parent (especially if parent is far from NICU)

Ways to stay in touch or keep friends and family updated (Web cameras, hospital Web page for family)

Policy regarding parent access to baby's chart

People Parents Need to Know

Primary nurse

Parent contact person (nurse manager, clinical nurse specialist, case manager)

Names of medical providers managing baby's care: how to contact, who covers when managing medical provider is unavailable

Lactation specialist or resource person for lactation support

Social worker assigned to baby

Other caregivers (physical therapist, development therapist, and so on): when they visit, how parents can participate

Other Useful Information for Parents

Classes and support groups for parents, siblings, grandparents

Discharge criteria

Discharge planning options (rooming-in, day pass to go home briefly before discharge)

Telephone numbers for medical records, financial counselor, business office

Information Nursery Needs About Parents

Telephone numbers (best daytime phone, nighttime phone; who else to call in an emergency)

Special needs of parents (hearing or visual impairment, literacy or language barrier)

Cultural or spiritual values that will affect baby's care or parents' involvement in caregiving

Social situation that might affect protection of baby, staff, or other NICU patients (restraining order against partner or others, child custody problems, history of unstable or violent behavior on part of significant other or family members, and so on)

84

Learning Checklist for NICU Parents

Parents Learn About

NICU Equipment

Basic

Gloves
Warmer
Incubator or isolette
Cardiorespiratory (heart/breathing) monitor
Pulse oximeter
Transcutaneous monitor
Phototherapy equipment
Infant scales
Diaper scale
Suction equipment
Other: _____

Respiratory

Oxygen
Endotracheal (breathing) tube and ventilator
Continuous positive airway pressure (CPAP)
Oxyhood
Nasal cannula
Oxygen tent
Oxygen analyzers
Chest tube
Positive pressure ventilation device
Other: _____

Lines

Peripheral intravenous (IV)
Umbilical catheter (arterial and venous)
Peripherally inserted central catheter
    (PICC) line (central)
Percutaneous line
Other: _____

Feeding

Gavage/tube
Cup/dropper
Gastrostomy tube
Pump
Infant formula (types)
Breast milk additives
Other: _____

NICU Medications

Intravenous (IV)
Endotracheal (ET)
Intramuscular (IM)
Aerosol (breathing)
Oral
Topical
Other: _____

NICU Procedures

Glucose test strip
X-ray
Sepsis workup
Ultrasound
Computed tomography (CT) scan
Echocardiogram (ECG)
Magnetic resonance imaging (MRI)
Electroencephalogram (EEG)
Other: _____

NICU Lab Work

Blood glucose
Complete blood count (CBC)/hematocrit (Hct)
Arterial blood gas (ABG)/
Capillary blood gas (CBG)
Electrolytes
Culture and sensitivity
Bilirubin
Metabolic screening
Medication levels
Other: _____

Parents Learn to

**Understand infant behavior/
    developmental care**

Hold and position baby correctly
Take baby's temperature
Change baby's diaper
Dress baby
Perform umbilical cord care if necessary
Perform skin care
Bathe baby

Learning Checklist for NICU Parents	
Parents Learn to (continued)	**Parents Know How to Access Referrals to**
Use kangaroo care if desired/appropriate	
Perform infant massage as appropriate	Support groups
Use breast pump; store and use breast milk safely	Specialty medical care (cardiac, gastroenterology, and so on)
Breastfeed and/or bottle feed	Hearing tests
Use bulb syringe; perform mouth care	Eye examinations
Administer medications	Occupational and/or developmental therapy
Use car safety seat correctly	
Perform infant cardiopulmonary resuscitation (CPR)	Public health nurse
Use home monitor and equipment if necessary	Home health nurse
Perform special care tasks	Social services
Recognize signs of illness	Other: _____
Immunize baby against preventable illness	
Other: _____	

Protecting Your Baby From Infection

Hand washing is the best way to protect your baby from infection. Each time you come to the NICU, you will be asked to scrub your hands at a sink, and you may be asked to remove your coat before entering the unit or cover your clothes with a clean hospital gown. Many NICUs supply waterless hand cleaner (alcohol gel) at each bedside for quick cleanups after you touch potentially unclean surfaces, such as the telephone, your baby's chart, or a wet diaper. Each NICU has its own policies for preventing infection, so ask your NICU nurse what to expect in your unit.

Some NICUs limit visitors to the baby's parents and perhaps, occasionally, grandparents. Policies for sibling visitation (by the baby's brothers and sisters) also vary from unit to unit. Siblings may be required not only to scrub and gown, but to wear a surgical mask to prevent respiratory viruses from infecting the babies in the nursery. Some units require immunization records of young children before they are allowed in the NICU. Do not allow children to visit if they have a fever, diarrhea, a common cold, or an ear infection, or if they have recently been exposed to an illness such as chickenpox. If you or your family members are experiencing any of the above symptoms, consult with your baby's nurse or health care provider before coming to the NICU. In some cases, it may be better to get well before visiting your baby again to decrease the risk of exposing your baby to infection.

Understanding Your Baby

As you become more accustomed to the NICU environment, and as your baby grows and heals, her capabilities will begin to emerge. What are these capabilities? What is being done to promote your baby's development, and what can you do to help? How can you understand what your baby is telling you?

Infant Capabilities

The sensory system is your baby's ability to see, hear, feel, taste, and touch. You may be quite concerned with your baby's capabilities in these areas, asking such questions as "Can my baby see? Can my baby hear? Can my baby feel pain?"

Sight

Newborn infants generally have poor eyesight and little ability to focus beyond 6 or 10 inches away. The amount of color vision is not known for certain, but infants probably do not see subtle differences in color until 2 to 3 months of age.

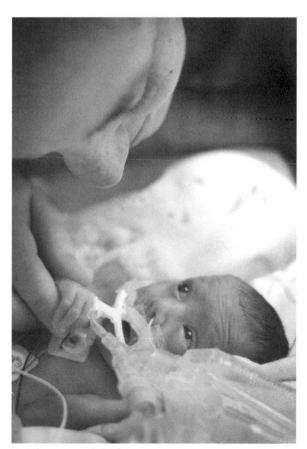

Getting acquainted.
Seeing Mother's face, hearing her voice, and feeling her touch are important and rewarding modes of communication for both mother and baby.

Courtesy of Gigi O'Dea.

The fetus's eyelids fuse (close) during week 10 of gestation and remain closed until about 26 weeks' gestation. If your baby is born with closed eyelids, no special precautions or treatments are necessary. The lids will open on their own within a short time, or by around 26 weeks. If your baby is born with fused eyelids, waiting for the lids to open can be frustrating. Although this may take only a short time to happen, it can seem like forever when you are anxiously waiting to make eye contact with your baby.

It is so wonderful to see your baby with her eyes open. There is something very real, very magical, and very life affirming about a baby with open eyes. Parents in the newborn nursery as well as in the NICU are frequently overheard saying, "Open your eyes, so I can see you and say hello." Seeing your baby's eyes open for the first time can be a really special way to connect with your baby.

Initially, your baby may not be able to look at you and follow your face, but as she grows and remains awake for longer periods, her eyesight will improve. Position your baby face-to-face about 6 to 10 inches away. This is where your baby can see the best, and faces are a baby's favorite visual stimulation.

Babies also like objects with high contrast, such as black-and-white bull's-eye patterns, checkerboards, and concentric circles of contrasting colors. It is good for your baby to have different things to look at, and she enjoys it when you occasionally change the objects in her environment. Before birth, your baby was accustomed to a dark, muted environment. To reduce stress to the newborns in their care, many NICUs use soft lighting. They may also place blankets over your baby's incubator or bed to create a dim, soothing, and nurturing environment for your ill or premature newborn.

"The first time my daughter looked at me it was as if a window had opened. I knew there was a little person in there, and I knew she was mine."

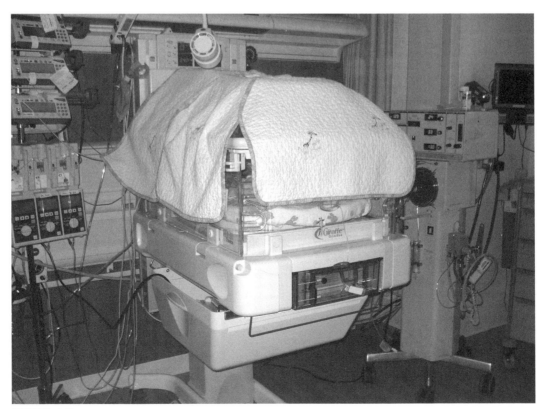

NICU lighting.
To reduce stress to the newborns in their care, many NICUs use soft lighting. They may also place blankets over your baby's incubator to create a dim, soothing, and nurturing environment.

Courtesy of Providence Regional Medical Center, Everett, WA.

Hearing

The ears begin to develop in the fourth week of gestation, and the sense of hearing continues to develop until the baby reaches term. As your baby grew during pregnancy, she was exposed to a variety of sounds, such as your heartbeat, sounds of digestion, blood pulsing through your vessels, and external sounds including others' voices.

Although the premature infant can hear quite well, the sense of hearing is still quite vulnerable. Continuous loud noises can not only harm your baby's hearing, but also produce stress, as seen by changes in heart rate, breathing, blood pressure, and oxygen needs.

Monitor alarms and caregiving activities that create unwanted noise are necessary for your baby's care. Many NICUs try to reduce unwanted noise by creating a soothing environment that helps protect your baby's hearing. Some of the things you may see in the NICU that help to reduce noise include

- Playing only soft, soothing music
- Talking quietly near infants and away from areas where infants are sleeping
- Placing reminder signs near babies who are very sensitive to noise
- Covering the top of the bed with a blanket to muffle the sound of anything placed on top of it
- Closing incubator portholes and doors carefully and quietly
- Placing earmuffs over your baby's ears to help decrease noise
- Removing telephones or silencing the ringer in patient areas
- Providing special "quiet rooms" or areas for babies who are especially sensitive to noise

As your baby grows and begins to heal, more sound can be introduced. How that stimulation is introduced will depend on your baby. It may mean moving your baby out of the "quiet room," removing earmuffs, or providing sounds for your baby to hear. It is so important for you to talk to your baby. Your baby can recognize your voice and will turn toward you when you speak as she gains strength and heals. Some parents find it helpful to provide audiotapes of themselves reading or talking, and some include soft music. Many NICU staff find that parents' voice recordings often help the baby to quiet and settle down to sleep.

Smell and Taste

Your baby also has a well developed sense of smell and taste. When feeding, she prefers the taste of your milk, and she recognizes your unique odor. Some families will place the mother's shirt or breast pad in their baby's bed to help comfort the baby and help the baby recognize the mother's smell in anticipation of breastfeeding. Ask your baby's nurse about the policy regarding placing items from home in your baby's bed.

Touch and Pain

The sense of touch develops very early in the fetus, and your baby is able to feel cloth against her skin, the warmth of your skin against hers, and heat and cold for the very first time after birth. Your baby's face, the area around the lips, and the hands are especially sensitive to your touch. Touching your baby is a wonderful way to connect and help care for your baby. You can help quiet your baby with soft, gentle stroking, or by holding her hand.

In addition to touching your baby, you can give her a sense of security by providing boundaries. Inside the uterus, your baby was surrounded and contained by the springy uterine wall. Now, outside the uterus, she has lost that form of body containment and may be unable to bring her arms and legs in close to her body without help. Your hand placed under your infant's feet or on top of your baby's head can serve as a boundary. As your baby matures, you may find that your hand under her feet and legs is all she needs to quiet her. Babies prefer boundaries, or a "nest," made of soft surfaces that yield to their movements. Some units use special buntings or enclosures resembling sleeping bags to provide containment, or your NICU nurses may place soft blankets under your baby. Your baby will transition away from these soft quilts and "nesting" materials in the weeks before she goes home. Unless your baby has unique sleep

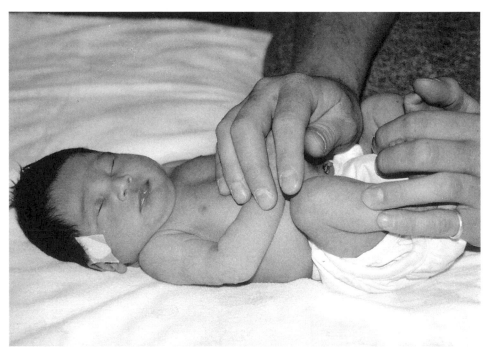

Containment.
Babies appreciate boundaries. This father can calm his baby by gently holding the baby's arms and legs securely against his body.

position requirements, your baby will sleep on her back on a firm mattress without any extra bedding or blankets to reduce the risk of sudden infant death syndrome (SIDS) (see Chapter 15).

You may also wonder if your baby can feel pain. Historically, it was believed that an infant's nervous system was too "disorganized" to recognize pain and that an infant's brain did not perceive conditions to be painful. Current research demonstrates that infants do indeed experience pain. Studies show definite physiological (physical) changes—such as increased heart rate, respiratory rate, and blood pressure, as well as increased oxygen use—during painful procedures. Based on this research, pain control is now an important part of NICU practice. Your baby may be given local anesthesia for painful procedures, and may also be given medication for general discomfort or agitation. You may find that your baby is less responsive and alert if she is receiving pain medication to keep her comfortable.

Individual Temperament

Your baby was born with a unique temperament or communication style. You may notice that your baby is more (or less) active than others in the nursery. You may observe that your baby favors a particular position. Your baby may prefer a pacifier, whereas her brother or sister may have preferred their thumb. As you spend more time with your baby, you will become aware of her unique personality and methods for communicating likes and dislikes. To understand your baby's behavior, you may find it helpful to understand infant behavioral states and communication cues.

Behavioral States

All newborns experience 6 different levels of awareness. These are called *behavioral states.* The 6 states are deep sleep, light sleep, drowsy, quiet alert, active alert, and crying. Your baby's state influences how she responds to people and the environment. By learning to recognize these states, you can begin to understand your infant's behavior and know when to best interact with her. An ill or premature baby will show the same behavioral states as a healthy term baby, but these states may not be as easily recognized and transition from state to state may not be as smooth. Also, your baby's state can be affected by internal stress factors, such as pain; hunger; illness; medication; or outside factors including noise, light, temperature, and activity. It may take you time to learn to recognize and respond to your baby's states. You and your baby have a special bond, and you will learn her unique temperament as she grows and heals.

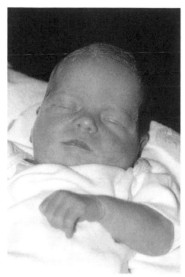

Deep sleep.
The baby is very difficult to awaken from deep sleep.

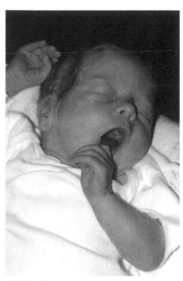

Light sleep.
The baby may move around, even fuss a little in this state, but she is not fully awake.

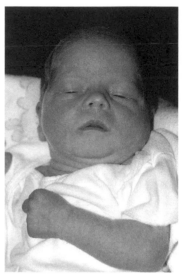

Drowsy.
The baby may open and close her eyes and move her arms and legs. By holding her upright and talking to her, you may be able to alert her. If left alone, she may go back to sleep.

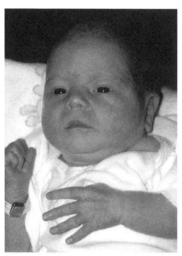

Quiet alert.
The baby "brightens" and focuses her attention on your face or voice. As your preterm baby matures, her quiet alert periods will increase.

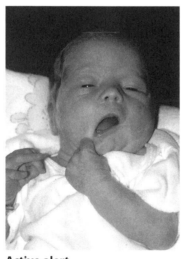

Active alert.
The baby is still alert but is easily distracted and unable to focus her attention. She may become fussy and overwhelmed. If you decrease stimulation, she may recover and return to a quiet alert state.

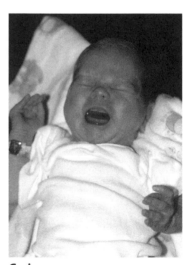

Crying.
The baby has had enough! She may calm down if held securely in quiet surroundings, given a pacifier or her fingers to suck on, or fed if she is hungry.

Deep Sleep

In deep sleep, your baby breathes regularly. Her eyes are closed, with no noticeable eye movements. Your baby does not move spontaneously but may occasionally startle or jerk. While in deep sleep, your baby is difficult to arouse, unable to respond to most external stimulation, and is not interested in eating.

Light Sleep

In light sleep—also known as *rapid eye movement (REM) sleep*—your baby may breathe irregularly. Her eyes remain closed, but eye movements can be seen beneath the lids. Some activities as well as intermittent sucking movements are common in light sleep. Your baby may fuss during this state and, although not fully awake, can be awakened enough to feed. This state is seen more clearly beginning at 36 weeks' gestation.

Drowsy

When in the drowsy state, your baby may open and shut her eyes, or her eyelids may flutter. She may move her arms and legs, and her breathing may become more rapid and shallow. If you speak to her or hold her in an upright position, your baby may move from drowsiness into the quiet alert state. If you leave your baby alone, she may go back to sleep.

Quiet Alert

In the quiet alert state, your baby has a "bright" look and is able to focus her attention. She does not move around much because she is paying attention to her surroundings. This is the ideal state for interacting with your baby because she is receptive to stimulation. Preterm babies can reach the quiet alert state, but often only for seconds. As your baby matures, her periods of quiet alertness will increase.

Active Alert

Your baby's activity increases in the active alert state. Reacting to sound, touch, or movement, she may startle and thrust her arms and legs. Her breathing can be irregular, and she may or may not be fussy. During this state, your baby is unable to focus attention for very long and has a decreased tolerance for continued interaction. If you continue to speak to your baby or try to make eye contact, she may start to cry. If you offer rest and containment, she may return to the quiet alert state.

Crying

Crying tells you that your baby has exhausted her coping skills. Her breathing may be irregular, shallow, and rapid. Crying indicates that your baby needs to rest, or needs relief from pain, discomfort, or hunger.

"I really wanted to be with my sleepy little baby! But the more I tried to get her to look at me or stay awake, the more sleepy and limp she became. Then I learned to be patient and watch for her cues—and she would slowly wake up and look into my eyes...it was magical."

Infant Cues

Your baby not only has sleep-awake states, but can also provide cues to her needs. For years, most infant behavior was assumed to be random and without meaning. Researchers now think that this behavior is meaningful and is an infant's means of communicating with parents and caregivers.

When you learn to recognize your baby's state, you will begin to recognize the best times to interact or play with your baby. Recognizing your baby's cues takes you one step further; it lets you interpret your infant's reaction to and tolerance for play. While spending time with your baby in the NICU, there may be periods where your baby does not show invitation cues and is not ready to interact. This can occur if your baby is ill or simply needs extra rest to grow and heal. Your baby is unique and will respond to stimulation in her own way. She will be able to tell you when she has had enough and when it's time for more.

Invitation Cues

Invitation, or "ready," cues are the behaviors your baby demonstrates when she wants to interact. These cues say, in effect, "I'm ready." Your baby usually shows invitation cues when in the quiet alert state.

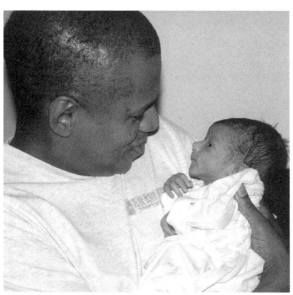

Invitation cues.
This baby is in a quiet alert state and enjoys interaction with his father. The baby encourages his father to continue talking with him with invitation cues such as his bright expression, good eye contact, and relaxed hand position.

Invitation cues include a relaxed appearance (especially of the arms and legs); a "bright" look; and regular, slow breathing. Some babies move their hands to their mouth. Additional invitation cues include

- Having pink color around the mouth
- Moving head, arms, and legs smoothly
- Maintaining position without squirming
- Actively doing things to keep self calm, such as bracing legs or feet against the bed or your lap
- Holding feet one on top of or next to the other
- Holding fingers or holding one hand in the other
- Sucking on fingers or fist
- Grasping blankets or a caregiver's fingers
- Curling up into a ball on one side
- Using help offered by a caregiver to stay calm (using a pacifier, holding onto a caregiver's hands, looking at a face or an object)
- Enjoying being held; calming when held
- Focusing eyes; watching faces or objects
- Making an "ooh" face by pursing lips when looking at a face
- Trying to smile or coo
- Looking eye-to-eye, listening, and following for sustained (but brief) periods

Stress Cues

Not only will babies tell you when they are ready to interact, but they will tell you when they have had enough or are not in the mood to interact. Infants show stress, or "take a break," cues when they have grown uncomfortable or are tired. Sometimes these cues mean only that your baby needs a short break from interaction; in this case, simply move your face or other stimulation out of view. At other times, your baby is telling you that she is ready to sleep or to be

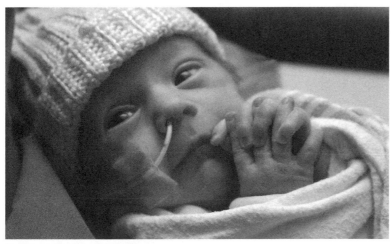

Self-comforting techniques.
By clasping his hands together and holding them near his face, this baby comforts himself and stays "organized" after feeding. With his eyes open, he may be able to sustain a quiet alert state and enjoy a quiet talk with his mother.

Courtesy of Gigi O'Dea.

left alone. By carefully reading your baby's stress cues, you can help her move to a lower state before she begins to cry. Stress cues include

- Changing breathing from a regular rate to faster, or pausing
- Changing color from pink to pale, white, or blue
- Hiccupping, gagging, or grunting
- Spitting up
- Straining as if to have a bowel movement
- Startling; tremoring; or twitching body (trunk), arms and legs, or face
- Coughing, sneezing, yawning, or sighing
- Squirming
- Having limp arms, legs, neck, face, or trunk
- Having stiff legs, arms, or fingers
- Sticking out tongue
- Arching back and neck
- Having a dull, tired, glassy-eyed appearance; staring; looking away; having a panicked or worried expression
- Crying weakly or being irritable
- Suddenly going to sleep
- Sleeping restlessly, with jerky movements or sounds, whimpering, or fussing
- Displaying frantic, ongoing, disorganized activity

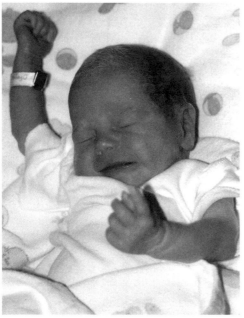

As you interact with your baby, you may begin to notice some of these stress cues. At first, after a brief rest, your infant may recover and invite more interaction. As your interaction continues you may see that your baby is not recovering as quickly after a break as she did earlier. At that point, your baby is telling you that it's time to stop interacting for now.

Stress cues.
This baby's closed eyes, frowning face, stiff arms, and squirming body are clear stress signals. If gently swaddled in a blanket and given a few moments of total quiet, she may settle down and recover a quieter state.

Mixed Messages

Your baby may demonstrate a mixture of cues. For example, your baby may appear to be in the quiet alert state, ready to interact, yet at the same time be hiccupping. This mixture of cues can be frustrating and confusing. Do you act on the invitation to interact, or do you stop what you are doing and give your baby a break?

If your baby is sending out mixed messages, look for other cues to help you decide whether to interact. For example, if your baby has sent out several invitation cues but then spits up, she may have just finished eating and needed to burp. Now that she has burped (which caused the spit-up), she is again ready for interaction. If, on the other hand, she burps and then begins to look pale and turns her gaze away from you, it's probably time for rest. With practice and experience, you'll learn what your baby is telling you in different situations.

Playing With Your Baby

Play fosters your infant's development—it is how babies and children learn. Although play is often seen as easy, natural, and requiring little thought, learning how to play with your baby may take some time. Initially you may feel awkward, but as you become more familiar with your baby and see positive responses, you will look forward to your time together.

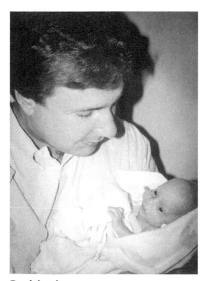

Positioning.
This father is trying to talk to his daughter, who is stressed and disorganized at this point. She waves her arms and has a panicked expression.

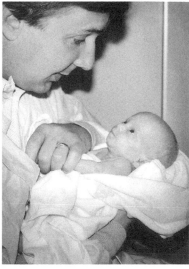

As the father gently holds the baby's arms and provides containment, she relaxes and focuses her attention on her father's face and voice.

Let Your Baby Lead

To make the best use of your time with your baby, learn her cues by observing closely. As you spend time at your baby's bedside, you will be especially aware of your baby's unique temperament and cues of engagement or stress. Notice what your baby is doing before any caregiving begins. Then observe your baby during and after caregiving.

Discuss and compare your observations with the nursing staff. The nursing staff appreciates knowing about your observations and insights into your baby's preferences and communication style.

Follow your baby's lead. If your baby is showing you ready signs, let her look at your face or hear your voice. *Introduce only one stimulus at a time* so your baby can concentrate and attend more effectively. Too many stimuli may overload your baby and lead to stress.

Introducing only one stimulus at a time takes practice. Speaking into a baby's face is instinctive for most of us, for example, but provides both auditory and visual stimulation. Speak to your baby first, then watch for the reaction. When your baby hears your voice, her eyes may brighten, and she may turn her head to find you. At that point, she is ready to see your face. If your baby is very premature or ill, she may not tolerate seeing a face and hearing a voice or hearing a voice and being touched at the same time. She may respond rapidly with physical signs of stress. As she stabilizes medically and grows, she will gradually learn to handle more interaction.

In some units, your baby may receive an Assessment of Preterm Infant Behavior (APIB), an evaluation by a specially trained nurse or developmental specialist. This information can give you a wealth of knowledge about your baby's developmental progress. An APIB evaluates how your baby reacts to stimulation and which cues she uses most often. The evaluation is usually repeated periodically to assess your baby's growing tolerance to stimulation and to identify activities that will foster development. Ask your baby's nurse if she has received a behavioral evaluation.

Use Nonnutritive Sucking

Another important developmental activity for your baby is nonnutritive sucking. This type of sucking does not provide nutrition; rather, your baby sucks on her finger or thumb, a pacifier, or your own clean finger. Nonnutritive sucking has been shown to help your baby gain weight, improve her ability to handle feedings, and decrease her oxygen needs. If your baby is being gavage fed (fed by a tube through her mouth or nose into her stomach), a pacifier may be provided during the feeding to offer pleasurable sucking sensations associated with the meal. (See more information about nonnutritive sucking in Chapter 5.)

Positioning

Positioning may be used to help your baby stay calm, focused, and "organized" in her behavioral states. A premature or ill infant's muscle tone is different from that of a healthy term infant. Term infants prefer to curl up in a flexed position. Because of their immaturity or illness, premature infants cannot flex their limbs and keep them flexed independently. If left to position themselves, preterm infants extend their arms and legs in a sprawling position.

Maintaining this extended posture for long periods can cause serious bone and muscle problems for your baby, such as problems with shoulder mobility and persistent arching of the neck and back. Flexing your baby forward and bringing her arms and legs to the center of her body can help prevent some of these problems and makes it easier for her to discover consoling behaviors, such as finger or hand sucking. Body containment, by swaddling and nesting, helps your baby feel safe and secure and facilitates normal growth and development. Your nursing staff will teach you how to hold and position your baby properly.

Ask About Skin-to-Skin Care

You may be able to hold your baby in the NICU as soon as she is stable and before she is ready to begin feedings. If so, you may be interested in skin-to-skin care, also called *kangaroo care*. Kangaroo care was developed in South America as a way to keep premature infants warm so that they could be released early from overcrowded hospitals. Mothers were instructed to hold their diaper-clad premature infants beneath their clothing, skin-to-skin, snuggled between their warm breasts.

The surprising benefits of kangaroo care for the infant include warmth, stability of heartbeat and breathing, increased time spent in the deep sleep and quiet alert states, decreased crying, increased weight gain, and increased breastfeeding (see Chapter 5). These benefits are apparent even when kangaroo care occurs for only a few minutes each day.

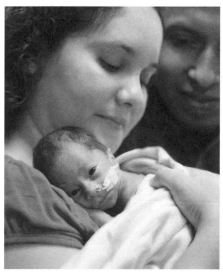

Kangaroo care.
Holding your baby skin to skin against your chest provides moments of closeness and belonging for parents and baby.

Courtesy of Gigi O'Dea.

Both mothers and fathers can give kangaroo care. Most nurseries have comfortable rocking chairs and screens that can be placed around your chair or the baby's care area. Simply wear a layer of clothing that opens down the front, and sit behind the screen or with your back to the room. Don't bother to dress your baby or wrap her in a blanket—all she needs is a diaper because she will stay warm next to your body. You may notice that your infant tolerates these holding sessions much better when they are not preceded by undressing, diaper changing, temperature taking, dressing again, and swaddling in blankets. Snuggle your baby upright on your chest, or lay your baby with her head against your chest.

Kangaroo care is a nice way for you to get acquainted with your baby in the NICU. The feeling of your baby's warm skin against yours is a special closeness and comfort for you both. At a time when so many people are caring for your baby, kangaroo care provides special moments of belonging that only you can experience with your baby.

Growing With Your Baby

During your baby's stay in the NICU, you'll notice how she is growing—physically as well as developmentally. During that time, parents will grow as well. Each time you spend time in the NICU, you'll become more familiar with the environment, the routine, the technology, and the staff. As your comfort level in the NICU increases, you'll be more at ease with your baby and her capabilities. You will soon be able to recognize your baby's unique language and respond appropriately to that language. With each visit you will gain confidence and comfort in the NICU.

At times you may feel extremely stressed or think that your baby's progress is slow. At those times, especially, focus on the special moments you share with your baby. Celebrate accomplishments and "firsts"—the first time you hold your baby, the first time you bathe her, the first time you feed her. You may wish to capture these moments in a special baby book of photos and memories that mark progress during your baby's NICU stay. Those milestones are important for your baby and for you and are part of your new vision for your baby and your family. Not only is your baby making progress, but with each milestone you are growing as well.

Enjoy the special time you have with your baby. Although this is probably not the way you had imagined becoming acquainted, it can be a memorable and special experience. You are the parents of this baby, and the nurses, physicians, and care providers are there to help you along this journey.

Chapter 5
Feeding Your Baby

"Then Tigger looked up at the ceiling,
and closed his eyes, and his tongue went
round and round his chops, in case he had
left any outside, and a peaceful smile
came over his face as he said,
"So *that's* what Tiggers like!"

Cindy C. Martin, MSN, RN, IBCLC, CKC
Jeanette Zaichkin, RN, MN, NNP-BC

Feeding your baby is an important parenting task and a satisfying activity you will want to share with your child.

Although few neonatal intensive care unit (NICU) babies can feed directly from the breast or bottle until some time after birth, special care infants still need nourishment. For a while, they get it in different ways than healthy term infants do.

This chapter begins by explaining the special advantages of providing breast milk for your NICU baby. Then we take a close look at feeding approaches used early in your baby's NICU stay. It goes on to teach you about techniques you can use to help your baby learn to feed—either from your breast or from a bottle.

Benefits of Breast Milk and Breastfeeding the NICU Infant

"Making the decision to breastfeed your very sick or low birth weight baby is not a decision about feeding. It's a health care decision that influences your baby's health for a lifetime."

If you have just given birth to a sick or premature baby, you may be thinking that you can't breastfeed your newborn. Take heart, because in almost all cases, you'll be able to feed your breast milk to your baby until he is able to suckle. Breastfeeding is by far the best choice for your baby. Your milk is perfectly suited to nourish your baby and to provide protection from infections, allergies, and other diseases. Nothing that scientists can create in a laboratory from cow's milk or soybeans can compare with human milk. Providing breast milk to a special care baby can be challenging during the NICU experience, but looking back, NICU parents feel the advantages were worth the extra effort.

The nutrients (protein, carbohydrates, fats, vitamins, and minerals) in human milk are present in the perfect proportions for a human baby. The proteins are made up of just the right amino acids, and the fats are a unique blend of cholesterol, omega-3 fatty acids, and other essential fats that are important for brain growth and development. All of these nutrients are in forms that your baby can absorb more easily than the nutrients made from cow's milk or soybeans.

However, there is more than just good nutrition in human milk. It is literally alive with cells that fight germs that can cause infections in your baby. Human milk has components in it that encourage the growth of beneficial bacteria (such as *Lactobacillus bifidus)* in your baby's stomach and intestines and inhibit the growth of harmful bacteria (such as *Escherichia coli).* It also contains enzymes that enhance your baby's digestion and make it easier for his body to use the nutrients present in milk. Most important, breast milk contains hormones and growth factors that promote optimal growth in human infants. Scientists have isolated more than 100 of these and other beneficial components in human milk—all of which are missing from infant formulas.

Many studies show that babies who are breastfed have lower rates of lymphoma, leukemia, and Hodgkin disease; overweight and obesity; asthma; ear infections; respiratory tract infections; urinary tract infections; diarrhea; and allergies than formula-fed babies. The illnesses of breastfed babies also tend to be less severe—and less likely to result in hospitalization. Children who were breastfed as infants are also less likely to have dental problems (such as decay and improper bite), juvenile-onset diabetes, and inflammatory bowel diseases (such as ulcerative colitis or Crohn disease).

Another advantage of breastfeeding is that it provides your baby the warmth and physical closeness of skin-to-skin contact when he is ready to nurse. You are probably keenly aware that the amount of time you can spend holding, rocking, and cuddling your baby may be limited because he is in the intensive care nursery. As soon as your baby is ready to breastfeed, you'll get to hold your newborn against your body. If you bottle feed, you can make an effort to hold your baby skin to skin—but when you breastfeed, you automatically have that contact at every feeding.

Advantages of Breast Milk for Preterm Infants

In the last 3 months of pregnancy, large protein molecules called *immunoglobulins* cross the placenta and are stored in the growing fetus. These immunoglobulins protect a newborn against the infections that the mother is immune to—for up to 5 or 6 months after birth. Although a premature baby misses out on some of this special protection because of the timing of birth, you can still provide him with immunoglobulins through breast milk. The milk you produce in the first few days after giving birth (colostrum) has the highest concentration of immunoglobulins, but you continue to give your baby extra immunoglobulins for as long as you give him your breast milk.

Human milk is important for the optimal growth and development of full-term babies, but it is even more important for babies born prematurely. If your baby is preterm, his stomach and intestines (which the NICU staff will refer to as his *gastrointestinal tract, GI tract,* or *gut)* are even smaller and less mature than the tiny, immature gut of a full-term baby.

If your NICU baby is premature, your milk will be different for the first few weeks than the breast milk of a mother who gives birth at term. Your body knows that your baby came early, and it provides milk that is better for the baby's needs. For the first 2 to 4 weeks after birth, your milk will contain more protein, fat calories, calcium, phosphorus, magnesium, zinc, sodium, and chloride than full-term milk. This early milk also has a laxative effect on your baby's bowels, helping him to pass the first stools (called *meconium*). Stooling is an important sign that the GI tract is working; it also helps resolve jaundice (see Chapter 9). Nurses notice that babies fed their mother's milk tolerate feedings better than those fed formula. Human milk is easy to digest, with very little left over in the baby's stomach. Because formula forms larger curds during the digestive process than breast milk, babies given formula commonly have undigested milk in their stomach 2 to 3 hours after feeding.

Brain growth and development are rapid in the final 3 months of gestation. During the latter part of pregnancy, the fetal brain more than doubles in size and weight, and nearly doubles again in the first year of life and well into the second year. Several studies have suggested that breastfeeding improves mental development. In fact, greater amounts of breast milk intake (compared with formula) have been correlated with higher developmental outcomes among the smallest preterm babies.

Although breastfeeding requires skill and maturity on your baby's part, it can be less stressful than bottle feeding. Possible difficulties of bottle feeding (because of the fast flow of milk from a bottle) are so common that doctors and nurses have come to think of them as "normal" responses to feeding: irregular or pauses in breathing (apnea) with a resulting drop in oxygen saturation, slowed heart rate (bradycardia), and blue skin color (cyanosis). Research has demonstrated that breastfeeding is less stressful than bottle feeding because the baby can "pace" the feeding, controlling the flow of milk and pausing when necessary. During breastfeeding, a baby stays warm, his heart rate remains regular, and oxygen levels stabilize (or even improve). Most healthy preterm babies begin breastfeeding between 32 and 34 weeks' gestation but do not begin bottle feeding until at least 34 weeks' gestation.

Your Baby's First Nutrition

You may be amazed at the strength with which your tiny newborn can suck on your finger or a pacifier shortly after birth. Your baby's ability to suck is incredible, but it doesn't mean he is ready to begin breastfeeding or bottle feeding. Feeding by breast or bottle is possible if your baby is clinically stable, has a respiratory rate (breathing rate) of less than 60 to 70 breaths per minute, and is at least 34 weeks' gestation. Babies between 32 and 34 weeks' gestation might be able to breastfeed or bottle feed if they have developed the skills to suck, swallow, and breathe in a coordinated way, but this is unlikely. Feeding a sick or premature baby in the NICU is a slow and deliberate process with risks and potential complications. Until breastfeeding or bottle feeding is safe, your baby will be nourished in other ways.

Intravenous Feeding

Your baby may not be fed by mouth immediately after birth. Instead, he may be fed through a peripheral or central intravenous (IV) line (see Chapter 2). At first, this type of feeding usually consists of glucose (sugar) water, and some babies receive added electrolytes—substances or elements that are essential for the proper functioning of each cell of the body. Electrolytes include sodium, chloride, calcium, potassium, and magnesium. All babies have sodium, potassium, and chloride added to their IV by a few days of age. Other electrolytes may be added depending on the baby's individual situation. Very small babies may receive total parenteral nutrition (TPN) (see below) within the first few days of life.

As your baby's physical condition improves, he will be given the opportunity to get started on nipple (breast or bottle) feedings. When this occurs depends on the maturity of your baby's feeding reflexes (sucking, gagging, and swallowing) and on his ability to coordinate those reflexes. While your baby's reflexes and coordination remain immature, feedings will be primarily by gavage (see below).

Parenteral Nutrition

If your baby cannot begin oral feedings for a long period (perhaps because of gastrointestinal problems, surgery, extreme immaturity, or chronic respiratory problems) or if your baby does not grow on standard feedings, an approach called *parenteral nutrition* will be used. The term *parenteral* refers to food that enters the body through a blood vessel. In TPN, all of the essential nutrients (carbohydrates, protein, fat, vitamins, and minerals) and water are provided in special solutions delivered through an IV line directly into one of the baby's veins. When a baby receives nutrients that exceed the normal requirements for nutrition, the fluid is called *hyperalimentation.*

Gavage Feeding

Babies are able to suck long before they are able to coordinate the process of sucking, swallowing, and breathing. Most infants younger than 32 to 34 weeks cannot suck and swallow effectively. They receive breast milk or formula through a tube (called a *gavage* or *feeding tube)* inserted through the nose or mouth and advanced down into the stomach. Sometimes the feeding tube is placed in the intestine (transpyloric feeding) rather than in the stomach.

Because babies who need gavage feeding generally do not have a strong gag reflex, insertion of the tube is usually easy on the baby. The most common methods of gavage feed-

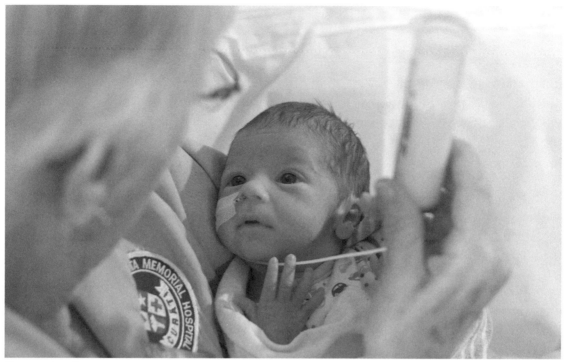

Gavage feeding.
A soft feeding tube goes through this baby's nose and into his stomach during a gavage feeding. The milk drips by gravity into the baby's stomach from a syringe held by the care provider. Ideally, the baby is given a pacifier to suck during the feeding.

Courtesy of Gigi O'Dea.

ing are orogastric (tube through the mouth into the stomach) and nasogastric (tube through the nose into the stomach). The tube may be inserted for each feeding or left in place for a time. Giving your baby a pacifier to suck on during gavage feeding (an approach called *nonnutritive sucking)* may enhance digestion and absorption of food.

Your baby may receive small amounts of milk on a regular schedule, such as every 2 or 3 hours (intermittent gavage feeding), or may receive milk from a feeding pump that provides a steady infusion through the gavage tube (continuous gavage feeding). With continuous gavage feedings, the feeding tube is inserted and left in for a time. Milk is slowly dripped down the tube at a set rate (such as 1–2 milliliters [or about 1/5–2/5 teaspoon] every hour).

The type of gavage feeding selected for each baby depends on many factors, including health status, size, and maturity. Infants who are gavage fed are carefully monitored to make sure that they are taking and absorbing (tolerating) the whole feeding. Tolerance of gavage feedings is assessed by observing for distention (enlargement) of the abdomen, for spitting up, and for the amount of food remaining in the stomach (called *residuals)* just before the next gavage feeding. Residuals do not necessarily indicate a problem;

however, increasing amounts of residuals over time may indicate an intestinal problem such as slow transit or necrotizing enterocolitis (see Chapter 9).

Each type of gavage feeding has advantages and disadvantages. Intermittent gavage feeding produces normal cyclic variations in digestive hormones and helps to stimulate the normal hunger cycle and stomach emptying. It is also easier to monitor for signs of feeding problems such as delayed emptying of the stomach (transfer of the feeding from the stomach to the intestines). Disadvantages of this type of feeding include risks of effects on breathing patterns and risk of feeding problems such as vomiting.

Continuous gavage feeding is often used for very small or ill infants. Advantages include reduced effects of the feeding on breathing patterns, reduced risk of stomach distention (enlargement), and less need to handle a baby who does not tolerate handling. Disadvantages include difficulty in monitoring feeding problems, lack of the normal cyclic changes in digestive hormones, and risk of tube dislodgement.

Transpyloric feeding (continuous feeding into the pylorus, a narrow channel between the stomach and upper intestine) is used less frequently than the other methods. This type of feeding may reduce problems such as markedly delayed stomach emptying or severe spitting up, help the infant tolerate larger amounts of feeding, and have less effect on breathing patterns. Disadvantages of transpyloric feeding include increased difficulty in placing and securing the tube; need for x-rays to check tube location; and risks of complications such as diarrhea, tube obstruction, abdominal distention, and intestinal perforation.

As your baby becomes ready, he gradually gets larger amounts of milk. Nurses watch for signs that your baby is tolerating the feedings (no vomiting, little or no milk left over in the stomach, a soft and undistended tummy, and no blood in the stools). As the amount of milk is gradually increased, the amount of IV fluid or TPN is gradually decreased. When your baby is taking all of the milk he needs for growth, he is said to be on "full feedings." At that point, he no longer needs an IV, except perhaps for medications.

Help Your Baby Get Ready for the Breast or Bottle

In the early weeks of life, before your baby is ready for breastfeeding or bottle feeding, much of the oral stimulation he receives is unpleasant. Endotracheal intubation and suctioning, gavage tubes, and even a nasal cannula taped to the cheeks provide unpleasant sensory stimulation to your baby's face and mouth. You can make it your job to offer some pleasant forms of oral stimulation for your baby. For example, gentle, loving stroking of your baby's lips and the area around his mouth can improve success at feeding. In addition, you can help your baby develop oral feeding skills by using the following techniques.

Nonnutritive Sucking

Sucking that does not supply nutrition is called *nonnutritive sucking*. This kind of sucking is not only good sucking practice, but helps weight gain and digestion. Nonnutritive sucking also helps develop self-calming skills and "state organization," which means moving smoothly through behavioral states, such as drowsy, quiet alert, and active alert (see Chapter 4).

The nurses will make sure that your baby gets opportunities for sucking during gavage feedings. This helps prepare preterm babies for successful nipple feeding. Offer your baby a pacifier or his fingers to suck. You can also offer opportunities for nonnutritive sucking when you notice signs that your baby would like to suck. These "feeding cues" include bringing his hands close to his mouth, turning his head and opening his mouth, and making sucking motions. Even if you don't see these cues, the next time you're holding your baby, try slipping your clean finger into his mouth (nail bed down) and gently stroking the roof of his mouth with the pad of your finger.

Skin-to-Skin Care

Skin-to-skin care, also called *kangaroo care,* is simple, safe, and beneficial for most babies. This technique of mom or her partner holding the baby skin to skin offers every baby the benefits of parent-infant bonding, temperature regulation, and preparation for breast-feeding. For as little as 20 minutes a day, or as much as several hours a day, snuggle your baby against your chest, between your breasts. You wear clothing that opens in the front (moms do not wear a bra during kangaroo care) and your baby wears only a diaper. Warm blankets are draped over both of you; sometimes your baby will wear a hat as well. If your baby is stable enough to be held in your arms, he can (and should, if you are planning to breastfeed) be held skin to skin. Some NICUs will allow skin-to-skin care even if the baby is on a ventilator, or nasal continuous positive airway pressure (CPAP) as pictured on page 227. Ask for this opportunity if the staff doesn't suggest it. Breastfeeding babies can nuzzle the mother's breasts during kangaroo care. This nuzzling (a form of nonnutritive sucking) may progress to attempts to suckle during gavage feedings. Mothers with an abundant milk supply may need to pump to remove milk from the breasts before allowing the baby to root at the breast during gavage feeding to prevent leaking large amounts of milk.

In studies comparing mothers and babies who were given the opportunity to use skin-to-skin care with mothers and babies who were not offered this opportunity, the effects of kangaroo care on breastfeeding were dramatic.

- Breastfeeding incidence is increased by at least 25% and up to 50%.
- Mothers' average daily milk production is higher.
- Mothers and babies breastfeed more often per day.
- Mothers and babies breastfeed for more weeks.

- Babies have better sleep, which supports weight gain.
- Babies have better weight gain.
- Babies have better thermal regulation.
- Babies have fewer episodes of apnea and bradycardia.

Kangaroo care can also support the bottle feeding baby's preparation for nipple feeding by stimulating feeding cues. Your baby may begin to root at the breast, searching with his mouth for something to suckle. The infant may also demonstrate hand-to-mouth movement, which indicates feeding readiness. Although the focus of skin-to-skin care is for premature babies who will breastfeed and for mothers to increase their milk supply, term babies and those who will bottle feed also benefit from this skin-to-skin closeness.

Using the Sense of Smell

Even very premature babies have a well developed sense of smell. Your baby recognizes your unique odor. Some NICUs will help ready a baby for breastfeeding by asking the mother to put a breast pad inside her bra, against her nipple. Then the pad is placed in the incubator, under or near the baby's head, to get the baby ready for breastfeeding through the sense of smell.

Patience and Practice

Depending on your baby's gestational age and health status, he may be fed solely by gavage for several days, weeks, or even months. You may watch your baby sucking on his fingers or a pacifier and wonder, "Why can't I just feed him? Why does he need those gavage feedings?" Staff in the NICU know from experience that if you let a preterm baby less than 36 weeks' gestation try to get all of his nourishment by breastfeeding or bottle feeding, he will soon become tired, lose weight, and have more difficulty staying warm as he uses all his energy to eat. This transition stage from gavage feeding to breastfeeding or bottle feeding is frustrating and requires patience as your baby learns and grows.

As he begins to develop the skills and reflexes necessary for nipple feeding, you will offer the breast or bottle for "practice." When your baby is ready to "begin" to nipple feed, he will try the breast or bottle once, the nurse will evaluate the baby's ability to feed, and try another feeding later. Some nurseries have protocols to provide incremental increases in oral feeding or nippling. Some feedings will go well; others will be more difficult. The nurses can help you to recognize those times of day when your baby is most awake, alert, and showing signs of readiness to breastfeed.

Learning to eat takes time—it doesn't happen overnight. As your NICU baby approaches this age, keep your expectations in line. Although a baby at 32 weeks may nurse well once, he probably won't be able to do it again for at least another day. In addition, keep in mind that 32 to 34 weeks is the earliest age at which babies are capable of breastfeeding. If your baby has health problems or other complications, the first feeding at your breast may have to be delayed. The average preterm baby learns to breastfeed fairly well by the time he is 36 to 38 weeks post-menstrual age (approaching what would have been his full-term due date). Most premature babies go home on some combination of breast-feeding and bottle feeding.

Ensuring Adequate Nutrition

At birth, the organ systems of all babies—particularly the stomach and intestines, the liver, and the kidneys—are immature. This is even truer of preterm infants. When medical illness is combined with organ immaturity, nutritional support becomes difficult. Providing adequate nutrition for special care babies is a complex process, one in which the NICU team carefully assesses the best approaches to helping your baby grow and get well.

Most NICU babies need additional calories during their hospitalization if they are preterm or critically ill whether breastfeeding or formula feeding. Sick or preterm infants weighing less than about 1,500 grams (3 pounds, 5 ounces) run out of fat and carbohydrate fuel within a few days after birth and begin to use up vital body protein unless they receive adequate nutritional support. In addition, babies who have long-term respiratory problems, such as bronchopulmonary dysplasia (chronic lung disease), need increased calories and nutrition to ensure growth throughout their first year of life. Babies with congenital heart disease also require expert nutritional support to ensure nutrition and adequate weight gain. For these babies, unfortified breast milk or standard infant formulas may not be enough. These babies often need extra nutrients to grow well, not only in weight and head circumference but in length and bone density.

Extensive evidence shows improvement in growth and nutritional status when premature and/or sick babies receive fortified human milk, preterm infant formulas, or a combination of the two. If you are breastfeeding your baby, this means extra protein, calories, calcium, phosphorus, vitamins, and other necessary nutrients will be added to your milk, either in a powder mixed into it or in equal volumes of breast milk and a liquid formula made especially for this purpose.

When premature infants cannot receive breast milk, they are fed specially designed preterm formulas that also contain extra protein, calories, sodium, calcium, phosphorus, copper, zinc, and selected micronutrients. Many experts recommend the inclusion of DHA and ARA (essential fatty acids) in both term and preterm infant formulas. New research supports that the higher levels of DHA (already in human breast milk and now added to infant formulas) provide better protection against infection and allergies than infant formulas and breast milk levels below 0.2 milligrams of DHA. These benefits seem to continue long after the child is weaned.

Glucose polymers and medium-chain triglyceride oil (MCT) may be added to breast milk or to preterm formula to provide extra energy. Glucose polymers contain sugars in a form that immature preterm newborns can easily digest and absorb. The fats in MCT oil are well absorbed and can be digested without the enzymes and bile salts these infants lack. Both provide extra calories. As your baby grows, a vitamin and mineral supplement may also be added to the diet.

Gaining and Growing

"Parents must be care partners when it comes to feeding. Breast, bottle, gavage...sometimes all are used in the same 24 hours."

Your baby's birth weight, length, and head circumference reflect the amount of growth and development during pregnancy. The relationship between your baby's birth weight and gestational age indicates how well he grew before birth and whether he is small, appropriate, or large for gestational age (see Chapter 8). After birth, weight gain and growth are closely monitored to ensure adequate nutrition, which affects brain growth and developmental outcome. Your baby's caregivers may plot your baby's growth—weight, length, and head circumference changes—on standard charts specific for preterm babies. These charts assume that a preterm infant will grow at a rate similar to that of a fetus until he reaches the gestational age of a full-term infant. Note, though, that research has not confirmed that this assumption is correct. The extrauterine world is much different from the world of the uterus, and a baby's growth is affected by many factors.

Weight Gain

Weighing your baby is important for monitoring his growth. In the nursery, your infant's weight is usually measured in grams. Because a gram is a smaller unit than an ounce, it gives a more precise measurement than pounds and ounces and makes it easier to recognize small changes in your infant's weight. One ounce equals 28 grams, although many nurseries count 1 ounce as 30 grams because it is mathematically easier to work with and makes no big difference in nutritional outcome. Appendix A contains a chart to help you convert grams to pounds and ounces.

Babies in the NICU are weighed daily or every few days, depending on their health status. The nurses will usually try to weigh your baby on the same scale each time because scales can differ from one nursery to another or even within the same nursery. However, daily variances in weight, while important for the health care team, can be frustrating and confusing to parents. Usually it is better for parents to look at weights once a week to see the trend in their baby's weight pattern.

After birth, all infants lose some weight. This is a normal process that reflects changes in water balance. The fetus is composed of large amounts of water and sodium (salt). After birth, your baby must excrete extra water and salt that he no longer needs. Term infants may lose up to 7% to 10% of their birth weight after birth; preterm babies may lose up to 12% to 15%. For example, if your son is preterm, weighs 1,200 grams at birth, and loses 15% of his birth weight, his weight would fall to 1,020 grams (15% of 1,200 is 180 grams). Smaller or sicker babies tend to lose the most weight.

Term infants usually lose weight only for the first few days of life. Sick preterm infants may lose weight for a few days to several weeks before starting to gain it back. At first, your baby may not gain weight regularly. His weight may increase on some days, stay the same on others, and occasionally go down. Even when your baby does begin to gain weight regularly, there will be occasional days of no gain or even a slight loss. This can be normal.

The average daily expected weight gain in a healthy growing preterm infant is about 15 grams for each kilogram of body weight. To convert grams to kilograms, divide the grams by 1,000. For example, a 900-gram baby weighs 0.9 kilogram. The daily expected weight gain for this baby would be about 13 grams ($15 \times 0.9 = 13.5$). An 1,800-gram baby weighs 1.8 kilograms, so this baby's daily expected weight gain would be 1.8×15, or about 27 grams. When your baby is on full feeds and "catching up" on his growth, the goal for weight gain is about 15 to 30 grams per day.

Remember, however, that each baby is unique and will establish his individual weight gain pattern. In addition, few babies gain exactly the expected daily amount each day. One day the baby may gain more, another less, and another none at all, or he may even lose a little weight. Factors that can influence weight gain include health status, activity level, energy needs, discomfort or pain, fluids and nutrients, temperature regulation, and calorie intake, as well as urine output and stools. It's interesting to note that the calorie count per ounce is standardized in infant formula, but the calories per ounce in breast milk change with every pumping throughout the day. To assess your baby's progress against the expected weight gain, average his actual daily weight gain or loss over a few days to a week. You may wish to review your infant's growth curves with your baby's medical provider.

Length and Head Circumference

Weight is not the only measure of growth and development. Your infant's body length and head circumference are also important and will be measured periodically. Increase in a healthy baby's head circumference usually means brain growth, which is a good thing. Length and head circumference are usually measured in centimeters. Appendix A provides a chart for converting centimeters to inches. Overall, the goal is to increase length and head circumference by about 0.9 cm (0.4 inch) per week.

Breastfeeding Basics

As detailed at the beginning of this chapter, providing breast milk for your baby is undoubtedly one of the most important things you can do to contribute to your baby's health. Unlike formula, breast milk provides protection from infections, allergies, and other diseases. It also contributes to your baby's long-term developmental outcome. If you had not planned to breastfeed, consider pumping your breast milk until your baby is well and ready for discharge from the hospital, or until your premature baby has reached term gestation. The advantages of breast milk, sometimes referred to by health care professionals as "liquid gold," are indisputable and have far-reaching consequences for your baby at this vulnerable time.

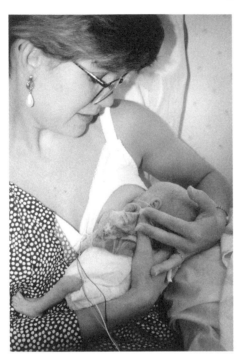

Breastfeeding.
This very small baby (actually born at 29 weeks' gestation and 6 weeks old here) breastfeeds well for short periods. The mother pumps breast milk for the baby's supplemental gavage feedings.

Advantages for Mothers

Breastfeeding has decided advantages for the mother too. Breastfeeding causes the uterus to contract, decreasing the chance of postpartum hemorrhage (bleeding). Women who breastfeed may have a decreased risk of breast cancer and ovarian cancer, an earlier return to pre-pregnancy weight, and possibly a decreased risk of hip fractures and osteoporosis after menopause.

But most NICU moms say that the best thing about breastfeeding is that it is something they (and they alone) can do for their baby. When your baby's survival depends to a great degree on the expertise of doctors and nurses, you may feel insignificant—as if your role doesn't matter. When you bring your breast milk to the NICU, you declare loudly and clearly that you are your baby's mother. You know you are making an important and tangible contribution to your baby's well-being and you feel confident that your baby needs you.

Breastfeeding also restores a sense of normalcy to your birth experience. One mother said, "I never got to wear pretty maternity dresses or go to childbirth classes. Then when the baby was born, I did not get to hold her right away or room-in like the other mothers on the maternity unit. I did find it fulfilling to pump my breasts and offer my daughter breast milk. I felt special that my milk was providing her nutrition."

So, although it may be challenging to provide breast milk for your special care baby, consider the good feelings it can provide.

- Reassurance of your role as the baby's mother
- A sense of normalcy about the pregnancy and birth
- The satisfaction of providing something tangible ("liquid gold") for your baby
- The knowledge that you are important to your baby's medical care, health, and survival
- The joy that comes from providing some physical comfort to your baby
- Greater confidence when it's time to take your baby home
- Pride in accomplishing something worthwhile

Taking Care of Yourself

Breastfeeding is a big commitment while your baby is in the NICU and requires a considerable amount of self-care. Your care provider and the lactation specialist and may offer more information about ways to ensure that you stay healthy during this time in your life. The information below will get you started and prompt discussion and questions about diet, rest, and family planning methods.

Diet

Breastfeeding burns calories—an estimated 600 to 900 calories to produce a liter (about a quart) of breast milk per day, or the equivalent of playing basketball for an hour and a half. Therefore, most lactating women need about 2,700 calories per day, which means adding about 250 to 500 calories per day to a normal diet. Recommendations for additional calories range between 250 and 500 calories per day because each mother's metabolism, milk production, and calorie usage will vary.

The commonsense approach is to eat more than you did when you were pregnant, or a normal healthy diet of fruits and vegetables, protein, and grains. Some mothers get adequate nutrition by "grazing" throughout the day with small frequent meals. An extra simple peanut butter sandwich can provide the added calories to support daily activities and milk production. When weaning occurs, calorie intake should be reduced to prevent unexpected weight gain.

The breastfeeding mother's diet plays an important role in the DHA and essential fatty acid content of her breast milk. The American Dietetic Association and the Dietitians of Canada have reviewed the evidenced-based research and recommend that the DHA and essential fatty acid in breast milk should be at least 0.2 milligrams or higher for term infants and even higher for preterm infants. The breastfeeding mother can easily meet this recommendation by eating 2 servings per week of fish or by taking a fish oil supplement of 200 milligrams of DHA per day. Fish that are not recommended include shark,

115

Healthy Fish Guide[a]
Eat Fish, Be Smart, Choose Wisely

SAFE TO EAT **2-3 MEALS** PER WEEK		SAFE TO EAT **1 MEAL** PER WEEK		**AVOID** DUE TO MERCURY
Follow this advice to reduce your exposure to mercury, PCBs, and other toxics:				Women who are or may become **PREGNANT, NURSING MOTHERS, and CHILDREN** should NOT eat:
♥ Anchovies Butterfish Catfish Clams Cod *(Pacific) (Atlantic)* Crab *(Blue, King, Snow) (US, CAN) (Imported King)* Crab-Imitation Crayfish *(imported farmed)* Flounder/Sole *(Pacific) (Atlantic)* ♥ Herring ♥ Mackerel *(canned)* ♥ Oysters Pollock/ Fish sticks	♥ Salmon *(fresh, canned)* ♥ Chinook *(King) (coastal, AK)* ♥ Chum *(Keta)* ♥ Coho *(Silver)* ♥ Farmed * ♥ Pink *(Humpy)* ♥ Sockeye *(Red)* ♥ Sardines Scallops Shrimp/Prawns *(US, CAN) (imported)* Squid/Calamari Tilapia *(US, Central/ South America) (China, Taiwan)* ♥ Trout Tuna *(canned light)*	♥ Black seas bass Chilean sea bass ♥ Chinook salmon *(Puget Sound)* Croaker Halibut *(Pacific) (Atlantic)* Lobster *(US, CAN) (imported Spiny Caribbean)*	Mahi mahi *(imported longline)* Monkfish Rockfish/Red snapper *(trawl-caught)* ♥ Sablefish/ Black cod ♥ Tuna, Albacore *(fresh, canned white) (WA, OR, CA troll/ pole) (longline – except Hawaii)* ★ **A seafood serving or "meal" is about the size and thickness of your hand, or 1 oz. for every 20 lbs. of body weight.** **160 lb. Adult = 8 oz.** **80 lb. Child = 4 oz.**	Mackerel *(King)* Marlin *(imported)* Shark Swordfish *(imported)* Tilefish *(Gulf of Mexico, South Atlantic)* Tuna Steak Bluefin Bigeye *(imported longline)* Yellowfin *(imported longline)*

♥ Highest in healthy omega-3 fatty acids
Underlined text: Overfished, farmed, or caught using methods harmful to marine life and/or environment
*For environmental and health information, visit www.doh.gov/fish/farmedsalmon
[a] Source: Washington State Department of Health. *Healthy Fish Guide.* Olympia, WA: Washington State Department of Health; 2009.
For more information, contact Washington State Department of Health at www.doh.wa.gov/fish or call toll free: 1-877-485-7316

mackerel, and tile fish because they pose a higher risk of mercury exposure. The Healthy Fish Guide (page 116) will help you decide how much to eat of different fish, and which fish choices reduce your risk of exposure to mercury and other contaminants.

Fluids

The recommendation for a breastfeeding mother's fluid requirement is probably familiar to you: drink about 8 glasses of fluid—which should be mostly water—every 24 hours. This is not difficult for most breastfeeding mothers because each time you pump or nurse you will feel thirsty. Nursing is the perfect time for a glass of water or other healthy beverage. Drink each time you are thirsty and keep the color of your urine a clear yellow, not cloudy or a dark concentrated yellow color.

Alcohol

Many mothers have questions about drinking alcohol now that pregnancy is over. The American Academy of Pediatrics (AAP) considers an occasional celebratory single alcoholic beverage compatible with breastfeeding. Because alcohol levels in breast milk parallel those in your bloodstream, most health care providers would encourage mothers to nurse or pump/express their milk immediately before having a drink and avoid breastfeeding for 2 hours after the drink to avoid transferring alcohol to the infant through the breast milk.

Caffeine

Caffeine, in the form of coffee, tea, and soda, does not usually cause a problem for breastfeeding babies. Remember that chocolate also contains caffeine, and so do some pain relievers and cold medications. Some experts recommend limiting caffeine intake to less than 750 milliliters—about the same amount in five 5-ounce cups of coffee. Your coffee cup probably holds 8 to 12 ounces or more. Caffeine accumulates in breast milk, and the baby who is over-caffeinated may be wakeful and possibly irritable. Caffeine intake in mothers of preterm babies does not seem to be as much of a problem for their babies as for mothers of term babies.

Rest

Rest is important for healing after childbirth. You are at risk for sleep deprivation due to the stress of having a NICU baby, and the additional work of splitting time between home and the NICU. Milk production requires energy too, so it is not surprising if you feel exhausted. Try to nap at least once during the day. You may need to put a special message on your phone and purposefully not answer the phone during the day.

Talk to your lactation specialist about the need to wake up once or twice during the night to pump. On the occasional night when you're especially tired, it may be more important to sleep well and pump more frequently the next day. Do not do this very often. If a mother lets her breasts get full, this slows milk production. She should pump and empty her breasts around-the-clock whenever possible. Failing to pump at night is one of the most common reasons for decreased milk supply.

Prescription Medications, Over-the-Counter Medications, and Herbs

It is important to talk with a lactation specialist, your health care provider, and the neonatologist about every prescription medication, every over-the-counter medication (such as cold remedies and antacids), and any other herbs or supplements that you take to ensure that they are compatible with breastfeeding. Usually the benefits of breast milk outweigh the risk of a trace of prescription drug in your breast milk, but a few medications are considered unsafe during lactation. Others, although safe, may cause symptoms in your baby; the staff need to know to watch for these symptoms.

Your medical provider, nurse practitioner, physician assistant, or lactation specialist will have access to an appropriate resource to check substances and their compatibility with breastfeeding. Credible useful references include *Medications and Mother's Milk: A Manual of Lactation Pharmacology* by Thomas Hale; *Breastfeeding Handbook for Physicians* from the American Academy of Pediatrics; or *Drugs in Pregnancy and Lactation* by Briggs, Freeman, and Yaffe. The NICU pharmacist, if your NICU has one, can also be a good resource for assessing the safety of medications while breastfeeding.

Drugs, Alcohol, and Nicotine Dependence

Don't be afraid to tell a trusted member of the NICU staff if you have issues with street drugs, alcohol abuse, or prescription drug abuse. These substances all pass through your breast milk to your baby and sometimes produce tragic side effects. Your health care providers should act as your advocate. Your well-being and the health of your baby are their top priorities. Let your team help you find assistance so that you can be the best parent possible.

Smoking cigarettes leaves nicotine in your breast milk, which will be ingested by your baby. Seek help from a smoking cessation specialist. Your baby may be the motivation you need to kick the habit. Most experts feel that the use of a nicotine patch is compatible with breastfeeding, and the benefit of decreased cigarette exposure outweighs the risk of exposure to the nicotine patch. In addition, smoking cigarettes exposes your baby to secondhand and thirdhand smoke and increases your baby's risk of sudden infant death syndrome (SIDS). See Chapter 16 for more information about reducing SIDS risk.

Contraception

Breastfeeding delays the return of menstrual periods for several months after childbirth—which allows the body to rebuild its store of iron and is a nice convenience. It also has a contraceptive effect.

However, breastfeeding is not a reliable method of contraception. You can become pregnant if you have unprotected sex around the time of your first ovulation following delivery, which means you will not even have had your first period. Hormonal methods of birth control, such as the pill, cannot be used for about 6 weeks postpartum (see below), and a diaphragm is not refitted for 4 to 6 weeks after delivery. If family planning is important to you, be prepared with spermicidal foam, condoms, or another form of birth control recommended by your care provider.

Exclusive Breastfeeding

If you are *exclusively* breastfeeding (feeding or expressing your milk every couple of hours around the clock), have had *no vaginal bleeding* after the 56th postpartum day, and are less than 6 months postpartum, your risk of getting pregnant is greatly reduced, but not 100% foolproof, in the first 6 months of breastfeeding. Pregnancy can occur, so don't depend on breastfeeding as a primary method of birth control if family planning is important to you.

Lactational Amenorrhea Method

Another method is called the *lactational amenorrhea method*. This method was developed by the Institute for Reproductive Health in 1996 and is fairly simple. It consists of 3 questions. If you answer yes to any of the questions, your chance of pregnancy increases and another form of birth control should be considered to prevent pregnancy. The 3 questions are

1. Has your menses (period or blood flow) returned?
2. Are you allowing long periods (4–6 hours) without pumping or breastfeeding (during the day or night) or supplementing regularly?
3. Is your baby older than 6 months?

If you have answered yes to any of these questions, then using breastfeeding as your only birth control method is very risky.

Hormonal Methods

Hormonal methods of contraception, such as the pill, an intrauterine device (IUD), or vaginal ring, are not recommended until 6 weeks postpartum if breastfeeding exclusively. Hormonal contraception use is delayed after childbirth because of risk of blood clots associated with pregnancy and hormonal methods of birth control and because most of them decrease breast milk production.

Contraceptive methods that use the hormone progestin are considered compatible with breastfeeding. Progestin-only methods include a variety of contraceptives, including the minipill, progestin IUDs, progestin-releasing vaginal rings, injections, and implants. Small amounts of progestin do pass into the mother's milk, but research has found no long-term effects on children of mothers using this form of contraception.

Use of hormonal contraception can begin at approximately 6 to 8 weeks postpartum. Early introduction of progestin (in the first couple of days) usually causes a negative effect on milk supply and the baby's ability to metabolize the hormone. Estrogen-based hormonal contraceptives are compatible with breastfeeding but are not considered the best choice for lactating women. Estrogen has a greater effect than progestin in reducing milk supply. You may notice a change in volume when pumping and that your baby has fewer wet diapers, is not satisfied after feedings, or sleeps for shorter periods. These signs indicate a reduction in milk supply. Talk with your baby's medical provider about the possible need for supplementation with formula to ensure adequate growth and development.

When Not to Breastfeed

Most babies benefit from their mother's breast milk; however, in some situations, it may not be safe to breastfeed your newborn. Mothers who should not breastfeed include those with

- **Human immunodeficiency virus (HIV):** In the United States, the Centers for Disease Control and Prevention and the AAP recommend that women who test positive for HIV use formula instead of giving their breast milk to their babies.
- **Human T-cell lymphotrophic virus type I or II.**
- **Untreated active tuberculosis.**
- **Cytomegalovirus (CMV):** Almost half of all adults test positive for CMV, meaning they have had this viral infection at some time in their life. During the active stage of this infection, this virus is shed in the throat, urine, genital tract, and breast milk. In theory, infants who are born very premature could become infected by breast milk from a CMV-positive mother because they did not receive the transplacental immunity the mother would have provided to them in the final 3 months of the pregnancy. Most NICUs do not screen for CMV, however, nor do they restrict CMV-positive mothers from providing breast milk. A few NICUs have adopted the practice of freezing all breast milk for the premature infant to reduce the possibilities of CMV exposure, although this is not a totally reliable method. If you know you are CMV-positive and your baby was born before 28 weeks' gestation, ask your baby's medical team for advice.

- **Herpes:** Some women get recurrent herpes lesions on their breasts. Just like the virus that causes cold sores on the lips (herpes type 1) or genital herpes (herpes type 2), the virus that causes these sores is life-threatening for newborns. If you have a herpes sore on your breast, discard the milk from that side, and don't breastfeed on that side until the sore is completely healed. Also note that the herpesvirus is shed before the appearance of a sore; you may wish to weigh the risks and benefits of breastfeeding in this situation. Ask your lactation specialist and physician for advice. Some women who experience recurrent herpes on one breast will choose to nurse their baby only from the unaffected breast. Although this takes more planning on the mother's part, the baby can usually breastfeed successfully from one breast. Similarly, if you have active cold sores anywhere on your mouth or lips, do not kiss your baby, as this may spread the virus.

In addition, breastfeeding is contraindicated for

- Mothers who have received radioactive materials for a nuclear medicine scan (for a certain period until the radioactivity has cleared from the milk; the lactation specialist or your doctor can determine the period)
- Mothers receiving chemotherapy or antimetabolites (until the medication has cleared from the milk)
- Mothers who use illegal drugs (or abuse prescription drugs)
- A newborn with galactosemia (who must receive lactose-free formula)

You may also need to stop providing milk or breastfeeding temporarily because of breast milk jaundice (different than physiological jaundice explained in Chapter 9). Some babies have such high blood levels of the substance called *bilirubin* that the doctor, nurse practitioner, or physician assistant may recommend discontinuing breastfeeding for a day or two. In most cases, the bilirubin level will come down when breastfeeding is temporarily discontinued. This does not mean that anything is wrong with your milk; you can resume breastfeeding without fear as soon as the baby's bilirubin drops to a reasonable level.

Providing Breast Milk for Your Special Care Baby

"My pregnancy was difficult. My baby's birth was complicated and frightening. Thank goodness my body made breast milk perfectly."

Every family has a lot to think about after labor and birth are over. You'll receive an overwhelming amount of information. Amid all the excitement, if you have decided to breastfeed, be sure to tell your nurse and the NICU nurse.

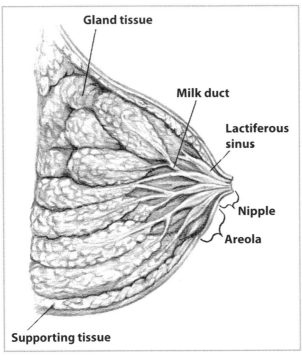

Gland tissue

Milk duct

Lactiferous sinus

Nipple

Areola

Supporting tissue

How the breasts make milk.
The fatty and supportive tissues that normally make up most of the volume of the breast are replaced by glandular tissue necessary to produce milk.

From: American Academy of Pediatrics. New Mother's Guide to Breastfeeding. *Elk Grove Village, IL: American Academy of Pediatrics; 2002.*

How the Breasts Make Milk

To appreciate the importance of emptying your breasts frequently and completely, it helps to have an understanding of how the breasts work.

By week 16 of pregnancy, your breasts start producing a thick, clear or yellow-gold secretion called *colostrum*. Within 2 or 3 days after you give birth, the colostrum begins to change to a thinner, whiter milk called *mature milk*. The amount of milk your breasts produce also increases dramatically at this time, and you may notice that your breasts are swollen, hard, and painful. This happens as a result of the hormonal changes that accompany birth—whether your baby is born early or on time and whether you breastfeed or not.

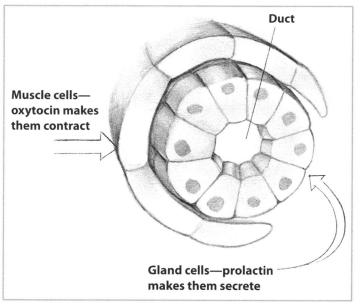

Hormonal changes.
Breastfeeding stimulates the increase of oxytocin and prolactin, hormones that cause the milk ducts to contract and secrete milk.

From: American Academy of Pediatrics. New Mother's Guide to Breastfeeding. *Elk Grove Village, IL: American Academy of Pediatrics; 2002.*

When a baby nurses, you manually express your milk, or a pump exerts suction and extracts the milk, your brain releases 2 hormones: prolactin and oxytocin. Prolactin causes the milk glands in your breasts to start secreting milk. You may notice sleepiness or peacefulness—side effects of prolactin release in your bloodstream.

The other hormone, oxytocin, may be familiar to you as the hormone of labor. Just as it causes the muscles of the uterus to contract, it also causes contractions of tiny muscles that surround the milk glands in your breasts. These contractions squeeze the milk down into small reservoirs just behind the nipples. This is called the *milk-ejection reflex* or the *let-down reflex*. An early sign that this is occurring may be menstrual-like cramps in your uterus. You'll notice these cramps only in the first week or two after birth, and you may not notice them at all if this is your first baby. After a week or so, you may notice a feeling of thirst a few minutes after you begin to pump, a tingling sensation or a sensation of "pins and needles" in your breasts, or milk dripping from your nipples. After pumping, you may notice distinct softening of your breasts (like deflated balloons). These are all reassuring signs that the oxytocin-induced milk-ejection reflex has occurred.

Prolactin is released every time your nipples are stimulated and only when your nipples are stimulated. Nothing else signals your body to make and keep on making milk. Oxytocin is released in response to sucking, but it can be released in response to other psychological stimuli too—such as sitting in the same chair to nurse or to pump your breasts, hearing the sound of the pump or your baby's cry (or another baby's cry), or just relaxing. This is called a *conditioned response.*

If You Have Had Breast Surgery

Breast implants usually do not interfere with breastfeeding. However, it is important to let your health care professional, nurse, and or the lactation specialist know that you have had surgery on your breasts. Care of the breasts with implants requires prevention of engorgement or overfullness of the breasts. Preventing engorgement decreases the pressure on the implants. Unless breast damage has already occurred from the surgery or other aspect of the implants, breastfeeding should proceed normally.

Breast reduction always influences milk production. If you have had breast reduction surgery, it is extremely important to share this information with your lactation specialist and your infant's health care provider. You may be able to produce some milk depending on the type of surgery that was performed. You will probably need to supplement your breast milk with formula to ensure enough nutrition for your growing infant. Frequent weight checks and recording the infant's intake and output will help determine if other interventions are needed. An experienced lactation specialist should work with you and your infant to help ensure a successful feeding experience.

What to Expect in the First Few Days

Soon after you give birth, your nurse will bring a breast pump to your room. (If your medical condition allows, ask for it within the first 6 hours after birth.) She'll show you how to hold the milk collecting cups up to your breasts and turn on the pump. Many mothers laugh about feeling "like a dairy cow." You may feel awkard and embarrassed—and possibly discouraged when only a drop or two of milk appears on your nipple. But every drop is precious, the NICU team calls it "liquid gold." Try to save whatever you can in a small container. The volume of your baby's first feeding is very small, perhaps only 1 to 2 milliliters (about 1/5–2/5 teaspoon).

In the first few hours after giving birth, especially with everything happening to your baby, trying to learn about expressing and storing your milk may feel overwhelming. Admittedly, this is not the best time to take in new information. Don't be ashamed to ask questions and repeat them until you understand the answers. Watch videos or DVDs if they are available, and ask for written materials that you can take home with you. Arrange to have your partner, a family member, or a friend in the room when the nurse or lactation consultant is explaining everything; chances are that between you, you'll remember the important points.

Practice pumping every 3 hours, even if little milk comes out. Your milk supply will increase dramatically by the third to fifth day, and for a few days you may need to pump more often to keep up with the production. It is normal for one breast to produce more milk than the other. In addition, you may observe that one breast has a faster flow of milk than the other. This is normal too. Do not worry about producing too much milk; it is much easier to reduce a plentiful milk supply than to build up one that is flagging.

The Breast Pump

Breast pumping can bring mixed emotions for new mothers who need to use an electric breast pump. The first thing is to remember that this is temporary and that soon your baby will be skin to skin with you—nuzzling at first, and then nursing in most circumstances. Breast pumping is the link between you and your baby. Think of your breast pump as a valuable machine helping you and your baby. Many mothers find that pumping at their infant's bedside helps their milk supply.

"I was so embarrassed to use the breast pump at first. But when I saw the containers filling up, and I saw the nurses giving my milk to Ryan, I got over it. The breast pump is a great tool for NICU mothers who want to breastfeed their babies."

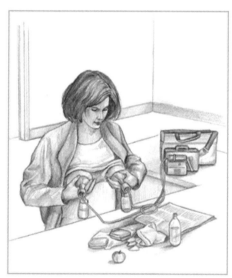

Using the breast pump.
A double breast pump expresses milk from both breasts at the same time. This not only saves time pumping, but produces more milk than if the mother pumps each breast separately. A hospital-grade pump is larger than the portable pump pictured here.

From: American Academy of Pediatrics. Breastfeeding Handbook for Physicians. Elk Grove Village, IL: American Academy of Pediatrics; 2006:162.

Stay Motivated

If pumping seems like too much trouble, try to focus on why you are expressing your milk. The medical benefits for your baby are huge. You are pumping to help your baby get and stay healthy. You are pumping not only to give your baby your milk now, but also to preserve your ability to make milk until your baby is ready to breastfeed. Make this your goal.

Talk to other breastfeeding mothers in the special care nursery. Ask your baby's nurse if there is a parent support group, or call one of the national support groups listed in Appendix D. If you are lucky enough to have a lactation consultant at your hospital or a private practice lactation consultant, she can give you the support you need. Breast pumping requires commitment on your part and encouragement from the people around you. Remember: *It is worth it.*

Considerations for Electric Breast Pump Rental

To establish and maintain a milk supply, you cannot depend on small hand-operated or battery-powered pumps. Only hospital-quality, fully automatic electric breast pumps are adequate for the job. You should pump both breasts at the same time. This not only saves time but also increases your prolactin levels. To use a pump of this sort, you hold 2 plastic, funnel-shaped cups over your breasts, and the pump automatically collects your milk in bottles attached to the cups. These collection kits are attached to the pump by tubing, which should not collect moisture. The pump has an on/off switch and a dial for adjusting the suction.

The NICU will have breast pumps for your use while you are spending time in the NICU. When selecting the type of breast pump for use at home, it is important to note a couple of design features that protect the milk from self-contamination. This includes a breast pump with a viral barrier close to the funnel-shaped cups that is placed between the funnel-shaped cups and the tubing that attaches to the pump. A pump that allows condensation is not recommended either, as this could pose the risk of mold, fungus, and other bacteria growing inside the tubing and contaminating the breast milk. The Human Milk Banking Association has outlined these features as recommendations for breast milk collection. Your lactation consultant can answer your questions about the features of the breast pump you use. The cost of renting an electric breast pump—from $1.00 to $3.50 per day—may also be a concern. At a time when you are rightfully concerned about medical bills, eliminating the breast pump may seem like one way to cut costs. Keep in mind, though, that having a breast pump at home saves time, simplifies the milk removal process, and builds your milk supply. In addition, formula costs more than breastfeeding and formula will be necessary throughout the first year for a formula-feeding infant. Check to see if insurance or Medicaid will cover the cost of breast pump rental. It is worth a call to your local WIC program (Special Supplemental Nutrition Program for Women, Infants, and Children) or public health department to see if they have a pump lending program; many do.

How Long and How Often to Pump

The guidelines that follow are general. Your NICU may have slightly different or more detailed instructions. Your nurse or the lactation specialist should be able to answer your questions.

Most experts agree that a mother should express (or pump) her milk 6 to 8 times in a 24-hour period. For mothers of preterm infants, at least 100 total minutes of pumping per day is required to maintain an adequate supply. Providing breast milk for your special care baby usually means pumping milk from your breasts every 2 to 3 hours. Most NICUs recommend that you pump your milk at least 8 times per day, and preferably more. Pumping both breasts simultaneously (which requires a double pump setup) with a hospital-quality electric pump usually takes only 10 to 20 minutes (15 minutes average). Short, frequent pumping sessions are necessary to keep up your milk supply.

In the beginning, before your milk supply is established, you will need to pump for about 10 minutes. Once your milk supply is established, you can use the flow of milk as your guide: Pump until the flow slows down or stops. If you are trying to increase your milk supply, pump more often—not longer. It's much more effective to pump every 3 hours for 10 to 20 minutes than to pump for a longer time but at wider intervals. Do not let your breasts feel "full" in between pumping, as this can further decrease your milk supply. Whether to pump during the night depends on several things: Are you awake anyway? Are you trying to build your milk supply? Are you trying to maintain your milk supply? Is your baby coming home soon? An answer of yes to any of these questions is a good reason to pump at night. If you decide that uninterrupted sleep is more important than pumping, don't let more than 6 hours go by without emptying your breasts, and pump at least 8 times during your waking hours. Do not skip pumping at night very often.

Keeping Milk and Equipment Clean

Breast milk is not sterile. The bacteria in the milk probably help the development of beneficial microorganisms in a healthy newborn. Before your NICU baby receives your milk, however, it will have been expressed, stored, exposed to light, handled by nurses, and sent through feeding tubes, so it makes sense to be extra careful about keeping it clean. Although some NICU protocols ask mothers to clean their breasts prior to pumping, most will tell mothers that breasts do not require cleaning, other than with soap and water in your bath or shower.

The best way to keep your breast milk safe and clean is to wash your hands before you pump and maintain proper cleaning of your breast pump parts. Only those parts of the pump that actually are exposed to your milk require cleaning after each use. Rinse them well in cold water, wash them with hot, soapy water, and rinse again—or wash them in the dishwasher. Some special care nurseries may ask you to sterilize your breast pump parts once each day. To sterilize, boil them in water for at least 5 minutes. Allow clean pump parts to air-dry; touch only the outside of the parts; and store them in a clean, covered container between uses.

A breast pump that allows condensation to occur in the tubing should be inspected after every use to avoid mold, fungus, or bacterial growth in the tubing. Be sure to read and follow the breast pump manufacturer's cleaning instructions carefully.

If your hospital has different equipment than what is recommended here, it is most likely efficient for milk removal. Do your part by cleaning your breast pump parts thoroughly, washing your hands, and following the instructions provided. Even with all of the handling your breast milk goes through in the NICU, it has working cells (phagocytes) that help protect your milk from germs and bacteria. If you are unsure about any cleaning or pumping procedures, ask for help from the lactation specialist, nurse, or health care professional in the NICU.

Storing and Labeling Your Milk

Your hospital may provide a supply of sterilized containers for storing and transporting your milk. Plastic bags are not used in the NICU due to higher risk of contamination than glass or hard plastic. You may use glass or hard plastic containers but be aware of the risk of injury with glass if the bottle is dropped or broken.

Many food and liquid containers are made of polycarbonate, or lined with an epoxy that contains the chemical bisphenol-A (BPA). Bisphenol-A is used to harden plastics, keep bacteria from contaminating foods, and prevent cans from rusting. There are concerns, though, over the possible harmful effects BPA may have on humans, particularly on infants and children. As research continues, you can look for "BPA free" when selecting containers for storing breast milk or bottle feeding.

Immediately after pumping, label the container with your baby's name and the date and time you pumped the milk. The NICU staff may give you a premade label used for your baby with a bar code to use on the containers. They will then check the bar code every time before giving the milk to your baby. This reduces the chances of giving your baby another mother's breast milk. If you are thawing frozen milk, also write on the label the date and time you took the container out of the freezer.

Several studies have been done on the effects of various methods of storing human milk, but more research is needed. You may get conflicting advice about storage. A general rule is that the longer breast milk is stored, the more nutrients and immunologic properties it loses. Some NICUs are more conservative than others in trying to preserve and protect milk quality. Most allow breast milk to be stored in the refrigerator for at least 24 to 48 hours, in the freezer compartment of a refrigerator for 2 to 3 weeks, or in a deep freeze (at -4°F plus or minus 3.6°F) for up to 6 months. For older babies, it's probably safe to hold milk for up to 5 days in the refrigerator and 6 months in the freezer. Once frozen milk is thawed, most NICUs like to use it within 24 hours (Table 1).

Each NICU will have a different method for thawing and warming breast milk in their NICU. Ask the lactation specialist or nurse how they recommend thawing and warming your breast milk. A few things to remember

- The higher the heat, the more of the living cells will be destroyed.
- At home, using hot water from the sink will thaw and warm the milk for home use, or use a bottle-warming device. Do not heat milk in a pot on the stove; this heat is too hot and can destroy the antibodies in the breast milk.
- **Never** warm milk in a microwave. Hot spots in the milk can burn the baby's throat and cause choking.

Table 1. Milk Storage Guide

Storage Time for Human Milk[a]	Deep Freeze (0°F/-18°C)	Refrigerator Freezer (variable 0°F/-18°C)	Refrigerator (39°F/4°C)	Cooler With Ice Packs Frozen (59°F/15°C)	Room Temperature	
					(66°F–72°F) (19°C–22°C)	(72°F–79°F) (22°C–26°C)
Fresh	Up to 12 months	3–4 months	8 days	24 hours	6–10 hours	4 hours
Frozen, thawed in fridge	Do not refreeze	Do not refreeze	24 hours	Do not store	4 hours	4 hours
Thawed, warmed, not fed	Do not refreeze	Do not refreeze	4 hours	Do not store	Until feeding ends	Until feeding ends
Warmed, fed	Discard	Discard	Discard	Discard	Until feeding ends	Until feeding ends

[a]Storage times may vary for premature or sick babies. Sources: Jones F, Tully MR. *Best Practice for Expressing, Storing and Handling Human Milk in Hospitals, Homes and Child Care Settings.* Raleigh, NC: Human Milk Banking Association of North America; 2006 and Mohrbacher N, Stock J. *The Breastfeeding Answer Book.* Schaumburg, IL: La Leche League International; 2003.

"I was proud of my accomplishment as I produced milk for my baby. My partner was proud, and we felt like we were working as a team. I pumped and labeled and he cleaned and stored the equipment. He was also very helpful in rotating the breast milk stock to bring to the NICU. He became the 'milk manager.'"

Transporting Your Milk to the Hospital

To take your milk to the hospital, pack it in a small cooler or an insulated bag. If you must transport frozen milk a long distance (requiring 24 hours out of the freezer), pack it in dry ice in a sturdy, insulated container. You may wish to ask your nurse or lactation specialist for advice on transporting milk safely.

Learning to Breastfeed

Getting comfortable enough to breastfeed in an intensive care setting is not easy. Nursing or pumping amid bright lights and alarms takes getting used to. Give yourself a lot of time to learn to relax. You may find that one chair fits you better than the others and that it helps to rest your feet on a small footstool. Experiment with pillows; one on your lap usually helps. There are special U-shaped pillows designed for feeding twins simultaneously. Privacy screens may be available in some nurseries.

While you and your baby are learning to breastfeed, keep pumping your breasts on your regular routine. Many mothers think they should skip pumping on the days they feed their babies. They want to be sure to have plenty of milk for the baby. What happens instead is that they arrive in the NICU with engorged breasts and nipples that are hard to compress and latch onto—and, later, their milk supply decreases. Instead, keep your pumping schedule. Help to open the breast ducts and increase the milk flow by applying a warm, moist compress and gently massaging the breast before and during pumping. Massaging your breasts for a few minutes right before and during the feeding not only softens your nipples and makes it easier for the baby to latch on, but also stimulates your milk-ejection reflex.

Position Your Baby and Your Breast

Two common positions for breastfeeding work especially well for preterm babies. Try the cross-cradle hold by laying your baby on the pillow, on his side facing you, with his

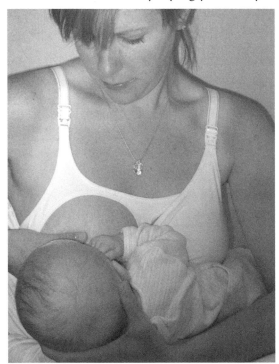

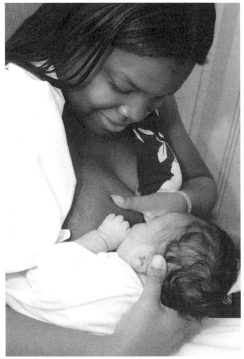

Cross-cradle hold.
This hold works well for nursing a premature infant. Hold the baby across your chest. Use the hand on the same side as the breast to support the breast. A pillow or two on your lap will help support the baby at the level of your breast and is less tiring than holding the baby without support.

Football hold or clutch hold.
Hold the baby at your side, with his mouth in front of your breast and his feet pointing toward your back. Your opposite hand supports the breast and guides the nipple into the baby's mouth.

Courtesy of Gigi O'Dea.

mouth right beside your nipple. Add pillows to bring the baby's mouth to the level of your nipple rather than trying to lift or lower your breast. Encircle your baby's body with the arm opposite the breast that your baby is about to nurse from, and grasp the back of the baby's lower head, neck, and shoulder blades in your hand. With the same-side hand (left hand on left breast, for example), cup your breast and present the nipple to your baby. Place your 4 fingers underneath and your thumb on top of your breast.

When using the football or clutch position, place a pillow on the same side as the breast you plan to offer. Place the baby with his legs pointing toward the back of the chair or bed. The same hand as the side of the breast you plan to offer will support the baby's head, neck, and shoulder. The infant is brought up to the breast in a gentle motion toward the nipple. The opposite hand is used to lift and guide the breast for the infant.

Compress Your Breast

With your fingers cupping your breast, you can shape your areola (the dark area around the nipple) to fit your baby's mouth. Although the mouth forms a circle when open wide, as soon as it clamps onto your areola and nipple, the lips and gums form a flattened oval. If you gently compress your breast in that same oval shape, your baby is likely to be able to suck longer. Consider this technique especially if your baby latches onto your nipple just fine and sucks 3 or 4 times, but then quits. If the concept seems hard to understand, think about how you squeeze a very thick sandwich just before you take a bite or how you turn an oval peg to fit it into an oval hole. Be sure that your thumb is parallel to your baby's upper lip and your index finger is parallel to your baby's lower lip. Some mothers find a U-shaped hold works better than a C-shaped hold. To do this, slide your fingers toward the center of your body and your thumb toward the outside of your breast. Your nurse or lactation consultant can help you with positioning. Finding a comfortable position to support your breast is important because not supporting the weight of your breast can also cause the breast to pull from your baby's mouth. Some breasts weigh as much as or more than the baby, so supporting the breast can make it easier for your baby to breastfeed.

Tickle Your Baby's Lower Lip

It is important to learn this next step so that you can use it when your baby is mature enough to respond, but it rarely works before 34 to 36 weeks' gestation. The idea is to get your baby to open his mouth using his natural rooting reflex. To do this, stroke the center of your baby's lower lip with the tip of your nipple. Brush your nipple lightly, delicately, and repeatedly over the lower lip, as if giving a signal. If you are able, express a few drops of breast milk to offer a familiar taste and smell. This can also encourage your baby to open and search for the nipple. When your baby is older and more experienced, this technique of touching your baby's lip with your nipple will be a powerful cue: Your baby will open his mouth wide. Then, with a forward movement of the arm encircling your baby, you'll place and guide him onto your breast. When you are both learning about feeding, though, your baby will probably not participate in the feeding as much as you do. Many babies in the early days seem to sleep through the experience. It may seem like you need another set of hands and arms. The lactation specialist or nurse can gently apply slight pressure to his chin to help him open wide or help to shape your nipple and aim it toward the roof of your baby's mouth.

Bring Your Baby to Your Breast

With one hand shaping your areola and the other hand holding your baby's head, you are in a perfect position to bring your baby onto your breast. As you do so, aim your nipple up toward the roof of the baby's mouth. This helps ensure that you get your nipple above your baby's tongue. Pull him in so close that the tip of his nose touches your breast. Continue to gently compress and support the weight of your breast throughout the *entire* feeding. You'll notice that your hand gets tired. That hints at why this technique works so well with premature babies: It probably keeps the tiny muscles around the mouth from getting fatigued.

Making Sure Your Baby Is Properly Latched On

You can tell that your baby is well latched on by looking for these signs.

- A wide-open mouth with lips spread out around your breast
- Your baby's mouth covers your entire nipple and some of the areola
- A firm tug on your breast every time your baby sucks
- Your baby can suckle for more than 3 or 4 sucks in a row
- Your baby can hang onto your nipple during pauses between bursts of sucks

Is Your Baby Getting Milk?

Once your baby is latched on well, he will suck in small, quick bursts until your milk begins to flow. Then the sucking pattern will change to slower, deeper, more rhythmic sucks. If the NICU is quiet enough, you may be able to hear your baby swallow. This is a sure sign that he is getting milk. If you cannot hear the swallowing, observe the throat area for swallowing. If you are still unsure, ask for the staff nurse or lactation specialist to observe you breastfeeding and confirm that your baby is swallowing.

When you first begin to breastfeed, your milk-ejection reflex may not occur until after your baby has tired of sucking and fallen asleep. But, just as your body became conditioned to respond to the breast pump, you will learn to respond to your baby's suck. One clever mother brought the breast pump to her baby's bedside for the first few feedings. She knew that her milk would let down as soon as she heard the sound of the pump.

You can assess how well the breastfeeding is going by counting the number of sucks and listening for the swallowing sounds. Every baby has a unique "suck signature." You will soon learn your baby's. Maybe your baby always sucks 10 times in a row and then pauses. In general, the more sucks a baby takes before pausing, the more milk he is taking. Also, if your baby swallows with every suck, he is obviously getting a lot of milk. For premature babies, the pressure with which he sucks, the number of sucks per minute, and the amount of milk extracted from the breast all increase as your baby gets older and stronger.

After a few minutes of sustained, rhythmic sucks, your baby will revert to bursts of little sucks with long pauses in between. The swallowing sounds will be further and further apart. It's time to take your baby off your breast (few mothers need to break the suction with a preterm baby by putting their finger in the baby's mouth to interrupt sucking), burp him, and switch to the other breast. On the second side, watch again for the sucking pattern to slow down and swallowing to become less frequent.

During early feedings, your baby may not be able to tolerate this "burp and switch" technique. Taking your baby off of the breast and switching him back and forth several times usually does not arouse a preterm baby to take more milk, but tires him. He'll do better if you let him nurse on only one breast at a feeding. To encourage your baby to stay awake, you can gently massage your breast when the sucking pattern slows down. Breastfeeding on only one side at a feeding may also improve your baby's weight gain, because the milk that comes at the end of the feeding (called *hindmilk)* is higher in fat and calories than the first milk. This is good to remember if you're producing much more milk than your baby can take at one feeding. In fact, if your baby is having trouble gaining weight, you may want to pump before nursing and freeze the thinner "foremilk" for later feedings. Talk to your baby's medical provider about how and when to collect foremilk and hindmilk. One-sided nursing is also a good approach if it takes a long time (10 or more minutes) to get your baby latched on. If you interrupt the baby's suction to switch sides, he may be too tired to resume nursing. It's better for your baby to nurse well on one breast than to nurse ineffectively on both.

Each NICU will have its own methods and philosophy for assessing the infant's intake. The only accurate way to determine how much milk your baby is getting is to weigh the baby on an electronic scale before and after feeding (called *test weights);* however, not all NICUs support the pre- and post-weight method of assessing the infant's intake. If your NICU uses pre- and post-weights to determine intake, ask your baby's nurse when this procedure begins. When you feel confident that your baby is getting milk and you would like these breastfeeding sessions to "count," it's probably time to ask the nurse to help you weigh the baby before your next feeding session. Then breastfeed until the baby's sucking and swallowing slows down, and put the baby back on the scale without changing his diaper or clothes.

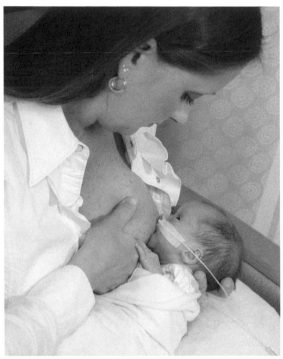

Nutrition from a nasogastric tube and bottle.
This baby seems alert and begins this feeding at the breast. When he tires, the remainder of the feeding will be given through his gavage tube.

Courtesy of Gigi O'Dea.

Each gram of weight gain is equal to approximately 1 milliliter of milk. If your baby's pre-feeding weight was 1,285 grams, and his post-feeding weight is 1,300 grams, your baby took 15 milliliters (about ½ ounce). If your baby took less than the amount needed, the nurse will probably supplement the breastfeeding with a gavage feeding. In time, the amount your baby takes from the breast will gradually increase until he is taking all he needs from your breast.

At first, you will be able to breastfeed only once or twice a day. Few babies under 36 to 37 weeks are able to suck more than this. They become tired and begin to lose weight if you push them to suckle more than they are developmentally capable. Your baby's other feedings will be by gavage. Continue to pump immediately after each nursing until supplemental feedings are no longer necessary. Although it's tempting to say, "I breastfed the baby, so I don't need to pump," if you don't keep pumping after every breastfeeding, you risk losing your milk supply.

As your baby matures, he will start to wake up and show signs that it's time for a feeding. At that point, gavage feeding is no longer appropriate. If you have been breastfeeding for a few days, bottle feeding by the nursing staff when your baby is awake and hungry (and you are not there) does not usually interfere with breastfeeding success.

Nipple Preference

Sometimes NICU parents and staff worry about nipple preference (sometimes called *nipple confusion),* in which a baby develops difficulty with breastfeeding after exposure to bottles. To avoid giving bottles to breastfeeding babies, some nurseries use techniques such as finger feeding or cup feeding. With finger feeding, the baby is encouraged to suck on a clean, gloved finger (nail bed down, pad up toward the roof of the baby's mouth), and a feeding device that has a small thin feeding tube that is slipped into the baby's mouth along with the caregiver's finger. With cup feeding, the baby is held upright, and small amounts of milk are placed on the baby's tongue with a small cup (medicine cup) or spoon. Finger feeding and cup feeding preterm infants are methods commonly used in developing countries. These methods have been researched and they do, to some extent, enhance breastfeeding success. They may also prolong total hospital stay; however, many mothers and breastfeeding specialists who have tried these methods believe that they do help prevent nipple preference.

Because bottles are a routine part of a breastfed baby's care in most NICUs, observe for difficulties with breastfeeding after bottles are introduced. If you notice that breastfeeding is not going as well now that your baby is being bottle fed, your best alternative is to spend more time at the hospital so that you can be there for most of his feedings. If this is impossible and you'd like to try finger feeding or cup feeding, discuss it with your baby's health care provider, doctor, nurse, or lactation specialist.

Breastfeeding Challenges

Breastfeeding can be especially challenging for NICU mothers and babies. In the beginning it may seem like you are participating in the feeding process and your baby is not. This is normal. Your NICU baby will need more time than a healthy term baby to participate in the feeding process. Give yourself and him time to learn, and ask for help when you encounter problems.

"Sticking to your decision to breastfeed is tough when your baby is in the NICU. It really helped me to talk to a mother who had been pumping for eight weeks. It can be done."

Helping Baby Latch On

If you can't get your baby latched onto your breast, ask for help. Your baby may be turning his head to reach your nipple, or the weight of your breast may be pulling the nipple out of your baby's mouth. Another position might work better (a football hold, for example, with the baby tucked under your arm at your side). An extra pair of helping hands, from a knowledgeable nurse or a lactation specialist, can help you through the awkwardness of learning what works for you and your baby.

Perhaps your baby is holding his tongue against the roof of his mouth. First check to be sure that your baby's head and neck are well supported. Then let your baby suck on your clean or gloved finger for a few minutes before feeding. Gently stroke the roof of his mouth several times to elicit the sucking reflex. Let your baby suck on your finger until the suck becomes rhythmical. The baby's tongue will drop down, and its sides will cup around your finger, forming a channel or "trough" for your finger to lie in. This technique works like warming up a pitcher in a bullpen. It seems to help babies get organized, which improves their suck.

In some cases, your nipple can be difficult for your baby to latch onto. If your nipple is short or inverted (does not protrude), first try pulling it outward with your fingers, then rolling it between your thumb and forefinger to make it erect. If that does not work, try pumping for 5 to 10 minutes before the feeding to soften the areola and elongate the nipple. Don't worry about removing milk that your baby might have taken at the feeding. The first step is to get your baby latched on; milk intake can come later. Wearing breast shells (a plastic dome with a center hole that allows the nipple to come forward) inside your bra before feedings can also encourage your nipples to stand out.

When these techniques do not work, a thin silicone nipple shield (an artificial nipple placed over your own nipple) sometimes helps. Some premature babies can extract more milk from a breast with a nipple shield than without one. However, the use of a nipple shield requires support and management from an experienced lactation specialist. When a nipple shield is used incorrectly, it can cause more harm than good. Ask the lactation specialist for assistance. A nipple shield is a *temporary* device that is meant to be used only for days to weeks, and not throughout your entire breastfeeding experience. The infant is eventually weaned from the nipple shield with guidance from a lactation specialist.

A few conditions make it difficult or nearly impossible for a baby to latch on. Infants with cleft lip may learn to breastfeed, but those with a cleft of the gum or palate (roof of the mouth) are unable to create suction. Babies with abnormalities of the skull and face may be unable to latch on effectively. A very small, recessed chin (a condition called *micrognathia)* may also interfere with breastfeeding. A very short frenulum (a baby with this condition is sometimes called "tongue-tied" because of the unusually short tissue attached to the base of the baby's tongue), may interfere with breastfeeding, but not always. If necessary, the physician can alleviate this problem by clipping the frenulum. Some babies with nervous system or heart problems don't have enough strength or coordination to suck effectively. Consult with the NICU lactation specialist or occupational or physical therapist with experience in infant feeding issues—many of these experts are trained to assess and treat infant feeding problems such as these.

Increasing Your Milk Supply

You might notice that you are producing less milk after the second or third week of pumping. This is less likely to happen if you have a hospital-quality electric pump in good working order, are using the double pumping kit, are using breast massage before and/or during pumping, and are pumping at least 8 times a day. If you skip a pumping session and let your breasts become overly full, your milk supply will decrease. Pumping frequency is important. If 2 women each spend 100 minutes a day pumping but one does ten 10-minute sessions and the other does five 20-minute sessions, the first mother will have a larger milk supply.

On the other hand, some mothers who pump religiously have trouble making enough milk. If you are one of them, you will find it frustrating to ask for advice and to be told only, "Pump more often." Feeling anxious about your baby's condition, feeling exhausted, taking some types of birth control pills, not eating or drinking enough, and coming down with a cold can all have an adverse effect on your milk supply. Ask your health care professional, lactation specialist, or pharmacist if any drugs you are taking might be affecting your milk supply. Consider low milk supply a signal to take extraordinarily good care of yourself. Read up on and practice stress management techniques. Spending more time skin to skin with your baby is the best way to help a diminishing milk supply.

As a last resort, you might ask your physician to prescribe metoclopramide hydrochloride (Reglan), which some studies have shown may improve milk supply. If Reglan is prescribed, follow instructions carefully and work with an experienced lactation consultant throughout the course of the medication trial. As with any body system, recognize that individuals vary; some women cannot make more than a limited amount of milk. If you have tried everything and still cannot build your milk supply, consider the possibility that it is a system (not a personal) issue. Another alternative may be herbal support. Many mothers believe that taking fenugreek boosts milk supply, but its positive effects have not been documented scientifically. Contact your local lactation specialist for more information. Be sure to make your baby's health care provider aware of any herbs you take to increase milk production.

Enhancing Your Milk-Ejection Reflex

If you feel as if your breasts are very full with milk but nothing comes out when you pump or feed your baby, you may need some supportive measures to enhance your milk-ejection (let-down) reflex.

Sometimes in the beginning, the let-down response is a little slow to respond. You can condition your milk-ejection reflex to respond, but this may take a little time. When you pump or feed in the NICU, sit in the same comfortable chair, sip the same beverage, apply a warm washcloth to your breasts, and massage them beforehand. If you are having difficulty releasing the milk at home, try taking a warm shower and massage the breasts in the shower. The milk may run down the shower drain, but this is OK. Immediately after the shower, sit down and use your electric double breast pump. If you get no results within 24 hours, ask your lactation specialist for help.

Sore Nipples

If your nipples become sore from pumping, try turning the pump's suction down, temporarily limiting pumping time to no more than 10 minutes, and applying modified lanolin around the areola before pumping. In addition, you may use a soft, flexible insert made for the electric pump that helps take the pressure off of your sore spot. Preterm babies exert much less pressure when they suckle than a pump or a full-term baby exerts and rarely cause sore nipples.

Yeast Infection (Thrush)

If your nipples suddenly become sore after being pain-free, or if your nipple pain is not associated with feeding or pumping, you may have a yeast infection. Babies often get yeast infections, called *thrush,* which appears as a milky white coating on the tongue and inner cheeks or as a persistent bright-red diaper rash. Thrush is particularly common in babies who have been on antibiotics. In mothers, the symptoms of thrush are very sore nipples—which may look perfectly normal or be quite pink—and burning/shooting/stabbing pains in the breasts. Check your baby's mouth periodically for signs of thrush on the tongue and roof of the mouth.

To treat the yeast infection, both you and your baby must be treated together, at the same time. You'll need prescriptions for antifungal medicine: an oral suspension for your baby and a topical cream for your nipples. During the treatment, you and your baby's caregivers must sterilize pacifiers, breast pump parts, bottle nipples, and anything else that might reinfect your baby's mouth and your breasts. You can continue to breast-feed during treatment. For some mothers, topical treatment alone will not suffice. They will then need a 2- to 3-week course of an oral antifungal medication such as fluconazole. This medicine is safe to take while breastfeeding or expressing milk for a premature infant.

Mastitis

If you develop fever, chills, and flu-like symptoms, along with a hot, red, tender area on your breast, you probably have a breast infection called *mastitis.* You'll be given an antibiotic to treat the infection. Make sure that your health care provider gives you a medication that will cover both "staph" and "strep," 2 germs that most often cause mastitis. Most cases of mastitis require 2 to 3 weeks of treatment to fully resolve. Under ordinary circumstances (a healthy full-term baby), women with mastitis should continue to breastfeed or pump; the baby probably has the germ in his mouth already. In fact, the baby probably brought the germ to your breast. In the special care nursery, if your baby has not yet suckled at your breast, it is probably a good idea to discard the milk from the infected breast(s) until the antibiotic starts to work and you feel better. Although you should discard your milk in this case, continue to pump your breasts so you can resume breastfeeding as soon as the infection clears up. Please let your baby's medical provider know that you have mastitis, as some germs in your milk could, for a short time only, be infectious to your premature or sick infant. However, there is usually no need for your baby's doctor to culture your milk.

In rare cases, mastitis can lead to a breast abscess. This is a serious condition that requires not only long-term antibiotic treatment but also surgical drainage.

Clogged Ducts

A clogged duct produces a red, hot, tender lump on one breast. A mother with a clogged duct has a tender lump that can reduce in size and discomfort within about 24 to 48 hours. Unlike mastitis, there is no fever associated with a clogged duct. However, if left untreated it could progress to mastitis (described previously).

Treat yourself as if you were coming down with a cold: Take it easy for a couple of days, rest in bed, and drink extra fluids. In addition, soak your breast several times a day in a tub of warm water, massage it gently (squeezing is painful and not helpful), and pump more frequently. The clogged duct may take 2 days, and sometimes 3, to resolve. Sometimes, as the clog moves down the duct, a painful white spot develops on the tip of the nipple. This will go way after the clogged duct is clear again.

Clogged ducts are sometimes caused by a mechanical obstruction—an underwire bra that presses in on the breast, a shoulder strap, or your sleep position, for example. Talk to a lactation specialist if you get clogged ducts repeatedly.

An Overabundant Supply of Breast Milk

Sometimes a mother will make so much milk she is in a position to donate her milk to help other mothers and infants in need. On a much sadder note, a mother who loses her baby may also consider donating her milk. The Human Milk Banking Association of North America regulates the milk banks and will accept donor milk from healthy mothers. By contacting them (see Appendix D), a mother can determine if her milk will be accepted into the donor pool of breast milk.

Making the Change to Home Feeding

A few common concerns parents have about breastfeeding at home are addressed here. Chapter 16 provides more information on home feeding. Once you are breastfeeding independently, you may have many more questions. Call your hospital's lactation specialist or a private practice lactation consultant with your questions, or find a support group in your community to help you stay inspired and confident in your abilities.

When your baby is finally ready to go home from the hospital, your biggest concern may be whether he is getting enough milk by breastfeeding. How are you going to manage breastfeeding at home, away from the scale, the staff, and the security of the NICU? In preparation for discharge, you need to know 2 things: (1) whether your baby's suck is effectively extracting (removing) milk from your breasts and (2) whether your milk supply is adequate for your baby to gain weight consistently.

How will you know the answers to these questions? Ask your baby's nurse how much milk the baby needs at each feeding. For example, a baby who weighs 5 1/2 pounds (about 2,500 grams) usually requires approximately 2 ounces (56 milliliters) every 3 hours. If you have not been weighing your baby on an electronic scale before and after each breastfeeding, ask for this to be done now, in the final days of hospitalization, so that you can know the effectiveness of your baby's suck. Is he capable of taking his minimum requirement directly from your breast by breastfeeding? Observing weight gain for approximately 5 days prior to discharge can indicate if your baby has been receiving enough milk through breastfeeding. Again, remember that not all NICUs will follow this practice of pre- and post-feeding weights. Some care providers estimate that the infant requires about 5 ounces of milk per kilogram of body weight per day. Therefore, if the baby weighs 3 kilograms, he will need about 15 ounces of milk per day. Note what his total intake and output was as charted in the medical record for a 24-hour period. Talk with the health care provider and confirm how the baby's intake is being assessed.

For several days before your baby comes home, keep track of the amount of milk you produce. Consult your health care provider and lactation specialist within a couple of days of going home and schedule weight checks at your health care provider's office. Exclusive breastfeeding depends on your ability to produce adequate milk supply and your baby's ability, strength, and stamina at the breast. Your health care professional and you should have the same goal regarding breastfeeding and work toward that goal. Some mothers are more comfortable renting an electronic scale to use at home as they are transitioning their baby over to full breastfeeding.

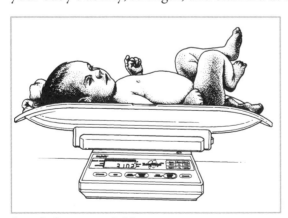

A scale for test weighing.
Your health care professional may recommend an electronic scale to determine if your baby needs supplemental feedings.

Courtesy of Medela, Inc. ©1999.

Effective Suck/High Supply

If your baby is sucking well when he is discharged from the hospital and your milk supply is high, you'll quickly progress to complete breastfeeding. How glad you'll be to get rid of that pump! But usually your baby's suck is not consistently strong immediately after discharge, and you'll need to depend on the pump for a few more weeks.

To find out whether your baby is getting enough milk, you have a few options.

1. Stay in the hospital with your baby for 24 hours prior to discharge, feeding exclusively by breast around the clock. See if your baby gains weight an average of 1/2 to 1 ounce per day or about 15 to 30 grams each day on breastfeeding alone.
2. Stop at your pediatric office on the way home from the hospital. Get a baseline weight on the office scale (scales are often slightly different). Make an appointment to go back in a day or two for another weight check to confirm that your baby is gaining the required 15 to 30 grams per day.
3. Count the average number of wet and dirty diapers your baby produced each day in the week prior to discharge. Use this number as a guide at home. A baby who was gaining steadily in the hospital with an average of 7 wet diapers and 3 bowel movements per day, for example, is likely to be gaining well if he keeps up this pattern at home. Get a weight check right away if his output drops.

Ineffective Suck/High Supply

Sometimes, despite a high supply of breast milk, test weights reveal that your baby doesn't take his required amount of milk by breastfeeding. Perhaps he bottle feeds well but hasn't mastered breastfeeding yet. (This is very typical, and very temporary, for premature babies). Or perhaps he was on a higher calorie formula or breast milk additive that gave him added calories for weight gain during hospitalization. So now you are taking him home, knowing that you have a good supply of milk but with a baby who is not able to breastfeed effectively to remove the breast milk. Try some of the following suggestions:

- Pump before nursing to stretch out your nipple, soften the areola, and get the milk flowing. If you notice that your baby chokes when your milk begins to flow, try pumping before nursing to help remove enough milk so that your initial let-down is not too forceful.
- If your baby takes a bottle well but can't seem to latch onto your breast, contact a lactation specialist. This consultant might suggest trying a nipple shield. If you use a nipple shield, you will need close follow-up to make sure that your baby is getting enough milk through the shield and to help wean your baby from the shield. This usually takes several weeks.
- To determine whether supplements are needed, rent an electronic scale for home use. Your lactation specialist can recommend a scale suited for this use.

Effective Suck/Low Supply

If your milk supply is low even when your baby sucks effectively, your baby will need supplements at home. During breastfeeding, massage your breast whenever your baby's sucking slows down. Use a nursing supplementer at your breast to give the extra milk your baby needs. This device, a bottle or bag that delivers milk to your baby through a tube that can be taped alongside your nipple, has special benefits.

- It gives your baby the necessary supplement at your breast rather than from a bottle, teaching your baby the correct way to suck and avoiding nipple preference.
- It makes for a 1-step feeding process: breastfeeding only, rather than breastfeeding followed by bottle feeding.
- It gives your breasts more stimulation, which should help you produce more milk.

Pump after every breastfeeding. Test weights are the only accurate means of knowing how much milk your baby is taking from your breast. Without weight checks, you have no idea when to stop giving supplements. Either rent a scale for home use or arrange for frequent weight check appointments (every 2–3 days) with a health care provider who is knowledgeable about both breastfeeding challenges and NICU graduates. The health care provider can advise you when you can safely stop giving supplements, refer you to other infant feeding specialists if needed, and counsel you about your chances of regaining a full milk supply if things don't improve within a week. You might also refer to the section Diminishing Milk Supply earlier in this chapter.

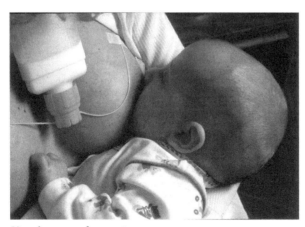

Nursing supplementer.
Your breast milk or formula is delivered to the baby from a tube taped alongside your nipple. This way, your baby receives supplemental feeding while nursing at your breast.

Courtesy of Medela, Inc. ©1999.

Ineffective Suck/Low Supply

If your baby is not effectively breastfeeding at discharge and your milk supply is low, pump religiously—8 to 12 times a day. Don't depend on breastfeeding to bring in a good milk supply. You will need to pump for at least 2 weeks after discharge. Use whatever milk you can express plus stored breast milk or formula to feed your baby the amount specified by the NICU team. If you can get your baby latched on, a nursing supplementer at your breast is the best way to accomplish your 2 goals of teaching your baby how to nurse and building your milk supply. Massage your breasts whenever the baby's sucking slows down. Adjust the supplementer so that the milk flows easily. If you cannot get your baby latched on, get help from a lactation specialist and ask about alternative methods of feeding your baby. Sometimes cup or finger feeding may keep your baby from becoming completely bottle fed while you increase your milk supply. Breastfeeding a premature infant can be a lot of hard work. Don't attempt to go it alone; arrange for frequent appointments with a lactation specialist.

Watching for Feeding Cues

If your baby doesn't demand to be fed at least 8 times a day, you'll need to encourage more frequent nursing. During the day, if your baby sleeps for more than 2 or 3 hours at a time, look for subtle signs that he is ready to feed: rooting, bringing his hands to his mouth, making sucking motions, licking his lips or sticking out his tongue, or simply moving about in his sleep. When you see these signs, called *feeding cues,* pick up your baby and encourage breastfeeding.

A good way to bring your preterm baby to a quiet alert state (the best state for feeding) is to allow him time to be skin to skin with you. Remove blankets and allow him free movement of his arms and legs, talk to him, stroke his face, and offer a drop of breast milk on your clean finger or a pacifier dipped in breast milk for 1 minute before breastfeeding. This may help him organize his sucking and breathing coordination and ready him for breastfeeding.

Meeting Your Baby's Needs

Learning to breastfeed your special care baby may be one of the most challenging things you'll ever do—but the rewards are worth it. You'll look back on this experience as something to be proud of. After weeks of pumping and days of awkwardness at breastfeeding, you'll finally take your baby home. This leap of faith—leaving behind the monitors, scales, and professional consultants in the NICU—requires courage and a commitment to breastfeeding. Eventually all of the pumps, tubes, and devices will be gone, and you will be feeding your baby on your own.

If You Need to Stop Breastfeeding

Even under the best of circumstances, not all mothers and babies can breastfeed. It's normal to grieve the loss of something you looked forward to and valued. If you pumped for even a few days, you truly did "breastfeed." Your baby will experience some long-lasting health benefits if he received even a little of your milk. Give yourself credit for your hard work. Don't let anyone make you feel guilty that you didn't try hard enough or long enough. Recognize that you made the best decision for yourself, your baby, and your family under very difficult circumstances.

Emotional Responses

For a while, you may feel waves of guilt or sadness about not breastfeeding. Also, expect to feel angry if you believe you didn't get the help or support you needed to breastfeed successfully. On the other hand, you may take on the task of learning to bottle feed without much emotional response to the "loss" of breastfeeding. A mother's response usually depends on how much discrepancy there was between what happened and what she had hoped would happen. In other words, if breastfeeding meant a great deal to you, expect to feel a sense of loss.

Physical Responses

If you are able to stop breastfeeding over a period of days or a few weeks, your milk supply will gradually diminish and cause little discomfort. But if you have an abundant milk supply and stop breastfeeding suddenly, the physical pain may be very uncomfortable. One mother whose baby died said that her continued milk supply was a sad and painful reminder that she had lost her baby: "It was like salt in a wound." If you, too, experience painfully full breasts when you stop breastfeeding, read ahead to the section titled Breast Engorgement.

Bottle Feeding Basics

Families formula feed their special care babies for many different reasons. Sometimes a mother tries and is unable to produce enough breast milk, or the baby is not able to breastfeed. Sometimes medical complications make breastfeeding inadvisable. For most women, formula feeding is a personal choice, perhaps influenced by culture and background. Unless there is a medical reason for not breastfeeding, the NICU team will probably encourage you to be a part of helping your baby get well by providing breast milk. Consider the pros and cons carefully and make the choice that is right for you and your baby. The NICU staff will support your decision and encourage your active participation in feeding your new baby.

Even though you have decided to bottle feed your baby, your body naturally begins to produce milk. This may become an uncomfortable condition called *breast engorgement*. The following information will help you cope with your milk production.

Breast Engorgement

After you give birth, your body experiences a dramatic hormonal shift. Levels of estrogen and progesterone, the major hormones of pregnancy, fall. Prolactin, the hormone that tells your body to make milk, rises. The effect of this shift is seen approximately 48 to 60 hours after birth, when your breasts swell with milk. If you don't remove the milk by nursing your baby or by pumping, your breasts may become rock hard and painful. The swelling may extend up into your armpits, making even simple movements uncomfortable. You may develop a mild fever. This combination of symptoms is called *postpartum engorgement.*

Your mother or grandmother may mention a medication that "dries up" your milk and wonder why your doctor doesn't prescribe it for you. Physicians no longer prescribe bromocriptine mesylate (Parlodel) and related drugs to suppress milk production because these drugs can have dangerous side effects. Stroke, heart problems, urinary system changes, and seizures have been reported. In addition, many women reported that their breasts became engorged when the medicine wore off—a phenomenon called *rebound engorgement.* For these reasons, doctors recommend letting the breast milk diminish naturally.

When milk is not removed from the breasts, your body stops making it. Pressure from the excess milk inside the mammary glands signals the pituitary gland to shut down the hormones that stimulate the milk supply. Many breastfeeding mothers learn this only after they have skipped a pumping session and let their breasts get overly full—their milk supply drops dramatically. Also, the absence of nipple stimulation—no baby sucking, no pump pumping—means that you will not have regular surges of prolactin and oxytocin. These 2 hormones signal your milk glands to continue making and releasing milk.

Comfort Measures

While you wait for the engorgement to resolve naturally, try these comfort measures.

- Apply cold compresses. Use gel-packs made for this purpose, a bag of frozen peas, wet washcloths chilled in the freezer, or the classic Australian remedy of cold raw cabbage leaves.
- Wear a bra if it fits well and feels good. Don't wear one if it digs into you and leaves red marks. If you have a stretch bra designed for athletic exercise, try that. Wear it to bed if the pain is keeping you awake at night.
- Take a pain reliever containing acetaminophen (such as Tylenol) or ibuprofen (Advil or Motrin). These not only relieve pain but also reduce swelling. (While you're still bleeding vaginally, avoid aspirin. It reduces blood-clotting ability.)
- Try heat to relieve the pain. Wrap your breasts in warm, wet washcloths (covered with plastic wrap to keep the heat in), dip your breasts in a basin of warm water, or take a warm shower, allowing any milk produced to flow down the drain.
- If you are comfortable with the idea, use a breast pump or hand express (remove milk using only your hands) to remove some of the milk. Don't worry that this will increase your milk supply. Express just enough to relieve the pain, and only as often as you need to. You can either discard the milk or ask the hospital staff for sterile containers in which to store it so that it can be given to your baby for these few days. As the swelling subsides, gradually pump or express less often. In a few days, you'll be able to stop altogether.

After 2 or 3 days of engorgement, you'll notice that your breasts are getting softer and more comfortable. They won't return to their pre-pregnancy size for several weeks. Until then, you may notice milk leaking from the nipples. Some women continue to notice leaking for several months after giving birth. This is normal, but leaking can be prolonged by anything that causes nipple stimulation—for example, running or other exercise that causes your breasts to bounce and sexual foreplay that involves your breasts and nipples. If you still have milk 6 to 12 months after giving birth, or if you think the leaking is excessive (and you've tried reducing the amount of nipple stimulation), talk to your health care provider.

Bottles and Nipples

Bottles designed for feeding babies in special care nurseries usually hold 1 1/2 or 2 ounces, and measurements are marked on the side of the bottle in tiny increments. The NICU staff measure formula using the more accurate metric system. You may hear the terms mL (pronounced "em-el" [which stands for milliliter]) and cc (pronounced "see-see" [for cubic centimeter]) used interchangeably. One ounce contains about 30 milliliters or cubic centimeters. A preterm infant's first feeding is usually 1 to 2 milliliters (about 1/5–2/5 teaspoon).

The nipples for bottles come in a variety of shapes and sizes. The smallest, softest, most pliable nipples—called *preemie nipples*—were originally designed to make feeding easier for babies with a weak or immature suck. It now seems that these nipples may actually make feeding more difficult for some babies because even a slight movement of the baby's mouth results in a flow of milk. This may be more milk than the baby can cope with. Ordinary nipples (designed for full-term babies) often work just fine for preterm babies and for babies with breathing problems.

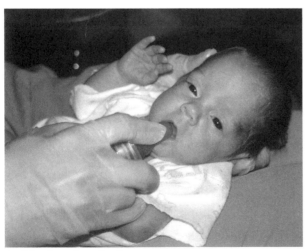

Positioning the nipple.
A preterm baby may try to bottle feed with his tongue on top of the nipple. You can help position the nipple correctly by guiding the nipple, with your finger on top of it, into his mouth.

Learning to Bottle Feed

Feeding a NICU baby offers many challenges. Here are some tips for bottle feeding your newborn when the time comes. Chapter 16 offers suggestions for successful bottle feeding after your baby comes home.

Watch Your Baby's Feeding Cues

Do what you can to help your baby be alert and ready when you offer the bottle. If you notice that preparations for feeding (diapering, dressing) seem to tire your baby, for example, next time feed him first, straight from the bed. Save the diapering for later.

Position Your Baby Properly

Hold your baby comfortably in your arms and close to your body, with his head slightly raised. You may wish to ask about warming the formula; however, most babies accept room temperature formula just fine. If your baby's arms and legs are limp, bend them into a flexed position to imitate the feeding posture of a healthy full-term baby. Hold your baby in your right arm at one feeding and in your left arm at the next to help him develop strong eye muscles and a symmetrical body. Don't sit where bright lights will

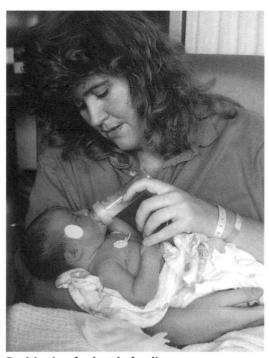

Positioning for bottle feeding.
Hold your baby close during bottle feeding. Flex the baby's hips, and hold his head higher than his bottom. This mother is helping the baby keep his hands in midline by supporting the baby's right hand with her little finger.

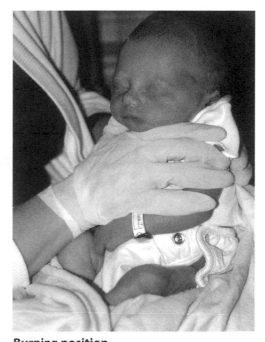

Burping position.
Your baby can rest and burp in the middle of the feeding by sitting upright on your lap. He is also more likely to stay awake when held upright. Support his head and neck, and pat his back gently. A lot of patting, jiggling, and position changing may cause your baby to spit up his feeding.

shine in your baby's face, and take a break if the noise in the NICU becomes too loud. Never prop the bottle. Your baby could choke or could spit up the milk and breathe it back into his lungs.

Establish a Bond

Even if you are bottle feeding, you need to take primary responsibility for your baby's feedings. Resist the temptation to let others feed your baby too often—so that you can "get something done." Breastfeeding mothers know that feeding is a great excuse to take a break, relax, put their feet up, and focus on their baby. Babies who are bottle fed also need this one-on-one time with a consistent person. Bottle feeding mothers, too, need extra rest to recover from childbirth. In addition, cues such as smell, taste, sound, sight, and touch from the person who feeds the baby may be important to the baby's feeding success. Babies who have difficulty feeding with many different nurses will sometimes feed better if one person (mother or her partner) does most of the feeds. Therefore, if the baby is past 34 weeks and doesn't have any apparent reason for not taking a bottle well, it may help to have the mother or her partner room-in and feed the baby the most often. In this case, sometimes the baby will progress with feedings more quickly than a baby who is fed by many different nurses.

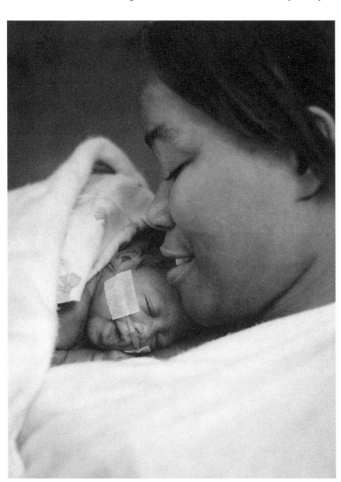

Kangaroo care for parents and babies.
Snuggling your baby skin to skin provides special moments of intimacy for you and your baby.

Courtesy of Gigi O'Dea.

Ask your baby's nurse about kangaroo (skin-to-skin) care (page 109). This method of skin-to-skin holding is not just for breastfeeding mothers. Most NICUs encourage parents and babies to enjoy the skin-to-skin warmth of kangaroo care, and parents appreciate the family closeness it offers. Providing skin-to-skin time with your baby in the NICU is helpful for bonding and establishing caregiving confidence. After you take your baby home, find times to hold him right next to your skin during bottle feeding—for example, after a bath or first thing in the morning. Allow yourself and your baby the pleasure and the tactile stimulation of skin-to-skin contact during feedings.

Let Your Baby Set the Pace

Relax, and let your baby set the pace during bottle feeding. Don't try to hurry the process by manipulating the nipple in your baby's mouth. If your baby stops sucking, let him rest. Prodding the baby to take more milk by jiggling the nipple, moving it back and forth, or twisting and turning it may result in what seems like a successful feeding. In the past, NICU staff took pride in their success at using these techniques to get the required amount of milk into very young premature babies. But they now know that forcing milk into a baby's mouth without the baby's active participation can make the feeding more stressful for the baby. In fact, pauses in breathing (apnea) and slowing of the heart rate (bradycardia) often result from this type of feeding. If the baby can't control the fast flow of milk from the bottle, there is also an increased risk that he will breathe the milk into the lungs (aspirate).

On the other hand, a feeding that lasts longer than 30 minutes may leave your baby exhausted. You will learn to interpret your baby's cues; they will tell you whether to stop feeding or to continue. Developing this partnership with your baby—this mutual understanding—takes time, but it is basic to successful feeding.

Your Baby's Need for You

Feeding is a common area of concern for the families of both full-term and preterm infants, for parents of babies who are healthy at birth and of those who need special care. Not only is nourishment vital to your baby's well-being, but feeding is closely related to many other areas of your baby's care and developmental progress. Whatever your concerns, questions, or struggles as you take on more of the responsibilities for nourishing your baby, specialists in the NICU will help you find the best approaches.

Chapter 6
Parenting in the NICU

"A little Consideration, a little Thought for Others,

makes all the difference."

—Eeyore

Lauren Thorngate, PhD(c), RN, CCRN

Terrie Lockridge, MSN, RNC-NIC

You are an important part of your baby's life in the neonatal intensive care unit (NICU) and a valuable member of your baby's health care team.

You may feel intimidated by the technology and outnumbered by the NICU staff, but you have a bond with your baby that no other member of the NICU team can match. You will learn how to care for your baby in a context of love that will continue long after the NICU stay is behind you.

Parents of healthy newborns have time to gain confidence before they must give up some control to the child care providers, teachers, and coaches who are an inevitable part of most children's lives. When your baby is admitted to the NICU, however, you are immediately forced to collaborate with others and trust them with your baby's welfare. Keep in mind that the NICU team members are only the first of many people you'll work with as your child grows to adulthood. These professionals present you with an early opportunity to learn how to work with those who will influence the course of your child's life.

The challenges of NICU parenting are great, but you can meet them. A positive NICU experience depends on forming a working partnership with the NICU health care team. Involvement helps you grow in your role as parent, learn about your baby, and prepare for a happy homecoming.

Overwhelming Beginnings

Even when you are prepared for the birth of a sick newborn, the actual event can be overwhelming. Some things may turn out better than expected; other complications may come as a surprise. The first hours or even days after your baby's birth may be chaotic and filled with unexpected events and emotions. You may feel off balance and out of control.

Family Imbalance

Separation is one contributor to this feeling of imbalance. It is not uncommon for the mother to be in the postpartum unit; the baby in the NICU; and the father, grandparent, or other support person running between units in the same hospital or even between hospitals. The support person's role becomes that of an information gatherer and messenger. This person is also expected to keep the rest of the family informed and, often at the same time, to care for other children, manage the household, and keep up with work demands.

Family dimensions vary widely; however, this chapter will try to describe aspects of parenting and family dynamics that encompass everyone. Your situation may be different than described here. Whether you are single, married, have a life partner, are supported by good friends and extended family, or have few allies, you will need to lean on others during this important time. You may have specific ethnic, cultural, or religious requirements. It is important to make the NICU staff aware of these needs so that they can work with you to support your requests.

The support person may be as stressed as the mother but feel a lack of support. Furthermore, the partner may try to protect the mother by minimizing a bleak prognosis and maintaining a cool exterior, or take the opposite approach by being totally honest about the prognosis. In some cases, the mother may think that her partner and others are holding back information. Other family members may feel, at times, that they are not hearing the whole story. Support people, especially grandparents, fathers, and others, also need nurturing and may have no one available to provide that support.

Some couples offer each other remarkable support, growing closer and strengthening their bond through this experience. More typically, though, this is a highly stressful time for parents, marked by feelings of both physical and emotional separation. You and your partner may feel separated by anger, guilt, denial, blame, or feelings of failure and ambivalence. Mothers and fathers, as well as other family members, may be using all of the resources they can muster to cope with the situation and not have any energy left over to support each other. In these cases, stress and misunderstandings can multiply because all parties are too exhausted to sort things out.

People Cope Differently

"We were on very different pages. He saw an undercooked but healthy baby, and I saw only tubes, wires, and a plastic tub. I could only think that our baby should still be tucked safely inside my body."

Individuals are different; fathers and mothers often use dissimilar coping strategies to deal with the situation. These variations in perspective can create difficulties between partners and cause problems that are difficult to resolve on your own. Many parents say that they don't tell each other what they are thinking or feeling. When issues are not discussed, marriages, partnerships, and family relationships can suffer.

Separation across hospital units can be difficult, especially if the mother has ongoing health problems during the postpartum time. It can be hard to be the one left in the hospital room (or in the birth hospital) recovering from childbirth while others are with the baby in the NICU (on another floor or farther away in another hospital). Feelings of

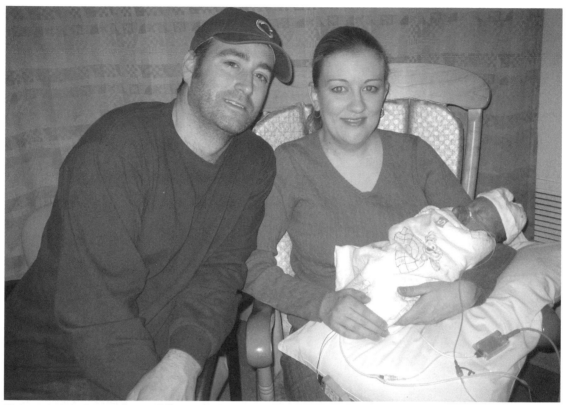

Moms and dads may have different NICU experiences.
Because men and women are different, mothers and fathers often react differently to the NICU experience. It is important to keep talking to each other during this stressful time.

jealousy and guilt can occur along with gratitude that your family can be with the baby. Mom might feel better if some family members or friends stay near her for support while others are in the NICU. In this way, support roles are assigned that allow both parents to be available to each other and to the baby, and friends or family members will know exactly how they can be involved and helpful.

It is also common for parents to experience different levels of optimism or despair when hearing the same information or seeing the same thing. One mother described her depression when seeing her baby connected to so many medical devices while the father was happy to imagine that the beautiful baby would someday be coming home. Even though the prognosis was good for their 33-week preemie, the mother felt devastated and the father was pleased that there were so few complications.

As a NICU mother, you may be getting less sleep than you need and catching meals on the run. You may feel that you have more responsibilities than your partner—and no time for yourself or the rest of your family. You may be making daily trips to the NICU and wonder why your partner does not seem more involved.

Some fathers cope by backing off, leaving the mother to assume the predominant parenting role. Many men busy themselves at work in an attempt to feel productive and to restore normalcy and control to their lives. Fathers and others who feel uncomfortable in the NICU may cope with their sense of powerlessness by avoiding the situation. Some parents naturally embrace the NICU environment and activities with interest in knowing about all the equipment and medical issues, while others prefer to spend quiet time with the baby.

On the other hand, the parent who touches and cares for the baby early on usually feels comfortable and more quickly becomes an active participant in the baby's care. However, the daily responsibilities of work and home cannot be ignored for long. Even the strongest partnership can become tense as you reposition and balance the new responsibilities of NICU parenting.

If parents are feeling stressed but coping in very different ways, it is no wonder that their relationship can become strained. When you are in crisis, you may not have the energy to help others. It can be difficult to talk to one another and understand the other's point of view.

Although open, expressive communication may be difficult, it is important to maintain your relationships. Seek help from other parents who have experienced the NICU, from your pastoral counselor, or from caring professionals. Many couples find that they need emotional support and professional assistance to work through difficulties and keep their relationships strong.

It may be hard to take time out for yourself, as well as ask for help; however, taking time is important to restore the energy you need to deal with the NICU. As soon as you feel you are able, take a day off from the NICU, make a date with your partner, and meet your own personal needs. This time-out is essential for your well-being. Don't think of it as taking time away from your baby.

Drugs and alcohol may temporarily help you forget your problems, but they only complicate things in the long run. If you have a substance abuse problem, you will not likely be able to face the realities of parenting without professional help. If your problems seem overwhelming, seek help from a trusted professional who has experience working with substance abuse problems.

What to Tell Siblings

If you have other children, they will want to know when the baby is coming home or where the baby is. Tell them as simply as you can about "their baby." Be honest, and try to answer your children's questions at their level. Remember that for younger children, a baby they cannot see is difficult to imagine. Showing them pictures of the baby can help them see her as a real person.

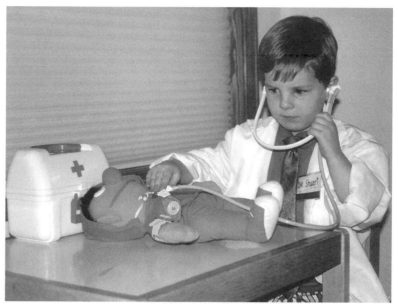

Figuring it out.
This big brother plays hospital with his doll in order to figure out the NICU experience. This is a good opportunity for parents to answer questions and give information at the child's level of understanding.

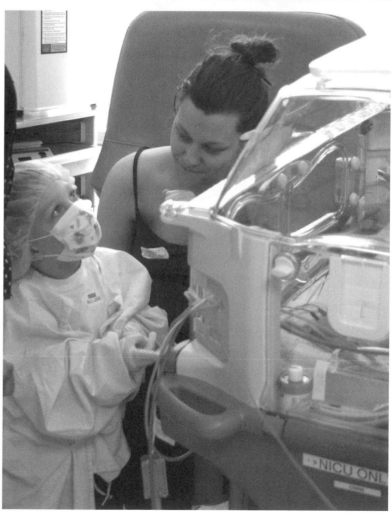

Getting acquainted.
Take advantage of sibling visitation in the NICU. This big brother will feel more involved and less anxious now that he has seen and held the new baby. Not all NICUs gown, glove, and mask siblings. You will learn the visitation rules and policies of your NICU.

Courtesy of University of Washington Medical Center, Seattle, WA.

It can be especially difficult for toddlers and preschoolers to understand what is happening. They need to be reassured that the baby's illness is not their fault. Young children may be jealous of the new baby and say things like, "I hate that baby." These feelings are normal.

Simple explanations and "exchanging" gifts with the baby help small children to feel important and involved. Parents can also tell a sibling, "When you're sick, Dad and I are worried and sad about it. Now your new baby sister is sick, and we're worried and sad about her." Some NICUs have sibling support classes, and attendance with you can help even toddlers.

You will be understandably upset by the birth of a sick baby, and even young children will know something is wrong. If you leave your children out of this experience or neglect to discuss everyone's feelings, they are likely to respond with regressive, acting-out behavior. These behaviors can include temper tantrums, crying episodes, clinging behaviors, or acting on fears that had previously been resolved. Your children know no other way to compete for your attention. Reassure them that you will still be able to care for them, and keep them safe and well, despite the current situation. They are likely to manage better if you keep them informed without overwhelming them with complex information.

If the NICU encourages siblings to come, take advantage so that your children can see the baby. Older children, especially, benefit from visiting the NICU. Rarely are they overwhelmed by the sights and sounds that bother adults. They tend to focus on the little human being that they, too, have been planning for. Actually seeing the baby and the place that is the NICU, along with updates about your baby's progress, will help make the baby real and make siblings feel involved.

Involving Grandparents

"Both of his grandmothers met my son before I did, and I'm having some jealousy over that. I don't want to put them off, but I need to talk with them about my need to have 'first-time' experiences with him, like giving his bath and being there when he gets his breathing tube out."

Grandparents often feel they should not voice their frustrations or fears. One grandmother said, "It is so hard to watch my daughter suffer and know there is nothing I can do to make it better. I don't know what to say. I am too far away to care for the other children, so all I can do is listen." A mother-in-law stated, "We have never had a close relationship. I know she thinks I blame her, but I don't at all. I just don't know how to

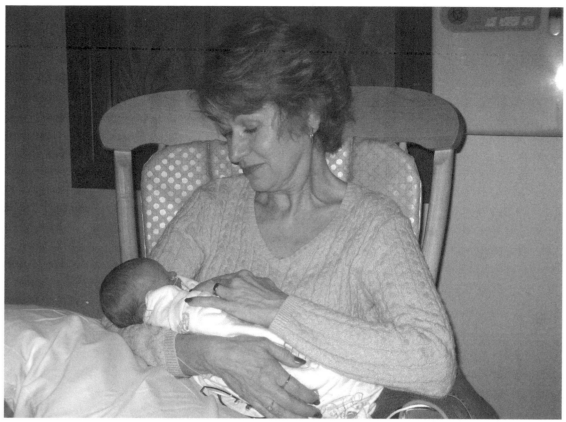

Grandparents may seek involvement.
Grandparents worry about their new grandchild and about the baby's parents too. By visiting the NICU, this grandmother gains an understanding of the challenges facing NICU parents and can provide better support for the family.

tell her so she will believe me. I can't talk to my son about this because he has enough on his mind." One mom expressed concern that both grandmothers met her son before she did, and still remembers her jealousy over not being there at the beginning. Feelings such as these should be addressed before the infant's discharge, or the relationship between parents and grandparents may never be the same. You may be reluctant to rely on grandparents for help after your baby's discharge unless you work things out before the baby comes home.

Parents should think carefully about their own needs when inviting the participation of their parents. Relationships between generations may be strained even before the baby comes along, and the pressure of NICU care may add layers of stress. Some grandparents are more assertive or wish to play roles different than those imagined by the parents. If setting boundaries is an issue within the family, parents and grandparents will benefit from discussing this, despite the difficulty that comes with uncomfortable conversations. Part of successful family management is knowing when to ask family members for help and support, and when to ask them to back off.

Grandparents benefit from talking with other grandparents who have gone through the NICU experience. Referral to a support group, even when the grandparents live in another city, may be beneficial. Photos and video can be shared across the distances and can help extended family develop attachments as well.

Experiencing the NICU when possible helps grandparents understand the true situation. Their fears about the child are often worse than the reality. During their time in the NICU, you and your nurses may be able to find concrete tasks that will make grandparents feel helpful, without interfering. In some families, putting the grandparents in charge of family communication helps ease the pressure on parents and gives the grandparents an active role to play. Grandparents can also be helpful in caring for other children and keeping up with the daily household routine so you are able to spend more time in the NICU.

Keeping Others Informed

There are many ways to keep family members and friends informed of your progress, of good times and hard ones. Some strategies include assigning a person close to you to check in and distribute the message or information that you choose to share; leaving an updated message on your phone or in a secure place so that people can hear what's going on without calling you directly; and using electronic communication such as e-mail, blogs, or Web pages, which can also be useful for sharing photographs and up-to-date information. Some hospitals have services that support development of a Web page or update page just for patients and families—these can be easy to build, are secure, and you invite only those you wish to view them. Ask the staff in your NICU about options that may be available and what has worked for other families. It is not your responsibility to return calls to all your family members, friends, and work colleagues during your busy NICU days.

Where to Find Support

Your Partner

No matter how well-meaning, those closest to you cannot always provide the support you need. Your partner's support can be important in coping with the NICU experience. As discussed, people cope differently, and depending on individual needs, communication with your partner may be difficult at times and may not meet all of your desires.

Others Who Can Help

Other sources of support include extended family members, friends, nurses, social workers, the NICU staff, and other NICU parents. You may find that as your needs change over time, so do your support people.

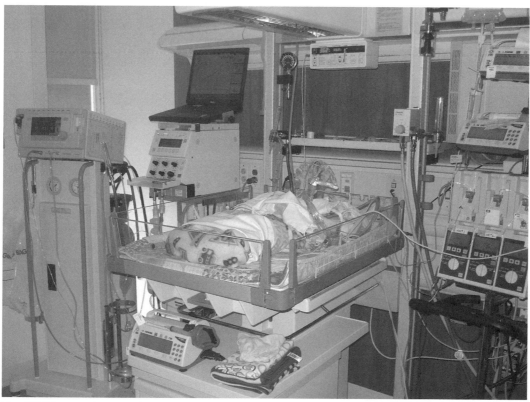

The NICU as parents see it.
The NICU setting presents many barriers to parenting. As you get acquainted with NICU staff and learn about NICU equipment, you will focus less on the technology and more on your baby.

Courtesy of Providence Regional Medical Center, Everett, WA.

Friends can be a source of stress as well as support. If they fear saying the wrong thing, they may cope by avoiding you and the NICU situation at a time when their support would be helpful. Pregnant friends or childbirth class buddies may feel guilty for being pregnant or having a healthy baby. Just when you need their support, they seem to pull away. Health care professionals can help you realize that this avoidance reflects your friends' feelings of inadequacy, rather than lack of caring. If you feel awkward or do not have the energy to do so, a steadfast friend, your partner, or your parents or partner's parents can tell your friends exactly what you need or how they can help. It can help to spend a little time thinking about what is actually supportive for you. Is it a friendly call or hug, is it someone who just knows what you need done for your family, or is it an afternoon of pampering for you? Friends usually have to be told only once, and then they'll make dinner, pick up your children at child care, run errands, or help in other directed ways. Don't concern yourself with those who cannot seem to help. Accept help from those who can.

Support Groups

At some point in your NICU experience, you may need to talk to someone about questions that your baby's caregivers cannot answer. "Why do I hear different opinions about how to care for my baby?" is one example. These questions can often be addressed in support groups that are offered at the hospital or in your community. It may also be possible to talk with another parent who has been through the experience. If there is someone who had a child of the same gestation, or with similar medical issues, you can often validate your feelings or questions. Ask the staff if there is a way to meet such families.

Many parents and families feel that support groups organized by nonprofessionals but led by a professional not directly associated with the NICU provide the "safest" and most supportive setting for sharing feelings. Some couples find that one of them does better in a group and the other does better with a one-on-one relationship. Seek the support that works for each of you, then share the benefits of that support with one another.

Challenges of NICU Parenting

Early parenthood is difficult even when pregnancy and childbirth go smoothly, but it may seem especially overwhelming within the unfamiliar surroundings of the NICU. Be assured that you will feel more comfortable in this busy environment with time. Even so, the NICU presents challenges to parenting. Here are some tips for dealing with some of these barriers.

Geographic Barriers

If your baby is in a NICU some distance from your home, family members may be separated from one another. It may be difficult to find an affordable place to stay near your baby. Low-cost temporary housing such as the Ronald McDonald House is sometimes available for parents. Some hospitals may make rooms available, or have arrangements with nearby hotels for parents and family. Ask about these resources and use them when you are able.

Physical and Mechanical Barriers

Many parents find the overall atmosphere of the NICU overwhelming. Bright lights and excessive noise, coupled with unfamiliar sights and situations, can make it difficult to manage an already stressful and exhausting experience.

Rest is essential to maternal healing and milk production, as well as to the emotional well-being of both parents. New parents need to be able to lie down or put their feet up when they become tired or overwhelmed. Meeting those physical needs is not always

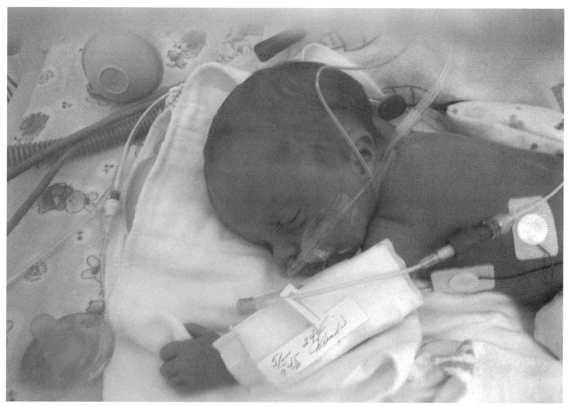

Tubes and wires.
A collection of tubes and wires sometimes makes parents hesitate to touch or hold their baby. You will learn to manage these attachments.

easy, however. Your orientation to the NICU should provide you with information about the locations of telephones, restrooms, and parent lounges.

Many mechanical barriers come between you and your baby in the NICU. Your baby's incubator can be intimidating at first. You may hesitate to break through this barrier and touch your baby. Intravenous tubing and monitor wires can tangle like vines in the jungle, and you don't want to risk pulling something loose. All of these barriers make caring for your baby a challenge, but the NICU nurses can work with you to learn how to overcome these obstacles. Remember that your baby will be comforted by your soft touch, gentle voice, and familiar aroma.

Psychological Barriers

When coming into the NICU, it may seem as if you have entered a foreign land. You may feel uncertain, and wonder about any unspoken "rules" or expectations. You may fear that if you ask too many questions or become demanding, you will put off the staff, and your baby may not receive as high a quality of care as she otherwise would. These fears are normal, but unfounded. They will lessen as you become more familiar and involved with the staff and with the NICU routine.

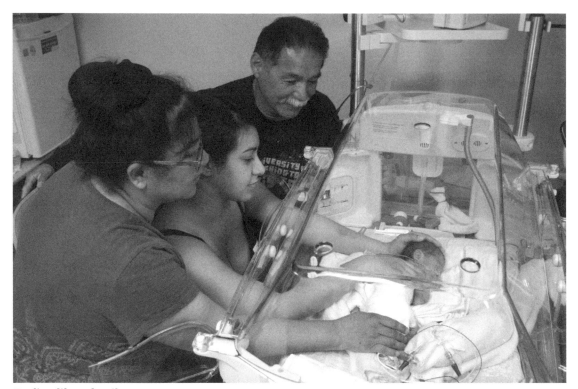

Feeling like a family.
Moments of togetherness are difficult to come by in the NICU, but your baby's nurse will help you find opportunities.

Courtesy of University of Washington Medical Center, Seattle, WA.

You may need to ask who may come with you into the NICU to provide support. Some NICU policies limit bedside presence to grandparents, but you may find better support from a neighbor or friend. A skilled NICU nurse or social worker can help you define your "family" and allow you to work out your own plan for family participation. This cooperation helps you feel more in control and fosters a partnership between you and the NICU team.

Psychological barriers may also include lack of privacy to spend quiet time together as a family. Some families report that they just can't be themselves in the NICU. Parenting within the NICU fishbowl creates stress; you may feel your caregiving skills are under constant scrutiny and are inferior to those of the nurses. You may feel shy and rigid as a family, with your usual warm, spontaneous family interactions inhibited. In part, these feelings resolve with time and experience.

Attachment Barriers

You want your baby's nurses to have both a professional and an affectionate bond with your baby, but it can be difficult when the nurses seem to know your baby better than you do. You may hear the nurses refer to your baby as "my baby." Some parents admit feeling jealousy toward their baby's nurses because the nurses do everything well and seem to meet their baby's needs better than they themselves can. Be assured that as you spend time with your new baby, you will find yourself becoming "the expert" about her cues. Actively participating in her care will help you feel more like a parent and resolve many of those feelings.

Another barrier to attachment may be the lingering fear that your baby may die or get sick again after discharge. Grief for the loss of the hoped for, healthy infant you pictured during pregnancy may delay feelings of love for and attachment to your special care baby. Give yourself some time to sort out your feelings, and remember that you are building a relationship with your baby that will grow stronger over time. You may find it helpful to discuss your concerns with your baby's nurse, the social worker, or another support person.

The Baby Blues

Pregnancy and childbirth bring about tremendous physical and emotional change, with dramatic fluctuations in hormone levels. These changes may affect brain function and can lead to depression. This is more common than many people realize, and many new mothers experience the "baby blues" to some extent. Symptoms may begin in the early days after the baby's birth and include feeling anxious or irritable, with mood swings. Many mothers find themselves suddenly tearful, and there may be unwelcome changes in appetite or sleep patterns. The "baby blues" should subside within 2 weeks, but sometimes symptoms will come later or extend beyond that time frame. These feelings usually go away on their own, and usually do not last for more than 2 weeks.

Postpartum depression is a more serious concern and can occur anytime during the first year after childbirth. It is more common in mothers who experience additional stresses such as those of special care parenting. Adoptive mothers who have not actually birthed their babies may also find themselves struggling with this common condition. Your new baby needs you to be at your best during this time, so it is vitally important to seek expert help if symptoms last longer than 2 weeks. Persistent symptoms that signal the need for professional intervention include feeling depressed and disinterested in activities that are usually enjoyable; having a hard time concentrating; and continued feelings of anxiety, guilt, unworthiness, or hopelessness. Some mothers may become so troubled that they consider harming themselves or others. If you find yourself feeling this way, it is essential to ask for help immediately.

Some mothers may develop a rare mental illness known as *postpartum psychosis.* In such situations, a mother may find herself feeling extremely agitated and unable to sleep. She may experience hallucinations and delusions, and her behavior may seem bizarre or irrational. This situation usually develops within a few weeks of delivery. Postpartum psychosis is a true psychiatric emergency and calls for urgent professional attention.

Whether symptoms are mild or severe, postpartum depression can be successfully managed. Talk to your own physician, your NICU nurse, or a social worker about seeking professional assistance. Your baby will benefit from a mom who has taken care of herself first and foremost.

Forming a Partnership With the NICU Team

Time and familiarity with the NICU routine eliminates much of the discomfort of NICU parenting. But your NICU experience will be much more positive when you and the NICU team work as partners to care for your baby. Because your baby requires intensive care, immediate decision-making and interventions in the best interest of your baby are often necessary. Obviously, parents are not included in every medical or nursing care decision on a moment-to-moment basis. However, the NICU team should strive for a working partnership with parents, which means that parents are included in the baby's overall plan of care. For this to occur, you need to learn appropriate skills that allow you to participate in your baby's daily care, and you need to be involved in any decision-making that affects your ability to care for your baby when her hospital stay is over. By working together, you and the NICU team achieve 2 important goals.

1. You help your baby reach her highest level of wellness.
2. You gain the confidence and skills you'll need to parent your special care baby.

You are an essential member of your baby's health care team. Your input and involvement are important in planning and carrying out your baby's NICU care. In a successful partnership, planning for your baby's discharge begins early in the NICU stay.

The Nurse-Parent Partnership

Nurses in the NICU have chosen a career that enables them to make a difference in the lives of families. However, NICU nurses must budget their time carefully so that they can meet the needs of each family. Nurses are typically assigned 1 or 2 "vents" (infants who require mechanical ventilation) or 3 or 4 "feeders" (babies who are growing and doing well). Time constraints usually don't reflect the nurses' lack of commitment to you, but rather represent the reality of a hospital budget.

Even in the face of nurses' heavy workloads, many parents form close and significant relationships with members of the NICU team. Your baby's nurses usually become your main source of information and insights, and gain your trust. Nurses also act as liaisons between you and other members of the health care team. They are individuals who explain your baby's condition in understandable terms and answer your questions as they arise.

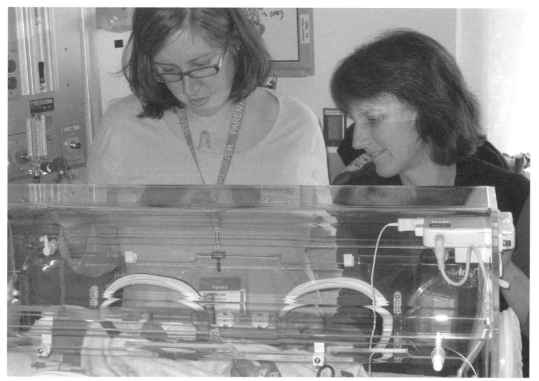

Parent and nurse.
Nurses and parents often form a bond by caring for the baby together. A team approach involves parents at the bedside who participate in the baby's plan of care.

Courtesy of Seattle Children's Hospital.

The better acquainted you are with your baby's nurses, the more likely you are to form trusting bonds with them. Units that assign primary nurses (one nurse or a nurse team assigned to coordinate the family and infant's care throughout the entire NICU stay) or a neonatal nurse practitioner to direct your baby's care encourage this type of relationship. Whatever their approach may be, most NICUs will try to assign the same team of nurses to your baby. This is most satisfying for you and for the nurses because it gives you the chance to learn about each other and form a good working partnership.

Black Cloud Days

Just as nurses learn to tune in to parents' moods, parents soon become attuned to those of the nurses. You'll begin to notice that during the best days, everyone works as a team, and the unit functions smoothly. There are times, however, when the unit is very busy or the overall mood is down, and families may pick up on stress felt by the staff.

On these "black cloud" days, you may feel in the way, both physically and psychologically. Although your baby's nurse will try to make you feel comfortable and included, you may notice that she has less time or her patience is strained on these days. Sometimes it helps to tell your nurse that you've noticed the unit is extra busy. This opens communication and allows both of you to discuss what you can realistically accomplish during your time there. Regardless of the unit environment, your baby will benefit from your comforting presence. These black cloud days should not be frequent, but they do occur.

Communication as a Building Block

"When we were confronted by a very capable nurse and my own feelings of inferiority, we felt better by reminding ourselves that we were learning valuable skills from an expert to help us when we go home."

Open, honest, and clear communication between parents and the NICU staff is the key to a caring partnership. This takes effort on everyone's part. Chapter 3 addresses many communication issues. Here are some other points to keep in mind.

Clarifying What You Overhear

"The nurses became our anchors. We will never forget how they helped us get through this experience."

You want to be valued as unique individuals. As consumers of health care services, you feel your needs deserve attention. It's common for NICU parents to believe that everything they see or overhear has something to do with them. Innocent comments taken out of context can sound frightening. Ask for clarification about anything you overhear that worries you. Your nurses can correct misconceptions and allay unnecessary fears; however, nurses and hospital staff can comment only on your baby due to privacy laws.

For example, a mother overheard one nurse reporting to another that housekeeping had not had time to clean the empty incubators. This mother did not realize that this was part of the change-of-shift report and that the nurse was passing on the information so that the next shift would clean the beds. Instead, the mother worried that her baby had been placed in a "dirty" bed and that perhaps that was why her baby had an infection. In addition to increasing her stress, misinterpreting these comments increased her fear of leaving her baby with strangers.

Don't feel shy about voicing your concerns. Tell the staff about any worries you have about your baby's quality of care—both for your peace of mind and to maintain good communication with the NICU team.

Getting Your Questions Answered

You need information. You want to know about your baby's medical condition and general status. You may also want to know the unknown. For example, you may ask, "Will my baby be OK?" or "When will my baby be able to go home?" Lack of concrete answers is frustrating for parents and health care providers alike.

You may also encounter different viewpoints. Some nurses may reassure you that your baby is OK. Others may not commit. Then you become suspicious: Does the nurse who won't commit know something the optimistic nurse doesn't? Is someone hiding something from us?

No one withholds information on purpose, but members of the NICU team may choose not to offer their own opinions. Nurses don't always feel comfortable sharing their personal thoughts about how your baby is doing. They may intuitively "feel" your baby is doing well but have no solid evidence to back up their hunch. Rather than sharing those vague feelings with you, they may say nothing. If you are not getting all of the information you want, you need to ask for it. Chapter 3 offers some suggestions.

Be wary of filling in the blanks yourself. Imagination is often more frightening than reality. Parents are commonly frightened when they see an intravenous (IV) line in their baby's scalp, for example. They may worry that the IV fluid is going directly to the baby's brain. In truth, some NICU nurses prefer a scalp site because it frees the baby's hands from IV tape and tubings and allows the baby to bring her hands to her mouth. By asking about the IV placement, you learn that the IV fluid does not go directly to your baby's brain. You become more knowledgeable about her treatment and more confident of the nurse's abilities. You may also feel more comfortable about asking your next question.

The language that health care professionals use when they talk to you can be a source of support or stress. If the language is simple and easy to understand, you're less likely to be intimidated and more likely to ask further questions. But if NICU staff answer a simple question with a long and complicated response, they create confusion and put up barriers to communication.

You should expect the NICU team to simplify complex information for you, to get to the point, and to reinforce what they tell you with written information whenever possible. They should validate their explanations with you—that is, they should make sure you understand what they have told you. They may do this by asking you to repeat what they have told you in your own words. If an explanation you receive from a care provider does not make sense to you, ask for clarification. If a care provider uses an abbreviation you don't understand, ask for the entire words and the explanation. The NICU staff often communicate using abbreviations (IVH, PDA, RDS, etc) and may use this language with you not meaning to confuse you. The NICU team also understands that it is difficult to absorb a lot of information during this period of great stress. They expect that you might ask for information to be repeated, or that you might ask the same question more than once. This is completely normal.

"Our four-year-old daughter was there when the doctor first told us, in very big words, about respiratory problems, infections, and other problems our baby could face. My daughter summed up the whole thing when she broke in and said, 'The baby's not done yet, Mom. Just put it back in.' "

Making Your Needs Known

Developing open and honest communication requires that you tell your baby's nurses about your needs and feelings. Although NICU staff members should anticipate your needs, they are human and sometimes miss your signals. Help those helping you by asking for what you need and being honest about what you don't understand. Clear communication establishes the basis for an ongoing partnership.

Learning Care Skills

Parenting in the fishbowl of the NICU is intimidating. At first, you may believe that your caregiving skills can never measure up to those of the nurses. The first step to active parenting is to recognize that your role is different from that of the nurses, but just as important to your baby's health. You are the center of the baby's universe. The nurses and staff are there to help support the baby's medical needs and to prepare you for a lifetime of parenting.

Your involvement in your baby's care is essential from the very beginning and may begin on a basic level. When you first meet your baby, the NICU team provides you with information and perhaps encourages you to touch your baby. This gentle beginning gives you a chance to recover from the stress surrounding the birth and learn about the NICU routine.

Later, when you are more comfortable in the NICU, your involvement moves to a different level. The information you take in becomes more detailed, and you begin to participate more in your baby's care. You may help by changing your baby's diaper or assist in changing the bed. This is a beginning. Because health professionals are individuals, the degree to which parents and family participate in care depends, to a certain extent, on each nurse's assessment of your baby's needs, your readiness, and on her own style of working with families.

Your participation in your baby's care may help parenting feel "real." You'll be encouraged to call your baby by name and talk to her about your day or play audiotapes of your voice or soothing songs. Changing your baby's diaper or perhaps bringing baby clothes from home may bring some normalcy to your relationship. Ask if you can personalize your baby's bed with name and birth date cutouts, family pictures, and special items from home.

As you spend more time with your baby, she will become responsive to you and will recognize you with all her senses: touch, sound, smell, sight, and taste. At the same time, you will start to recognize what your baby likes and dislikes. For instance, you may notice that your baby sleeps more soundly on the right side or spits up less when stroked and calmed after feeding. These "little" things are subtle but just as important to your baby's care as things the nurse may note about the baby. Talk about the cues you see, and encourage the health care team to use these suggestions during caregiving. This little person is your child, and nurses are her guest caretakers for a short while. In some ways, this is more support than families of healthy newborns get before they leave the hospital.

You will learn new things about your baby every day that will help ease the transition from hospital to home. Some aspects of your baby's care will make perfect sense and come easily to you. Others may be more complicated and take longer to learn. Here are some things to keep in mind as you learn care skills in the NICU.

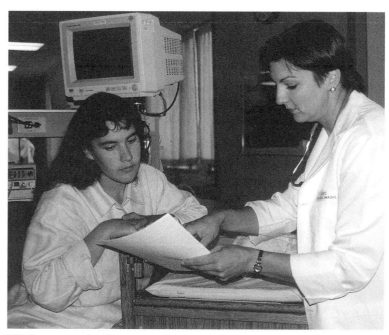

Vital communication.
Ask questions and be clear about what you want to know. The NICU team should keep you informed and involved in your baby's care.

Keep Focused for Learning

It's very hard to pay attention or to understand new information if you are distracted by pain, hunger, fear, or exhaustion. Take care of yourself so that you can give your baby your best. This means you must spend some time away from the NICU to rest. Similarly, your baby won't respond well to care if she is in pain, tired, or uncomfortable. If you are learning something with your newborn and she begins to cry or show signs of distress, the teaching session will include slowing down and learning how best to support or console your baby. The same holds true for you. If you feel "weepy" or sad, stop and take a break. Share your feelings with a nurse who can help you sort out your feelings and provide support. When you feel better, you will have more confidence in your ability to learn about your baby. It is common for parents to be emotional during this time, and they often have high expectations about naturally knowing what to do for their baby.

Figure Out What You Know and How You Learn

The NICU team will spend a lot of time asking you questions before they give you information or begin formal instruction. This process may seem time-consuming, but assessing what you already know is an important first step in the learning process. Some people feel better if they take notes or write down tips from the nurses or details about things they are learning. Still others will want to repeat the material more than once. If you know how you learn best, share this with the staff and jointly plan your teaching times and methods to best meet your learning style.

Parents may hesitate to ask for clarification or to admit they don't understand something. As a result, the NICU staff often give plenty of basic information. They aren't talking down to you; they just want to be sure they are not talking over your head. It is important to develop a relationship that supports both the teacher and the learner. Even if this is your second or third baby, most NICU nurses won't assume that you know everything there is to know about newborn care. Unless you tell them otherwise, your NICU team will teach you the basics first.

Ask Questions and Learn As You Go

No question is silly or unnecessary. Take as much time as you need to discuss your concerns and questions. Don't be afraid to say that you just don't understand something or need the information presented in a different way. People learn in many different ways and at different paces. The NICU team expects you to have plenty of questions. Many times you can watch a video or DVD to help you learn. Take notes if doing so helps you learn, or ask for a demonstration.

Most NICU parents report thinking, "I know the nurse gave me that information, but I have no idea what she said." Not remembering everything you're told is normal when you're distracted by the NICU environment. Printed information, videos for review, and your own notes may help the information sink in. Don't be embarrassed or afraid to ask for the information again. The nurses are there to help you learn about your baby. Write down questions that come up later, often when you least expect them, and review them with the staff when you are back at the bedside.

It is also important to let nurses know if there is something that makes you anxious or afraid. You may not need to learn every skill, as some will not be needed after your baby goes home. Some technical skills may be part of her care while in the hospital, but not at home. Some things look more complicated than they are and can be easily performed by a parent who has been properly instructed and supervised. It will be up to you and the nurses to determine what skills are needed to care for your baby.

Get On-the-Job Training

At first you may be hesitant to dive in and care for your new baby. Most parents begin to learn by watching the nurse provide care and then asking the nurse questions about what she is doing. Observing care is a comfortable way to begin to learn. While you observe caregiving, ask questions. Encourage your baby's nurse to talk with you about how your baby is doing, how to know when to stop what you're doing and help the baby to rest, why certain procedures are necessary, and how much care you can provide as a parent.

As you become more comfortable touching your baby, you should have opportunities to provide more care, such as taking your baby's temperature. When it's time for diapering or bathing, for example, the nurse may first demonstrate the procedure and then ask you to do the same

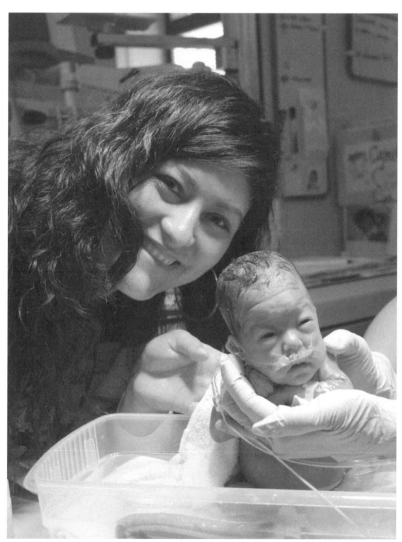

Ready to learn.
The NICU team encourages you to care for your baby as soon as you and the baby are ready. This mother is learning about bathing her baby.

Courtesy of University of Washington Medical Center, Seattle, WA.

task, either immediately or later. As you care for your baby, your nurse will probably coach you through the procedure and stand ready to help if you need it.

During your baby's NICU stay, you'll learn to do much of your baby's care. Some parents are immediately comfortable with activities such as diaper changing, bathing, and feeding; others require some practice. When you and your baby are ready, ask your baby's nurse to plan feeding, bathing, and other care activities for when you can be there. This helps you learn to manage your baby's care before you take her home, helps define you as the parent, and allows you to maintain some control over certain areas of your baby's life.

Give as much of your baby's care as possible. Caring for your baby builds your self-confidence for her homecoming. Even though you may continue to think of questions about each skill you learn, don't by shy about asking the nurse to teach you the next skill. For example, if you know how to take your baby's temperature, ask if you may learn how to give the bath. Continue learning new skills as your confidence builds. If your baby will need a special type of feeding at home, such as tube feeding, watch the feeding and ask questions. The next time, ask to do the feeding with the nurse as she supervises. When the nurse watches you care for your baby, she is better able to assess what else you need to know before discharge. As you cooperate together, you strengthen your partnership.

Be Flexible

Some nurses are stronger teachers than others. Each will have a style that is different from others and not all will match up with your style of learning. Ideally, your nurse will be diplomatic as she makes constructive comments or corrects you if your technique is not safe. You will also encounter nurses who have different opinions on how certain things should be done. Listen for the reasons each one gives for doing the task in a certain way, then do what makes sense to you based on those principles.

Your ability to be flexible is also appreciated when an expected baby care activity, such as feeding, doesn't work out according to plan. Occasionally your baby will awaken and fuss "off schedule," and if you are a distance away, the nurse may go ahead and feed her for you. If this happens, cuddle or stroke your baby when you arrive. Such a missed opportunity is disappointing, but this type of occurrence should not happen often. If it does happen often, discuss the problem with the primary nurse or the NICU charge nurse.

Be an Involved Long-Distance Parent

If you are parenting from a long distance, set up a phone call schedule and communicate frequently with your baby's nurses, physicians, nurse practitioners, and physician assistants. Some nurseries have strategies to help you cope with long-distance parenting. These may include sending you postcards, e-mails, and photos to update you on your baby's progress and involve you in your baby's life. Try not to feel guilty if you are not able to be there as much as you would like. Keep in touch with your baby's nurses—they know that you care. For parents at a distance, the opportunity to room in with your baby before she is discharged is very valuable. Ask the team about the possibilities.

Continue to Learn After Your Baby Comes Home

The NICU staff will try to teach you what you need to know to care for your baby after discharge. However, until you're home with your baby, anticipating what you don't know or will need to know can be difficult. Learning about some aspects of your baby's special care is like being asked if you have any questions about driving before you get behind the wheel of a car. You can expect to have questions long after your baby leaves the NICU.

If you are offered a home visit, public health nurse referral, or phone follow-up after discharge, take advantage of this important service. Home visits are most effective during the first week after discharge, when most questions and concerns arise. The visiting nurse can reinforce previous teaching, help you troubleshoot potential problems, and guide you in solving real ones. Families of newly discharged babies are under tremendous stress and may need to cope with new situations, sometimes daily. A home visit can reassure you that many things are going well, building your confidence. It can also help you address any difficulties you may encounter.

The Parenting Process

It may take some time for you to feel that you are truly your baby's parent. Getting to know the NICU staff and the routine and providing care for your baby helps break down some of the barriers to NICU parenting. Open and honest communication within the health care team creates trusting partnerships. Mutual respect and understanding of each person's contribution to your baby's care is a starting point. Everyone involved has a common goal: the health and well-being of your new baby. When parents and the NICU staff work together toward this goal, each member of the care team helps the others achieve success. The days and hours before you leave the familiar NICU are very busy and can be as stressful as the first few when you arrived. Just as you trusted the hospital staff to care for your baby, you will need to trust that they know the timing of when you and the baby are ready to go home. The staff will ensure that you have the skills needed and the support in place, and that your baby is medically ready to transition to the next phase of life—with you as competent and loving parents.

Special thanks for careful review, important insights, and feedback from Karen Emmerman Mazner, NICU parent, Seattle, WA.

Chapter 7
Organizing Your Finances

"Nobody knows anything about this....

This is a Surprise."

—Eeyore

Katie Stiver, MSW, LICSW

Along with your concern for your baby's physical well-being, you are probably also very anxious about the financial aspects of your baby's neonatal intensive care unit (NICU) hospitalization.

Your concern is merited because the costs of neonatal care are quite high. Whether or not your baby's care is covered by insurance, there are many important points to consider. We offer this information about finances to help calm your fears and reduce your stress about the cost of your baby's hospitalization. Because programs and funding sources vary greatly from state to state, it is difficult to provide one-size-fits-all financial information that would meet the needs of every family in every NICU. The most important step is identifying the person (or persons) on your NICU team who can address your individual financial needs and has knowledge of the resources available to you and your baby in your state. This person is often a social worker, care coordinator, or financial counselor.

Financial Survival Basics

First and foremost, rest assured that your baby will not be denied the medical and nursing care he needs in the NICU. The well-being of your baby, not your personal finances, is the primary concern of everyone involved with your baby's care. Your baby's health insurance status is not the focus of any of his caregivers. In fact, most of the nurses, respiratory therapists, other health professionals, and staff such as chaplains who care for your baby have no idea whether he is covered by private insurance, Medicaid, or nothing at all.

Some NICUs have financial counselors available to work with you about any financial issues. In other units, individuals with other titles may help you in different ways. Take advantage of any resources available to you, such as a social worker, case manager, patient representative, billing department staff, or information from a parent support group. Reach out by expressing your concerns. Doing so will let these individuals know that you and your family want their help.

If either parent is employed, consider talking with your work supervisor(s) and/or with someone in your employer's human resources department. Your employer can share information with you regarding the Family and Medical Leave Act of 1993 (FMLA). The FMLA, also known as Public Law 103-3, was enacted by the US Congress on February 5, 1993, to ensure that certain employers grant family and temporary medical leave under certain circumstances, including the birth, adoption, and/or care of a child. The FMLA allows eligible employees to take job-protected, unpaid leave or to substitute earned or accrued paid leave for up to 12 workweeks in any 12-month period. The employer must continue the employee's health insurance benefits during FMLA leave on the same terms as if the employee had continued to work. One purpose of the FMLA is to promote stability and economic security for your family.

When You Have Insurance Coverage

When your baby was admitted to the NICU, you may have been asked for your insurance or Medicaid information. Often the parent who first sees the baby after his NICU admission is the one to whom these questions about insurance are addressed. Compiling this information is the responsibility of different individuals at different hospitals. Sometimes administrative support staff in the NICU will ask the questions; at other institutions, data collection is the responsibility of staff from the admissions, registration, or billing office. You may have been asked for your insurance or Medicaid card so that it could be photocopied. The purpose of photocopying the information is to avoid mistakes in transcribing numbers or letters.

"With all the other issues we're trying to face at this time, we just can't believe this insurance coverage is one more stressor. We filled out the papers my employer sent us to add our baby to the policy, then found out they had sent us the wrong forms. We just made the cutoff for adding her to our policy!"

Private Health Insurance

Some parents and families are fortunate enough to have private health insurance. Typically, there are specific requirements for adding your new baby to your health insurance policy. You may need to change from single coverage to single with dependents or to family coverage. Direct telephone communication with the member services department at the insurance company will facilitate the process of adding your baby to your policy. Check your insurance card for the telephone number of the member services department. It's important that you quickly find out what steps are necessary to insure your new baby and then take them to avoid complications or lack of insurance coverage.

The great variety of health insurance plans makes it difficult to generalize about coverage. Different types of plans cover different health care services and require different premiums, copayments, and deductibles each year. If this is your first experience with the hospitalization of a family member, you may not be familiar with the specifics of your insurance plan. Request a copy of your health insurance policy or plan information, and take the time to read it to find out what benefits you are entitled to. Following the policy or plan guidelines can minimize the out-of-pocket costs of your baby's care to you and your family. Many insurance companies employ case managers and/or care coordinators to ensure efficient, cost-effective coordination of needed services. When a case manager/care coordinator is available, communicate with that individual to get help managing your baby's insurance coverage.

Some parents and families do not have private health insurance. Other parents have health insurance but cannot add the new baby to their policy. In these situations, it may help to consider applying for Medicaid or for the Children's Health Insurance Program.

Medicaid

Medicaid is an assistance program for families with low and limited assets that can help pay your baby's hospital and doctor bills. The Medicaid program is operated by the individual states and funded by both the federal and state governments. Each state's eligibility guidelines differ, so you will need to contact your Medicaid state agency for more information about Medicaid. If you currently receive Medicaid yourself and plan to pursue Medicaid for your new baby, contact your caseworker to add your baby to your preexisting case. This process varies depending on where you live. In your state, you may be able to do this by telephone, you may need to go to an office and do this in person, or a representative may meet with you at the hospital. In any case, add your baby to your preexisting case as soon as possible after the baby's birth.

Children's Health Insurance Program

Although it is state administered, the Children's Health Insurance Program (CHIP or SCHIP) is, like Medicaid, a federally funded program. Also known as Title XXI, it was part of the Balanced Budget Act of 1997. The Children's Health Insurance Program is intended to provide support to families who do not qualify for Medicaid but earn a modest income. Establishment of a state CHIP is an important opportunity for a state to expand insurance coverage to a large portion of uninsured children. The Children's Health Insurance Program availability and guidelines vary by state.

Billing/Dual Coverage/Certification

Bills for your baby's NICU care may be sent to your home or may be sent directly to your state Medicaid program or insurance company. If the hospital bills you directly, be sure to review the bills for accuracy and contact the hospital billing office with all questions and concerns and for help interpreting any confusing information. Take the time to open and examine each bill when it arrives, rather than putting the bills aside for too long.

Some families may have health insurance coverage under more than one policy. Dual coverage can be a wonderful asset as well as an additional burden. Having a secondary insurance carrier provides another potential source of coverage for hospital and doctor bills. The downside can be disagreement between the administrators for the 2 insurance companies regarding which is the "primary" insurance coverage and which is the "secondary" coverage. Primary coverage refers to the policy that will be billed first for services provided during hospitalization. The secondary insurer will be billed for the remainder of the costs after the primary insurer has paid the portion required by the terms of its policy.

Some families are eligible for Medicaid as a secondary insurance. Some programs offer secondary Medicaid insurance coverage based on presumptive disability criteria or length of hospital stay. Availability and eligibility vary by state, so be sure to speak with your social worker to determine whether or not your baby qualifies for this type of secondary insurance coverage.

Throughout the course of your baby's NICU hospitalization, the hospital's utilization review department will provide clinical updates to your baby's insurer. The insurer will then certify each day of your baby's hospital stay based on these clinical updates. Your baby's insurer may send you documentation of days certified. This documentation may cause you some concern because it will not reflect the most current status of hospital days covered. Also, the certified days may end on a certain date that is well before you think your baby is ready for discharge. But don't worry; the date for the end of certified days just triggers another review in which additional days are certified. Be assured that it is not your responsibility to pursue certification of hospitalized days. This process occurs through communication between the hospital and your insurance company.

Transport Charges/Special Home Care Needs

For a variety of reasons, your baby may be in a NICU with which your insurer does not contract. This can be a concern if you are insured by a managed care plan. Staff in the NICU are responsible for checking into this issue for you. Your insurer's utilization review staff and/or insurance case managers will communicate with the NICU staff and will typically request transport of your baby to a contracted provider once your baby is stable enough for the transport. Clarification by NICU staff of the medical necessity for your baby's NICU admission will ensure coverage at the noncontracted hospital. Your insurer will probably cover the costs of transport because it is being performed at the insurer's request.

Perhaps you delivered out of state, either electively or unexpectedly. Once your baby is medically stable, he may be transported to a NICU closer to your home provided that your insurance company authorizes the transport. If your baby is covered by Medicaid, transport across state borders can be difficult because of the issue of which state Medicaid program will assume responsibility for the transportation costs.

In preparation for your baby's discharge from the NICU with home care, it is essential that NICU staff obtain authorization for the special services that will be needed in the home. Every insurance policy has different benefits for skilled nursing visits, speech and occupational therapy, and durable medical equipment. Medicaid programs often cover special services needed in the home. Some insurance plans restrict benefits for home care. Negotiations between the NICU staff and the insurance company may convince the insurer to provide coverage, especially if authorizing home care will reduce the length of your baby's NICU stay.

Your choice of a provider for your baby's primary care after discharge may depend on the type of insurance plan you have for your baby. Managed care plans attempt to control the rising cost of medical care by specifying that those they insure select a plan-affiliated provider if they wish the insurer to cover services at the highest benefit level. In the case of health maintenance organization (HMO) plans, a referral from the baby's primary care physician is required for any services received after discharge from the NICU.

Covering Your Expenses

"My baby's dad cannot take any more time off work. He may lose his job because of the days he's missed already, when it was important for us to be together with our baby."

The costs of your baby's hospitalization itself are only part of the expenses your family will incur as a result of your baby's NICU stay. Other potential expenses may include

- Transportation to the hospital to visit your baby
- Parking at the hospital
- Housing costs if your baby is in a NICU far from your home
- Meals at the hospital or at nearby restaurants
- Child care for your other children while you are at the hospital

Ask your social worker about Medicaid-funded assistance that may be available to your family to offset some of these costs.

The mothers of some NICU babies require days, weeks, or even months of bed rest, either in the hospital or at home, after they give birth. In addition, parents who are employed may lose hours or days from work as a result of the mother's and/or the baby's hospitalization, reducing the family's income substantially.

When your baby is discharged home with special needs, additional expenses may include

- Medications
- Special infant formulas
- Transportation to and from subspecialist appointments
- Increased utility bills as a result of the use of durable medical equipment (equipment that is not disposable, such as a suction machine or a ventilator)

You can recover some exceptional expenses you incur throughout the year for your baby's medical care or related to your baby's care through deductions on your federal and state income taxes. To take advantage of these tax savings, you will need to itemize your income tax deductions. Be sure to save all receipts associated with your baby's medical care and related expenses. Allowable income tax deductions depend on income tax regulations and legislation. Your tax accountant, a low-cost tax preparation service, your federal Internal Revenue Service district office, and your state Department of Revenue office can assist you with the specifics of income tax preparation.

Special Public Assistance Programs

Numerous programs are offered both nationally and at the state level that may benefit your family. Sources of financial support can be found through special public assistance programs at your state and local human service agencies and public health departments, as well as through local charitable foundations.

Special Supplemental Nutrition Program for Women, Infants, and Children

Popularly known as WIC, the Special Supplemental Nutrition Program for Women, Infants, and Children is a program administered at the federal level by the Food and Nutrition Service of the US Department of Agriculture. The WIC program provides federal grants to individual states for supplemental foods, nutrition education, and health care referrals for pregnant and postpartum women, infants, and children up to age 5 who are in need. Eligibility for WIC is based on income guidelines, state residency requirements, and a "nutritional risk" determination by a health professional. Two major types of nutritional risk are recognized: (1) medical based, such as anemia, underweight, or pregnancy complications, and (2) diet based, such as inadequate dietary pattern. Most state WIC programs distribute vouchers for use at authorized food stores for the purchase of iron-fortified infant formula and infant cereal, prescribed therapeutic infant formulas for specific medical conditions, as well as special food packages high in protein, calcium, iron, and vitamins A and C for mothers and children. The NICU may have copies of the WIC referral form, which usually requires a physician's signature. When the form is completed, you take it to the local WIC office, which is often affiliated with the county public health department.

Temporary Assistance for Needy Families

Previously and more commonly known as welfare, TANF, or Temporary Assistance for Needy Families, is a program created by the Welfare Reform Law of 1996. Effective July 1, 1997, TANF replaced what was known up to that time as welfare: Aid to Families with Dependent Children (AFDC) and the Job Opportunities and Basic Skills Training (JOBS) programs. The TANF program is overseen by the Office of Family Assistance, located in the US Department of Health and Human Services, Administration for Children and Families. The program provides federal grants to individual states for assistance and work opportunities for families in need. The individual states are granted wide flexibility to develop and implement their own welfare programs.

Enrollment in TANF may automatically provide eligibility for the Medicaid program as well as for WIC. This varies by state, so it's important to check with your local human services agency.

Supplemental Security Income

Many babies in the NICU qualify for a federal assistance program called Supplemental Security Income (SSI). This program is run by the Social Security Administration and is financed by the general revenue funds of the US Treasury. As its name implies, SSI pays monthly benefits to *supplement* your income up to a certain level. After approval, the first SSI payment will be made for the first full month following the application filing date.

To sign up for SSI, you can visit your local Social Security office, or you can call the Social Security Administration at 800/772-1213 to arrange an appointment with a Social Security Administration representative, who can assist with the application. Some NICUs have made special arrangements with local Social Security Administration representatives to meet with eligible families at the hospital.

Although parents and children may be eligible for benefits under both SSI and TANF, recipients cannot receive payments from both programs simultaneously. If you qualify, you will need to select which of the 2 programs offers the most advantages.

Local Charitable Foundations

A variety of religious and civic organizations assist individuals and families in financial difficulty. Some churches also have emergency cash assistance and loan funds for families in need. Multidenominational ministries may sponsor families by providing short- or long-term financial support. Many civic organizations sponsor specific charitable programs at the local, state, or national level. Organizations that help those with specific diseases or disabilities, such as the Easter Seal Society or the Spina Bifida Association, may offer emergency cash assistance to children with special health care needs.

Staying Financially Healthy

Many resources and programs are available to help your family through the financial stress of your baby's NICU hospitalization. Remember to communicate your concerns to the appropriate individuals on your NICU team so that they can make the referrals that can alleviate some of your financial concerns.

Telephone calls and written requests can take time and effort, but your persistence will be key to getting the help your family needs. It takes practice to learn the best ways to seek information and diplomacy to challenge an agency's decisions in a way that is most likely to benefit you. See page 187 for examples of what to say in a telephone conversation and page 189 for points to cover if you are writing a letter. These tips may help you get started if you need to call a health care coverage agency or write for information or services.

Families are often drawn to the Internet in search of information about available resources. If you would like to seek information in this way to supplement the information provided to you by your baby's team, a great way to start is by typing in your state's name followed by "children with special health care needs." This can be a great way to find information specific to your neighborhood and information specific to your child's diagnosis. If you need assistance, plenty of people in your NICU can help you search for these local resources in this way.

Communicating With Your Health Care Coverage Agency[a]

Sample Phone Call

Below are some examples of how you might talk with plan representatives if you need information or disagree with a decision.

If You Need a Second Opinion

1. *Call your Health Plan's customer service number, and explain the situation.*

   Parent: "Hello, my name is Susan Jones and I am calling about my son, John Jones. His chart (or member) number is 111-22-333. My son is a year old and I am worried about his growth and development. I talked to our doctor, Dr. Smith, at the First Street Clinic. He wants to wait and see but I don't want to wait any longer to find out what is happening."

2. *Tell the plan representative that you disagree. Ask for a second opinion.*

   Parent: "I don't agree with this decision and am very concerned about my son. I want to see another doctor who specializes in the care of children. Under Washington law, I am entitled to a second opinion."

3. *Ask what the plan will do to help resolve the issue.*

   Parent: "Does this plan have other doctors who specialize in this area? What other options are available to me?"
   Plan Representative: "I will send you a list of pediatricians in your area who can give you a second opinion. The list will include phone numbers for the clinics."

4. *Be sure to find out how long it will take to get information or services.*

   Parent: "I need to schedule an appointment soon. When can I expect the information?"
   Plan Representative: "I will mail the list today. You should receive it by Friday. If you haven't received it, please call me. My name is Mary Harris and my direct line is 555-0000."

5. *Be courteous and let them know you are writing down information about the call.*
   Parent: "Thank you for your help. I have written down your name and phone number to call if I don't receive the information."

Communicating With Your Health Care Coverage Agency[a], continued

If You Disagree With a Decision

1. ***Give your name, your child's name and chart number as in the sample above. Then tell why you are calling.***

   Parent: "I received a letter from ABC Health Plan that said my request for physical therapy for my daughter was not approved. It did not explain why the request was denied or how I can appeal the decision. I have reviewed my policy and do not find a reason that the request sent by our doctor was denied."

2. ***Clearly say what you want to happen***

   Parent: "Please tell me in words that I can understand, why the request was declined and how I can appeal this decision."

   Plan Representative: "I will have to look up your benefits and find out why your request was not approved. I will send you the rules you need to follow to appeal this decision."

3. ***Ask how long it will take them to get information or answers to you.***

   Parent: "When can I expect your call? It is important that we continue therapy. I will appeal this decision. I know that Washington law protects our rights to continue services during an appeal."

   Plan representative: "It will take some time to study your file. I will call you back within seven business days. I will also mail you a booklet that tells you how to file an appeal. You should receive it in three days."

4. ***Be sure to write down what was said, the name of the person you spoke with and what you talked about.***

   Parent: "I have noted your name and phone number in my records. I prefer to have you send a letter telling me why our request was not approved. I will expect the letter and a copy of your appeals guidelines within seven business days so that I can begin the appeal. Thank you for your help."

Communicating With Your Health Care Coverage Agency[a], continued

Helpful Hints for Writing a Letter of Appeal

1. It is better to address your letter to a specific person instead of a general department or the managed care plan itself. Try to find out who will be making the decision and send the letter directly to that person.

2. Be sure to show your child's name and chart or account number within the plan, your address, and phone number.

3. Begin your letter with a brief statement of who you are and why you are writing.

4. If you are requesting a written explanation of the reason for denial, state that you have reviewed your contract and can't find a valid reason for the denial in your policy. Ask for specifics, not just a response that states "not a covered benefit" or "not medically necessary."

5. If you are appealing a denial, state your understanding of the denial and explain why you feel the services are necessary and/or should not be denied. Use any articles, research, or other supporting professional opinions.

6. Include dates and names of people in the managed care plan you have already talked with.

7. Ask for a response (a letter, meeting, or phone call) within a reasonable time. State a date that you want to hear back from the plan. Don't wait too long. Your plan may have very limited time periods to file an appeal.

8. Have someone proofread your letters.

9. Keep a copy for your personal records.

10. Send copies to other important people who have helped you.

[a]Reprinted from: *Finding Your Way In Managed Care: A Guide for Washington Families of Children with Special Health Care Needs* (Washington State Dept of Health: http://www.doh.wa.gov/cfh/mch/documents/FYWayinEnglish.pdf (pages 43–46).

Chapter 8

Mother-Baby Factors: Effects on Newborn Health

"It is hard to be brave," said Piglet, sniffing slightly, "when
you're only a Very Small Animal." Rabbit, who had
begun to write very busily, looked up and said:
"It is because you are a very small animal that you
will be Useful in the adventure before us."

Debbie Fraser Askin, MN, RNC-NIC

After birth, babies may need the kind of special care provided by a neonatal intensive care unit (NICU) for many different reasons. One of the most common reasons newborns need intensive care is that they are born early (premature or preterm).

The first section of this chapter explains the relationship between the length of the pregnancy and the infant's size and weight at birth. It also describes how premature infants differ from term infants in their appearance and level of maturity at birth. Chapter 9 describes specific problems common to premature infants.

Other factors, explained later in this chapter, determine whether your newborn will need special care and include

- The mother's health before and/or during pregnancy (called *maternal factors)*
- The health of your unborn baby as she grows and develops in the uterus (called *fetal factors)*
- How the baby is affected by factors associated with labor and delivery

Gestational Age and Growth Patterns

As a new parent, the first question you usually hear from relatives and friends is, "How much does your baby weigh?" This information is important, but weight alone does not give a complete picture of your newborn's growth, development, and maturity status. A newborn's weight is important in relation to the length of the mother's pregnancy—the period called *gestation*—which is the period of development from conception until birth. So to a care provider in the NICU, an equally important question is, "How many weeks' gestation is this newborn?" The answer tells the caregiver if the baby is term (on time), preterm (premature), or post-term (overdue).

Health care providers sometimes have difficulty identifying the length of a pregnancy from the information parents can provide (such as the date of the mother's last menstrual period, which is sometimes uncertain). A physical examination of the newborn, however, is a reliable way to identify gestational age (the number of weeks from the mother's last menstrual period before conception to birth). As a pregnancy progresses, the baby's brain, nerves, and muscles develop, as do many physical characteristics, in a predictable fashion. These indicators of maturity can be used to pinpoint your baby's gestational age (such as "26 weeks' gestation") plus or minus 2 weeks. Gestational age is correlated with your baby's birth weight, length, and measurement of head circumference to categorize your newborn's size as appropriate for gestational age (AGA), small for gestational age (SGA), or large for gestational age (LGA). The growth chart on page 198 will help you find your baby's classification of size based on gestational age.

Small for Gestational Age

A newborn can be small for her gestational age whether born at term (after a full-length pregnancy) or prematurely (before the end of the 37th week of pregnancy). If a fetus is significantly underweight for gestational age, the condition is called *intrauterine growth restriction* (IUGR). Slow growth in the uterus can occur either throughout the entire pregnancy or just during the last portion, both of which are responsible for low birth weight. Slow growth can occur because of maternal problems during pregnancy (including smoking, kidney disease, and hypertension), fetal development problems (viral infection, multiple gestation, and genetic defects), or placental problems (reduced blood flow to the fetus). It is also possible for a newborn's weight to be low at birth simply because both parents are small.

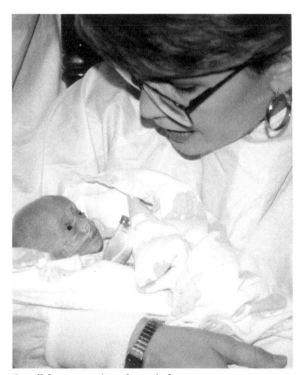

Small for gestational age infant.
This baby's tiny size is deceptive. Although she is preterm, she is more mature than her size would indicate. About 6 weeks old in this photograph, she was born at 29 weeks' gestation and weighed 1 pound, 9 ounces (about 710 grams).

Newborns who have IUGR and who have experienced slow growth and development throughout the pregnancy often appear "old looking" for their tiny birth size. They are generally short in length and have a small head. This is referred to as *symmetric growth restriction*. Infants whose growth and development slowed only during the final weeks of the pregnancy often appear scrawny, but their length and head size are normal. This is referred to as *asymmetric growth restriction*. The skin of post-term newborns with IUGR is often loose, dry, and scaly. Babies with IUGR have little fat and muscle tissue development. These infants are usually alert and active, however, and seem very hungry.

Because there are many causes of fetal growth restriction, it is impossible to generalize about complications. However, an SGA infant often develops low blood sugar (hypoglycemia) after birth because of higher energy needs and lower glucose stores than larger infants. The baby with IUGR had a smaller placenta that was unable to transfer enough glucose before birth or the baby used up existing stores or did not build up enough stores during labor and birth. The increased energy use of a baby who required resuscitation at birth can also deplete glucose stores and increase the risk of hypoglycemia. Hypoglycemia is monitored by checking the baby's blood glucose frequently and often requires an intravenous (IV) line.

In many cases, growth and development of SGA babies after birth is normal. If there are no serious medical problems, these babies may not lose weight after birth as most babies do, and catch-up growth will occur. Newborns who are both SGA and preterm may experience complications related to their prematurity (see Chapter 9). In addition to the risk of hypoglycemia, complications may include

- Problems related to the stress of the birth process such as meconium in the amniotic fluid (see Chapter 10)
- High red blood cell count
- Low body temperature
- Infection
- Neurologic problems (especially if both the head and body are small)

Large for Gestational Age

Some babies grow larger than usual during gestation and so weigh more at birth than the average baby of the same gestational age. These babies are called LGA. The infants may be born preterm, at term, or post-term. Fast growth often occurs in babies whose mothers have diabetes, babies whose parents are larger than average, and babies who have certain congenital (genetic) syndromes. Infants who are LGA show the physical characteristics appropriate for their gestational age—that is, they do not develop and mature faster than AGA babies—but they have above-average amounts of fat tissue at birth.

The size of a preterm LGA baby can be deceptive because she may weigh as much as an "older" baby who is born closer to term. But the preterm LGA baby can experience many complications of prematurity. Preterm LGA babies, especially those of diabetic mothers, are at high risk of respiratory problems, including respiratory distress syndrome (see Chapter 9) and persistent pulmonary hypertension of the newborn (see Chapter 10). Large for gestational age babies are also at risk for the following:

- Complications related to the stress of the birth process such as meconium in the amniotic fluid (see Chapter 10)
- Birth injuries like a fractured clavicle (collarbone)
- Low blood sugar and calcium levels
- High red blood cell count
- Immature lung development

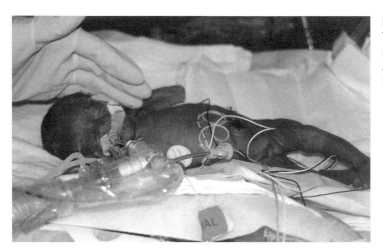

Baby at 25 weeks' gestation.
This baby is very premature and requires a ventilator for breathing assistance. The umbilical catheter is also visible in this photograph.

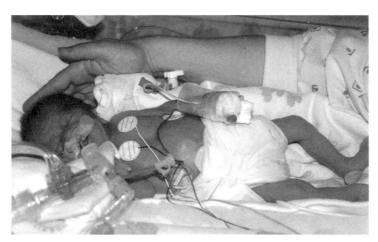

Baby at 28 weeks' gestation.
This baby is premature and also requires ventilator assistance. Note the round leads for the cardiorespiratory monitor placed on her chest and the IV line in her left hand.

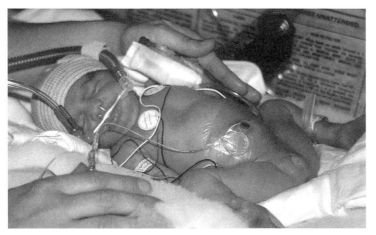

Baby at 32 weeks' gestation.
This premature baby receives breathing assistance from nasal CPAP (see Chapter 9). She also has an IV line in her left hand and an umbilical catheter.

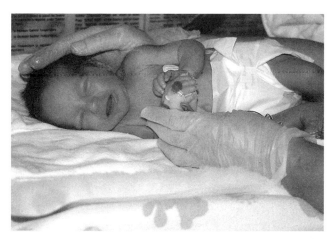

Baby at 35 weeks' gestation. Although still considered premature, this baby does not require breathing assistance or supplemental oxygen at this time. She has an IV line in her right hand.

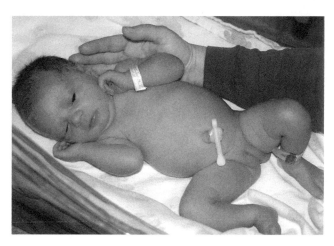

Baby at 38 weeks' gestation. This baby is considered full term. Note the rounded appearance of this mature newborn, her flexed position, and her good muscle tone.

The Term Newborn

A term (or full-term) baby is one who is born between weeks 38 and 42 of gestation. Term babies who are AGA average about 19 1/2 inches (49 centimeters) long and weigh about 7 pounds (3,200 grams) (see growth chart on page 198), but term newborns may also be SGA or LGA. The skin of term newborns is soft, and the blood vessels underneath do not show through. Vernix (a greasy white or yellow material made up of secretions and dead skin cells) is usually present at delivery only in skin creases. There may be a bit of soft, downy hair—called *lanugo*—on the newborn's shoulders and upper back.

The hair covering a term newborn's head is rich and silky. The nails may extend past the tips of the fingers, and the soles of the feet show creases on the entire length of the sole. Term newborns have strong muscle tone, and healthy term newborns readily curl up into the familiar fetal position. A term newborn's cry is strong and sounds healthy.

The Premature Newborn

"I looked at my baby and wanted to say how beautiful she was. But she wasn't beautiful. She was long and skinny and furry. She was not very cute for quite a while."

A premature—or preterm—baby is one who is born before week 38 of gestation. Premature babies can be SGA, AGA, or LGA, but most are either small or appropriate weight for their gestational age.

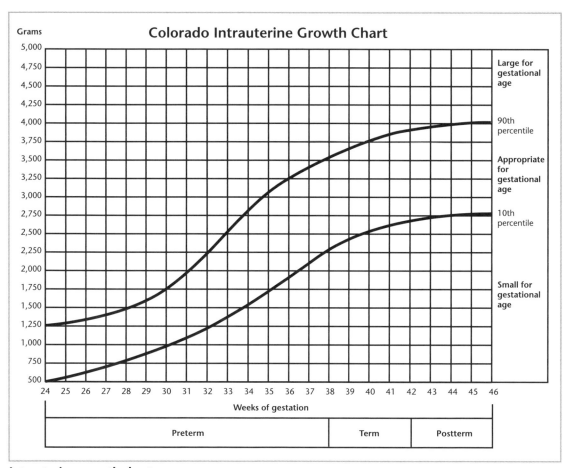

Intrauterine growth chart.
Find your baby's gestational age in weeks on the bottom line of the chart. Then find her weight on the side of the chart. The intersection of the 2 lines determines whether your baby's weight is small for gestational age, appropriate for gestational age, or large for gestational age. For example, a baby born at 32 weeks' gestation and weighing 1,100 grams would be classified as small for gestational age.

From: Battaglia FC, Lubchenco LO. A practical classification of newborn infants by weight and gestational age. J Pediatr. 1967;71(2):159–163. Reprinted by permission of Mosby-Year Book.

The gestational age of a baby born prematurely determines the problems for which she is at risk. In general, the earlier in the gestational period your infant is born, the higher the risk of complications—and the higher the level of care she will likely need. Your baby's appearance at birth is directly related to length of gestation. Your infant's level of maturity at birth determines how she will interact with her new environment outside the uterus.

A baby born at 24 weeks' gestation usually weighs about 1 pound, 12 ounces (800 grams) and is about 12 1/2 inches (32 centimeters) long. The skin is red and immature, with a shiny, transparent appearance that allows the blood vessels beneath to be seen easily. The skin is often described as gelatinous. There may be traces of lanugo, and some vernix is visible at delivery. There are no creases on the soles of the newborn's feet. The eyelids are fused (closed), and the earlobes are flat and soft and can be folded easily. This newborn has little fat or muscle tissue beneath her skin. Because muscle tone has not yet developed, a baby born at 24 weeks' gestation has limited ability to bend her arms and legs and does not breathe regularly on her own.

The fetal weight doubles between 24 and 28 weeks' gestation. A baby born at 28 weeks' gestation usually weighs about 2 pounds, 7 ounces (1,100 grams) and is about 15 inches (38 centimeters) long. The skin is less red now and more pink* because it is becoming less transparent, although the veins can be seen through it. Thick vernix covers the skin at birth, and long, thick lanugo is present, especially on the back. The nails on the fingers and toes are developed. There are faint red marks (the beginnings of creases) on the soles of the feet near the toes. The eyelids are now open. The earlobes are soft and easily folded but are beginning to spring back on their own if folded. The baby has developed some fat and muscle tissue under the skin and can bend her arms and legs a bit.

A baby born at 32 weeks' gestation usually weighs about 3 pounds, 10 ounces (1,650 grams) and is about 16 inches (41 centimeters) long. The skin is pale pink and thickening and may be peeling. Only a few of the larger blood vessels (in the abdominal area) can be seen through the skin. Vernix covers the skin at birth, but lanugo (especially over the lower back) is thinning. This newborn has definite sole creases near her toes, with red marks reaching the middle of her soles. The eyelids are open. The earlobes are soft but show some cartilage development; they will spring back if folded. At this age, the newborn has developed some muscle tone and can keep her arms and legs slightly bent at rest.

---

* Pink refers to the color of the skin's undertones. Term newborns of dark complexion are pink over their palms, soles, and mucous membranes (especially inner lips and gums). Very preterm babies may lack the dark complexion of their parents until close to term gestation.

A baby born at 36 weeks' gestation usually weighs about 5 pounds, 12 ounces (2,600 grams) and is about 19 inches (48 centimeters) long. Her skin is pale overall, appearing pink only over the ears, lips, palms, and soles. The skin has thickened and has begun to crack and peel on the hands and feet. Only a few large blood vessels can be seen faintly in the abdominal area. Lanugo has diminished, and areas without it are visible. Hair on the head is fuzzy or woolly and sticks together. The skin is covered with vernix at birth. Creases extend to the middle of the soles of the feet. The earlobes are firm, with well-formed cartilage, and spring back immediately if folded. Muscle tone is quite developed; the newborn's legs are usually in a frog-like position, and the arms are bent at the elbow.

The Post-term Newborn

Babies born later than week 42 of gestation are called *post-term newborns.* Most are healthy, but as the pregnancy continues past 42 weeks, the placenta becomes less efficient at supplying the fetus's nutritional needs, which increase as the baby continues to grow. The baby may actually lose weight when the pregnancy goes beyond term. Many of the physical characteristics post-term newborns show are associated with this decline in nutritional sustenance. Sometimes called the *syndrome of post-maturity,* these charac-

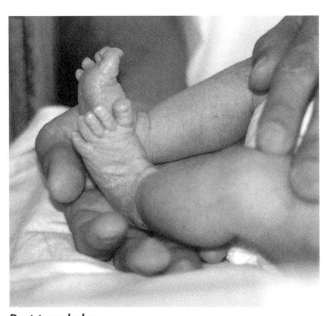

teristics include a somewhat malnourished appearance (despite large size) caused by loss of fat tissue. The post-term newborn's skin appears dry, cracked, peeling, loose, and wrinkled (especially at the ankles and wrists and on the palms of the hands and soles of the feet). The post-term baby may be meconium stained. Meconium, a sterile, dark-green substance produced in the fetus's bowel that may be released into the amniotic fluid before birth, will color ("stain") the skin and umbilical cord.

Post-term baby.
This baby has the typical peeling skin of an "overdue" newborn.

Post-term infants are at risk for the following:

- Complications resulting from the stress of labor and delivery, including meconium in the amniotic fluid or meconium aspiration syndrome (see Chapter 10)
- Birth injuries
- Low blood sugar and calcium levels
- High red blood cell count
- Feeding difficulties (baby feeds slowly, tires easily)
- Difficulty making the transition from fetal to newborn blood circulation (See persistent pulmonary hypertension of the newborn in Chapter 10.)

Maternal Factors That May Affect Your Baby

An unborn baby grows and develops within the complex environment of the mother's uterus. This is called the baby's *prenatal environment.* The fetus depends on its mother for oxygen and nutrition. During development, the fetus does not easily adapt to stress or changes in the surroundings. This dependence means that a mother's health and well-being are very important to her growing baby.

A mother's medical condition both before and during her pregnancy affects the prenatal environment in which her baby grows and develops. Use of alcohol, substance abuse (including misuse of prescription drugs), and cigarettes creates a hazardous environment for a growing fetus. Certain medical conditions, most of which are outside anyone's control, can cause specific problems for the developing baby or produce effects seen only after birth. Health care providers who have cared for the woman during her pregnancy, labor, and delivery generally inform the pediatrician or neonatologist about her health during her pregnancy so that the health care team can anticipate any immediate or long-term consequences her condition might produce in her newborn. Many maternal conditions can affect a developing baby. The most commonly monitored conditions include

- Diabetes
- Heart disease
- High blood pressure
- Bleeding
- Infection
- Blood type incompatibilities

Diabetes and How It Might Affect Your Baby

Pregnancy changes the way a woman's body uses sugar. Diabetes happens when the body either does not make enough insulin (a hormone produced by the pancreas) or does not use insulin normally. Insulin is necessary to maintain normal blood sugar levels. Some women already have diabetes when they become pregnant. Others are unable to produce enough insulin during pregnancy, a condition called *gestational diabetes.* Whether the condition exists before pregnancy or develops during it, the increased sugar available to the fetus from the mother's blood alters the environment for fetal development. If you are diabetic, the key factor to the well-being of your baby is keeping your blood sugar at a safe level throughout your pregnancy.

Your baby uses glucose (sugar) to produce energy for cells, to drive chemical reactions within the body, and to build new tissue for growth. Before birth, the fetus gets a constant supply of glucose from the mother across the placenta. The fetus also stores some of the glucose as a reserve for use during birth, when energy needs are high. Immediately after birth, the infant depends on 2 sources of glucose: the stored glucose (called *glycogen)* and the glucose in breast milk or formula or in the IV fluid if the infant is not being fed orally. In all infants, the blood glucose level falls during the first few hours after birth. In healthy term infants, the blood glucose level stabilizes. However, infants of diabetic mothers are at risk for a blood glucose level that becomes too low (a condition called *hypoglycemia).*

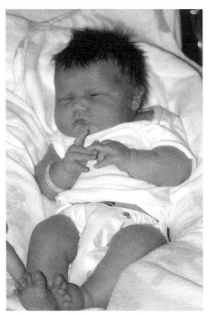

Infant of a diabetic mother.
This large baby is actually about 35 to 36 weeks' gestation. Infants of diabetic mothers are often preterm and large for gestational age.

Infants of diabetic mothers develop hypoglycemia because these infants produce too much insulin (a condition called *hyperinsulinemia).* If a baby has too much insulin, too much glucose may be removed from the blood. The result is hypoglycemia, a temporary condition that lasts a few hours or days until the baby's pancreas readjusts and produces the correct amount of insulin to maintain a normal blood glucose level.

Why do some babies of diabetic mothers produce too much insulin? This may occur if these babies had higher than normal glucose levels (hyperglycemia) during fetal development. Glucose rapidly crosses the placenta from mother to fetus. If a mother has above-normal glucose levels (as is the case for many diabetic women whose blood sugar is high), her fetus will also develop hyperglycemia because the fetus's blood glucose level is just slightly lower than the mother's level.

Maternal insulin itself does not cross the placenta to the fetus. The fetus's pancreas is stimulated to produce a lot of insulin because of the higher than normal glucose levels in the fetal blood.

At birth, the umbilical cord is cut and the newborn stops receiving glucose from the mother through the placenta. Her blood glucose falls, but her pancreas continues to produce extra insulin. The extra insulin causes too much glucose to move out of the baby's blood, which can cause hypoglycemia.

Babies who are hypoglycemic may or may not have obvious signs. Even when signs are present, however, it can be difficult to know whether hypoglycemia is causing them. This is because the signs of hypoglycemia are often nonspecific. Many of them are also indicative of other disorders. Signs of hypoglycemia may include tremors or jitteriness, irregular breathing, decreased muscle tone, decreased temperature, and cyanosis (a bluish skin color). Hypoglycemia can be dangerous because it can deprive the baby's brain cells of glucose and lead to seizures (convulsions).

If you have diabetes you should work carefully with your care provider to keep the glucose levels as close to normal as possible during your pregnancy. This may mean giving yourself insulin shots several times a day. After birth, care providers will monitor your newborn closely. Because the signs of hypoglycemia are nonspecific or may be absent, any baby at risk for hypoglycemia is carefully monitored. A digital glucose meter analyzes a drop of blood and gives a number value. If the test indicates that an infant's blood glucose level is low, a blood sample will be sent to the laboratory to determine the exact level so that therapy can be started if necessary. Therapy consists of additional glucose provided to the baby through an IV line. After a few days, the baby's insulin level usually stabilizes at a normal level, and hypoglycemia is no longer a problem.

In addition to hypoglycemia, possible complications for the baby of a mother whose blood sugar levels are difficult to control include

- Low calcium
- Low magnesium
- Respiratory distress syndrome (see Chapter 9)
- Jaundice (see Chapter 9)
- Increased number of red blood cells
- Increased birth weight, which can increase the risk of birth injuries
- Premature birth (see Chapter 9)
- Small size for gestational age (if maternal diabetes is chronic and advanced)
- Increased incidence of birth defects (affecting the heart, kidneys, stomach and intestines, brain and spinal cord, and/or bones)

Maternal Heart Disease and How It Might Affect Your Baby

When you are pregnant, your heart and circulatory system must work harder than when you are not pregnant. The amount of blood in your system increases, raising the rate at which your heart beats and the amount of work it must do. These changes provide adequate blood flow through the placenta, supplying the developing fetus with the oxygen and nutrition necessary for healthy growth and development. If you have heart disease, pregnancy can have important medical consequences for you and for your baby.

Although your heart disease may not worsen during pregnancy, the increased work your heart must do may cause your symptoms to worsen. To cope with the increased work of pregnancy, your heart may reduce blood flow to your placenta and baby so that it can provide enough blood flow to your brain, liver, and heart. These disturbances in blood flow to the placenta can result in loss of the pregnancy (spontaneous abortion), premature birth, abnormal fetal growth and development, and/or an inadequate supply of oxygen to the baby at various times during development.

Babies of mothers with serious heart disease are also at risk because of the medications their mothers must take to manage their condition. Many drugs are used to manage cardiovascular disease in pregnant women. Although some can affect the developing infant, most can be used safely during pregnancy.

If a pregnant woman has congenital heart disease, she will probably have a procedure called a *fetal echocardiogram* (heart ultrasound) during pregnancy to examine the infant's heart. Evaluations after birth may include a chest x-ray, an electrocardiogram, and an echocardiogram. The baby of a mother with heart disease is more likely to be preterm and/or SGA depending on the mother's heart condition. The NICU team will perform a detailed physical examination and manage complications related to these problems. Chapter 9 discusses heart conditions that may affect a premature baby. Chapter 10 covers congenital heart defects.

High Blood Pressure and How It Might Affect Your Baby

"This was our first baby who made it as far as the NICU.

For us, this was a joyful birth."

Blood pressure does not usually increase during pregnancy, but high blood pressure does complicate about 6% to 8% of pregnancies in the United States. A woman who has high blood pressure before she becomes pregnant, or develops high blood pressure before the 20th week of gestation, is said to have *chronic hypertension.* A woman who develops high blood pressure after 20 weeks' gestation is said to have *gestational hypertension.* Some women with gestational hypertension go on to develop an additional complication of pregnancy known as *preeclampsia.* This occurs when, in addition to high blood pressure, protein leaks from the kidneys into the urine. Women with chronic hypertension are more at risk for developing preeclampsia than women who do not have chronic hypertension. If gestational hypertension leads to seizures in the pregnant woman, the disease may be called *eclampsia.* If gestational hypertension leads to serious problems with blood clotting abilities and liver function, it is called HELLP syndrome. HELLP is an acronym that stands for hemolysis (breakdown of red blood cells), elevated liver enzymes, and low platelets.

If you develop gestational hypertension, you will probably respond to medications to lower your blood pressure so that you can continue your pregnancy. If your blood pressure stays high, however, blood flow to your kidneys, liver, brain, and uterus can be reduced. This can limit your baby's supply of oxygen and nutrients. If your hypertension does not respond to medical treatment, the only solution is delivery of your baby.

Because they lower the mother's blood pressure, the drugs used to treat hypertension—among them methyldopa (Aldomet), propranolol hydrochloride (Inderal), and magnesium sulfate—may also reduce blood flow through the placenta. The risks of preeclampsia to your developing baby are generally associated with this reduction in blood flow. An additional risk of preeclampsia is that you may not be able to carry your baby to term; many mothers with preeclampsia begin labor and deliver their babies prematurely. Because babies of mothers with preeclampsia experience periods of decreased blood flow during their growth and development in the uterus, they are frequently underweight at birth; this is evidence of slow fetal growth.

Blood tests after delivery may also show your newborn to have a high red blood cell count, a lower than normal number of platelets and white blood cells, and a higher than normal level of electrolytes. Babies of mothers treated with magnesium sulfate for preeclampsia may have high levels of magnesium in their blood. Symptoms of high magnesium levels in the baby include poor feeding, intolerance to feedings (vomiting, food left in the stomach from a previous feeding, abdominal swelling), failure to pass stools, easy tiring, muscle weakness, and/or apnea (pauses in breathing). If apnea is severe (which is rare in this case), your baby may need breathing assistance. As long as your baby's kidneys are functioning normally, the magnesium level usually decreases on its own.

Bleeding During Pregnancy and How It Might Affect Your Baby

Some women experience vaginal bleeding during pregnancy. This bleeding can be ongoing (chronic) or a one-time event (acute). Chronic bleeding can lead to anemia (a low red blood cell count) in the mother, decreasing the oxygen available to her developing baby. Acute bleeding decreases the mother's blood volume, which reduces blood flow (and thus oxygen and nutrients) to her developing fetus.

Bleeding during pregnancy occurs for 2 common reasons. The first, called *placenta previa,* occurs when the placenta lies abnormally low in the uterus, near to or covering the cervical opening. Placenta previa may cause occasional painless bleeding and often results in premature labor. Precautions regarding sexual activity during pregnancy may be necessary if placenta previa is diagnosed by your care providers. *Placental abruption,* separation of the placenta from the uterine wall before delivery, is life-threatening for both mother and baby. This separation limits the flow of blood and oxygen the baby needs to survive and can cause severe maternal and fetal hemorrhage. A woman with placental abruption usually experiences abdominal pain and rigidity. Vaginal bleeding may occur, or it may be hidden if the blood from the placental site stays within the uterus. When significant placental abruption occurs, the baby must be delivered as rapidly as possible. A baby born following placental abruption can be severely ill, requiring a high degree of breathing and blood pressure support. The newborn's red blood cell count may be low, and she may need emergency blood transfusions. Lack of oxygen may cause damage to all major organs (brain, kidneys, liver). Care providers will evaluate the infant's brain, kidneys, liver, and heart to determine whether they are functioning normally.

"We had good prenatal care. We simply had really bad luck."

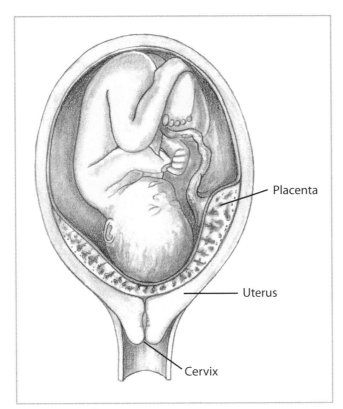

Placenta

Uterus

Cervix

Placenta previa.
The placenta normally lies near the top of the uterus. With placenta previa, painless vaginal bleeding may occur when the placenta partially or completely covers the cervix. This bleeding is potentially dangerous for the mother or her baby.

From: American College of Obstetricians and Gynecologists. Your Pregnancy and Birth. 4th ed. Washington, DC: ACOG; 2005. Reprinted by permission.

Infection During Pregnancy and How It Might Affect Your Baby

When a pregnant woman develops an infection it is cause for concern. Infections can be caused by viruses, bacteria, or fungi—and you can pass an infection to your developing baby. Among the risks of maternal infection are premature birth, stillbirth, abnormal fetal growth and development, abnormal blood cell count in the baby's blood, jaundice, seizures, pneumonia, and infection of the fluid that surrounds your baby's brain.

Certain infections are most threatening.

- TORCH—A group of viral infections that may affect a baby while in the uterus and/or during the birth process. The letters in TORCH stand for **t**oxoplasmosis, **o**ther, **r**ubella virus, **c**ytomegalovirus, and **h**erpes simplex virus.
- Group B streptococcus (GBS)—Ten percent to 30% of women carry GBS bacteria in their vaginas or rectums. Although usually harmless to the woman, the bacteria can cause serious illness in the newborn. Women are screened for GBS at about 36 weeks' gestation; those who test positive receive antibiotics during labor to help protect the baby from GBS infection.
- Human immunodeficiency virus (HIV)—The virus that causes acquired immuno-deficiency disease syndrome (AIDS).
- Any infection of the female reproductive or urinary tract, including sexually trans-mitted infections such as chlamydia, gonorrhea, or syphilis.

Chapters 9 and 10 discuss these and other infections—including those a mother can pass to her baby before or during birth. These chapters also explain why newborns are especially susceptible to infection when exposed and detail the consequences of infection for the baby.

Blood Type Incompatibility and How It Might Affect Your Baby

To understand blood type incompatibility, you need to know something about human blood cells. Blood cells have substances called *antigens* attached to their surface. Blood type identification is based on these antigens. Our immune system (which protects our bodies from invasion by "foreign" cells) recognizes antigens as either "friendly" (compatible) or "foreign" (incompatible). Foreign bodies are usually bacteria or viruses that cause infection. If the immune system recognizes a blood cell carrying a foreign antigen, it takes the same action it would for an infection-causing agent—it produces antibodies to destroy or deactivate the antigen. When that happens, the antibody destroys the blood cell carrying the antigen along with the antigen itself. Antibodies can affect 2 types of blood cells: red blood cells and platelets.

Red Blood Cells

All human beings have a blood type, which depends on the type of red blood cells they have. Blood types are identified by the ABO system: type O (the most common), type A, type B, and type AB. Blood types are either compatible or incompatible when mixed—that is why any blood used for transfusion must be tested carefully (typed and cross-matched) to be sure it is compatible with the blood of the person who is to receive the transfusion.

In addition to your blood type, human blood also has an Rh factor—a positive or negative designation (for example, blood type A positive or A negative). Both your blood type and your Rh factor are determined by genes that are passed from mother and father to child. It is possible for a mother and her fetus to have incompatibilities because of a difference in their blood types and/or a difference in their Rh factors. This is due to the fact that the fetus gets half of her genes from her father.

A blood type incompatibility between the mother and her baby is often referred to as *ABO incompatibility,* or an ABO "setup." This complication occurs most often when the mother's blood type is O and the baby's blood type is A or B. Incompatibilities of this type are rare for mothers whose blood type is A or B. ABO blood type incompatibility does not present as great a threat to the fetus and newborn as Rh incompatibility. The newborn with the ABO type incompatibility is at risk for jaundice and hyperbilirubinemia soon after birth. (See Chapter 9 for information about hyperbilirubinemia.)

Problems caused by Rh incompatibility are usually more serious for the fetus and newborn than ABO problems. Rh incompatibility is possible if the mother is Rh negative and the father is Rh positive. This is because the fetus could be Rh positive, having inherited this factor from the father. Problems are possible when the Rh-negative mother carries an Rh-positive fetus.

Pregnancy complications that are caused by Rh incompatibility are not a concern if the mother is Rh positive or if the mother and father are both Rh negative.

The problems of blood type/Rh incompatibility occur when the fetal red blood cells cross the placenta and enter the mother's circulation. This happens commonly during birth, but can occur during pregnancy or may have occurred during a previous pregnancy, miscarriage, previous blood transfusion, or at the mother's birth. This introduction of Rh-positive blood cells or an incompatible blood type sensitizes the mother to this type of cell. The mother's immune system then produces antibodies against the fetus's "foreign" blood antigens. When the antibodies travel back into the fetal circulation, the maternal antibodies destroy the fetus's red blood cells. If this incompatibility occurs in future pregnancies, the mother's body quickly produces this antibody and puts the fetus at risk for red blood cell destruction.

The medical term for destruction of red blood cells is *hemolysis.* In the case of ABO incompatibility, the fetus usually compensates for hemolysis by increasing its production of red blood cells. After birth, a newborn whose blood type is not compatible with her mother's may develop anemia (a low red blood cell count) because hemolysis continues after birth, but the newborn cannot produce red blood cells fast enough to keep up with their destruction. With red blood cell destruction, a waste product of destroyed red blood cells (bilirubin) may build up more quickly than it can be eliminated, causing jaundice (see Chapter 9). The baby's blood type will be checked, and red blood cell and bilirubin counts will be monitored frequently. The baby may require phototherapy (treatment with light) to reduce jaundice and IV fluids to prevent dehydration. In rare cases, the baby may require an exchange transfusion. This transfusion removes some of the baby's blood containing antibodies and replaces it with donor blood that is of the same type as the baby's.

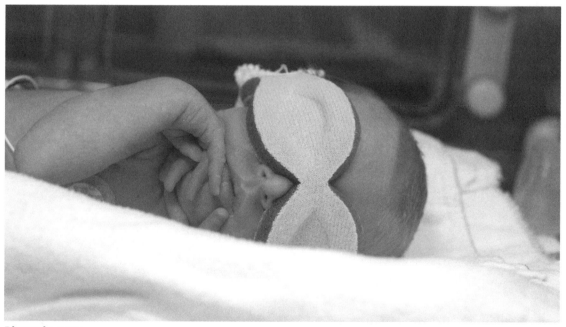

Phototherapy.
This baby requires phototherapy (treatment with light) to reduce jaundice. Babies wear protective shields over their eyes while the lights are on.

Courtesy of University of Washington Medical Center, Seattle, WA.

If the mother's antibody response against her fetus is particularly strong, as is often the case with Rh incompatibility, hemolysis may result in severe fetal anemia and jaundice. Sometimes the fetus can receive a blood transfusion while within the womb. This type of fetal therapy can be lifesaving for the unborn baby because a severely affected fetus can be born with heart failure, edema (swelling), shock, an enlarged liver, and bleeding problems. These babies usually require help breathing (with a ventilator), IV fluids, blood transfusions, and medications to maintain an adequate blood pressure, and antibiotics to fight infections.

To anticipate any potential incompatibility problems, pregnant women have a blood test early in prenatal care that determines their blood type and Rh factor and determines the presence of blood antibodies. Because Rh incompatibility produces more serious complications for the fetus and newborn baby than does ABO (blood type) incompatibility, mothers who are Rh negative are followed very closely throughout their pregnancies. In most cases, the first pregnancy is not affected; however, sometimes the fetal red blood cells cross the placenta and enter the mother's circulation before delivery. Rh-negative mothers usually receive a medication called RhoGAM (called WinRho in Canada) at the beginning of the third trimester of pregnancy (at about 28 weeks' gestation) and again right after they give birth. RhoGAM destroys fetal cells in the mother's circulation and therefore blocks the production of antibodies against Rh-positive red blood cells. (RhoGAM is effective only for women who have not already formed antibodies against the Rh-positive factor.) RhoGAM is given to protect not only this baby, but also future fetuses. Unless the antibody-producing response is blocked with medication, an Rh-negative mother begins to make antibodies against the fetus's Rh-positive cells. If a future fetus is Rh-positive, the mother's immune system may begin to produce antibodies quickly, even before she knows she is pregnant, putting her growing fetus at high risk for complications of Rh incompatibility.

"We knew that pregnancy was a risk to my health. But we planned carefully, got excellent prenatal care, and everything turned out fine. We were lucky."

Platelets

Blood cells that control bleeding are called *platelets*. Platelets have antigens on their surfaces; these antigens determine the platelet "type." The antigen system that identifies platelet type is known as the *PLA system*. Platelet type is determined by genes that are inherited in the same way that red blood cell type is. You and your baby may have the same platelet type (platelet compatibility) or 2 different platelet types (platelet incompatibility). The latter condition is again caused by the inheritance of PLA factors from the baby's father.

Your developing baby's platelets can cross the placenta and circulate in your bloodstream if there is a leak in the tiny vessels in the placenta. If the fetus's platelet type and your own are not the same (incompatible), your body will produce antibodies against your fetus's platelets. When these antibodies return to your fetus through the placenta, they can destroy the fetus's platelets and cause low platelet counts.

A maternal disease called *idiopathic thrombocytopenic purpura* can also cause destruction of fetal platelets. Some women who have this disease produce antibodies directed against all platelets. These women have frequent problems with low platelet counts because the antibodies their immune systems make destroy even their own platelets. During pregnancy, these antibodies cross the placenta and destroy the fetus's platelets. The babies of these women may be born with low platelet counts.

The medical term for low platelets is *thrombocytopenia*. Babies with a low platelet count may look healthy or may show bruising; a purplish, speckled "rash" (called *petechiae* and pronounced pe-TEE-kee-eye) that actually results from tiny hemorrhages of the blood vessels just under the skin surface; and bleeding that is difficult to control because of the decreased number of platelets. Sometime this bleeding can occur in or around the brain. Some of these babies require only protection from injury that could cause bleeding. Others may need transfusions of platelets or medications to reduce platelet destruction. Blood tests to check blood and platelet type, red blood cell count, and platelet count will be done. The baby's platelets will be low only until the antibodies from the mother are eliminated from her system. This can take a few days to a few weeks. When the antibodies have been eliminated, the baby's platelet count will be normal.

Although blood typing is a routine part of prenatal care, platelet typing is not. If your newborn baby has low platelets, the physician may want to test your blood and the baby's father's blood to see if you have platelet antibodies or to determine your platelet types. Knowing if you carry antibodies against platelets or if your platelet type is incompatible with your newborn's can give the NICU team certain clues about how to treat your newborn's low platelet count. This information will also be important to your obstetrician for future pregnancies.

Fetal Factors That Affect Your Baby

As babies grow and develop throughout pregnancy, they interact with their environment. That environment is their mother's uterus and the amniotic fluid surrounding them in the uterus. The rate of growth of your uterus and the amount of amniotic fluid surrounding your baby are valuable clues to your baby's growth and development status.

Multiple Pregnancies

"The ultrasound technician discovered our triplets. She was very quiet, staring at the screen; then she cleared her throat and asked, 'Are you and your husband planning a large family?'"

If you are pregnant with more than one fetus (called a *multiple-gestation pregnancy),* lack of uterine space can affect your fetuses' weight gain in the final third of your pregnancy. Through week 29 of a healthy pregnancy, the growth rate of more than one fetus is nearly the same as it is for one. But at 30 weeks and later, multiple fetuses do not gain weight as rapidly as a single fetus does. In fact, with more than one fetus, the babies may not gain weight or grow in length at all after week 37 or 38 of pregnancy. In contrast, a single fetus is able to gain weight and grow until term.

A second risk associated with more than one fetus is abnormal blood flow through the placenta. If your multiple-gestation pregnancy resulted from a single egg, the fetuses are called *identical* and usually share one placenta. If more than one egg was fertilized, the fetuses are *fraternal,* and each has its own placenta. With more than one fetus, the connection of the umbilical cords to the placenta (in the case of identical fetuses) can develop abnormally, or the separate placentas (in the case of fraternal and some identical fetuses) can connect to one another abnormally. These abnormal connections can cause differences in blood flow between or among the fetuses. This is known as a *twin-to-twin transfusion.* Newborns who have reduced blood flow during pregnancy (this baby is called the *donor)* can show signs of low birth weight, low red blood cell count, reduced blood volume, and perhaps altered kidney function and congestive heart failure. Newborns who have received greater than normal blood flow during pregnancy (called the *recipient)* are generally sicker than those who have received limited amounts. They often show a high red blood cell count, signs of jaundice, an overworked heart, a high blood volume, and abnormal liver function.

If you are pregnant with more than one fetus, you are at risk for developing gestational diabetes, gestational hypertension, and anemia. These conditions were discussed previously in this chapter—and all can be problematic for your developing babies. An additional risk with multiple births is the presence of above-normal amounts of amniotic fluid (see the next section). More than one infant also increases the risk of premature birth and/or injury during labor and delivery for both mother and babies.

Amniotic Fluid and Its Effects on Your Baby

Your developing baby is surrounded by amniotic fluid in your uterus. This fluid cushions your fetus against jolts and bumps, helps control fetal temperature, protects the umbilical cord, and prevents infection.

Amniotic fluid is made up of fetal urine and lung fluids, as well as fluid made by the lining of the sac that holds your baby. The fetus regulates the amount of amniotic fluid present by swallowing, "breathing" (the amniotic fluid moves in and out of the fetus's lungs), and urinating. Presence of a normal amount of amniotic fluid indicates that the fetus's lungs, esophagus, nervous system, and kidneys are developing normally. If a fetus has problems swallowing (or if there is an obstruction in the fetal intestinal tract), "breathing," or making urine, greater or less than normal amounts of amniotic fluid will likely be present.

Oligohydramnios is the medical name for a lower than normal amount of amniotic fluid surrounding the fetus. This condition is most commonly the result of a pregnancy that extends beyond 40 weeks' gestation; in this case, a combination of fetal, placental, and maternal factors contributes to the reduced volume. Oligohydramnios may also occur if the fetus's kidneys are improperly formed or improperly functioning. Severe oligohydramnios may be the result of absent or nonfunctioning fetal kidneys. Maternal causes of oligohydramnios include a small tear in the amniotic sac, permitting a slow leak of fluid over time, and inadequate maternal nutrition.

When the fetus is not surrounded by enough amniotic fluid during development, the environment is cramped and constricted, causing compression (pressure) and dehydration. The newborn may display physical features characteristic of this environment: a set of facial features that develop because of the compressive forces around the baby's head (short neck; tiny nose; wide-set eyes; small chin; large, low-set ears); small, undeveloped lungs; wrinkled skin; stiff joints; and bone problems. In addition, the umbilical cord can become compressed during labor and delivery because of the restricted space and lack of cushioning fluid. This can limit blood flow to and from the fetus, placing her at risk for complications during labor.

If oligohydramnios has been a problem during pregnancy, your newborn's NICU team will observe her closely to see whether her kidneys are working properly. They will monitor the relationship between fluid intake and urine output and will also check the level of electrolytes in her urine and blood. Ultrasound evaluation of the kidneys may be used to determine kidney structure. Newborns whose kidneys are not functioning normally often require bladder catheterization (insertion of a tube into the bladder) for accurate measurement and/or collection of urine. Newborns who have developed in less than normal amounts of amniotic fluid may also have underdeveloped lungs, called *pulmonary hypoplasia* (see Chapter 10). They need help breathing. Chest x-rays and measurement of blood gases will likely play a part in the assessment of your newborn's lung development.

A greater than normal amount of amniotic fluid—a condition called *polyhydramnios*—may also occur during pregnancy. Causes of polyhydramnios include an improperly formed or improperly functioning gastrointestinal tract (stomach and intestines) or an improperly formed or malfunctioning brain and spinal cord. Fluid builds up when the fetus cannot swallow effectively because of a blockage in the gastrointestinal tract or a problem in the nervous system. It also increases if the fetus cannot absorb the amniotic fluid it swallows. Finally, fluid volume can grow if the fetus's nervous system is leaking cerebrospinal fluid. This occurs with conditions such as spina bifida. Multiple gestations and maternal diabetes are also associated with polyhydramnios.

When polyhydramnios is present, the baby is often in either the breech (buttocks or feet first) or oblique (shoulder first) position at delivery. These infants rarely show any physical features indicating their developmental condition. Care providers will assess the newborn's breathing patterns, muscle tone, and response to stimuli (to determine nervous system status) and her ability to suck and swallow, tolerate feedings, and pass stool (to determine the condition of the gastrointestinal tract).

Birth Defects

Some newborns show physical abnormalities at birth. The medical term for these abnormalities is *congenital* (meaning "existing at birth") *anomalies,* and they are more commonly called *birth defects.* For information on specific birth defects, see Chapter 10.

Structural malformations are seen when organs or organ systems develop in an unusual fashion. The changes may be genetic (inherited) or may be caused by some environmental or maternal factor. Structural malformations often occur early in the pregnancy (between the third and eighth weeks), before many women are even aware that they are pregnant. They include heart defects, cleft lip/cleft palate, a defect of the spine called *spina bifida,* and defects of the abdomen in which internal organs protrude outside the body (for example, omphalocele and gastroschisis). Structural malformations require medical, surgical, and/or cosmetic treatment.

Many babies are born with minor anomalies (small variations in appearance), which are caused by mechanical pressure on the fetus in the uterus. For example, bowed legs or a turned-in foot can be caused by positioning in the uterus and usually resolves without treatment. Other variations include skin tags (small outgrowths of the skin) on the earlobes, extra fingers or toes, or partially fused toes (called *syndactyly*). These variations can occur in families as a hereditary trait.

Malformations may appear singly or in patterns (several defects together). Many congenital malformations are discovered only after birth, during the first physical examination, but more are now detected during pregnancy through ultrasonography. Sometimes internal malformations (such as certain heart defects) are not apparent in the newborn period and will be discovered days or weeks later.

How Your Baby Is Affected by Factors Associated With Labor and Delivery

The process of labor and birth is greatly influenced by the health of the mother and her unborn baby. Many of these factors have been discussed previously in this chapter. The birth process involves an amazing chain of events that are all interrelated and dependent on the healthy functioning of the mother's body and on her baby's ability to tolerate the stresses of labor and the transition to extrauterine life. A healthy fetus will be able to withstand the normal stresses of labor and delivery with no ill effects. A fetus that has developed in a problematic environment (and thus is at risk even before the birth experience) or a baby who experiences a greater than normal degree of stress during labor and delivery may need special care immediately after birth.

Major risk factors for mother and baby are usually anticipated prior to labor and birth. Appropriate prenatal care and ongoing assessment during labor enable your health care team to make decisions that result in the best possible outcome for you and your new baby. Chapter 1 discusses what you may expect if you experience a complicated labor. This section discusses some of the occurrences of labor and birth that may result in a newborn who requires special care.

Problems With Oxygen Supply and Delivery

The unborn baby must have a sufficient supply of oxygen during labor and birth. If the mother's own oxygen supply is at risk (perhaps because of cardiac or respiratory problems or serious blood loss), the fetal supply is also in jeopardy. Problems with placental function (perhaps because of infection, poor placental development, partial separation of the placenta from the uterine wall, or decreased efficiency late in pregnancy) as happens with hypertension can influence oxygen supply to the unborn baby. The fetus can also have heart or circulation problems before labor that further stress abilities to use oxygen efficiently.

Maternal, placental, and fetal problems are usually discovered before the baby's birth. Adequate prenatal care is important for discovery and management of these conditions. In some cases, newborn intensive care may be inevitable, but good prenatal care and close monitoring before and/or during labor enable the health care team to deliver the baby in the best possible condition.

The oxygen supply to the fetus is decreased during labor contractions—this is a normal and expected part of the labor process. Even a healthy baby can experience distress. However, sometimes the mother experiences unusually forceful contractions, contractions that are too close together, or contractions that last an unusually long time. These abnormalities in the labor process can cause an inadequate oxygen supply to the baby. The health care team takes steps as necessary to ensure an oxygen supply to the fetus by administering extra oxygen to the mother, increasing the circulating blood volume to the fetus by giving the mother a large amount of IV fluid (called a *bolus),* and by attempting to restore normal labor contractions.

The unborn baby can also have problems with oxygen supply if the umbilical cord becomes squeezed or compressed. The cord can become trapped between the baby and the mother's uterine wall during contractions, or the baby's head or body may press on the cord, limiting oxygen supply to the baby. Compression can also occur if the cord slips past the baby and enters the mother's birth canal before the baby. This event is called *umbilical cord prolapse* and requires emergency delivery of the baby.

Newborns whose oxygen supply is inadequate during labor may require resuscitation at birth to breathe and to achieve or maintain an adequate heart rate (see Chapter 2). Infants have an amazing capacity to overcome serious problems at birth, but extended lack of oxygen during labor and birth can damage the infant's major organs. These complications are discussed in Chapter 10.

Lung Preparation During Labor and Birth

During labor, the fluid that has been in the fetus's lungs during growth and development begins to be absorbed. This process of fetal lung fluid absorption during labor prepares the newborn's lungs to breathe air and absorb oxygen immediately after birth. Lung preparation is believed to be an important function of labor.

Labor and vaginal birth also help prepare the lungs for breathing. Infants who do not experience labor (those born by scheduled cesarean section before the onset of labor, for example) or whose mothers have only a very brief labor can have problems breathing immediately after birth, called *transient tachypnea of the newborn* (see Chapter 10). If this respiratory distress is severe, it may require a brief stay in intensive care. The situation usually resolves rapidly, however.

Precipitous Labor and Delivery

A labor and delivery that lasts less than 3 hours is called a *precipitous labor.* In such labors, the mother's uterine contractions are very strong, and they push the fetus through the birth canal quickly. Problems associated with precipitous labor include reduced blood and oxygen flow to the baby (because of the strength of the uterine contractions). They may also include injury to the infant's head (because the cervix has not dilated sufficiently to allow the baby to pass through easily).

Birth Trauma and How It Might Affect Your Baby

Birth injuries—often called *birth trauma*—can occur during a difficult labor or birth. These injuries may be minor, with no long-term consequences for your baby, or they may be more serious. Birth injuries are more frequent among babies who are large in weight for their gestational age, babies who are born prematurely, those born following a precipitous labor (see previous section) or a lengthy labor, those not born headfirst or, rarely, those delivered with mechanical assistance (forceps or vacuum extraction).

There are 3 categories of birth injuries: (1) head and neck, (2) nerve, and (3) bone. The more common injuries are discussed here.

Head Injuries

A cephalhematoma occurs when blood from a broken blood vessel collects between the surface of the skull bone and the tough membrane that covers the skull bone. It is normally seen as a lump only on one side of the head. Most often, a cephalhematoma is small and resolves without causing the baby any problems, but in rare cases, it can become quite large. Bleeding from a large cephalhematoma in a newborn may cause your baby to become jaundiced. Cephalhematomas on both sides of the babies skull are sometimes associated with an underlying skull fracture. Cephalhematomas usually resolve without treatment over the first months of life. Bleeding can also occur in a space at the back of the neck called the *subgaleal space.* In some cases, a large amount of bleeding into the subgaleal space can occur. This is an emergency.

Rarely, fracture of the skull or bleeding underneath the skull can occur during birth and may cause a serious birth injury. In addition to the bone damage, the fracture can cause the brain to be bruised, or damage can occur to the blood vessels in the brain, causing bleeding. An x-ray and sometimes a computed tomography (CT) scan are performed to aid diagnosis. Superficial fractures that do not involve the brain heal without treatment or complications in 8 to 12 weeks. If the newborn's brain has been bruised or if bleeding in the brain has occurred, the baby's brain or nervous system development can be affected.

Nerve Damage

Brachial plexus palsy (sometimes call *Erb palsy)* is the most common birth injury affecting the nerves. It involves the roots of the nerves at the base of the newborn's neck. These nerves may swell, become irritated, or be damaged by stretching and twisting during delivery. Erb palsy usually affects only one side of the body and causes paralysis (lack of movement) of the arm, hand, and/or fingers only on the affected side. It is often seen with babies who are especially large at birth and may be associated with fracture of the clavicle (collarbone) on the same side. Healing generally occurs naturally, but range-of-motion exercises and maintenance of joint alignment can help. If the injury does not heal on its own, growth of the affected arm may be stunted.

Bell palsy involves damage to the newborn's facial nerve. It causes paralysis on one side of the face. The damage heals on its own without treatment or complications. During recovery, the infant may have difficulty sucking and may need eye drops to keep the eye on the affected side moist.

Damage to the phrenic nerve (another nerve root at the base of the baby's neck) during delivery can cause paralysis of the diaphragm. The diaphragm is the muscle under the lungs that assists in breathing. Because the phrenic nerve controls this muscle, damage to that nerve can cause paralysis of the diaphragm on one or both sides, affecting the infant's breathing. Some babies require assistance with breathing. An x-ray and an ultrasound examination are used to diagnose the problem. Recovery usually takes from 1 to 3 months. During recovery, caregivers focus on keeping the infant from developing pneumonia (an infection of the lungs).

Paralysis of the vocal cords can result from damage to the laryngeal nerve at the base of the baby's neck. Diagnosis of vocal cord paralysis is made by examining the newborn's vocal cords. One or both can be affected. During recovery, the newborn may receive help in breathing and feeding to prevent choking. If only one vocal cord is involved, the infant will usually recover in 4 to 6 weeks. When both are involved, the infant will need mechanical help to breathe, and recovery will likely take longer. The baby may have a hoarse cry for some time after delivery.

Bone Injuries

Term infants born in the breech position and term babies who weigh more than average for their age at birth are the most likely to sustain birth injuries to their bones. The causes of these injuries are stress to and twisting of the bones during birth. The most common location for bone breakage is the clavicle (collarbone). A newborn with a fracture of the clavicle may show limited movement of the arm on the side of the break and may also have muscle spasms. An x-ray may be taken to diagnose the injury. Care providers will limit the infant's arm movements during the healing period, which takes 7 to 10 days.

Your Baby's Special Needs

Most of the time, the circumstances that result in a NICU admission are beyond any-one's control. Even though your health care team is able to plan ahead for most factors that place the mother or fetus at risk, a NICU admission is sometimes inevitable. This is especially true for preterm birth. Other babies admitted to the NICU are those who have problems resulting from a complicated labor and birth, infection, birth defects, or maternal problems that affect the unborn baby's growth and development.

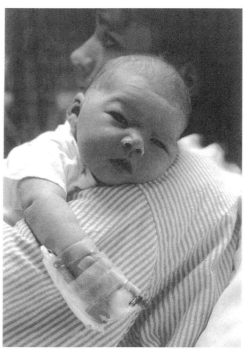

Relaxing with Mom.
The NICU cares for babies of all sizes with many different problems. But every baby needs a parent's special care.

The delivery of a newborn is a time of emotional highs and lows. If your baby needs intensive care, the joys and fears of this emotional roller coaster will be even more extreme. You will need some time to begin to understand why your baby is in the NICU. Soon you will realize the challenges facing your baby. Remember that even if your baby requires special care for the same reason as another baby, your child's needs will be unique. As parents, you will discover how to work with the NICU team to best meet those special needs.

Chapter 9
Problems Associated With Premature Birth

"Listen to this, Piglet," said Eeyore,

"and then you'll know what we're trying to do."

Gary M. Weiner, MD, FAAP

Babies delivered before 37 completed weeks of pregnancy are considered premature. In the United States, approximately 12% of all births are premature, with nearly 500,000 premature babies born each year.

Despite efforts to understand the cause of premature labor and develop methods to prevent premature birth, the premature birth rate has been steadily increasing in the United States since the early 1980s. Most premature births occur close to full term (34–36 weeks' gestation) and may be called *late preterm* infants. These infants may require additional monitoring and hospital care but are at lower risk of serious health complications. Nearly 3% of all births, however, occur before 34 weeks of pregnancy and are at risk for multiple health problems. By the time your baby is born, even if he is born very prematurely, all the major body systems have been formed but they are immature and still developing. These organ systems may not function the same way that they would in a full-term infant and are at risk of injury or abnormal development.

This chapter describes possible problems that premature babies may experience because of the immaturity of one or more of their major body systems. Your baby's health care providers know the wide range of problems that can affect premature infants, are trained to recognize early or subtle signs of developing problems, and can intervene to try to keep minor problems from becoming major crises. Keep in mind that even though a baby is *at risk* of developing a problem it does not mean that he *will* develop the problem. Talk with your baby's nurses and doctors about any concerns you have for your special baby.

Problems Affecting the Lungs

The lungs are part of the respiratory system. This system is responsible for maintaining the correct amount of oxygen and carbon dioxide in your baby's body. Health professionals sometimes call the air that we normally breathe *room air*. Oxygen is a gas that makes up approximately 21% (1/5th) of room air. Carbon dioxide is a waste product produced by cells during energy production and is removed from the body by exhaling. It is very important to maintain the correct balance of oxygen and carbon dioxide within the bloodstream; too much or too little of either gas is not healthy. When you breathe in, air travels into the lungs through a series of tubes that get progressively smaller until it reaches tiny sacs called *alveoli*. In the alveoli, oxygen moves into the bloodstream to be carried to the rest of the body. Carbon dioxide is brought to the lungs through the bloodstream and moves into the alveoli to be exhaled when you breathe out. Premature babies may have difficulty with many of the respiratory system's functions. These problems may begin in the delivery room and include difficulty beginning the process of breathing, keeping their lungs open, and controlling their breathing rate.

Respiratory Problems at Birth

Before delivery, a baby's lungs are full of fluid and are not responsible for providing oxygen to the body. Instead, oxygen moves from the mother's blood through the placenta to the fetus. At the time of delivery, babies must quickly remove the fluid from their lungs, begin breathing, inflate their lungs with air, and use their lungs to carry oxygen to the blood. Although many premature babies will cry in the delivery room and require little intervention from the health care team, more than half of babies delivered before 32 completed weeks of pregnancy will have trouble making this important transition and will require some assistance. The health care provider caring for your baby in the delivery room may use a face mask and positive pressure ventilation device (such as a resuscitation bag) to assist his first breaths. Babies born very prematurely may need to have a tube placed into their throat, directed into the windpipe (trachea), and attached to a breathing machine (respirator or ventilator) to provide more assistance with breathing (ventilation). Some premature infants may require even more intensive interventions

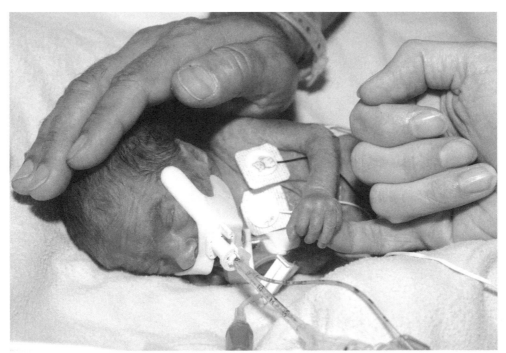

Premature infant with an oral endotracheal tube for respiratory support.
Babies born very prematurely may need to have a tube placed into their throat (intubation), directed into the windpipe (trachea), and attached to a breathing machine (respirator or ventilator) to provide assistance with breathing (ventilation).

Courtesy of Gigi O'Dea.

to stabilize their respiratory system immediately after birth. Additional details about delivery room resuscitation are provided in Chapter 2.

Respiratory Distress Syndrome

Respiratory distress syndrome (RDS) is the most common lung condition affecting premature babies. You may hear some health care providers use the term *hyaline membrane disease* (HMD) instead of RDS. Respiratory distress syndrome is a disease that primarily affects infants delivered before 35 weeks' gestation, although some more mature infants may develop RDS. More than half of babies delivered before 30 weeks' gestation will develop RDS. The earlier a baby is born, the more likely he is to have RDS, and the more severe the disease is likely to be.

Physical immaturity of the chest and lungs coupled with a decreased amount of a substance called *surfactant* are the causes of RDS. Surfactant is a soap-like substance that is produced by specialized cells in the lungs. Surfactant production begins around the 24th week of pregnancy, but the surfactant production system is not fully developed until 34 to 36 weeks of pregnancy. Respiratory distress syndrome is more common in males than females, white infants than black infants, and infants delivered by cesarean section without labor. Infants delivered to mothers with diabetes may have a delay in surfactant production.

Surfactant coats the inside of the tiny breathing sacs (alveoli) and helps to keep them open as the baby breathes in and out. Without enough surfactant, the alveoli tend to collapse during exhalation, and the baby must use additional effort to re-expand the alveoli with

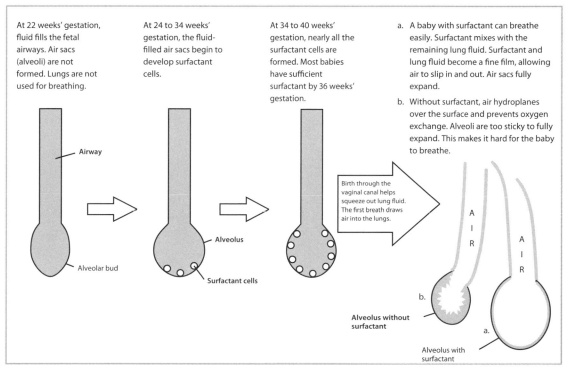

How lung surfactant helps a baby breathe.

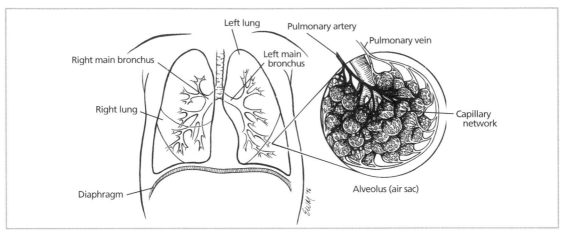

Breathing sacs in lungs.
An alveolus is an air sac in the lungs. Oxygen passes through the alveoli, into the tiny blood vessels called *capillaries,* and through the circulatory system to the body tissues. Alveoli are coated with surfactant, a soapy substance that keeps these tiny sacs open as the baby breathes in and out after birth. Surfactant production begins at about 24 weeks' gestation, but is incomplete until about 34 to 36 weeks' gestation; therefore, a baby born prior to this time faces the possibility of respiratory distress syndrome.

each breath. Collapse of the alveoli makes it difficult for the baby to maintain the correct balance of oxygen and carbon dioxide in his blood. The oxygen level may decrease and the carbon dioxide level may increase. Without enough surfactant, fluid and proteins may leak into the breathing sacs, causing the formation of an abnormal layer of debris. This abnormal layer is called a *hyaline membrane* when it is seen under a microscope.

Each baby's lungs mature at a different rate. Health care providers can help speed up the production of surfactant in some babies by giving steroids to the mother before delivery. An obstetrician may be able to perform a test by sampling the amniotic fluid (amniocentesis) to identify how mature your baby's lungs are before delivery.

Signs of Respiratory Distress Syndrome

Premature babies may show signs of RDS within minutes after delivery or they may develop progressive breathing problems during the first few hours after birth. You may notice that your baby is breathing rapidly or that he appears to be working hard to breathe. He may have retractions (pulling in the skin and muscles between the ribs or just below the rib cage) or grunting (a moaning sound) when he breathes out. Your baby may have a dusky or bluish color around his lips called *cyanosis* or a pale and mottled appearance to his skin. If your baby is working hard to breathe and begins to tire, his breathing rate may become irregular and he may take pauses in his breathing, called *apnea.* In addition to the breathing signs, he may not produce much urine in the first 2 days of life, leading to puffy swelling around the eyes, hands, feet, and back.

Diagnosis of Respiratory Distress Syndrome

If RDS is suspected, your baby's health care providers may order a chest x-ray and a blood gas for further evaluation (see Chapter 2). Infants with RDS frequently have a white, hazy, granular appearance to their chest x-ray. Their blood gas may show a relatively low oxygen level and an increased carbon dioxide level. There is, however, no definitive test for RDS. The x-ray findings of RDS are very similar to those found in congenital pneumonia. Respiratory distress syndrome is diagnosed based on the care provider's clinical judgment after considering the x-ray findings and blood tests in combination with the baby's history, physical examination, and progress over the first days of life.

Treatment of Respiratory Distress Syndrome

The options for treating RDS have changed over the last 20 years and continue to be an area of active research. Infants with mild RDS may only require additional oxygen

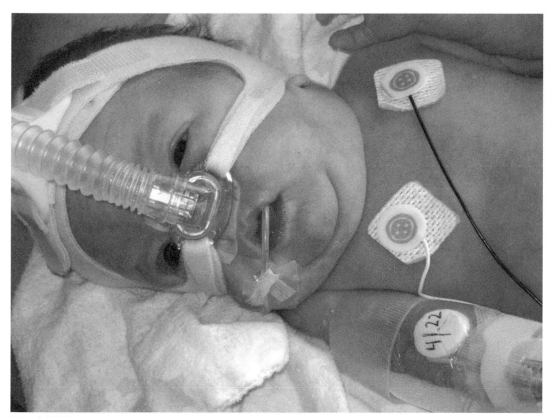

Nasal CPAP.
CPAP delivers pressurized air and oxygen to the baby's lungs to stabilize the alveoli and prevent them from collapsing. The baby continues to breathe on his own. Another device used to deliver CPAP is pictured on page 44.

Courtesy of Seattle Children's Hospital.

provided with an oxygen hood or through small plastic prongs, called a *nasal cannula,* placed in the baby's nose. If the baby has more significant RDS, he may receive oxygen through a device called *nasal continuous positive airway pressure* or *nasal CPAP.* Nasal CPAP delivers pressurized air and oxygen to the baby's lungs through tubes placed in the nose or a small mask placed over the nose. The CPAP pressure helps to stabilize the alveoli and prevent them from collapsing. Although the CPAP machine helps to keep the baby's lungs open, the machine does not provide any breaths, so the baby has to breathe on his own.

Babies with the most significant RDS may need surfactant replacement and a mechanical ventilator to temporarily assist their breathing while their lungs mature. If mechanical ventilation is needed, a small tube is placed in the baby's windpipe (trachea) in a procedure called *intubation.*

Surfactants, obtained from animals or produced in a laboratory, can be given through a tube placed in your baby's trachea (windpipe). The surfactant drains into the baby's lungs, coats the alveolar surface, and helps to stabilize the alveoli until he is able to make his own surfactant. A dose may be given within the first few minutes after birth (called *preventive* or *prophylactic treatment)* or only after signs of RDS appear (called *rescue treatment).* Depending on the baby's response, surfactant replacement may be repeated several times during the first 1 or 2 days of life.

Surfactant replacement therapy doesn't completely prevent RDS. It decreases the severity of the disease by stabilizing the alveoli. The goal of this therapy is to reduce the amount of extra oxygen and to lower the ventilator pressures that must be used to maintain normal levels of oxygen and carbon dioxide in your baby's blood. An associated goal is to be able to wean your baby from the ventilator sooner, which decreases the chances that he will develop complications associated with ventilator therapy.

Determining which babies should be treated with CPAP and which babies would benefit from surfactant replacement is a controversial topic that investigators around the world continue to research.

Possible Complications of Respiratory Distress Syndrome

The complications of RDS largely depend on the degree of prematurity at birth and the severity of the disease. Possible complications include air leaks, bronchopulmonary dysplasia, and infection. Decreased oxygen supply to the baby's tissues or hypoxia from severe RDS can contribute to problems in other body systems, including intraventricular hemorrhage, periventricular leukomalacia, patent ductus arteriosus, and necrotizing enterocolitis. All of these are explained later in this chapter.

Air Leaks

Babies with RDS have stiff lungs that don't open and close as easily as healthy lungs. When a baby with stiff lungs breathes or receives assistance from CPAP or a ventilator, one or more of the thin-walled alveoli can rupture. Air will leak out of the lung and collect in a space where it does not belong. A pneumothorax occurs when air collects in the space between the lung and the rib cage. A pneumomediastinum occurs when air leaks into the space in the center of the chest where the heart and major blood vessels lie and does not generally require treatment. Pulmonary interstitial emphysema, a more serious problem, occurs when air leaks into the structural spaces within the lung tissue. Term babies with respiratory problems are also at risk for this air leak. See Chapter 10 for more information about air leaks and how they are treated.

Bronchopulmonary Dysplasia

Bronchopulmonary dysplasia (BPD) is a chronic lung disease occurring primarily in infants delivered between 23 and 32 weeks. It may also be called *chronic lung disease* or *CLD*. The definition of BPD has varied over time. Recently it has been described as an infant delivered at less than 32 weeks' gestation who has required oxygen therapy for at least 4 weeks and continues to require oxygen supplementation at 36 weeks corrected gestational age.

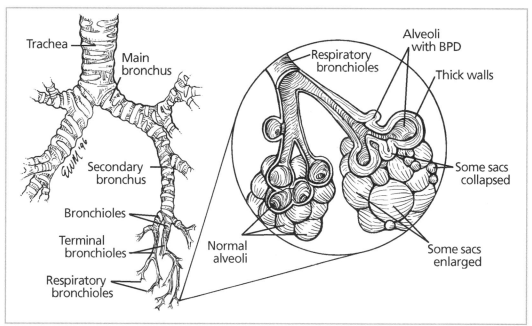

Lungs with BPD.
The enlarged portion of the diagram shows normal alveoli and alveoli with BPD. Alveoli with BPD have thick walls, making it more difficult to transfer oxygen through the alveoli into the circulatory system. Some of the alveolar sacs trap air and enlarge, and some collapse, forming areas of atelectasis (collapse).

Bronchopulmonary dysplasia occurs when the alveoli, blood vessels, and supporting structures in the immature lung are damaged during a vulnerable stage of their development. Premature newborn lungs are exposed to many potential injuries both before and after birth. Researchers are still trying to understand exactly what causes BPD and how it can be prevented. We currently believe that multiple related factors cause a decrease in the total number of both alveoli and blood vessels in affected lungs. Babies with BPD have fewer, larger alveoli and fewer blood vessels surrounding their alveoli. This decreases the total surface area available for exchanging gases within their lungs. In addition, some infants with BPD may have thickening, swelling, and scarring of the airways within their lungs. Some of the factors that may be involved include toxic substances created by oxygen in the lung, inflammatory substances made by the baby's immune system, and mechanical injury from repeated opening and closing of the tiny alveoli.

Risk Factors for Bronchopulmonary Dysplasia

Although the risk of developing BPD increases with the degree of prematurity, it is not clear why some premature babies develop BPD while others do not. Risk factors for BPD include infection of the amniotic fluid (chorioamnionitis), severe RDS, pneumonia, nutritional deficits, excess fluid in the lung, and a patent ductus arteriosus in the newborn period. Still, some infants who had only mild RDS will develop BPD. We believe that this is because their lungs were in such an early stage of development at the time of birth that even minimal injuries interfered with the complex development of their fragile alveoli and blood vessels. Genetics and family history may also play a role in the susceptibility to BPD because inherited genes can affect how your baby's lungs respond to injuries. Overall, BPD occurs in approximately 20% of babies that are delivered before 30 weeks' gestation, but the rate of BPD varies widely between different hospitals.

Diagnosis of Bronchopulmonary Dysplasia

Babies with RDS usually begin to wean from the ventilator after several days to a week of treatment. Infants who develop BPD often have more severe RDS initially, are slow to begin weaning, or may begin to wean and then stop making progress. Chest x-rays may show a diffusely hazy, bubbly, or cyst-like appearance in the lungs. The severity of BPD is classified by the amount of oxygen required at 36 weeks' corrected gestational age.

Treatment of Bronchopulmonary Dysplasia

At birth, term babies only have a fraction of the alveoli that they will have when they are full grown. The lung continues to grow, and new alveoli develop for several years. The goal of BPD treatment is to allow the infant's lung to heal while new, undamaged lung tissue develops. Treatment for BPD includes providing additional oxygen as needed, providing good nutrition with sufficient calories to promote growth, and avoiding excess fluid. The health care team will try to limit the amount of oxygen and mechanical pressure used while still maintaining a safe level of oxygen in your baby's blood. Several medications may also be used to help improve your baby's lung function. Diuretics like furosemide (Lasix), spironolactone (Aldactone), and chlorothiazide (Diuril) may help decrease the amount of fluid in the lungs. Inhaled medications like albuterol may help expand the breathing tubes if your baby has episodes of wheezing or bronchospasm. Additional vitamin A may be prescribed. Appendix B gives additional information about these medications.

Some babies with the most severe BPD may require treatment with a steroid to decrease the inflammation in their lung. Although steroids given to mothers before premature delivery are both safe and beneficial, steroids are not routinely given to premature babies after birth. They may offer short-term benefits by decreasing the severity of lung disease and allowing babies to wean off of a mechanical ventilator earlier; however, they may interfere with normal brain development and increase the risk of long-term neurodevelopmental handicaps. Because of this risk, health care providers avoid prescribing systemic steroids after premature delivery except in severe cases of respiratory failure.

Bronchopulmonary dysplasia is a chronic disease that can take months or occasionally years to heal. Because your baby could miss exploratory stages of a healthy infancy, it is important to provide him with opportunities to develop and grow. Your baby's nurse or therapist will work with you and your baby on a variety of exercises and activities designed to promote optimal growth and development.

Complications of Bronchopulmonary Dysplasia

Bronchopulmonary dysplasia represents a spectrum of illness. Mild BPD can mean that your baby requires oxygen for a month or longer but is able to go home without extra oxygen or medications. Babies with moderate BPD may need to go home with oxygen for a time and others may require home oxygen for several months. Babies with the most severe BPD may not be able to breathe effectively without a ventilator and may require a prolonged hospital stay and even a home ventilator program. Most babies will have mild or moderate BPD.

Babies with BPD may have increased production of mucus and episodes of wheezing or bronchospasm. Some infants with BPD develop "blue spells" or "desats." These spells can occur when the baby becomes upset or distressed. Sometimes these spells occur at a predictable time each day. During a spell, the baby may become cyanotic, have a decrease in heart rate and oxygen saturations, and become even more agitated. Parents and care providers can often identify the triggers that begin one of these episodes and learn how to decrease their severity. Bronchopulmonary dysplasia may place additional strain on the baby's heart and, in severe cases, may lead to signs of heart failure. Your baby's medical team can tell you if your baby is at risk of developing heart failure and explain how this is evaluated.

Babies with BPD frequently have difficulty tolerating oral feedings. They may develop a negative reaction to having things placed in their mouth, called *oral aversion*. Some babies with BPD may have slow emptying from their stomach, and feedings may flow backward into their esophagus. This backward flow is called *reflux*. Physical or occupational therapists may assist the NICU team in developing an oral stimulation plan for babies with BPD who have difficulty with feeding.

Most babies with BPD show gradual improvement in their lung function after discharge but may have some degree of abnormal lung function for a number of years. They may not tolerate exposure to pollutants in the air and should not be exposed to environmental tobacco smoke. Infants with BPD have an increased risk of developing asthma and pneumonia. If they develop viral respiratory illnesses like influenza or bronchiolitis, they may become very ill and require rehospitalization. Before discharge, your baby may receive an injection (palivizumab [Synagis]) to help prevent complications from a common viral respiratory infection called *RSV (respiratory syncytial virus)* bronchiolitis that commonly occurs during the fall and winter (see Chapter 15).

Apnea of Prematurity

Even though a fetus doesn't use his lungs for oxygen exchange, he does make breathing movements before birth. This breathing isn't continuous and doesn't have a regular pattern. After birth, babies rely on their lungs and must develop a regular breathing pattern, even when they are sleeping, in order to maintain a constant supply of oxygen. Premature babies frequently have irregular breathing patterns with episodes of shallow breathing or pauses. A prolonged breathing pause is called *apnea*. Apnea is one of the most common problems of premature infants occurring in 25% of all premature babies and in more than 80% of babies weighing less than 1,000 grams (about 2 pounds, 3 ounces).

Apnea of prematurity is caused by immaturity of the respiratory center in the baby's brain. The respiratory center is responsible for setting the pattern of breathing by sending signals to the chest muscles and diaphragm. When a premature baby has apnea, or becomes apneic, his heart rate may slow and his blood oxygen level may decrease. Slowing of the heart rate is called *bradycardia*. Decreases in oxygen levels are called *desaturations* and are recorded on a machine called a *pulse oximeter* or *pulse ox*. The NICU staff may call these events *As* and *Bs* for apneas and bradycardias or *A-B-Ds* for apneas, bradycardias, and desaturations.

If apnea begins suddenly or existing apnea worsens, it may be an early sign of other problems. Depending on the baby's condition, health care providers may look for a low body temperature (hypothermia), infection, low blood sugar (hypoglycemia), necrotizing enterocolitis, seizures, or intraventricular hemorrhage.

Management of Apnea

"Our nurse told us that apnea was a typical problem for a baby like Jason. My imagination ran wild. If turning blue was typical, what other death-defying tricks could we expect from Jason?"

Infants at risk for apnea have an electronic cardiorespiratory monitor that tracks their heart and breathing rates. They may also be monitored with a pulse oximeter that monitors the oxygen level in their blood. (Both monitors are described in Chapter 2.) Alarms on these machines are set to sound when the heart rate, breathing rate, or oxygen level falls below a specified level for a certain period. When the alarm sounds, a caregiver is alerted to the event. Apnea can be very frightening for parents, but many apneic spells end spontaneously and the baby begins to breathe again on his own. If the baby does not begin breathing on his own, the care provider may gently rub the baby's side or foot to stimulate respirations. This is known as *tactile stimulation*. Sometimes the care provider also needs to give the baby extra oxygen. If the baby doesn't start breathing after stimulation or the heart rate remains low, a caregiver may need to give several assisted breaths (positive pressure ventilation) with a face mask. Chapter 2 provides more information on both interventions.

Babies with frequent apnea episodes that lead to bradycardia and desaturation may require extra oxygen, airflow, or medications. Oxygen or airflow may be provided with a nasal cannula or nasal CPAP. As described previously, nasal CPAP helps keep the airways and alveoli open and it may provide some stimulation for breathing. Caffeine and theophylline are medications that stimulate the breathing center and may help to normalize the baby's breathing pattern. As the central nervous system and respiratory system mature, apnea of prematurity gradually improves and ultimately disappears. Apnea of prematurity resolves in most premature babies before they are discharged home. Once apnea of prematurity resolves, it does not come back. Very premature babies, delivered before 28 weeks' gestation, may not have fully mature breathing control until several weeks after their due date. These infants may require home apnea monitoring after discharge. Chapter 16 has additional information about these monitors.

Other Types of Apnea

Three main types of apnea are seen in premature infants: central apnea, obstructive apnea, and mixed apnea. Apnea of prematurity is a type of central apnea because it is caused by immaturity of the respiratory center in the baby's brain. Obstructive apnea occurs when the baby is trying to breathe but the airway becomes blocked. A premature baby has decreased muscle tone in the upper portions of the throat, making the airway more prone to becoming blocked. During sleep, these structures may partially collapse and block air movement into the lungs. Obstructive apnea may also occur while a baby is being held if the head falls either too far forward or backward and closes the airway. When babies have a combination of both central and obstructive apnea, it is called *mixed apnea*. Mixed apnea is very common.

Periodic Breathing

Periodic breathing is a cyclic pattern in which the infant takes repeated brief pauses in breathing (5–10 seconds) and then takes several regular breaths. Periodic breathing is a common pattern in premature infants and may last for many weeks after birth. Healthy term infants may also exhibit this pattern in the first few days after birth.

Apnea, Prematurity, and Sudden Infant Death Syndrome

Parents are often concerned about a possible relationship between apnea of prematurity and sudden infant death syndrome (SIDS) or crib death. Apnea of prematurity is a developmental event that disappears as the infant matures. Sudden infant death syndrome is a condition that is very rare in the first month of life. Apnea of prematurity is not the same as SIDS and is not considered to be a specific risk factor for SIDS. The cause of SIDS is unknown. Strategies for reducing the risk of SIDS are found in Chapter 16.

Problems Affecting the Heart

The heart and blood vessels make up the cardiovascular system. Development of the heart is complete very early in pregnancy. The heart is a 4-chambered pump that moves

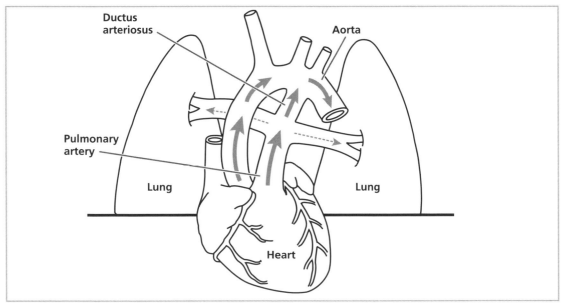

Normal circulation through the heart of the fetus.
Because fetal lungs are not used for breathing, blood is directed away from the lungs through a patent (open) ductus arteriosus into the aorta.

From: American Academy of Pediatrics, American Heart Association. Textbook of Neonatal Resuscitation. 5th ed. Kattwinkel J, ed. Elk Grove Village, IL: American Academy of Pediatrics; 2006: 1–4.

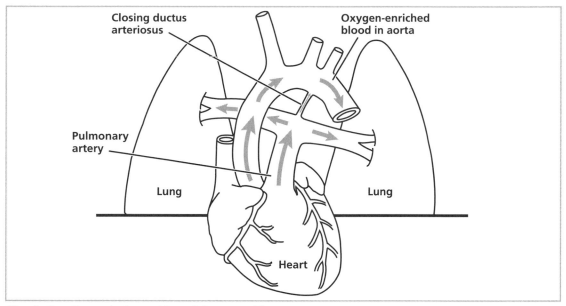

Circulation through the newborn's heart and lungs.
At birth, the full-term baby breathes and fills his lungs with air. Blood vessels relax in the lungs and the ductus arteriosus begins to close. Now blood is not diverted away from the lungs, but flows to the lungs and picks up oxygen for transport to body tissues.

From: American Academy of Pediatrics, American Heart Association. Textbook of Neonatal Resuscitation. 5th ed. Kattwinkel J, ed. Elk Grove Village, IL: American Academy of Pediatrics; 2006: 1-6.

blood through the lungs and the body. Arteries are vessels that carry blood rich with oxygen to the tissues, and veins are vessels that return blood back to the heart. Blood carrying oxygen leaves the left side of the heart and is pumped into a very large artery called the *aorta*. From there, it is distributed into smaller arteries throughout the body. When the blood arrives at the tissue, it delivers oxygen and picks up the waste gas (carbon dioxide). After making this exchange, blood returns through veins to the right side of your heart. Blood in the right side of the heart is pumped to the lungs through the pulmonary artery. In the lungs, the blood gets new oxygen and eliminates carbon dioxide. Finally, the blood returns to the left side of the heart to start the cycle over again. The most common heart problems seen in preterm babies are a patent ductus arteriosus and low blood pressure (hypotension).

Patent Ductus Arteriosus

When your baby was in the womb, the blood circulating through his heart followed a path that is slightly different from the mature path described above. This path, called *fetal circulation,* allows most blood to bypass the baby's lungs. The fetus doesn't use his lungs for exchanging oxygen and carbon dioxide, so it isn't necessary to send blood to the lungs. The mother's lungs and the placenta have already done this work. The baby's heart has 2 "short circuits" that allow blood to go directly from the right side of the heart to the left side of the heart without going through the lungs. The foramen ovale is a small opening with a "trap door" between the top 2 chambers of the heart. The ductus arteriosus is a short vessel that connects the pulmonary artery and aorta.

In full-term babies, the 2 paths that allowed blood to bypass the lungs normally start to close shortly after birth. In preterm babies, the ductus arteriosus may remain open after birth or reopen in the weeks following birth. This is referred to as a *patent* (open) *ductus arteriosus* or *PDA*. In the first few hours to days after birth, a PDA may still direct blood away from the lungs because the blood vessels in the lungs are relatively narrow. This is called a *right-to-left shunt* and is similar to the circulation pattern the baby had in the womb. As the blood vessels in the lungs relax and blood can enter them more easily, blood flows through the PDA in the opposite direction. Now the PDA allows blood to flow from the aorta back into the lungs (a left-to-right shunt). If too much blood enters the lungs, it can lead to both heart and breathing problems.

A PDA affects about nearly half of babies born at less than 30 weeks' gestation or weighing less than 1,000 grams (about 2 pounds, 3 ounces). The more premature a baby is at birth, the greater the risk of a symptomatic PDA. The signs of a PDA often occur toward the end of the first week.

Signs of Patent Ductus Arteriosus

The signs of a PDA depend on how widely open the ductus arteriosus is, how much blood is flowing through it, and the direction that the blood is flowing. The signs of a PDA may include a heart murmur, worsening respiratory problems, faster breathing, an enlarged heart, visible heart pulsations on the chest wall, throbbing pulses, decreased urine output, or increasing acid levels in the baby's blood. A heart murmur is a swooshing sound heard with a stethoscope. Heart murmurs are very common in newborns, sometimes come and go, and do not necessarily mean that there is a problem. Sometimes the largest PDAs have very soft murmurs or none at all, and very small PDAs may have loud murmurs. The signs of a PDA may vary over the course of several hours.

Diagnosis of Patent Ductus Arteriosus

If your baby's caregiver suspects a PDA, an echocardiogram may be ordered. An echocardiogram is an ultrasound of the heart that can show if the ductus arteriosus is open. It can estimate both its size and how much blood is moving through it. Echocardiograms use sound waves to create moving images. There is no radiation exposure from an echocardiogram. It is very similar to the ultrasound used by obstetricians to evaluate a fetus during pregnancy.

Treatment of Patent Ductus Arteriosus

The treatment of a PDA depends on its size and the amount of difficulty that it is causing your baby. A small PDA in an otherwise healthy premature baby may cause few if any problems and may not require any treatment. Many small premature babies, however, do not tolerate a PDA and will need treatment. In very tiny infants, the caregivers might routinely look for a PDA and may recommend treatment before it begins to cause any signs.

Medical treatment includes decreasing the amount of fluid given to your baby and adjusting the respiratory support as needed to help with the excess fluid in the lungs. One of 2 related medications, indomethacin or ibuprofen, may be given to try to close the PDA. They are both given intravenously and have similar functions. Both interfere with a chemical in the body called *prostaglandin*. The goal is to make the muscle that surrounds the ductus arteriosus squeeze tightly, close the ductus, and ultimately cause it to "glue" shut.

Both of the medications that are used to treat a PDA can cause a temporary decrease in kidney function. After receiving either of these medications, many babies will have a decrease in urine output and retain water. This type of water retention most often resolves within several days without any additional treatment. Until it resolves, care providers may need to limit the amount of fluid that is given to the baby. If the medication is unsuccessful or can't be used because of other problems, surgical closure may be needed. Surgery for a PDA may be performed in an operating room, in a special area within the NICU or, rarely, at the baby's bedside. Medications are used to put your baby to sleep during the surgery and provide pain relief. The surgeon makes an incision on the left side of your baby's chest wall. The ribs are spread apart and the lung is moved aside. The surgeon then places a stitch or clip around the ductus arteriosus. The surgery takes approximately 1 hour, and babies generally do well. When the surgery is completed, there will be a dressing over the incision and possibly a chest tube. The chest tube drains air and any fluid from the chest cavity and is usually removed within a day or two after surgery. Some babies may be sicker after the surgery than they were before surgery. They may have trouble with low blood pressure or more significant breathing problems until they fully recover from surgery.

Surgical closure of the PDA has a low risk of complications including air leak (pneumothorax), bleeding from the wound site, wound infection, damage to one of the large blood vessels in the chest, damage to a nerve that controls the vocal cords, or collection of either blood or fatty (lymphatic) fluid in the chest.

Congestive Heart Failure

Congestive heart failure (CHF) is any condition in which the heart is under strain and unable to meet the energy needs of the body. If untreated, a large PDA causes your baby's heart to work harder. The blood that was just pumped out of the heart returns through the short circuit and has to be pumped out again. This places a strain on your baby's heart, which can lead to CHF.

Congestive heart failure can result in increased pressures inside the heart and may cause blood to back up into the lungs or the liver. Extra blood in the lungs may cause fluid to leak into the lung tissue. This condition is called *pulmonary edema.* Your baby's work of breathing may increase and require additional oxygen or breathing support. While extra blood is flowing through the PDA it may divert blood intended for the kidneys and intestines. This may interfere with the functioning of these organs.

Treatment of Congestive Heart Failure

The ideal treatment for CHF is identification and elimination of the cause. If CHF is caused by a PDA, the PDA is treated, either with medication or surgery. If CHF comes from another cause, such as a different congenital heart defect, your baby's fluid intake will be restricted. Drugs called *diuretics* (furosemide, chlorothiazide, and the combination of spironolactone and hydrochlorothiazide [Aldactazide]) may be given to help your baby eliminate excess fluid and to reduce the load on the heart. Other drugs, such as dopamine or digoxin, may be used to strengthen the heart's contractions. Occasionally, medical or surgical treatment for a PDA must be delayed because of poor kidney function or an intervening infection. In this case, fluid limitation, diuretics, and drugs to improve the heart's function may be used until the PDA can be treated. (See Appendix B for more information on these medications.)

Other treatment includes supportive care—oxygen to maintain adequate levels in the blood and tissues, and maintenance of normal temperature. High-calorie formula or breast milk supplements and special feeding plans may be used for babies with chronic CHF to ensure adequate calories and nutrition while maintaining fluid restriction.

Low Blood Pressure (Hypotension)

Blood pressure is controlled by a combination of factors including the tone of the tiny muscles that surround arteries, how much fluid is inside of your blood vessels, and how hard your heart pumps. Babies have lower blood pressures than older children and adults. A healthy premature baby has even lower normal blood pressures than a healthy full-term baby. Defining exactly what blood pressure numbers are normal for any given baby is difficult and depends on the baby's gestational age, age after birth, and health condition. Although it seems like a very basic question, researchers are still trying to determine what a "normal" blood pressure is for a premature baby and how low a blood pressure can be before it needs treatment.

In the NICU, blood pressure is measured using a tiny blood pressure cuff attached to an electronic machine. If the health providers need to obtain frequent arterial blood samples or need continuous monitoring of your baby's blood pressure, they may place an arterial line. An arterial line is a special plastic catheter that is threaded into an artery and then attached to a continuous monitor. In the NICU, arterial lines are frequently placed into an artery in the wrist, ankle, or umbilical cord (see Chapter 2).

Treatment of Low Blood Pressure

If treatment is needed, your baby's medical providers will first try to identify which cause of low blood pressure is most likely. They may give additional fluid, called a *volume bolus,* in order to fill the blood vessels better. They may also give an intravenous (IV) medication like dopamine or dobutamine. These are medications that can increase tone in the tiny muscles around arteries, increase the strength of heart contractions, and increase the heart rate. These medications are often called *vasopressors* (or *pressors).* Occasionally, a premature infant's blood pressure remains very low despite receiving additional volume and vasopressors. In this case, a short course of IV steroids, such as hydrocortisone, may be used.

Problems Affecting the Gastrointestinal System

"We eventually figured out that Matthew would have good days and not-so-good days. On the good days, we would feel great. On the bad days, we knew we would just have to hold on until another good day came along."

The major organs of the gastrointestinal (GI) system are the stomach and the intestines (bowels). The GI system is responsible for processing food, absorbing nutrients, and removing waste in the baby's stool. Good nutrition is an essential component of your baby's care. Because the GI system is immature, your baby may have difficulty digesting food. Making sure that he can get enough food and fluid to support growth can be a challenge.

Fluid and Nutrition

The more premature a baby is, the more immature the GI function. These infants are born with limited protein and energy reserves. It is important to provide premature infants with good sources of nutrition, including protein, fat, carbohydrates (sugars), minerals, and vitamins, soon after birth. They use the proteins in their nutrition to build new tissues. Calories from fats and carbohydrates (sugars) provide the energy they need for the cells in their bodies to do their work. Minerals, like sodium, calcium, potassium, and magnesium, are important for all of the cells in the body to function normally. An infant's energy balance is the difference between the calories they receive from nutrition and the calories they use to make their body do its work. Whatever is left over can be stored for weight gain and future energy needs.

First "Feedings"

Each infant's fluid and nutrient needs are unique. Working from estimates of protein, carbohydrate, fat, vitamin, mineral, and water needs for infants of various gestational ages, care providers develop a plan for each baby. For example, some babies may lose more fluid through their thin skin and therefore need more water. Others may need more or less sugar to maintain a normal blood sugar level. Your baby may not be fed by mouth immediately after birth. Instead, he may receive all of his nutrition through an IV line. If a baby is not receiving feedings in their stomach, the health care team may say he is "NPO," which means "nothing by mouth."

Your baby's caregivers can put everything that he needs to grow into the IV line. At first, the IV may only include dextrose—a type of sugar. Premature infants often receive total parenteral nutrition (TPN). The word "parenteral" means that the nutrition enters the body through a blood vessel. Total parenteral nutrition includes a wide range of nutrients, including dextrose, protein, fat, minerals, and vitamins. Very premature infants may receive TPN on the very first day of life and others may receive TPN later if they cannot meet their nutritional needs with feedings alone. Additional information about IV fluids and TPN is provided in Chapter 5.

Beginning Oral Feedings

When your baby's physical condition is stable, he will start receiving nutrition from either breast milk or formula in his stomach. For some premature babies, this may occur on the first day of life. For others with more complicated problems it may be several days, a week, or even more. The initial feedings may be provided through a thin plastic or silicone tube placed in his nose or mouth and directed into his stomach. This method of feeding may be called *tube feeding* or *gavage feeding,* and the feeding tubes are frequently called *nasogastric* or *orogastric* tubes. Very premature infants may receive only tiny amounts of milk at first, less than a teaspoon, and their feedings may advance very slowly. Care providers may call these tiny feedings *minimal enteral nutrition, gut priming,* or *trophic feeds.* They are meant to prepare a baby's immature intestines for digesting nutrition. More mature infants without significant breathing problems (usually 33 weeks' gestation or more) may try nipple feeding by mouth, either breastfeeding or bottle feeding, shortly after birth.

Breast milk is the ideal nutrition for both full-term and premature infants. Although formulas have been developed to support the nutritional needs of premature infants, human breast milk has many unique properties that are particularly important for premature infants and cannot be replicated in formula. Some of the benefits of human breast milk include a lower risk of hospital-acquired infection, a lower risk of a serious GI complication (necrotizing enterocolitis), a lower risk of chronic lung disease, a shorter hospital stay, and improvements in developmental testing at school age. Recent studies have shown a relationship between the amount of breast milk that premature infants received and the

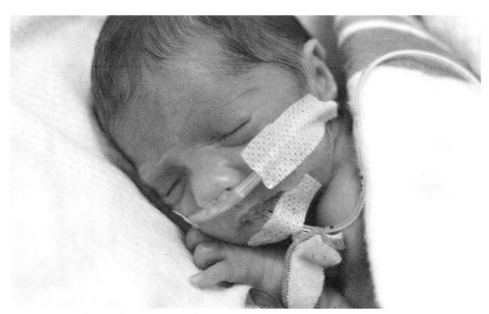

Orogastric tube and nasal cannula.
This narrow feeding tube is passed through the baby's mouth (orogastric tube) and into his stomach to provide gavage (tube) feedings. The tube is taped into place, eliminating the need for insertion and removal at every feeding. Also visible is the baby's nasal cannula, which delivers supplemental oxygen, secured over his cheek with tape.

Courtesy of Gigi O'Dea.

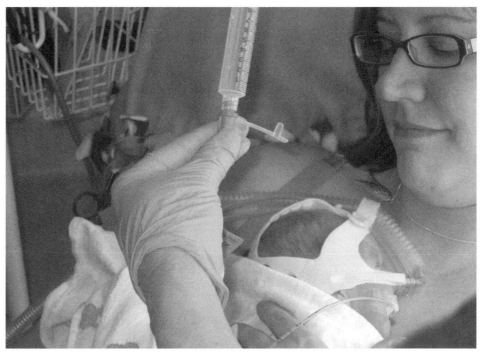

Gavage feeding during skin-to-skin care.
This baby finishes a gavage feeding through his orogastric tube while he and his mother enjoy skin-to-skin care. This baby is wearing a nasal CPAP device, pictured on page 227.

Courtesy of Seattle Children's Hospital.

degree of the potential benefits. Infants who received more breast milk had the lowest risk of serious complications. Because of these important benefits, the American Academy of Pediatrics strongly encourages mothers to breastfeed both full-term and premature infants. This can be more challenging for mothers of premature infants; however, there are significant benefits for your baby even if you can only provide a portion of his nutritional need with pumped (expressed) breast milk or if you can breastfeed only for a limited time. More details about feeding can be found in Chapter 5.

Feedings by Breast and Bottle

It is difficult to predict exactly when a premature baby will be successful with nipple feeding. It primarily depends on when your baby is able to coordinate sucking, swallowing, and breathing all at the same time. More premature babies and those that have ongoing breathing problems tend to have more difficulty learning to coordinate these steps. Even though twins are born at the same gestational age, they may master this skill at a different rate. Just as babies will learn to sit, stand, and walk at different ages, premature babies learn to feed by mouth at different ages. Your care providers may be able to give you an estimate based on his gestational age at birth, but remember that every baby is unique. Additional information about both breastfeeding and bottle feeding is provided in Chapter 5.

"I measured Katie's progress by how much weight she gained every week. I was so proud when she topped 3 pounds and her favorite nurse nicknamed her Cannonball."

Monitoring Growth

Weighing your baby is important for monitoring his growth. Factors that can influence weight gain include health status; activity level; energy needs; fluid, nutrient, and calorie intake; urine and stool output; and temperature regulation. Your infant's body length and head circumference are also important and will be measured periodically. Your baby's caregivers may plot your baby's growth—weight, length, and head circumference changes—on standard charts. Often, health care providers use the metric system for weights and length measurements because drug doses and other medical devices are based on this system. Appendix A contains a chart to help you convert grams to pounds and ounces and a chart for converting centimeters to inches. Chapter 5 has more information about feeding and growth, and Chapters 15 and 16 have information about feeding after your baby comes home.

Necrotizing Enterocolitis

Necrotizing enterocolitis (NEC) is an intestinal emergency where the cells lining the bowel wall become injured and swollen, and may die. The exact cause of NEC is unknown, but it primarily occurs in premature infants after they have started feeding. The initial injury

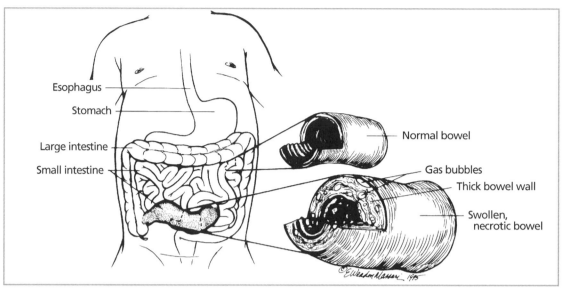

Necrotizing enterocolitis.
Enlargements of the gastrointestinal system show appearance of a section of normal bowel and a section of bowel with NEC. The bowel with NEC shows bubbles in the bowel wall, along with swelling and thickening of the bowel wall. Necrotizing enterocolitis can affect the small or large intestine.

may be caused by decreased blood flow or oxygen delivery to the premature bowel wall. Bacteria that are normally present in the bowel may invade the wall and cause further damage. Damage to the bowel wall may be minimal or quite extensive. In severe cases, the wall of the bowel may perforate (rupture), leading to peritonitis (infection of the abdominal cavity) and failure of multiple organ systems.

Risk Factors for Necrotizing Enterocolitis

Necrotizing enterocolitis is a disease that primarily affects premature infants; however, some term infants may also get NEC. The more premature an infant is at birth, the greater the risk of developing NEC. In the United States, NEC occurs in nearly 10% of babies with a birth weight less than 1,500 grams (3 pounds, 5 ounces). The reason that babies develop NEC is not completely understood, but NEC most often occurs after infants have begun feedings. Premature infants who receive breast milk have a significantly decreased risk of developing NEC. Infants who receive only breast milk seem to have a lower risk of NEC compared with those who receive either premature formula or a combination of formula and breast milk. Additional risk factors for NEC include

- Too little oxygen or blood reaching tissues (hypoxia and ischemia are discussed in Chapter 10)
- Low blood pressure
- Cold stress
- Receiving an exchange transfusion for high bilirubin
- PDA
- Polycythemia (high blood count)

Signs of Necrotizing Enterocolitis

Infants with NEC may show a variety of signs. The early signs of NEC may be very subtle, difficult to distinguish from other babies without NEC, and progress gradually. Other infants will have a sudden remarkable change in their abdomen and the signs will progress very quickly. Early signs include abdominal distention (swelling) and difficulty digesting feedings. Residuals from the previous feeding may remain in the stomach when it is time to start a new feeding. Feeding residuals, however, are very common among healthy premature infants, and the presence of a feeding residual by itself does not mean that your infant has or will develop NEC. Infants with NEC may have visibly enlarged loops of bowel, vomiting, blood in their stool, or decreased bowel sounds. There may be more general signs suggesting illness including a decrease in activity (lethargy), apnea, bradycardia, and abnormal body temperature.

Diagnosis of Necrotizing Enterocolitis

At the first signs of feeding problems, care providers will watch your baby very closely. They will check the amount of residuals in your baby's stomach and may test the stool for blood. If feeding problems continue or worsen, they will begin diagnostic tests for NEC.

The most common test for NEC is an abdominal x-ray. X-rays can identify bowel swelling and signs of gas in the bowel wall or the liver. Bacteria invading the injured bowel wall may produce gas, which appears as little bubbles on the x-ray. This sign is called *pneumatosis intestinalis* and confirms the diagnosis of NEC. Often, the x-ray shows mild abnormalities but does not definitely diagnose NEC. In this case, care providers may plan additional follow-up x-rays or an ultrasound in an attempt to confirm or rule out NEC. Caregivers may also obtain blood samples to check the blood count, platelet levels, blood gas tests, electrolytes (salts and minerals), and blood sugar levels. Samples of blood, urine, and spinal fluid may be sent to the laboratory in order to identify if an infection is present.

Treatment of Necrotizing Enterocolitis

Treatment for NEC depends on the severity of your baby's symptoms. If care providers have a suspicion of possible NEC without definite evidence, feedings may be stopped and antibiotics administered for 24 to 72 hours while additional tests are performed. When a baby is not receiving feedings in their stomach, caregivers may say he is "NPO." If the signs resolve and no evidence of NEC is found, feedings may be restarted and antibiotics stopped after this period of close observation. This is often called a *NEC scare*. If caregivers consider NEC to be likely, your baby may have feedings held and antibiotics administered for a week or longer. Initially, a tube will be passed through your baby's nose or mouth and into his stomach to drain any mucus or swallowed air and allow the

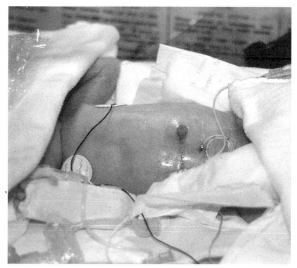

Ostomy site.
The dark circular opening on this baby's abdomen is the stoma (artificial opening) of his ostomy site. In this case, the ostomy (surgical opening into an organ) is into the intestine. The diseased portion of bowel has been removed, and a portion of the intestine has been brought to the surface and attached to the wall of the abdomen. An ostomy bag will fit over the opening to collect stool. An ostomy into the small intestine is called an *ileostomy*; into the large intestine, it is a *colostomy*.

bowel to rest. While he is NPO, your baby will receive TPN through an IV line or a central line.

Babies with NEC can be very ill and require close monitoring. X-rays may be done several times a day to check for rupture of the bowel wall ("free air"). Your baby may require additional oxygen or a ventilator for apnea. Additional fluids and medications (pressors) may be needed to maintain your baby's blood pressure. Blood and platelet transfusion may be required if your baby develops problems with blood clotting.

Most babies with NEC improve with medications alone. When babies respond to medications, they usually start to show signs of improvement within 48 to 72 hours. Approximately one-quarter to one-half of babies with NEC will continue to get sicker during the first 24 to 48 hours despite medications and will require surgical treatment.

Possible Complications of Necrotizing Enterocolitis

Rupture of the bowel wall is a serious complication of NEC that will require emergency surgery. Surgeons may initially place a small tube, called a *peritoneal drain,* in the abdomen to allow fluid and pus to drain out. Other infants may have an exploration of their abdomen where the surgeon opens the abdomen and removes portions of the bowel that are severely diseased or dead (necrotic). After surgery, babies may become very unstable and get progressively sicker. Despite antibiotics and surgery, some babies will not become better and will die.

After an open operation, your baby may come back from surgery with a temporary ostomy in place. An ostomy is a surgical opening on the surface of the baby's abdomen where the bowel has been attached so that it can drain and have more time to heal. Stool drains from the ostomy opening into a collecting bag. If the portion of bowel that is draining out of the abdominal wall comes from the large intestine, it is called a *colostomy*. If the opening is from the small intestine, it is called an *ileostomy* or *jejunostomy* (depending on the portion of small bowel that drains to the abdominal wall). The opening onto the abdominal skin surface is called a *stoma*. A second operation may be possible at a later time to reattach the healed portion of the bowel and close the ostomy. More information on colostomies, ileostomies, and jejunostomies can be found in Chapter 16.

Infants with severe NEC may need to have a large portion of their bowel removed. The amount of healthy bowel remaining after surgery may be quite short and unable to absorb enough nutrients and water from the baby's food. This is called *short bowel syndrome* or *short gut*. Babies with short gut require prolonged TPN and may need special formula and nutrient supplements. Short gut is a challenging problem with a high risk for serious complications.

Several weeks after NEC heals, the bowel wall that was diseased may develop scars that narrow the size of the bowel opening. Narrowing of the bowel is called a *stricture*. Infants with strictures will have difficulty tolerating their feedings. Their abdomen may become distended again and they may pass blood in their stool. These complications may require surgical treatment to remove the scarred and narrowed bowel segments.

Problems Affecting the Kidneys

Kidneys are the major organs in the renal system and are responsible for making urine. They play a major role in controlling how much water you have in your body and they help your body remove waste products and certain drugs from your bloodstream. Your kidneys also play a role in managing your blood pressure.

Kidney Function

At birth, your baby's kidneys do not function as well as yours do. In babies born after about 35 weeks' gestation, however, the kidneys mature rapidly during the first 2 weeks following birth. Kidney function takes longer to mature in babies born before 35 weeks' gestation because the kidney cells that adjust how urine is made are still in the process of forming.

"Wet" or "Dry"

Controlling the amount of water in the body can be a challenge for preterm infants. It is important to maintain just the right balance because having either too much water (fluid overload) or too little water (dehydration) can cause health problems. If a baby has too much water in the body, caregivers may say he is "wet." If he has too little water in the body, caregivers may say he is "dry."

Dehydration in premature babies has 2 main causes: (1) they lose water through their immature skin and (2) their kidneys cannot concentrate urine very well. Even when their bodies are running low on water, they continue to leak water out of their kidneys. Older infants and adults would make their urine very concentrated to save every drop of water. At the same time, premature infants also have difficulty getting rid of excess water—again, because of the immaturity of their renal system. To guard against both of these problems, care providers carefully measure how much fluid goes into your baby's body, how much urine comes out, and your baby's weight. Using all of this information, they calculate your baby's fluid needs carefully—to the drops needed per minute.

Electrolytes

Electrolytes or "lytes" are salts and minerals found in the blood, cells, and body fluids. They are critical to the functioning of all body cells. If the levels of electrolytes in the body are too high or too low, the cells will not function properly and the infant can become ill. Electrolytes are often referred to by their abbreviations: Na for sodium, K for potassium, Cl for chloride, HCO_3 for bicarbonate, Ca for calcium, P for phosphorus, and Mg for magnesium. Electrolytes enter the body from breast milk, formula, or IV fluids and are lost in the urine and stool. The kidney plays an important role in maintaining the right combination in blood by making adjustments to the amount of water and electrolytes lost in urine. The concentration of an electrolyte will be too low if the baby has either too much water in his blood or not enough of the electrolyte. Similarly, the concentration will be too high if the baby has either too little water or too much of the electrolyte in his blood. When referring to abnormal concentrations of an electrolyte, the staff may use the terms *hypo* (too low) or *hyper* (too high). For example, hypocalcemia means a low concentration of calcium in the blood. Very premature babies may lose excess water through their skin, making it more difficult for the kidneys to do their job correctly. Levels of electrolytes in your infant's blood will be monitored regularly so that care providers can make adjustments to your baby's feedings or IV fluids as needed.

Calcium

Calcium is a mineral that is critical for bone growth and development, heart function, blood clotting, muscle contraction, and other body processes. The fetus receives a steady supply of calcium from the mother, but the largest amount of calcium is transferred to the fetus during the last trimester of pregnancy. After birth, infant calcium levels fall over the first few days, then become stable. Your baby must now get calcium and other minerals from IV fluids or feedings.

Hypocalcemia

Hypocalcemia (low blood calcium) is a common finding during the first days of life in premature infants. It is most often caused by an interruption of the maternal supply of calcium across the placenta and relatively low levels of the hormone that controls calcium levels. Hypocalcemia occurring after the first week of life is less common and the causes are more complex. Late-onset hypocalcemia may be caused by abnormal hormone levels, renal failure, medications that cause the kidneys to lose calcium, and nutritional deficiencies.

Although hypocalcemia may be found during the first days of life by laboratory screening, most infants have no symptoms. Late onset hypocalcemia is more likely to be associated with symptoms, including low muscle tone, tremors, twitching, apnea, or seizures. Calcium levels tend to normalize after the first few days of life. Infants with very low calcium levels or with symptoms of hypocalcemia are treated with IV calcium.

Problems Affecting the Brain

The brain and nervous system begin developing during the third week of pregnancy, and their development continues well beyond the second year of life. The outer layer of the brain is called the *cerebral cortex* or *gray matter*. The gray matter houses the nuclei (central portions) for millions of cells called *neurons*. This is where thoughts begin and memories are stored. Underneath the cerebral cortex is the white matter where millions of thin filaments, called *axons*, carry electrical messages between neurons and into the spinal cord. You can think of the gray matter like computer chips and the white matter like the wires and cables carrying data. The lower portion of the brain is called the *brain stem*. It is responsible for many of our reflexes and vital body functions such as breathing. Ultimately, many of the messages that started in the gray matter and brain stem will be carried into the spinal cord and then out to nerves throughout the body. Messages from the body, such as temperature and pain sensations, are carried into the spinal cord along nerves and then find their way to the cerebral cortex. Deep within the brain are a series of chambers called *ventricles*. A clear fluid, called *cerebrospinal fluid* (spinal fluid) or *CSF,* is produced within the ventricles and circulates around the brain and spinal cord providing a cushion of protection. The brain uses a significant amount of energy and needs a constant supply of blood, nutrition, and oxygen. Because the brain is so complex and it is still developing at the time of premature birth, it is vulnerable to injury from many different causes.

Brain Hemorrhage

Hemorrhage is the medical term for bleeding. Germinal matrix and intraventricular hemorrhages are 2 types of bleeding within the baby's brain.

An area in the developing brain called the *germinal matrix,* near the floor of the ventricles, makes both new neurons and the cells that support them. This area may also be called the *subependymal region.* Blood vessels in the germinal matrix carry a large amount of blood and are very fragile. During the hours before and after premature birth, changes in blood flow may cause these vessels to break and bleed. When bleeding occurs, the blood initially collects in the germinal matrix and may spill into the adjacent ventricle.

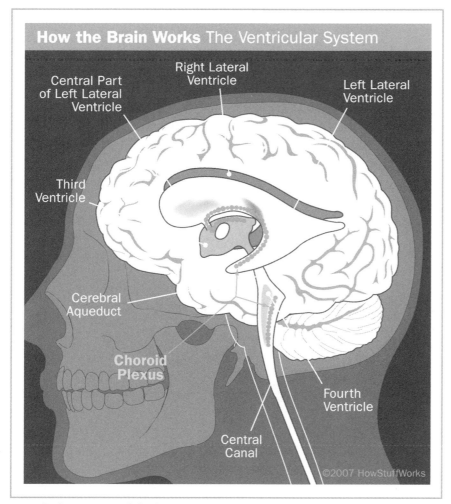

Ventricular system of the brain.
Chambers called *ventricles* are deep within the brain. Cerebrospinal fluid is produced within the ventricles. If the infant bleeds in his brain, blood may spill into the ventricles.

Reprinted courtesy of HowStuffWorks.com.

Risk Factors for Germinal Matrix Hemorrhage or Intraventricular Hemorrhage

The greatest risk of bleeding causing a germinal matrix (GM) or intraventricular hemorrhage (IVH) is on the first day of life, and nearly all bleeding (75%) occurs during the first 3 days of life. If a premature baby has not had a GM or IVH by the end of the first week of life, it is very unlikely that it will occur. The risk of GM/IVH is directly related to the degree of prematurity and birth weight. Babies born at 27 to 28 weeks' gestation or weighing 900 grams (2 pounds) to 1,200 grams (2 pounds, 10 ounces) have a risk near 20% to 25% (1 out of 4–5 chance) of developing a hemorrhage. Smaller and more premature babies have both a higher risk of bleeding and higher risk of the more severe grades of hemorrhage. The germinal matrix matures between 32 to 36 weeks' gestation, significantly decreasing the risk of this type of bleeding in the brain.

Symptoms of Germinal Matrix or Intraventricular Hemorrhage

Most commonly, babies with a developing GM/IVH have no symptoms. They may have subtle changes in their behavior, activity, or muscle tone, or a decrease in their hematocrit (blood count). Premature infants without hemorrhages may also have these symptoms, making it very hard to identify infants with an IVH by physical examination alone. If the hemorrhage is large, the baby may have a sudden change in his condition with seizures, loss of consciousness, apnea (breathing pauses), bradycardia (low heart rate), and a bulging fontanel (the soft spot on the top of the baby's head).

Diagnosis of Germinal Matrix or Intraventricular Hemorrhage

Germinal matrix and IVHs are diagnosed using an ultrasound scan of the brain. Many NICUs routinely perform an ultrasound during a very premature baby's first or second week of life even if there are no symptoms. The ultrasound scanner is placed over the baby's fontanel and sound waves are used to create images of the baby's brain. Ultrasound does not expose the baby to any radiation. These images can show the presence and extent of bleeding. If there is bleeding, it will be assigned a grade from 1 to 4 based on the amount of bleeding, its location, and the presence of dilation (swelling or enlargement) of the ventricles. Grade 1 is the smallest amount of bleeding (GM only), Grade 2 means that the bleeding has extended into the adjacent ventricle, and Grade 3 bleeding means that the blood has entered the ventricles and the ventricle is dilated. Bleeding into the substance of the brain that is separate from the GM and ventricle may be called an *intraparenchymal hemorrhage,* a *Grade 4 hemorrhage,* or *periventricular hemorrhagic infarction.* Babies with this type of bleeding frequently also have a large IVH. If bleeding is present, its progress and the reabsorption of blood will be monitored with additional ultrasounds.

Complications of Germinal Matrix or Intraventricular Hemorrhage

Most hemorrhages (75%) are mild (Grade 1) or moderate (Grade 2), and nearly 90% of these will resolve with few short-term problems. A small percentage of infants (less than 10%) with mild or moderate hemorrhages may develop a blockage of CSF in their brains causing dilation of their ventricles. This is called *hydrocephalus* or *water on the brain* (see page 252).

Some infants with mild or moderate hemorrhages (15%–25%) will go on to develop neurologic problems including cerebral palsy or learning disabilities. More severe hemorrhages result in more significant short- and long-term problems. Nearly 75% of babies (3 out of 4) with Grade 3 or 4 hemorrhages will develop hydrocephalus.

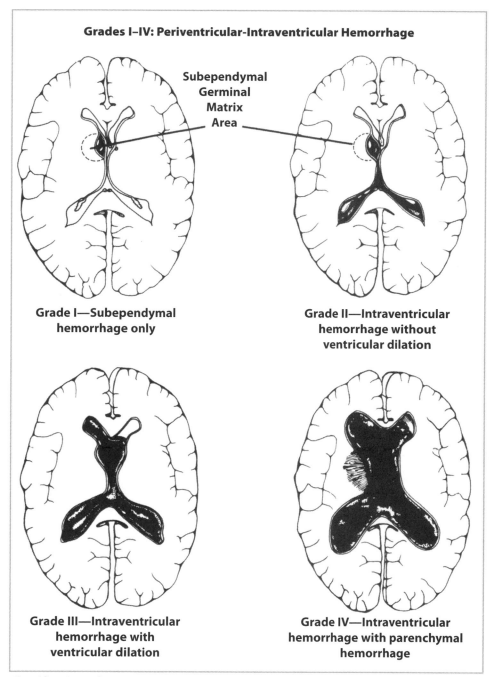

Grades I–IV: Periventricular-Intraventricular Hemorrhage

Subependymal
Germinal
Matrix
Area

Grade I—Subependymal
hemorrhage only

Grade II—Intraventricular
hemorrhage without
ventricular dilation

Grade III—Intraventricular
hemorrhage with
ventricular dilation

Grade IV—Intraventricular
hemorrhage with parenchymal
hemorrhage

Classification of IVH.
Diagrams show views of IVHs, looking down into the brain structure.

From: Rozmus C. Periventricular-intraventricular hemorrhage in the newborn. Matern Child Nurs. 1992;17:79. Reprinted by permission of Wolters/Kluwer Health.

Between 50% and 75% of babies (2–3 out of 4) with Grade 3 or 4 hemorrhages will develop long-term problems. Long-term problems may include cerebral palsy, hearing loss, vision loss, and learning disabilities.

Hydrocephalus

Your baby's brain and spinal cord are surrounded by CSF. This clear fluid is constantly made by spongy tissue inside of the ventricles. It circulates around the brain, drains through a series of canals, and then circulates around the spinal cord. Finally, the fluid is reabsorbed by a membrane in the nervous system called the *arachnoid*. Hydrocephalus literally means "water on the brain." It occurs when the circulation of CSF is blocked or when its reabsorption is impaired. Following an IVH, the blood in the CSF may block the drainage system or scar the membrane responsible for its reabsorption. The CSF backs up in the ventricles causing them to expand and push on the surrounding brain tissue. The baby's fontanel may bulge and the skull bones may enlarge. If left untreated, the continued accumulation of fluid and pressure can cause damage to the tissue of the brain. Treatment may include surgical placement of a ventricular shunt.

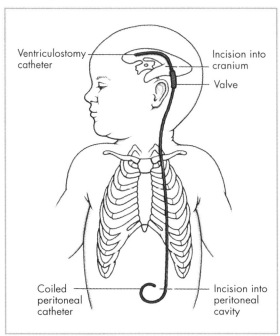

Ventricular shunt.
A ventricular shunt may be needed to drain excess CSF and relieve the pressure in the ventricles of the brain of a baby with hydrocephalus.

From: Hill CJ. Nursing Management of Children. Servonsky J, Opas SR, eds. Sudbury, MA: Jones & Bartlett; 1987:1297. www.jbpub.com. Reprinted by permission.

Hydrocephalus may also develop if the flow of CSF is blocked by a malformation (birth defect). See page 279 for additional information on treatment of hydrocephalus.

Periventricular Leukomalacia

Periventricular leukomalacia (PVL) means abnormal development of the white matter of the brain near the ventricles. The white portion of the brain is made of fibers that carry electrical messages between the brain cells and the nerves in the spinal cord. These fibers are prone to injury from a number of different causes including lack of blood flow or oxygen at a vulnerable time during development. Periventricular leukomalacia may be seen by ultrasound, computed tomography (CT) scan, or magnetic resonance imaging (MRI) and may look like small cysts or holes in the brain tissue. Even though the injury that caused PVL may have occurred before or shortly after birth, PVL may not appear on imaging for several weeks after birth. Infants with PVL have a high risk of developing cerebral palsy.

Cerebral Palsy

Cerebral palsy (CP) is not a disease. It is a general term that describes an abnormality of posture, tone, or coordination of body movements resulting from damage to the brain. Cerebral palsy specifically refers to motor (movement) problems, not cognition (thought) problems. However, many children who have CP also have seizures and mental deficiency. People with CP can have muscles that are either weak and floppy (hypotonic), or stiff and rigid (spastic).

The cause of CP is not always clear. Risk factors for the development of CP in some babies include lack of blood flow or oxygen to the brain, prematurity, severe IVH, infection, or PVL. Overall, approximately 5% to 10% of babies delivered weighing less than 1,500 grams (3 pounds, 5 ounces) will develop CP. The risk increases with the degree of prematurity and with evidence of brain injuries. Cerebral palsy also occurs in some term infants, even those with no risk factors, but the incidence is very low.

In premature babies, the portions of the brain that are most likely to be affected are the nerves that control movement in the lower legs. Affected babies may have tight leg muscles with poor coordination and brisk reflexes. As the degree of CP worsens, muscles controlling the neck, chest, and arms may be affected. Some babies may have involvement of the face, tongue, and speech area. Children with CP often have poor balance and difficulty walking. They may develop stiff joints (contractures), curving of the spine (scoliosis), turned out ankles, and problems with their hips. Although the presence of CP does not mean that there is a problem with intelligence, some infants with CP will also have learning disabilities.

Diagnosis of Cerebral Palsy

It is difficult to predict a baby's long-term outcome in the first year of life. The diagnosis of CP is not usually made until 12 to 18 months of age. Criteria for diagnosis are based on the baby's age. In the follow-up clinic, developmental clinic, or doctor's office, your premature baby will be tested for such things as muscle tone and strength, reflexes, posture and balance, quality and type of movements, ability to achieve normal gross motor milestones (sitting, crawling, walking), and fine motor movements (grasping). Some early motor problems will be monitored and may resolve on their own. Abnormalities that do not resolve may lead to the diagnosis of CP.

Treatment of Cerebral Palsy

If your baby is diagnosed with abnormal muscle tone, a team of health care professionals will follow him closely. Occupational or physical therapists may provide you with special exercises for your child and activities to aid with muscle development and to lessen complications. In some cases, surgery may be needed to correct muscle tightness. See Chapter 17 for more information about CP and developmental follow-up.

Problems Affecting the Eyes

Your baby's eyes begin to develop during the first month after conception, but the development is not complete until after birth. The eye functions like a camera. Light enters through a thin, clear membrane called the *cornea* and is focused by the lens. The middle of the eyeball is filled with a jelly-like substance that helps the eyeball maintain its shape. The back of the eye has a thin lining called the *retina* that works like the film in a camera. Messages from the retina are carried to a nerve at the back of the eye and then to the brain for processing.

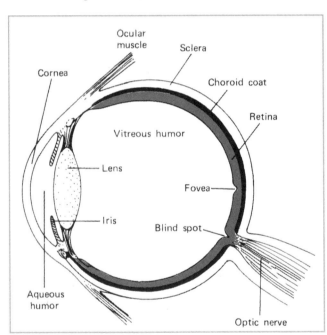

Normal eye anatomy.
The lens is at the front of the eye, on the left of the diagram. The retina lines the back of the eye, on the right of the diagram.

From: Burke S. Human Anatomy & Physiology in Health and Disease, *3E. ©1992 Delmar Learning, a part of Cengage Learning, Inc. Reproduced by permission. www.cengage.com/permissions.*

The eyelids in very preterm babies (less than 26 weeks) may be fused shut at birth but usually open within a few days to a week after delivery. Once open, your baby's eyes can see an object 8 to 10 inches away from his face but will be quite sensitive to bright light. All babies prefer the human face and black and white patterns, but premature babies may find visual stimulation overwhelming.

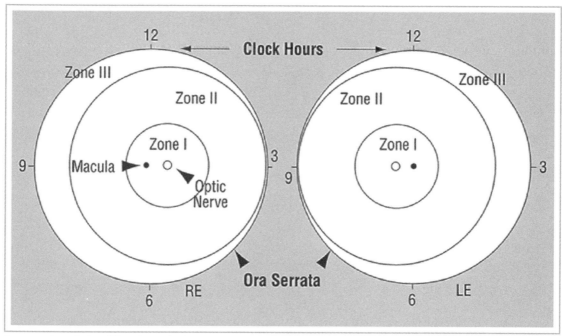

International classification of ROP.
This diagram describes the location and extent of ROP by dividing the retina into 3 circular zones. Immature retinal vessels begin growing near the optic disc in Zone I and gradually progress through Zones II and III. ROP in Zone I, the area of central vision, is more serious than ROP limited to Zones II or III.

From: Fleck BW, McIntosh N. Retinopathy of prematurity: recent developments. NeoReviews. *2009;10:e20–e30.*

Retinopathy of Prematurity

Retinopathy of prematurity (ROP) is a disease that occurs when abnormal blood vessels grow and spread throughout the developing retina. The retina begins developing around 16 weeks of gestation. It starts at the back of the eye and gradually spreads along the inside of the eyeball. The retina is made of living cells and needs a network of blood vessels to develop along with it. The process of retinal development continues until near a baby's due date.

Shortly after premature birth, the normal growth of the retina and its blood vessels temporarily stops. Although we do not fully understand why this happens, one factor is the rapid change in the amount of oxygen in the baby's blood that follows birth. Babies in the womb receive much less oxygen than after they are born. After several weeks, the retina and blood vessels begin to grow again but the blood vessels may not grow normally. There may be rapid irregular growth of new vessels. These abnormal blood vessels are fragile and can leak, scarring the retina and pulling it out of position. If the retina is pulled away from the back of the eye it is called a *retinal detachment*. Retinal detachment is the main cause of severe visual impairment and blindness in ROP.

Risk Factors for Retinopathy of Prematurity

Retinopathy of prematurity is usually seen only in babies less than 30 weeks' gestational age. After that, the retinal vessels have developed enough that they are not at risk. The risk of ROP increases with decreasing gestational age and birth weight. More than half of babies delivered less than 27 weeks' gestation will develop some degree of ROP. Other factors contributing to the risk of ROP include anemia, blood transfusions, respiratory distress, breathing difficulties, and the baby's overall health. Because the cause of ROP is not fully understood, it is not yet possible to keep babies from developing this disorder, nor is it possible to predict which babies will develop ROP.

Higher levels of blood oxygen are thought to play some role in the development of ROP. Because of this association, health care providers in the NICU carefully monitor the blood oxygen saturations for all premature babies receiving oxygen. They will try to ensure that the baby receives enough oxygen to support his body's needs while limiting excess oxygen that may contribute to ROP. Most NICUs have target oxygen saturations for each individual baby that they hope to maintain as long as the baby is receiving supplemental oxygen. In real life, this is very difficult to do as babies often have fluctuating oxygen levels.

Even still, ROP develops in some babies with lower oxygen levels and does not develop in some babies with higher oxygen levels. There have even been cases of ROP in babies who did not receive supplemental oxygen at all.

Diagnosis of Retinopathy of Prematurity

Babies born at less than 30 weeks' gestation or less than 1,500 grams (3 pounds, 5 ounces) usually have their eyes examined by an ophthalmologist (eye specialist) when they are approximately 4 weeks old. Some infants weighing 1,500 to 2,000 grams or delivered between

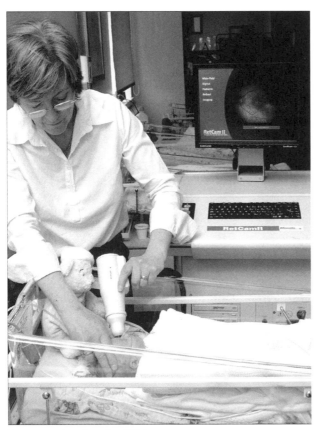

Eye examination for ROP.
Wide-field camera in use for ROP screening examination.

Reprinted with permission of NeoReviews. 2009;10(1):e20.

30 and 32 weeks will be examined if their physician thinks they are at risk. In some institutions, photographs of the retina are taken with a special camera and electronically sent to an ophthalmologist for evaluation. Before the eye examination, drops will be placed in the baby's eyes to enlarge (dilate) the pupils so that the retina can be viewed. The ophthalmologist uses a special lens to look into the eyes and evaluate the progress of retinal development. The ophthalmologist may simply say that the retina is still immature. This means that no ROP was seen; however, the retina and its blood vessels are still developing and are at risk of ROP. If abnormal blood vessels are seen, the ophthalmologist will describe the ROP according to a standard system. The description includes both a number that describes the severity of the condition (stage) and a description of which portion of the retina is involved (zone). The term *PLUS disease* is used if the ophthalmologist sees very aggressive ROP with thick and twisted blood vessels. Retinopathy of prematurity may involve only one eye or both. Depending on the maturity of the retina and the presence of ROP, the ophthalmologist will schedule additional follow-up examinations.

Treatment of Retinopathy of Prematurity

In mild cases, ROP resolves by itself and leaves no permanent damage. About 90% of all infants with ROP have mild disease and do not need treatment. Infants with mild ROP are still at risk of vision problems like myopia (nearsightedness), strabismus (crossed eyes), amblyopia (lazy eye), and glaucoma.

Infants with more severe disease can develop impaired vision or even blindness and may require intervention with laser surgery. With this treatment, a laser beam directed into the eye destroys the peripheral (outer) areas of the retina, slowing or reversing the abnormal vessel growth. By destroying the peripheral retina, the laser treatment will destroy some of the baby's peripheral vision. The goal of laser surgery, however, is to prevent retinal detachments and save the baby's most important central (straight ahead) vision. Infants who require laser surgery will receive sedatives to keep them calm and still during the treatment. Infants with the most advanced ROP who have suffered a retinal detachment may need additional surgery.

Problems Affecting the Immune System

Our immune system protects us from infection. The body has multiple defense mechanisms to prevent things like bacteria and viruses from invading. Because the defense mechanisms of babies are still immature, infants are at greater risk for developing an infection than are older children or adults. Also, because of their immature defense mechanisms, such as their skin and mucous membranes, babies tend to develop a general infection (sepsis) rather than a local (limited) infection. On the other hand, because the immune system is immature, babies are less likely to develop adverse reactions to drugs or blood transfusions.

Why Premature Babies Are at Risk

Physical barriers, including skin and the mucous membranes that line the respiratory and GI systems, help to keep potential invaders out. If foreign bodies get past these physical barriers, white blood cells, antibodies, and other substances in the blood are called to find and attack them. Premature infants are at greater risk of developing infections because all of these defense mechanisms are immature. Their skin does not form a complete barrier, their white blood cells are not as effective at killing invaders, and they have fewer antibodies in their blood. Babies receive antibodies from their mothers during the third trimester of pregnancy, and many premature babies are born before these antibodies are transferred across the placenta. Some of the medical equipment and procedures that premature babies need to survive, including plastic breathing tubes, feeding tubes, and IV lines, interfere with their protective barriers and increase the risk of infections.

Signs of Infection

Signs of infection in premature babies are often subtle and not very specific. Because the temperature regulating center in the brain is immature, premature babies frequently do not have a fever when they have an infection. They may have a low temperature (hypothermia) or no change in their temperature at all. Other signs associated with infection in premature infants include poor feeding, irritability, lethargy (lack of energy), respiratory distress, apnea, and abdominal distention. None of these signs are specific for infection; they may be a sign of another problem or just a temporary change in the baby's behavior. Sometimes it can be very difficult for care providers to decide if changes in a baby's condition are being caused by an infection or some other reason.

Hospital-Acquired (Nosocomial) Infections

While the equipment and invasive procedures used in the NICU can be lifesaving for very premature infants, they may also increase the risk of developing hospital-acquired (nosocomial) infections. Within hours of birth, all newborns' skin, respiratory, and GI tracts become covered or "colonized" with bacteria. Colonization with bacteria cannot be prevented and does not reflect either poor cleanliness in the NICU or inadequate nursing care. In most circumstances, colonizing bacteria don't cause infection because they are prevented from invading beyond the protective barriers of the skin and the mucous membranes lining the respiratory and GI tracts. When babies require invasive equipment or procedures, however, colonizing bacteria on the skin and mucous membranes have the opportunity to get past the defensive barriers and cause infection. Approximately one-third of babies delivered at less than 28 weeks' gestation will develop a hospital-acquired infection during their stay. Infants delivered more prematurely and at lower birth weights have the highest risk.

The most common cause of hospital-acquired bacterial infection in the NICU is a type of staphylococcus called *Staphylococcus epidermidis.* The NICU team may refer to these bacteria as *coag negative staph* or *CONS.* Infections due to *S epidermidis* can occur any time during a hospital stay, but tend to occur between the second and fourth week of life. Risk factors for this type of infection include the presence of central IV catheters, TPN, and mechanical ventilation. The bacteria colonize the baby's skin, contaminate the outer portion of IV lines, and may track down the catheter causing blood infection. *S epidermidis* can also cause pneumonia, meningitis (infection of the spinal fluid), and skin infections. Most infants with *S epidermidis* infection do not develop sudden or extreme signs of infection. Instead, they may gradually have more episodes of apnea or feeding intolerance. Sometimes parents and care providers say, "He just isn't acting right today." The NICU team may perform a "sepsis workup" where they obtain samples of blood, spinal fluid, and urine to send to the laboratory for culture. At times, it can be difficult to determine if a baby truly has an infection with *S epidermidis* if only a single blood culture becomes positive because the bacteria colonize the baby's skin and can contaminate the blood culture bottle resulting in a false-positive test. On the other hand, the blood culture may be negative but the baby appears to truly have an infection. A false-negative test may occur because the samples of blood are small and the bacteria may not always grow in a laboratory culture. The health care team must use their best judgment to determine which infants need treatment and how long the treatment will be continued.

S epidermidis infections are treated with an IV antibiotic called *vancomycin.* Frequently central IV catheters must be removed in order to successfully treat the infection. The risk of dying from an *S epidermidis* infection is approximately 10%. Although most infants recover from the infection, it is a setback in their progress and frequently increases the length of their hospital stay.

Other bacteria, viruses, and yeast can cause late-onset infections among premature babies in the NICU. Some of these infections can be quite severe, with a high risk of death or serious complications. Additional information about infections and the organisms that cause them can be found in Chapter 10 (beginning on page 322).

Problems Affecting the Blood

The hematologic system includes the blood, bone marrow, and liver. Whole blood includes many different components. Red blood cells (RBCs) carry oxygen from the lungs to the cells. White blood cells (WBCs) are important components of the body's defense against infection. Platelets play an important role in blood clotting. Plasma is the liquid portion of blood and contains proteins, electrolytes, and other substances. Bone marrow is the spongy substance in the middle of the bones that makes blood cells. During fetal life and the early portion of a very premature infant's life, the liver also makes blood cells. At birth, a premature infant's blood has all of these components. Their function and quantities, however, differ from those of full-term newborns and older children. The normal quantities of each blood component vary widely depending on your baby's gestational age at birth and continue to change during the first several weeks after birth.

Anemia

Anemia means that there is a decrease in the number of circulating RBCs in a baby's blood. Hemoglobin is the molecule within RBCs that actually carries oxygen. Health care providers often monitor the amount of RBCs in blood by measuring the hemoglobin level. Another way to describe the amount of hemoglobin in blood is *hematocrit* or *crit*. Hematocrit is the percentage of RBCs in whole blood.

Causes of Anemia

Anemia is a very common problem and has multiple causes. Newborns are particularly at risk of anemia because their RBCs have a shorter life span and their bone marrow has a limited ability to make new blood cells. In general, anemia is caused by either blood loss, destruction of blood cells within the body, or a decrease in blood production. In total, an infant's body contains approximately 80 milliliters of blood for every kilogram (2 pounds, 3 ounces) of body weight. Using this estimate, a 1.5-kilogram (3 pound, 5 ounce) baby has approximately 120 milliliters, or 4 ounces, of blood. Blood may be lost before or during delivery because of a problem with the placenta. Internal bleeding may cause sudden severe blood loss. During the first few weeks of life, blood may be gradually lost if a baby requires frequent laboratory tests. Infection, blood group incompatibility between the baby and mother (see Chapter 8), or inherited abnormalities of the blood cells can lead to blood destruction both before and after birth. A very common cause of anemia in premature infants is a decrease in RBC production called *anemia of prematurity*.

Anemia of Prematurity

Anemia of prematurity occurs because RBC production temporarily stops after birth. A hormone called *erythropoietin* (EPO) is made in your baby's liver and kidney. Erythropoietin stimulates RBC production in the bone marrow. Shortly after birth, EPO production stops and the bone marrow stops making RBCs. Hemoglobin levels gradually decrease over several weeks, reaching their lowest value between 4 to 10 weeks after birth. Eventually, the hemoglobin reaches a level where EPO is secreted again and RBC production resumes. This is a process that occurs even in full-term infants; however, it occurs earlier, lasts longer, and is more severe in premature infants.

Signs of Anemia

If anemia occurs very suddenly because of a rapid blood loss, babies may have signs of "shock" with a low blood pressure, fast heart rate, weak pulse, pale or ashen gray color, and respiratory distress. Anemia of prematurity causes a more gradual decrease in RBCs and may cause no symptoms at all. Infants with symptomatic anemia of prematurity may have a pale color to their skin and gums. They may have poor growth, decreased activity, a rapid heart rate, rapid breathing, an increase in apnea events, or feeding difficulties.

Diagnosis of Anemia

A blood sample is used to measure the hemoglobin or hematocrit. If the cause of anemia is not readily apparent, the NICU team may order additional diagnostic tests to look for evidence of bleeding or RBC destruction. Infants with anemia of prematurity may have their hemoglobin and hematocrit levels monitored regularly to ensure that their hemoglobin level does not fall too low. A blood reticulocyte level may be checked intermittently to monitor how quickly the bone marrow is making new RBCs.

Treatment of Anemia of Prematurity

Infants without symptoms may not require any treatment. They may receive additional iron in their diet to ensure enough iron stores to support RBC production once it begins. Some hospitals will give regular injections of EPO in order to prevent or treat anemia of prematurity; however, this practice remains controversial and is not routinely practiced in the United States. Infants with symptomatic anemia may require one or more blood transfusions.

The likelihood of requiring a blood transfusion is related to the degree of prematurity at birth. More premature infants, and those with more significant health problems, have a greater risk of requiring transfusions. There is no single criterion for receiving a blood transfusion. Researchers continue to investigate the risks and benefits of different blood transfusion practices. Currently, more than half of babies born under 28 weeks' gestation will receive at least one blood transfusion.

Jaundice

Red blood cells have a relatively short life span. When the body breaks down old RBCs, a substance called *bilirubin* is released. Before the body can dispose of the bilirubin, a chemical reaction in the liver must change (convert) the form released—called *indirect bilirubin*—into the form called *direct bilirubin*. A special protein, called an *enzyme*, speeds up the rate of this conversion process. Once direct bilirubin is formed, it is transferred to the intestines for removal with the baby's bowel movements. Some of the direct bilirubin that arrives in the intestine is converted back to indirect bilirubin and reabsorbed into the bloodstream. This is called *entero-hepatic circulation.* This recirculation of indirect bilirubin is increased in breastfed infants, infants who receive antibiotics, and those with delayed bowel movements.

Before birth, the fetus transfers indirect bilirubin across the placenta, and the mother's liver manages its disposal. The enzyme that the baby's liver requires for the conversion reaction is not very active at the time of birth. In other words, it takes a few days for the conversion reaction to "turn on." Until the liver can convert a large amount of indirect bilirubin into direct bilirubin, the indirect form may build up in a newborn's blood. Some of this bilirubin may leave the blood, deposit in the skin tissue, and cause jaundice (yellow skin color).

Physiologic Jaundice

In most infants, indirect bilirubin levels reach their peak toward the end of the first week of life and then gradually fall over the next 1 to 2 weeks. The peak level is higher in preterm infants and may remain elevated for longer. This type of jaundice is very common, occurring in nearly half of full-term infants and up to 80% of preterm infants. It is not the same type of jaundice that occurs in older individuals and it does not mean that something is wrong with your baby's liver. It is simply a result of your infant's immature liver function and is called *physiologic jaundice*. Physiologic jaundice does not require any treatment.

Hyperbilirubinemia

An infant whose indirect bilirubin level rises higher or faster than normal has a condition called *hyperbilirubinemia.* Hyperbilirubinemia may be caused simply by an exaggeration of the normal physiologic process that causes high bilirubin levels in the newborn. The enzyme controlling the speed of the conversion reaction in the liver takes longer to "turn on" in premature infants and may cause bilirubin to increase above "physiologic" levels. It may also be caused by excessive production of bilirubin, slower than normal conversion in the liver, or increased reabsorption in the intestines. Anything that causes more RBCs to break down, such as bruising during birth, increases the amount of bilirubin that the liver must handle. Blood type incompatibility between the mother and baby is

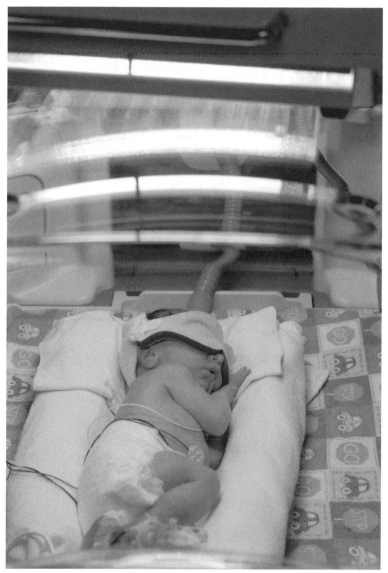

Phototherapy for hyperbilirubinemia.
The phototherapy light is a common sight in the NICU. (The hose at the end of the isolette is not attached to the baby.)

Courtesy of University of Washington Medical Center, Seattle, WA.

another cause of increased RBC breakdown. The most common type of incompatibility occurs when the mother is type O and the baby is type A. Antibodies created by the mother's immune system enter the baby's bloodstream and destroy RBCs. Other problems, such as infection, may alter liver function and cause a rapid increase in bilirubin levels. If your infant is at risk for hyperbilirubinemia, his bilirubin levels will be monitored.

If the bilirubin level reaches a point that requires treatment, phototherapy will be started. Phototherapy is a treatment that uses blue-green light waves to change the shape of the indirect bilirubin molecule so that it can be eliminated in the baby's urine or stool without requiring the conversion reaction.

Patches are commonly placed over a baby's eyes during phototherapy to shield them from the bright light. In very premature babies, phototherapy may be started shortly after birth to prevent bilirubin concentrations from reaching high levels. Most infants that require treatment for hyperbilirubinemia can be successfully treated with phototherapy. Infrequently, phototherapy cannot adequately control the bilirubin level. In this case, an exchange transfusion may be necessary. During this procedure, a calculated amount of the baby's blood is withdrawn through an umbilical catheter and replaced with fresh blood from a compatible blood donor.

With appropriate management, hyperbilirubinemia causes no long-term effects. The primary reason that hyperbilirubinemia is a concern is that bilirubin is a molecule that can cross the brain's protective barrier. If excessively high levels of bilirubin pass into the brain, it can cause a disorder called *kernicterus* and result in permanent brain damage. Kernicterus is a very rare problem in the United States.

Problems Affecting Metabolism

Metabolic processes refer to the chemical reactions in your body that convert the nutrients in foods into substances that cells can use to function. Premature babies frequently have trouble regulating portions of their metabolism. In particular, your baby may initially have trouble managing his blood sugar. Your baby uses glucose (sugar) to produce energy for cells. Before birth, mothers provide their fetus with a constant supply of glucose across the placenta. The fetus uses this glucose for energy and growth. During the last trimester of pregnancy, full-term infants have the chance to store some glucose, in a form called *glycogen,* as a reserve for use during and after birth. When the umbilical cord is cut, the supply of glucose is interrupted and the newborn has to depend on either stored glucose or glucose provided from breast milk, formula, or IV fluid. In full-term infants, the blood glucose level falls during the first few hours after birth and then stabilizes as their body forms glucose from substances like protein and fat. Premature infants often have difficulty stabilizing their blood sugar after birth. Infants of diabetic mothers are also at risk for blood sugar difficulties (see Chapter 8).

Hypoglycemia

Hypoglycemia means "low blood sugar." It develops in preterm babies for 2 major reasons: (1) they have smaller stores of glycogen (stored glucose) than full-term babies and (2) their immature livers cannot easily produce glucose from substances such as fat and protein. Premature infants whose mothers received medications to stop preterm labor occasionally develop hypoglycemia as a response to those drugs. Premature infants that required significant resuscitation at birth or became very cold also have an increased risk of hypoglycemia.

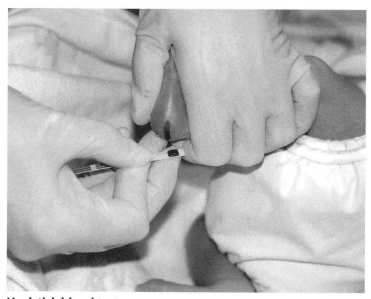

Heelstick blood test.
The baby's heel is pricked, and a drop or two of blood is used to screen his blood sugar.

Signs of Hypoglycemia

The signs of hypoglycemia can be very subtle and are not very specific. Some infants may not have any signs. The common signs of hypoglycemia include tremors or jitters, irregular breathing, and decreased muscle tone. Because the signs of hypoglycemia are nonspecific or may be absent, any baby who is at risk for hypoglycemia is carefully monitored. One monitoring method is to test a drop of blood from the baby's finger, heel, or toe using a small meter at the baby's bedside. If the test indicates a low blood sugar, an additional sample may be sent to the laboratory.

Treatment of Hypoglycemia

Hypoglycemia is treated with either feeding (breast milk or formula) or IV dextrose (sugar). If a preterm baby has persistent hypoglycemia, a high concentration of dextrose may be delivered through an IV placed in a large blood vessel (central line) instead of a peripheral IV.

Hyperglycemia

Hyperglycemia means "high blood sugar." Although low blood sugar is common immediately after birth in premature infants, they may have problems with hyperglycemia after they begin receiving IV fluids. Insulin is a hormone made by the pancreas that controls blood sugar. A very premature infant may develop hyperglycemia because his pancreas cannot produce enough insulin to manage the sugar contained in the IV fluids. Some premature infants make enough insulin but their tissues do not respond normally to the insulin. Some medications, like caffeine and steroids, can cause hyperglycemia. Premature infants may also develop hyperglycemia as a response to stress. New onset hyperglycemia may occur following surgery or it may be a sign of an infection.

Neonatal diabetes is very rare. When a premature infant has hyperglycemia, it does not mean that he has or will develop diabetes.

Hypertriglyceridemia

Triglycerides are a type of fat measured in the bloodstream. When infants are receiving TPN, they will usually be receiving a continuous IV infusion of fat. Premature infants frequently have difficulty fully metabolizing fats, and their blood triglyceride level may increase. Caregivers may need to temporarily decrease the dose of fat infused.

Newborn Metabolic Screen

All states require that newborns have a sample of blood sent to the state laboratory to screen for a wide range of metabolic and endocrine (hormone) diseases. The blood test is usually obtained within the first 3 days of life and is placed on a special piece of cardboard that is mailed to a state laboratory. Most of these diseases are rare, and it is important to identify them and begin treatment early. It is common for premature newborns to have an "abnormal" metabolic screen because the normal values are based on full-term newborns. Premature newborns have different normal values and frequently receive nutritional supplements in their TPN that appear abnormal on the metabolic screen. Most often, the abnormal metabolic screen is a false-positive and does not mean that the baby has any metabolic or endocrine disease. The state laboratory will usually request to have the screening test repeated at some time in the future and may recommend additional tests. If your infant has an abnormal newborn screen, talk to your health care provider to obtain more details about the specific test that was abnormal and their plans for follow-up testing.

Problems Affecting the Skin

The skin consists of 3 layers: an outer layer (the epidermis), a middle layer (the dermis), and an inner layer (the subcutaneous tissue). Intact skin is an important barrier. It protects the body from invading bacteria and viruses. It helps maintain fluid balance by preventing excessive water loss and provides insulation for temperature regulation. Premature skin is a less effective barrier and more prone to injury than fully mature skin. The epidermis is thin and less firmly attached to the dermis, and there is little insulating fat.

The Premature Baby's Skin

You may notice that a very premature baby's skin initially appears shiny, sticky, and gelatinous with visible veins. More mature babies have a dry, flaky layer covering the epidermis called the *stratum corneum.* After birth, premature skin matures quickly. Within 2 to 3 weeks, a preterm infant's epidermis and skin permeability are similar to those of a term infant. You will notice your baby's skin becoming dry and flaky. This is a normal and healthy change. At 28 weeks' gestation, the stratum corneum is only 2 or 3 cell layers thick. By 32 weeks, there are 15 layers, which is equivalent to adult skin.

Special Care for Premature Skin

To protect their skin and prevent skin breakdown, all premature babies receive special skin care. Skin care includes gentle handling; avoidance of lotions, ointments, or other substances (unless medically indicated); use of special tape that is gentle to the skin; avoidance of adhesives; and use of special transparent dressings. These dressings can be used over skin irritations to promote healing or over places where IV lines or catheters have been inserted to protect these sites and reduce the risk of infection. A soft, easy-to-remove barrier may be placed between the tape and the infant's skin. Even with careful attention to skin care, however, some premature infants may develop areas of irritation because of the immaturity of their skin. Preventing irritation and skin breakdown is an important but challenging goal for neonatal care providers. New research is constantly changing neonatal skin care practices, and each NICU may have its own skin care protocol.

The Importance of Touch

After birth, touch is an important way that parents can calm and soothe their premature baby. Through touch receptors in the skin, your baby interacts with and learns about the world. Touch sensation is one of the earliest senses to develop. The fetus begins to respond to touch early in development. Gentle touching—a hand placed on the infant's head or back—is soothing to many babies. Chapter 4 provides more information on the sensory capabilities of newborns.

Problems Affecting Temperature Control

At birth, an infant moves from the warm environment of his mother's uterus to the cooler delivery room. For the first time, the infant must control his own temperature.

Premature Infants and Temperature Control

Premature infants have a high risk of excessive heat loss, causing low body temperature (hypothermia). They lose heat through their skin in 4 ways: (1) when water evaporates from their skin (evaporation), (2) when air currents move across their skin (convection), (3) when they are in contact with a cool surface (conduction), and (4) when heat waves from their skin move toward cooler objects near them (radiation). Because they have less insulating fat and a relatively large expanse of skin compared with their body weight, premature infants can rapidly lose heat from all 4 mechanisms. Older infants can create additional heat by shivering or using a special kind of stored fat, called *brown fat,* to

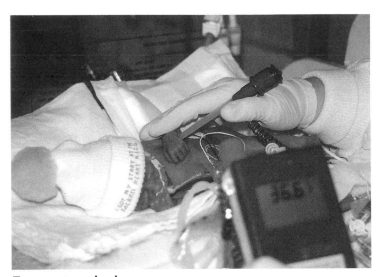

Temperature check.
Many body functions depend on temperature regulation. A baby's temperature is usually taken in the axilla (armpit) with a digital thermometer.

generate heat. Premature infants do not shiver, and their small supply of brown fat becomes exhausted quickly. Instead, premature infants will narrow blood vessels in an attempt to keep warm blood near their core and away from the skin where it can lose heat. They may try to use metabolic energy to produce heat when they are cold. Producing heat with metabolic energy uses up oxygen and sugar that infants need for other purposes. Once these few mechanisms have been used, premature infants cannot support their temperature and quickly become cold.

Complications of Low Body Temperature

Early in the history of neonatology, researchers found that carefully maintaining a normal body temperature improved survival for premature infants. Hypothermia may cause breathing problems and low blood sugar. If premature infants use metabolic energy for heat production, they may use up their glucose stores and develop hypoglycemia. Infants who are cold stressed over a period may not gain weight because they are using their energy for heat production rather than for growth.

Temperature Management in the NICU

Maintaining a normal body temperature is a major focus of care from the moment of birth. Strategies have been developed to address each of the 4 mechanisms of heat loss. In the delivery room, your baby will be placed under an electric (radiant) warmer. Warm cotton blankets may be placed around your baby so that he does not lie on cool metal surfaces. Very premature infants may be covered with a clear plastic sheet or bag similar to the plastic wrap that you use in your kitchen. Shortly after birth, premature infants may be moved to an incubator (isolette). The incubator keeps your baby warm by controlling the environmental temperature and blocking cool air currents that could move across his body. A second interior wall is built into the incubator as an additional heat insulator. Very premature infants may have humidity added to their incubator to prevent heat loss from water evaporation through their immature skin. Your baby's temperature and the temperature of the environment are measured regularly and adjustments are made to keep your baby's body temperature normal. Temperature may be measured in degrees centigrade or Fahrenheit. Appendix A provides a chart for converting centigrade temperatures to Fahrenheit.

Kangaroo Care

Kangaroo care is a method of warming a stable, growing premature baby that uses skin-to-skin contact with the mother or the mother's partner. The premature infant is held naked directly against his parent's skin and covered with a blanket to mimic being inside a kangaroo's pouch. First developed in South America, this method of warming has been shown to have benefits including improved success with breastfeeding, improved parental bonding, and more stable infant sleep patterns. During kangaroo care, premature infants frequently have fewer apnea events and less periodic breathing. Kangaroo care is also discussed in Chapter 5.

The Key: Knowledge

This chapter has described many of the common problems seen in premature infants. The wide range of potential problems may seem overwhelming. It is important, however, to remember that being at risk for a problem does not mean that a baby will certainly develop it. Most premature infants will experience one of the problems described in this chapter, many will experience several and, unfortunately, a few will experience many. Knowledge of your baby's risks for specific problems enables both you and your health care team to monitor your baby carefully, identify signs of developing problems, and begin treatment quickly. Your caregivers can provide more specific information about your baby's risks based on his gestational age, birth weight, and unique health condition.

Chapter 10
Major Medical Problems

"This is Serious," said Pooh.

"I must have an Escape."

Lori A. Markham, MSN, MBA, NNP-BC, CCRN

J. Craig Jackson, MD, MHA, FAAP

Some babies complete their neonatal intensive care unit (NICU) experience without many problems. Others face serious difficulty.

This chapter explains many of the major medical problems faced by infants needing intensive care. These problems can affect both preterm and term infants, but this chapter will focus on those that most commonly occur in babies born near their due date. Remember that no baby will experience more than a few of these problems. You may want to refer only to those sections that talk about your baby's current problems. Use these explanations as you prepare questions for your baby's health care team and interpret the information you're given.

The information in this chapter is meant to serve as a base on which to build your knowledge about your baby's special needs. Each child is unique (and none has read this book!), so your baby's situation may differ a little or a lot from the descriptions you read here. Above all, ask as many questions of your baby's care providers as you need to feel comfortable. There is no such thing as a bad question or a question asked too often.

Problems Affecting the Brain and Nervous System

Brain and nervous system development begins in the third week of pregnancy and continues well beyond the second year of life. When development is complete, the brain consists of many interconnected areas capable of performing all of the tasks that make us human.

The outer layer and largest part of the brain is the cerebral cortex. Made up of billions of nerve cells (neurons), the cerebral cortex is the nerve center of the brain. Underneath, white matter links the nerve cells of the brain and spinal cord.

The lower part of the brain is the cerebellum and brain stem. They are responsible for many of our reflexes and for vital body functions such as breathing. The spinal cord sends information the body feels or senses to the brain and carries action messages from the brain back to the body. Some reflexes are also controlled by the spinal cord.

Because of its complex nature, the developing brain is vulnerable to injury and to drugs and infections. Many factors play a part in brain development, both before and after birth. These include nutrition, oxygen and blood circulation, genetic makeup (cell structure), and cell function.

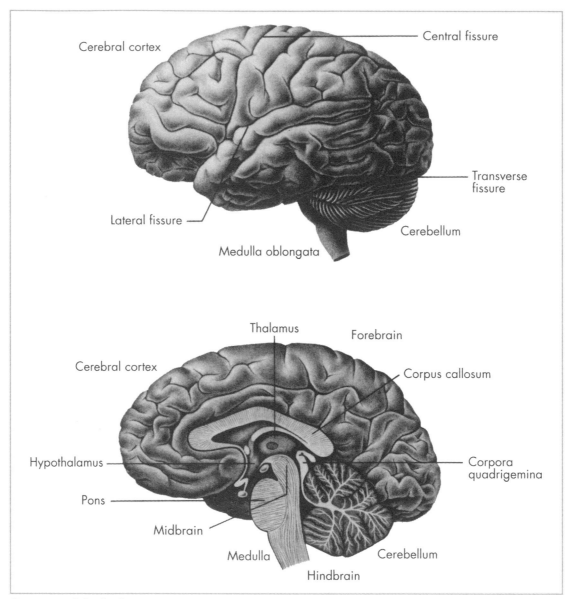

Structure of the brain.
Upper diagram shows the external surface of the brain. The folds and grooves of the surface are called *convolutions.* The lower diagram is a cross-section of the brain and shows important internal structures.

From Burke S. Human Anatomy & Physiology in Health and Disease, *3E. © 1992 Delmar Learning, a part of Cengage Learning, Inc. www.cengage.com/permissions. Reproduced by permission.*

If one or more of these factors are impaired or do not perform properly, the result can be brain injury. If brain injury occurs during fetal development, the tissue in the brain may not develop normally, producing a congenital malformation—commonly called a *birth defect.* Brain injury that occurs at or near the time of birth may be the result of insufficient oxygen delivery to brain tissue.

Asphyxia

Asphyxia occurs when the cells of the body do not receive enough oxygen because a life-threatening situation severely impairs oxygen delivery. The lack of blood flow is known as *ischemia*. The cells, said to be *hypoxic* (low oxygen) in this situation, cannot work properly without oxygen and begin to produce waste products in the form of acids. These acids build up, causing a condition called *acidosis,* which can temporarily or permanently damage many of the body's cells. The effect on the brain is called *encephalopathy,* and so the condition of asphyxia is sometimes called *hypoxic-ischemic encephalopathy* or *HIE*. Severe or prolonged lack of oxygen may result in permanent cell damage. The brain is especially sensitive to damage from asphyxia because its cells need a lot of oxygen.

Causes of Asphyxia

When the baby is in the uterus, asphyxia may occur at any time blood flow through the placenta is inadequate. Box 1 lists factors that can cause a critical lack of oxygen. Following delivery, babies who do not start to breathe and circulate oxygen-rich blood through their bodies for a prolonged period will experience asphyxia.

Box 1. Factors That Can Cause Critical Lack of Oxygen to the Fetus

- Separation of the placenta from the uterine wall (placental abruption)
- Compression of the umbilical cord during labor and delivery, a cord tightened around the baby's neck (nuchal cord), a cord trapped below the baby in the birth canal (prolapsed cord)
- Prolonged or difficult delivery
- Unusual presentation during vaginal birth, such as buttocks first or legs first (breech presentation)
- Life-threatening maternal or fetal infection
- Certain medical conditions of the mother, such as severe hypertension (high blood pressure), severe hypotension (low blood pressure, as in shock), or maternal hypoxia (lack of oxygen to the tissues related to acute asthma, severe pneumonia, or apnea during maternal seizures)
- Umbilical cord accident (a cord that knots in the uterus or tangles with a twin and cuts off circulation to the fetus, for example)
- Traumatic injury to the mother (from a motor vehicle accident, for example) causing maternal hypotension, maternal hypoxia, or placental abruption
- Severe anemia of the fetus due to infection, damage to the red blood cells, or hemorrhage into the mother's circulation or into a twin

Prevention of Asphyxia

One of the goals of the health care team is to identify pregnancies that may be at risk for asphyxia and to intervene, if possible, before the baby is in critical condition. When the potential for birth asphyxia is identified during pregnancy (if you have high blood pressure or diabetes, for example, or if the fetus is not growing or gaining weight appropriately), prenatal testing with frequent ultrasounds or electronic monitoring of the baby's heart rate may be done to measure fetal well-being. Induction of labor may be done or cesarean birth may be necessary if the health care team determines that the baby's chances for continued growth and survival are better outside the uterus or if the team determines that spontaneous labor could jeopardize fetal well-being. During labor and delivery, fetal heart rate monitoring is one tool that can help detect trouble. The goal of careful monitoring is to deliver the baby before a severe chemical imbalance (acidosis) occurs but not so early as to cause other medical problems.

Severe birth asphyxia is an unusual pregnancy complication, with most factors being outside anyone's control. Asphyxia is often undetected until a pregnant woman presents with a problem or complaint, such as decreased fetal movement or severe abdominal pain. During the mother's examination, the nurse or physician may detect a fetal heart rate that is tachycardic (unusually fast), bradycardic (unusually slow), or unusually steady and does not change in response to fetal movement or stimulation. On examination, the nurse or physician may find vaginal bleeding, unusual uterine tenderness, a prolapsed umbilical cord (part of the umbilical cord slips into the birth canal ahead of the baby), or the presence of meconium in the amniotic fluid (a sign of potential fetal distress, discussed later in this chapter).

If an emergency delivery is necessary, additional people may attend the birth to assess your baby and provide care as needed. (See Chapter 2 for information about newborn resuscitation.) Babies who are only mildly asphyxiated may be quickly revived by the resuscitation team by providing breathing support, using positive pressure ventilation with air and oxygen. After stabilization, such babies must be closely monitored.

Babies who are severely asphyxiated require a more complex and prolonged resuscitation. If the baby's blood oxygen level is very low, the blood carbon dioxide level very high, and the resulting chemical imbalance (acidosis) severe, the baby may need more than breathing support. Lifesaving techniques, such as intubation, cardiac compressions, and emergency fluids, and medications may be necessary. Your baby will require close monitoring in the NICU and may develop serious complications as a result of the asphyxia.

Complications of Asphyxia

When the oxygen supply begins to fall and if the body has time, it will try to restrict the blood supply in the bowel, kidneys, muscles, and skin. This helps to redistribute available oxygen to the heart and brain, where it is needed most. If the oxygen supply continues to be inadequate, and as the body continues to respond, the heart loses power and efficiency, also affecting the blood supply to the heart and brain. If the loss of oxygen is abrupt, the body may not have time to redistribute blood flow.

After delivery, the infant recovering from asphyxia may show signs of tissue injury. The severity of the symptoms and the length of time they last depend on the severity of the asphyxia. Mild asphyxia usually resolves without long-term problems. In the short term, though, hypoglycemia (low blood sugar) may mean your baby will need an intravenous (IV) line. Because the intestines are sensitive to lack of oxygen, feeding may be delayed for one or more days to allow the bowel to rest and recover. Sometimes the lung blood vessels don't relax properly, leading to a condition called *persistent pulmonary hypertension* (see page 315). Box 2 lists other complications of asphyxia.

Box 2. Complications of Asphyxia

- Seizures
- Swelling of the brain
- Temperature instability
- Low heart rate
- Changes in circulation
- Persistent pulmonary hypertension
- Congestive heart failure
- Respiratory distress
- Kidney damage
- Damage to the bowel
- Necrotizing enterocolitis
- Low blood sugar
- Hormone and chemical imbalances in the blood
- Blood clotting problems

Treatment of Asphyxia

Severely asphyxiated infants often need mechanical ventilation until their own respiratory effort is adequate. They need very careful management of glucose and fluids, especially if the kidneys have been injured. Some centers offer cooling of the head or the entire body in attempts to reduce further brain injury (see Chapter 12); this is sometimes called *therapeutic hypothermia.* It is common to need medications for seizures.

Many babies recover fully from mild or moderate asphyxia, but some will have life-long disabilities such as problems thinking, seeing, hearing, or walking. (See Cerebral Palsy on page 281.) It may be very difficult for the doctors to predict how well your baby will do until months or even years later. Sometimes hearing tests, brain imaging, and an electroencephalogram may provide clues.

Seizures

Seizures occur when the electrical signals in the brain short circuit. Seizures are a sign of brain injury or irritation. In term infants, seizures may be the first sign of brain injury.

In term babies, seizures may appear as jerking movements of the arms or legs; stiffening or arching of the back; or rhythmic movements of the eyes, lips, or tongue. Apnea and bradycardia (periods with no breathing and a low heart rate) may also occur. In preterm babies, the signs of seizures may be quite difficult to detect because premature babies are normally quite jerky or jittery. Normal jittery movement stops when a hand is placed on the baby's arms or legs; however, seizure activity does not.

Causes of Seizures

Many seizures are idiopathic—that is, no cause can be found. Others may result from asphyxia, infection, chemical imbalances in the blood (such as low blood sugar or low calcium), bleeding in the brain or surrounding tissues, swelling of the brain, or malformation of the brain.

Diagnosis of Seizures

If the NICU team suspects seizures, they will study your baby's brain waves using a painless test called an *electroencephalogram (EEG)* to help diagnose the problem. This test involves placing electrodes on the skin of the baby's scalp and recording the electrical activity in the baby's brain. Seizures appear as abnormal patterns of electrical activity on the brain-wave tracing.

Tests that may be done to determine the cause of seizures include

- An ultrasound of the brain to look for bleeding or abnormalities in the brain's structure
- Computed tomography (CT) scan or magnetic resonance imaging (MRI) to look for bleeding, swelling, or abnormalities in the brain's structure and/or blood vessels

- Blood tests to look for chemical imbalances (sugar, sodium, calcium, etc) or abnormalities in function of some of the body's cells
- Blood and spinal fluid tests to look for infection

A neurologist (doctor specializing in disorders of the brain and nervous system) may also examine your baby and help the NICU team manage your baby's problems.

Treatment for Seizures

Seizures cause the brain to use large amounts of sugar, oxygen, and other nutrients. Continued seizures may harm the cells of the brain and interfere with normal breathing patterns. Seizures are treated with medications such as phenobarbital (phenobarb for short), fosphenytoin (Cerebyx), and levetiracetam (Keppra) (see Appendix B). Often the medications are continued for several weeks or months, depending on the underlying problem, in an attempt to prevent a recurrence of the seizure activity.

Potential Outcome for a Baby With Seizures

The long-term prognosis for a baby who has seizures depends on what is causing them, how severe they are, and the number of days over which they occur. Many babies recover completely, with no long-term signs of brain damage, especially if the seizures are easily controlled. Seizures occurring because of severe asphyxia or disease of the brain may persist for a longer period. Follow-up visits with the neurologist or developmental specialists may be needed to evaluate your baby's progress.

Hydrocephalus

Your baby's brain and spinal cord are surrounded by cerebrospinal fluid (CSF). This clear fluid is produced constantly in the ventricles (small chambers in the brain) and circulated around the brain and cord. It is then reabsorbed by the membrane covering the outside of the brain. Cerebrospinal fluid acts as a shock absorber to cushion the nervous system.

Hydrocephalus (literally "water on the brain") occurs when the circulation of CSF is blocked or when the reabsorption of the fluid is delayed. The CSF then backs up in the ventricles, causing them to expand and push on the surrounding brain tissue. As the ventricles expand, they push on your baby's skull bones, causing the baby's head to enlarge. Continued accumulation of fluid and pressure may eventually result in damage to the tissue of your baby's brain.

Causes of Hydrocephalus

Some infants develop hydrocephalus before birth when the flow of CSF is blocked by a malformation. The blockage may occur in the spinal cord when there is a myelomeningocele (see page 281) or within the brain. In preterm babies with intraventricular hemorrhage (see Chapter 9), blood in the CSF may cause a blocking or scarring of the

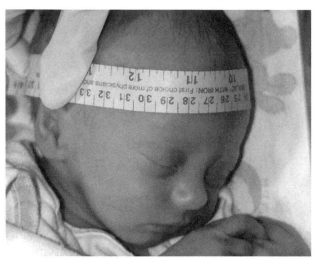

Measuring head circumference.
This measurement allows the health care professional to monitor normal growth and also to assess abnormal enlargement of the head caused by pressure within the brain from dilated ventricles or hydrocephalus.

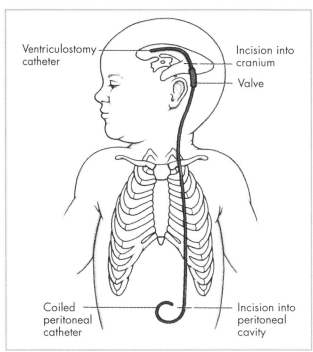

Ventricular shunt.
A ventriculoperitoneal shunt may be needed to drain excess CSF and relieve the pressure in the ventricles of the brain of a baby with hydrocephalus.

From: Hill CJ. Nursing Management of Children, Servonsky J, Opas SR, eds. Sudbury, MA: Jones & Bartlett; 1987:1297. www.jbpub.com. Reprinted by permission.

membranes responsible for reabsorption of the fluid, leading to hydrocephalus.

Diagnosis of Hydrocephalus

A brain ultrasound or a CT scan is used to diagnose dilated ventricles or hydrocephalus (see Chapter 12). The effects of pressure within the brain are also monitored by measuring your baby's head circumference and feeling the soft spot on the top of the head (anterior fontanelle).

Treatment for Hydrocephalus

In some cases, dilation of the ventricles may stop on its own. Treatment becomes necessary when the ventricles continue to expand. A lumbar puncture (spinal tap) or ventricular puncture can be done to remove CSF and may temporarily relieve the pressure on the brain. Medicines may also be used to decrease the production of spinal fluid. Surgery, to place a shunt for the fluid, will be needed if these measures fail to relieve the pressure in the ventricles.

During surgery, a thin tube known as a *shunt* is inserted through the skull and brain into your baby's ventricle. The other end of the tube is passed underneath the skin and drains into a reservoir outside the body, or into the scalp, the abdominal cavity, or the heart, where the body reabsorbs the CSF. Some shunts have a pump or reservoir, which can be felt as a circular bump under the skin on your baby's scalp. Once inserted, a shunt into the abdominal cavity usually remains in place and may need to be lengthened every few years as your child grows. Sometimes the shunt will be removed and no permanent shunt is necessary. Complications occurring with shunts include infection and blockages.

Cerebral Palsy

Cerebral palsy (CP) is defined as an abnormality of posture or movement resulting from damage to the brain. The cause of most cases of CP is unclear. Risk factors in the development of CP in some babies include asphyxia during pregnancy or shortly after birth, very high bilirubin levels, prematurity, severe intraventricular hemorrhage, or periventricular leukomalacia (the presence of brain cysts). Overall, approximately 10% of babies delivered weighing less than 1,500 grams (3 pounds, 5 ounces) will develop CP. The risk increases with the degree of prematurity and evidence of brain damage. For more information about CP, see Chapters 9 and 17.

Myelomeningocele

A type of spina bifida, myelomeningocele occurs during the third or fourth week of pregnancy. In this birth defect, the spinal column does not close completely, leaving a gap between the vertebrae. The covering of the spinal cord then pushes out through this gap, forming a sac. The sac can also contain spinal nerve fibers.

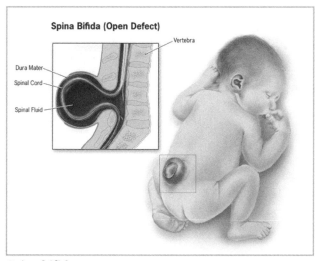

Spina bifida.
Babies born with spina bifida require surgery soon after birth to close the sac and to prevent infection.

From: Centers for Disease Control and Prevention, National Center on Birth Defects and Developmental Disabilities.

The incidence of myelomeningocele is 1 in 1,000 live births. Most defects occur in the lower back (lumbar region). Spina bifida often occurs with hydrocephalus, discussed earlier in this chapter. The location of the sac determines the types of problem that are likely to occur. Nerves supplying the areas below the defect are often damaged or nonfunctional, resulting in some loss of feeling and paralysis in the lower limbs. In addition, there may be a loss of bladder and bowel control.

Babies born with spina bifida require surgery very soon after birth to close the sac to prevent infection. If hydrocephalus is present, a shunt may need to be inserted. Extensive follow-up and ongoing treatments are required to optimize mobility and prevent bladder infections.

Problems Affecting the Heart

In adults, the heart is the size of a fist and consists of 4 muscular chambers that work together as a pump. The chambers are separated by valves, which control the flow of blood. Blood returns to the heart from the veins in the body. It first enters the right atrium and then flows into the right ventricle. From there, it is sent to the lungs, where it picks up oxygen. Then the blood returns to the heart, first to the left atrium and then to the left ventricle, the strongest of the 4 chambers of the heart. The left ventricle must pump blood, rich in oxygen, out to the rest of the body through the aorta.

Development of the heart is complex but is complete quite early in the pregnancy. When the heart or blood vessels near the heart don't develop normally during pregnancy, the baby is born with a congenital heart defect. Sometimes a viral infection, such as rubella (German measles) contracted by the mother during pregnancy, interferes with the heart's development. Other times genetic problems such as Down syndrome are associated with a

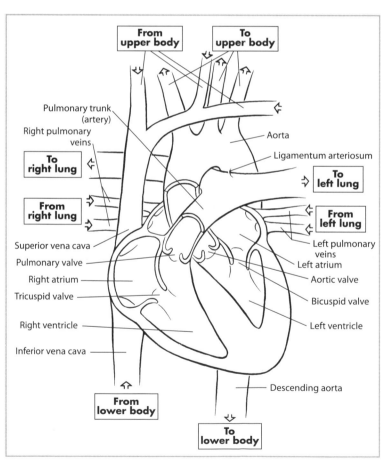

Chambers of the heart and heart valves.
The chambers of the heart are the left and right atria and left and right ventricles. The valves of the heart are the aortic valve, mitral valve, pulmonary valve, and tricuspid valve.

heart defect. The cause of a heart defect is most often unknown. Some defects may be small and may cause your baby few problems; others are life-threatening.

At least 1% of all live-born infants have a heart defect. A great deal of progress has been made in recent years in the treatment of congenital heart defects. See the pages listed below for a discussion of the more common heart defects.

Common Heart Defects[a]

Congenital heart defects are structural problems arising from abnormal formation of the heart or major blood vessels. At least 18 distinct types of congenital heart defects are recognized, with many additional anatomic variations. If your child is born with a heart defect today, the chances are better than ever that the problem can be overcome and that a normal adult life will follow. Recent progress in diagnosis and treatment (surgery and heart catheterization) makes it possible to fix most defects, even those once thought to be hopeless.

As diagnosis and treatment continue to advance, scientists will develop treatments for other defects. Your pediatric cardiologist will discuss your child's heart defect, treatment options and expected results. The descriptions and pictures of common heart defects that follow will help you understand your child's heart problem. These information sheets will also answer some common questions such as those about treatments, ongoing care your child might need, and activities your child can participate in.

[a] Reprinted with permission. www.americanheart.org ©2009, American Heart Association, Inc. To review the information on normal heart function see www.americanheart.org/presenter.jhtml?identifier=770 and for endocarditis see www.americanheart.org/presenter.jhtml?identifier-11078.

Atrial Septal Defect (ASD)

(Note: before reading the specific defect information and the images that are associated with them, it will be helpful to review normal heart function.)

What is it?

An ASD is an opening or hole *(defect)* in the wall *(septum)* between the heart's two upper chambers *(atria).*

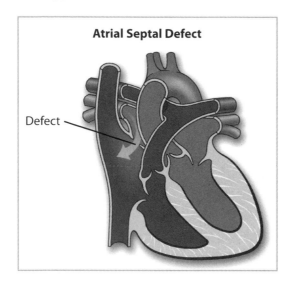

Atrial Septal Defect

Defect

What causes it?

Every child is born with an opening between the upper heart chambers. It's a normal fetal opening that allows blood to detour away from the lungs before birth. After birth, the opening is no longer needed and usually closes or becomes very small within several weeks or months.

Sometimes the opening is larger than normal and doesn't close after birth. In most children the cause isn't known. Some children can have other heart defects along with ASD.

How does it affect the heart?

Normally, the left side of the heart only pumps blood to the body, and the right side of the heart only pumps blood to the lungs. In a child with ASD, blood can travel across the hole from the left upper heart chamber (left atrium) to the right upper chamber (right atrium) and out into the lung arteries.

If the ASD is large, the extra blood being pumped into the lung arteries makes the heart and lungs work harder and the lung arteries can become gradually damaged.

If the hole is small, it may not cause symptoms or problems. Many healthy adults still have a small leftover opening in the wall between the atria, sometimes called a Patent Foramen Ovale (PFO).

How does the ASD affect my child?

Children with an ASD often have no symptoms. If the opening is small, it won't cause symptoms because the heart and lungs don't have to work harder. If the opening is large, the only abnormal finding may be a murmur (noise heard with a stethoscope) and other abnormal heart sounds. In children with a large ASD, the main risk is to the blood vessels in the lungs because more blood than normal is being pumped there. Over time, usually many years, this may cause permanent damage to the lung blood vessels.

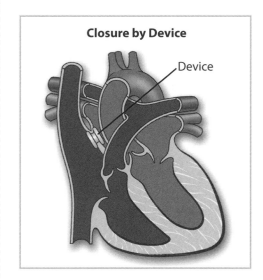

Closure by Device

Device

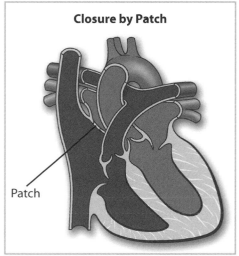

Closure by Patch

Patch

Can the ASD be repaired?

If the opening is small, it doesn't make the heart and lungs work harder. Surgery and other treatments may not be needed. Small ASDs that are discovered in infants often close or narrow on their own. There isn't any medicine that will make the ASD get smaller or close any faster than it might do naturally.

If the ASD is large, it can be closed with open-heart surgery, or by cardiac catheterization using a device inserted into the opening to plug it. Sometimes, if the ASD is an unusual position within the heart, or if there are other heart defects such as abnormal connections of the veins bringing blood from the lungs back to the heart (pulmonary veins), the ASD can't be closed with the catheter technique. Then surgery is needed.

Closing a large ASD by open-heart surgery usually is done in early childhood, even in patients with few symptoms, to prevent complications later. Many defects can be sewn closed without using a patch.

ª Reprinted with permission. www.americanheart.org ©2009, American Heart Association, Inc. To review the information on normal heart function see www.americanheart.org/presenter.jhtml?identifier=770 and for endocarditis see www.americanheart.org/presenter.jhtml?identifier-11078.

What activities can my child do?

Your child may not need any special precautions and may be able to participate in normal activities without increased risk. After surgery or catheter closure, your child's pediatric cardiologist may advise some activity changes for a short time. But after successful healing from surgery or catheter closure, no restrictions are usually needed. Sometimes medicines to prevent blood clots and infection are used for a few months after ASD closure.

What will my child need in the future?

Depending on the type of ASD, your child's pediatric cardiologist may examine your child periodically to look for uncommon problems. For a short time after surgery to close an ASD, a pediatric cardiologist must regularly examine the child. The long-term outlook is excellent, and usually no medicines and no additional surgery or catheterization are needed.

What about preventing endocarditis?

Most children with an ASD are not at increased risk for developing endocarditis. Your child's cardiologist may recommend that your child receive antibiotics before certain dental procedures for a period of time after ASD repair. See the section on Endocarditis for more information.

Atrioventricular Canal Defect

(Note: before reading the specific defect information and the images that are associated with them, it will be helpful to review normal heart function.)

What is it?

Many terms are used to describe this complex defect. They include atrioventricular (AV) canal, complete AV canal, complete common AV canal and endocardial cushion defect.

Atrioventricular (AV) canal defect is a large hole in the center of the heart. It's located where the wall (septum) between the upper chambers (atria) joins the wall between the lower chambers (ventricles). This septal defect involves both upper and lower chambers. Also, the tricuspid and mitral valves that normally separate the heart's upper and lower chambers aren't formed as individual valves. Instead,

ª Reprinted with permission. www.americanheart.org ©2009, American Heart Association, Inc. To review the information on normal heart function see www.americanheart.org/presenter.jhtml?identifier=770 and for endocarditis see www.americanheart.org/presenter.jhtml?identifier-11078.

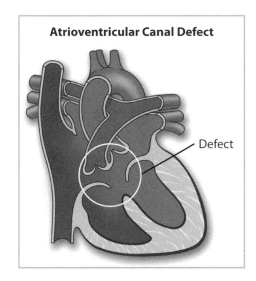

Atrioventricular Canal Defect

Defect

a single large valve forms that crosses the defect in the wall between the two sides of the heart.

What causes it?

In most children, the cause isn't known. It's a very common type of heart defect in children with a chromosome problem, Trisomy 21 (Down syndrome). Some children can have other heart defects along with AV canal.

How does it affect the heart?

Normally, the left side of the heart only pumps blood to the body, and the heart's right side only pumps blood to the lungs. In a child with AV canal defect, blood can travel across the holes from the left heart chambers to the right heart chambers and out into the lung arteries. The extra blood being pumped into the lung arteries makes the heart and lungs work harder and the lungs can become congested.

How does the AV canal defect affect my child?

A child with AV canal defect may breathe faster and harder than normal. Infants may have trouble feeding and growing at a normal rate. Symptoms may not occur until several weeks after birth. High pressure may occur in the blood vessels in the lungs because more blood than normal is being pumped there. Over time this causes permanent damage to the lung blood vessels.

In some infants, the common valve between the upper and lower chambers doesn't close properly. This lets blood leak backward from the heart's lower chambers to the upper ones. This leak, called regurgitation or insufficiency, can make the heart work harder, too.

What can be done about the defect?

An AV canal can be fixed. Open-heart surgery is needed to repair the defect. Unlike some other types of septal defects, the AV canal defect can't close on its own. Medicines may be used temporarily to help with symptoms, but they don't cure the defect or prevent permanent damage to the lung arteries.

ᵃ Reprinted with permission. www.americanheart.org ©2009, American Heart Association, Inc. To review the information on normal heart function see www.americanheart.org/presenter.jhtml?identifier=770 and for endocarditis see www.americanheart.org/presenter.jhtml?identifier-11078.

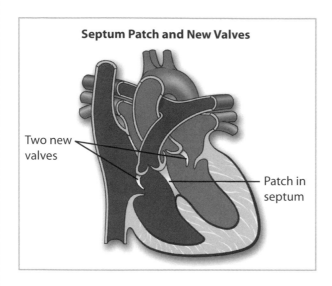

Septum Patch and New Valves

Two new valves

Patch in septum

In an infant with severe symptoms or high blood pressure in the lungs, surgery must usually be done in infancy. During the operation, the surgeon closes the large hole with one or two patches. Later the patch will become a permanent part of the heart as the heart's lining grows over it. The surgeon also divides the single valve between the heart's upper and lower chambers and makes two separate valves. These will be made as close to normal valves as possible.

If an infant is very ill, or has a defect that may be too complex to repair in infancy, a temporary operation to relieve symptoms and high pressure in the lungs may be needed. This procedure (pulmonary artery banding) narrows the pulmonary artery to reduce the blood flow to the lungs. When the child is older, an operation is done to remove the band and fix the AV canal defect with open-heart surgery.

What activities can my child do?

If the AV canal defect has been closed with surgery, your child may not need any special precautions regarding physical activities and may be able to participate in normal activities without increased risk. Being physically active is healthy for the cardiovascular system, but some children may need to limit their activity. Discuss this with your child's pediatric cardiologist.

What will my child need in the future?

After surgery your child must be examined regularly by a pediatric cardiologist. More medical or surgical treatment is sometimes needed.

Surgical repair of an AV canal usually restores the blood circulation to normal. However, the reconstructed valve may not work normally. The valve structures

ᵃ Reprinted with permission. www.americanheart.org ©2009, American Heart Association, Inc. To review the information on normal heart function see www.americanheart.org/presenter.jhtml?identifier=770 and for endocarditis see www.americanheart.org/presenter.jhtml?identifier-11078.

can leak or narrow. But, for many children, the long-term outlook is good, and usually no medicines or additional surgery are needed.

What about preventing endocarditis?

Children with AV canal defect may risk endocarditis both before and after repair. Ask about your child's risk of endocarditis and about your child's need to take antibiotics before certain dental procedures. See the section on Endocarditis for more information.

Coarctation of the Aorta (CoA)

(Note: before reading the specific defect information and the images that are associated with them, it will be helpful to review normal heart function.)

What is it?

In this condition the aorta (the main artery that carries blood from the heart to the body) is narrowed or constricted.

What causes it?

In most children, the cause isn't known. Some children can have other heart defects along with coarctation.

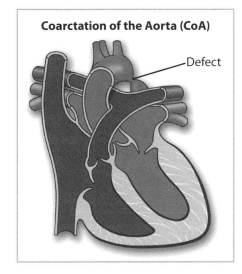

Coarctation of the Aorta (CoA)

Defect

How does it affect the heart?

Coarctation obstructs blood flow from the heart to the lower part of the body. Blood pressure increases above the constriction. The blood pressure is much higher than normal in the left pumping chamber (left ventricle) and the heart must work harder to pump blood through the constriction in the aorta. This can cause thickening (hypertrophy) and damage to the over-worked heart muscle.

ª Reprinted with permission. www.americanheart.org ©2009, American Heart Association, Inc. To review the information on normal heart function see www.americanheart.org/presenter.jhtml?identifier=770 and for endocarditis see www.americanheart.org/presenter.jhtml?identifier-11078.

How does the coarctation affect my child?

Usually no symptoms exist at birth, but they can develop as early as the first week after birth. A baby may develop congestive heart failure or high blood pressure.

If the obstruction is mild, the heart won't be very overworked and symptoms may not occur. In some children and adolescents, coarctation is discovered only after high blood pressure is found.

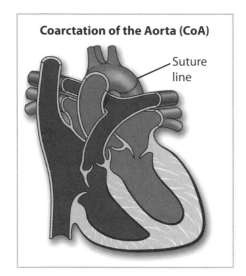

Coarctation of the Aorta (CoA)

Suture line

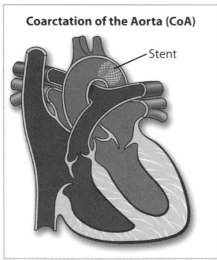

Coarctation of the Aorta (CoA)

Stent

What can be done about the coarctation?

The coarctation obstruction can be relieved using surgery or catheterization.

During cardiac catheterization a special catheter containing a balloon is placed in the constricted area. Then the balloon is inflated for a short time, stretching the constricted area open. The balloon and catheter are then removed.

Surgery is often used to repair coarctation. A surgeon doesn't have to open the heart to repair the coarctation. It can be fixed in several ways. One way is for the surgeon to remove the narrowed segment of aorta. Another option is to sew a patch over the narrowed section using part of the blood vessel to the arm or a graft of synthetic material.

An infant with a severe coarctation should have a procedure to relieve the obstruction. This may relieve heart failure in infancy and prevent problems later, such as developing high blood pressure as an adult because of the coarctation.

What activities can my child do?

If the coarctation has been repaired, there is no important leftover obstruction or high blood pressure, your child may not need any special precautions regarding physical activity, and may be able to participate in normal activities without increased risk.

Some children with obstruction, hypertension, heart muscle abnormalities or other heart defects may have to limit their physical activity. Check with your child's pediatric cardiologist about this.

What will my child need in the future?

The outlook after surgery is favorable, but long-term follow-up by a pediatric cardiologist is needed. Rarely, coarctation of the aorta may recur. Then another procedure to relieve the obstruction may be needed. Also, blood pressure may stay high even when the aorta's narrowing has been repaired.

What about preventing endocarditis?

Children with coarctation of the aorta may risk developing endocarditis. Your child's cardiologist may recommend that your child receive antibiotics before certain dental procedures for a period of time after coarctation repair. See the section on Endocarditis for more information.

Hypoplastic Left Heart Syndrome

(Note: before reading the specific defect information and the images that are associated with them, it will be helpful to review normal heart function.)

What is it?

In hypoplastic left heart syndrome (HLHS), the heart's left side—including the aorta, aortic valve, left ventricle and mitral valve—is underdeveloped.

What causes it?

In most children, the cause isn't known. Some children can have other heart defects along with HLHS.

How does it affect the heart?

In HLHS, blood returning from the lungs must flow through an opening in the wall between the atria (atrial septal defect). The right ventricle pumps the blood into the pulmonary artery and blood reaches the aorta through a patent ductus arteriosus (see diagram).

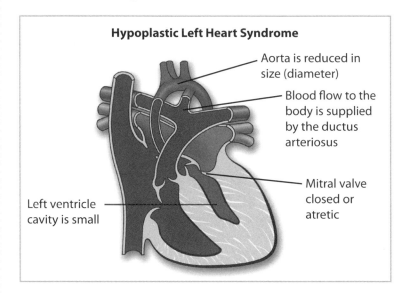

Hypoplastic Left Heart Syndrome

Aorta is reduced in size (diameter)

Blood flow to the body is supplied by the ductus arteriosus

Mitral valve closed or atretic

Left ventricle cavity is small

How does the defect affect my child?

The baby often seems normal at birth but comes to medical attention within a few days of birth as the ductus closes. The baby may appear ashen, have rapid and difficult breathing and have difficulty feeding. This heart defect is usually fatal within the first days or month of life unless it's treated.

What can be done about the defect?

This defect isn't correctable, but some babies can be treated with a series of operations, or heart transplantation. Until an operation is performed, the ductus is kept open by intravenous medication. Because these operations are complex and need to be adapted for each child, it's necessary to discuss all the medical and surgical options with your child's doctor.

If you and your child's doctor agree that surgery should be performed, it will be done in several stages. The first stage, referred to as the Norwood procedure, allows the right ventricle to pump blood to both the lungs and the body without the need for the ductus to be kept open. Blood is directed to the lungs through either a Blalock-Taussig (arrow on inserted picture) or Sano shunt. The Norwood procedure must be performed soon after birth. The second stage (bidirectional

ª Reprinted with permission. www.americanheart.org ©2009, American Heart Association, Inc. To review the information on normal heart function see www.americanheart.org/presenter.jhtml?identifier=770 and for endocarditis see www.americanheart.org/presenter.jhtml?identifier-11078.

Glenn or hemi-Fontan) is usually performed between 4 and 12 months and the third stage (lateral tunnel Fontan or extracardiac Fontan) is usually performed between 18 months and 3 years.

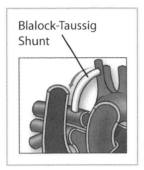

Blalock-Taussig Shunt

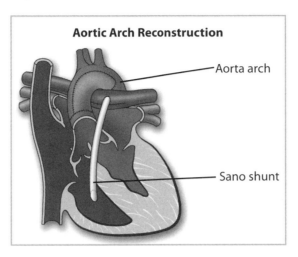

Aortic Arch Reconstruction

Aorta arch

Sano shunt

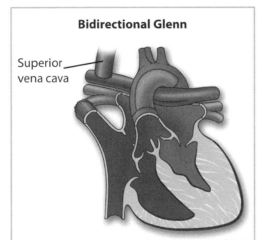

Bidirectional Glenn

Superior vena cava

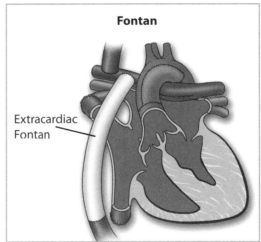

Fontan

Extracardiac Fontan

These operations create a connection between the veins returning low-oxygen (bluish) blood to the heart and the pulmonary artery. The goal is to allow the right ventricle to pump only oxygenated blood to the body and to prevent or reduce cyanosis (lower than normal blood oxygen levels). Some infants require several intermediate operations to achieve this.

ᵃ Reprinted with permission. www.americanheart.org ©2009, American Heart Association, Inc. To review the information on normal heart function see www.americanheart.org/presenter.jhtml?identifier=770 and for endocarditis see www.americanheart.org/presenter.jhtml?identifier-11078.

Some doctors recommend heart transplantation to treat HLHS. Although it can provide the infant with a heart that has normal structure, the infant will require life-long medications to prevent rejection. Many other transplant-related problems can develop, and these should be discussed with your child's doctor.

What activities can my child do?

Children with HLHS may be advised to limit their physical activities to their own endurance. Generally, many competitive sports pose greater risk. Your child's pediatric cardiologist will help determine the proper level of activity.

What will my child need in the future?

Children with HLHS require lifelong follow-up by a cardiologist for repeated checks of how their heart is working. Virtually all children with HLHS will require heart medicines, heart catheterization and additional surgery.

What about preventing endocarditis?

Children with HLHS are at increased risk for developing endocarditis. Ask your pediatric cardiologist about your child's need to take antibiotics before certain dental procedures to help prevent endocarditis. See the section on Endocarditis for more information.

Pulmonary Atresia

(Note: before reading the specific defect information and the image associated with it, it will be helpful to review normal heart function.)

What is it?

In pulmonary atresia, no pulmonary valve exists. Blood can't flow from the right ventricle into the pulmonary artery and on to the lungs. The right ventricle and tricuspid valve are often poorly developed.

What causes it?

In most children, the cause isn't known. Some children can have other heart defects along with pulmonary atresia. (Children with tetralogy of Fallot who also have pulmonary atresia may have treatment similar to others with tetralogy of Fallot.)

ª Reprinted with permission. www.americanheart.org ©2009, American Heart Association, Inc. To review the information on normal heart function see www.americanheart.org/presenter.jhtml?identifier=770 and for endocarditis see www.americanheart.org/presenter.jhtml?identifier-11078.

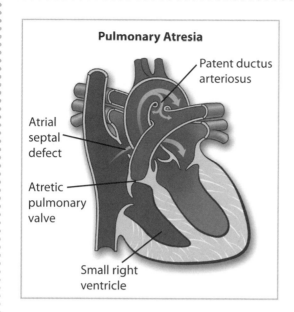

Pulmonary Atresia

- Patent ductus arteriosus
- Atrial septal defect
- Atretic pulmonary valve
- Small right ventricle

How does it affect the heart?

An opening in the atrial septum lets blood exit the right atrium, so low-oxygen (bluish) blood mixes with the oxygen-rich (red) blood in the left atrium. The left ventricle pumps this mixture of oxygen-poor blood into the aorta and out to the body. The infant appears blue (cyanotic) because there's less oxygen in the blood. The only source of lung blood flow is the patent ductus arteriosus (PDA), an open passageway between the pulmonary artery and the aorta.

How does pulmonary atresia affect my child?

If the PDA narrows or closes, the lung blood flow is reduced to critically low levels. This can cause very severe cyanosis. Symptoms may develop soon after birth.

What can be done about the defect?

Temporary treatment includes a drug to keep the PDA from closing. A surgeon can create a shunt between the aorta and the pulmonary artery that may help increase blood flow to the lungs.

A more complete repair depends on the size of the pulmonary artery and right ventricle. If the pulmonary artery and right ventricle are very small, it may not be possible to correct the defect with surgery. In some children, abnormal channels (sinusoids) form between the coronary arteries and the right ventricle. These sinusoids can also limit the type of surgery a child can have. In children where the pulmonary artery and right ventricle are more normal in size, open-heart surgery may help the heart work better.

If the right ventricle stays too small to be a good pumping chamber, the surgeon can connect the body veins directly to the pulmonary arteries. The atrial defect also can be closed to relieve the cyanosis. These surgeries are called the Glenn and Fontan procedures.

What activities can my child do?

Children with pulmonary atresia may be advised to limit their physical activities to their own endurance. Some competitive sports may pose greater risk. Your child's pediatric cardiologist will help determine the proper level of activity.

What will my child need in the future?

Children with pulmonary atresia need regular follow-up with a pediatric cardiologist and, once they reach adulthood, lifelong regular follow-up with a cardiologist who's had special training in congenital heart defects. Some children may need medicines, heart catheterization or additional surgery.

What about preventing endocarditis?

Children with pulmonary atresia are at increased risk for developing endocarditis. Ask your pediatric cardiologist about your child's need to take antibiotics before certain dental procedures to help prevent endocarditis. See the section on Endocarditis for more information.

Pulmonary Stenosis (PS)

(Note: before reading the specific defect information and the image that is associated with it, it will be helpful to review normal heart function.)

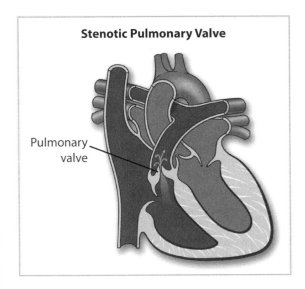

Stenotic Pulmonary Valve

Pulmonary
valve

What is it?

The pulmonary valve opens to let blood flow from the right ventricle to the lungs. Narrowing of the pulmonary valve (valvar pulmonary stenosis) causes the right ventricle to pump harder to get blood past the blockage.

What causes it?

In most children, the cause isn't known. It's a common type of heart defect. Some children can have other heart defects along with PS.

ª Reprinted with permission. www.americanheart.org ©2009, American Heart Association, Inc. To review the information on normal heart function see www.americanheart.org/presenter.jhtml?identifier=770 and for endocarditis see www.americanheart.org/presenter.jhtml?identifier-11078.

How does it affect the heart?

Normally the right side of the heart pumps blood to the lungs. In a child with PS, the pressure is much higher than normal in the right pumping chamber (right ventricle) and the heart must work harder to pump blood out into the lung arteries. Over time this can cause damage to the over-worked heart muscle.

How does the PS affect my child?

If the stenosis is severe, especially in babies, some cyanosis (blueness) may occur. Older children usually have no symptoms.

What can be done about the pulmonary valve?

The pulmonary valve can be treated to improve the obstruction and leak, but the valve can't be made normal.

Treatment is needed when the pressure in the right ventricle is high (even though there may be no symptoms). In most children the obstruction can be relieved during cardiac catheterization by balloon valvuloplasty. In this procedure, a special tool, a catheter containing a balloon, is placed across the pulmonary valve. The balloon is inflated for a short time to stretch open the valve. Some children may need surgery.

What activities can my child do?

If the obstruction is mild, or if the PS obstruction has mostly been relieved with a balloon or surgery, your child may not need any special precautions regarding physical activities, and can participate in normal activities without increased risk.

What will my child need in the future?

The long-term outlook after balloon valvuloplasty or surgery is excellent, and usually no medicines and no additional surgery are needed. Your child's pediatric cardiologist will examine your child periodically to look for uncommon problems such as worsening of the obstruction again.

What about preventing endocarditis?

Ask about your child's risk of developing endocarditis. Children who have had pulmonary valve replacement will need to receive antibiotics before certain dental procedures. See the section on Endocarditis for more information.

---

[a] Reprinted with permission. www.americanheart.org ©2009, American Heart Association, Inc. To review the information on normal heart function see www.americanheart.org/presenter.jhtml?identifier=770 and for endocarditis see www.americanheart.org/presenter.jhtml?identifier-11078.

Tetralogy of Fallot

(Note: before reading the specific defect information and the images that are associated with them, it will be helpful to review normal heart function.)

What is it?

Tetralogy of Fallot has four key features. A ventricular septal defect (VSD; a hole between the ventricles) and obstruction from the right ventricle to the lungs (pulmonary stenosis) are the most important. Also, the aorta (the major artery from the heart to the body) lies directly over the ventricular septal defect, and the right ventricle develops thickened muscle.

What causes it?

In most children, the cause of tetralogy of Fallot isn't known. It's a common type of heart defect. It may be seen more commonly in children with Down syndrome or DiGeorge syndrome. Some children can have other heart defects along with tetralogy of Fallot.

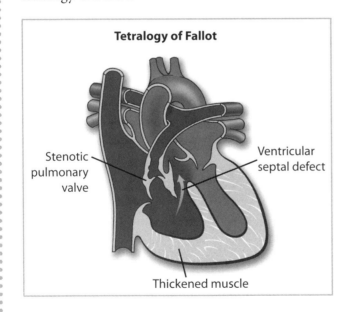

Tetralogy of Fallot

Stenotic pulmonary valve

Ventricular septal defect

Thickened muscle

How does it affect the heart?

Normally the left side of the heart only pumps blood to the body, and the heart's right side only pumps blood to the lungs. In a child with tetralogy of Fallot, blood can travel across the hole (VSD) from the right pumping chamber (right ventricle) to the left pumping chamber (left ventricle) and out into the body artery (aorta). Obstruction in the pulmonary valve leading from the right ventricle to the lung artery prevents the normal amount of blood from being pumped to the lungs. Sometimes the pulmonary valve is completely obstructed (pulmonary atresia).

How does tetralogy of Fallot affect my child?

Infants and young children with unrepaired tetralogy of Fallot are often blue (cyanotic). The reason is that some oxygen-poor blood is pumped to the body through the hole in the wall between the right and left ventricle instead of being pumped to the lungs.

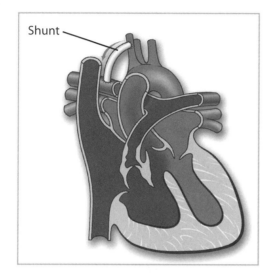

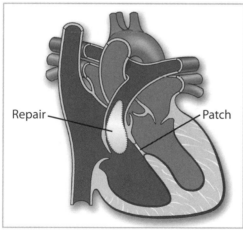

What can be done about tetralogy of Fallot?

Tetralogy of Fallot is treated surgically. A temporary operation may be done at first if the baby is small or if there are other problems. Complete repair comes later. Sometimes the first operation is a complete repair.

Temporary Operation

In some infants, a *shunt* operation may be done first to provide adequate blood flow to the lungs. This is not open-heart surgery and doesn't fix the inside of the heart. The shunt is usually a small tube of synthetic material sewn between a body artery (or the aorta) and the pulmonary artery. The shunt is closed when a complete repair is done later.

Complete Repair

Complete repair tends to be done early in life. The surgeon closes the ventricular septal defect with a patch and opens the right ventricular outflow tract by removing some thickened muscle below the pulmonary valve, repairing or removing the obstructed pulmonary valve and, if needed, enlarging the branch pulmonary arteries that go to each lung.

ª Reprinted with permission. www.americanheart.org ©2009, American Heart Association, Inc. To review the information on normal heart function see www.americanheart.org/presenter.jhtml?identifier=770 and for endocarditis see www.americanheart.org/presenter.jhtml?identifier-11078.

Sometimes a tube is placed between the right ventricle and the pulmonary artery. This is sometimes called a Rastelli repair. It's similar to the type of repair used for some other heart defects.

Will my child's activities be limited?

Your child may need to limit physical activity, particularly for competitive sports, if there is leftover obstruction or leak in the pulmonary valve, which is common after repair. Children with decreased heart function or rhythm disturbances may need to limit their activity more.

If the tetralogy has been repaired with surgery, and there's no obstruction or leak in the pulmonary valve, your child may be able to participate in normal activities without much increased risk.

Your child's pediatric cardiologist will help decide if your child needs limits on physical activity.

What will my child need in the future?

If your child has had tetralogy of Fallot repaired, he or she will need regular follow-up with a pediatric cardiologist. As an adult, your child will need lifelong regular follow-up with a cardiologist who's had special training in congenital heart defects.

Some long-term problems can include leftover or worsening obstruction between the right pumping chamber and the lung arteries. Children with repaired tetralogy of Fallot have a higher risk of heart rhythm disturbances called arrhythmias. Sometimes these may cause dizziness or fainting.

Generally, the long-term outlook is good, but some children may need medicines, heart catheterization or even more surgery.

What about preventing endocarditis?

Children with tetralogy of Fallot are at increased risk for endocarditis. Some children, including those have had a valve replacement, still have a shunt or have leaks around surgical patches, and need to take antibiotics before certain dental procedures to help prevent endocarditis. See the section on Endocarditis for more information.

[a] Reprinted with permission. www.americanheart.org ©2009, American Heart Association, Inc. To review the information on normal heart function see www.americanheart.org/presenter.jhtml?identifier=770 and for endocarditis see www.americanheart.org/presenter.jhtml?identifier-11078.

Total Anomalous Pulmonary Venous Connection (TAPVC)

(Note: before reading the specific defect information and the image that is associated with them, it will be helpful to review normal heart function.)

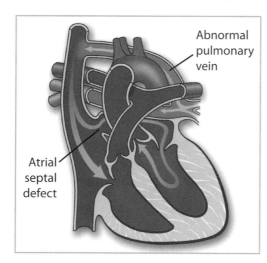

Abnormal pulmonary vein

Atrial septal defect

What is it?

In total anomalous pulmonary venous connection (drainage, return), the pulmonary veins that bring oxygen-rich (red) blood from the lungs back to the heart aren't connected to the left atrium. Instead, the pulmonary veins drain through abnormal connections to the right atrium.

What causes it?

In most children, the cause isn't known. Some children can have other heart defects along with TAPVC.

How does it affect the heart?

In the right atrium, oxygen-rich (red) blood from the pulmonary veins mixes with low-oxygen (bluish) blood from the body. Part of this mixture passes through the atrial septum (atrial septal defect) into the left atrium. From there it goes into the left ventricle, then into the aorta and out to the body. The rest of the blood flows through the right ventricle, into the pulmonary artery and on to the lungs. The blood passing through the aorta to the body doesn't have a normal amount of oxygen, which causes the child to look blue.

How does TAPVC affect my child?

Symptoms may develop soon after birth. In other children, symptoms may be delayed. This partly depends on whether the lung veins are blocked as they drain toward the right atrium. Severe obstruction of the pulmonary veins tends to make infants breathe harder and look bluer (have lower oxygen levels) than infants with little obstruction.

ª Reprinted with permission. www.americanheart.org ©2009, American Heart Association, Inc. To review the information on normal heart function see www.americanheart.org/presenter.jhtml?identifier=770 and for endocarditis see www.americanheart.org/presenter.jhtml?identifier-11078.

What can be done about the defect?

This defect must be surgically repaired in early infancy. At the time of open-heart surgery, the pulmonary veins are reconnected to the left atrium and the atrial septal defect is closed.

What activities can my child do?

Children with repaired TAPVC may be advised to limit their physical activities to their own endurance. Some competitive sports may have greater risk if there is leftover obstruction in the pulmonary veins, or if the child has heart rhythm problems. Your child's pediatric cardiologist will help determine the proper level of activity.

What will my child need in the future?

When surgical repair is done in early infancy, the long-term outlook is very good. However, your child will need regular follow-up with a pediatric cardiologist and, once your child reaches adulthood, lifelong regular follow-up with a cardiologist who's had special training in congenital heart defects. Follow-up is needed to make certain that any remaining problems, such as an obstruction in the pulmonary veins or irregularities in heart rhythm, are treated. Some children may need medicines, heart catheterization or even more surgery.

What about preventing endocarditis?

Children with TAPVC are at increased risk for developing endocarditis. Ask your pediatric cardiologist about your child's need to take antibiotics before certain dental procedures to help prevent endocarditis. See the section on Endocarditis for more information.

---

[a] Reprinted with permission. www.americanheart.org ©2009, American Heart Association, Inc. To review the information on normal heart function see www.americanheart.org/presenter.jhtml?identifier=770 and for endocarditis see www.americanheart.org/presenter.jhtml?identifier-11078.

Transposition of the Great Arteries

(Note: before reading the specific defect information and the images that are associated with them, it will be helpful to review normal heart function.)

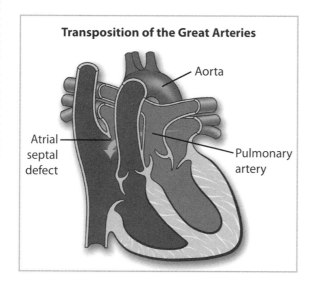

Transposition of the Great Arteries

Aorta

Atrial septal defect

Pulmonary artery

What is it?

In transposition of the great arteries, the aorta and pulmonary artery are reversed. The aorta receives the oxygen-poor blood from the right ventricle, but it's carried back to the body without receiving more oxygen. Likewise, the pulmonary artery receives the oxygen-rich blood from the left ventricle but carries it back to the lungs.

What about surgical treatment?

Patients with transposition of the great arteries require surgery early in life to

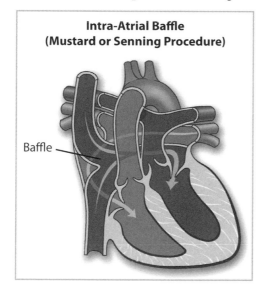

**Intra-Atrial Baffle
(Mustard or Senning Procedure)**

Baffle

survive. Many infants undergo a procedure in the catheterization laboratory to "buy time" and delay the surgery until they can handle it better. The procedure enlarges a naturally occurring connection between the right and left upper chambers (the atria). This lets the blood mix so some oxygen-rich and oxygen-poor blood can be pumped to the correct side.

Two major types of surgery can correct the transposition. The first creates a tunnel (a baffle) between the atria. This redirects the oxygen-rich blood to the right ventricle and aorta and the

---

ª Reprinted with permission. www.americanheart.org ©2009, American Heart Association, Inc. To review the information on normal heart function see www.americanheart.org/presenter.jhtml?identifier=770 and for endocarditis see www.americanheart.org/presenter.jhtml?identifier-11078.

oxygen-poor blood to the left ventricle and the pulmonary artery. This operation is called an atrial or venous switch. It's also called the Mustard procedure or the Senning procedure.

The second type is called the arterial switch operation. The aorta and pulmonary artery are switched back to their normal positions. The aorta is connected to the left ventricle, and the pulmonary artery is connected to the right ventricle. The coronary arteries, which carry the oxygen-rich blood that nourishes the heart muscle, also need to be re-attached to the new aorta.

What type of problems might my child have?

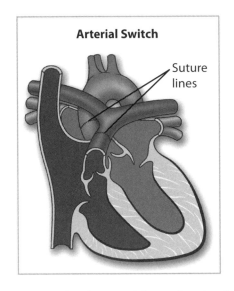

Arterial Switch

Suture lines

Heart function problems

Patients who've had an atrial switch (e.g., Mustard or Senning operation) may have a serious decline in heart muscle or heart valve function. This is because the right ventricle is pumping blood to the entire body instead of just the lungs. Medications to help the heart pump better, control fluid accumulation (diuretics) and control blood pressure may help. Patients who've had the arterial switch operation don't seem to have as great a risk of heart muscle decline. They may have valve leakage or coronary artery problems, however.

Heart rhythm problems (Arrhythmias)

People with repaired transposition, especially those who've had the Mustard or Senning operation, are at risk of developing heart rhythm abnormalities (arrhythmias). These arrhythmias often arise in the heart's upper chambers. Your child's heart rate may be too slow or too fast. If the heart rate is too slow, an artificial pacemaker can speed it up. If your child's heart rate is too fast, medication can slow it down. At times, your child may need a cardiac catheterization to study and treat these rhythm disturbances.

Will my child need more surgery?

Some patients need more surgery to help their heart pump better, repair abnormal valves or control heart rhythm disturbances. Patients who've had the Mustard or

ᵃ Reprinted with permission. www.americanheart.org ©2009, American Heart Association, Inc. To review the information on normal heart function see www.americanheart.org/presenter.jhtml?identifier=770 and for endocarditis see www.americanheart.org/presenter.jhtml?identifier-11078.

Senning operation may need surgery to correct abnormalities of the tunnel in the atria, repair abnormal valves or control rhythm disturbances.

Patients who had the arterial switch operation may need more surgery to relieve narrowings in the aorta or pulmonary artery where the original surgery was done, or to fix leaky valves.

Will my child's activities be limited?

Most cardiologists recommend that patients limit their physical activities to their endurance. They don't recommend competitive sports for high school and college students. Your child's cardiologist will help determine the proper level of activity restriction.

What will my child need in the future?

Patients with transposition will require lifelong follow-up with a cardiologist trained to care for patients with congenital heart disease. Your child may need to take medications to improve how his or her heart works. The cardiologist will track your child with a variety of non-invasive tests. These include electro-cardiograms, Holter monitors, exercise stress tests and echocardiograms.

What about preventing endocarditis?

Children who have transposition of the great arteries are at increased risk for endocarditis. Some children will need to take antibiotics before certain dental procedures. See the section on Endocarditis for more information.

Tricuspid Atresia

(Note: before reading the specific defect information and the images that are associated with them, it will be helpful to review normal heart function.)

What is it?

In this condition, there's no tricuspid valve so blood can't flow from the right atrium to the right ventricle. As a result, the right ventricle is small and not fully developed. The child's survival depends on there being an opening in the wall between the atria (atrial septal defect) and usually an opening in the wall between the two ventricles (ventricular septal defect). As a result, the low-oxygen (bluish) blood that returns from the body veins to the right atrium flows through the

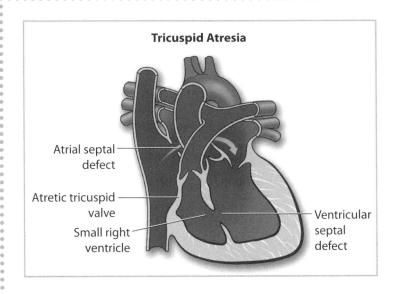

Tricuspid Atresia

Atrial septal defect

Atretic tricuspid valve

Small right ventricle

Ventricular septal defect

atrial septal defect and into the left atrium. There it mixes with oxygen-rich (red) blood from the lungs. Most of this partially oxygenated blood goes from the left ventricle into the aorta and on to the body. A smaller-than-normal amount flows through the ventricular septal defect into the small right ventricle, through the pulmonary artery, and back to the lungs. Because of this abnormal circulation, the child looks blue (cyanotic).

What can be done to treat it?

Often it's necessary to do a surgical procedure, called a shunt, to increase blood flow to the lungs. This improves the cyanosis. Some children with tricuspid atresia have too much blood flowing to the lungs. They may need a different type of surgery, called pulmonary artery banding, to decrease blood flow to the lungs. This is important to protect the lung blood vessels.

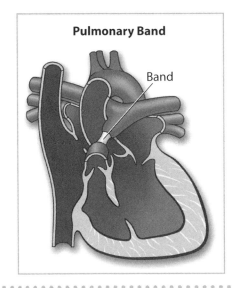

Pulmonary Band

Band

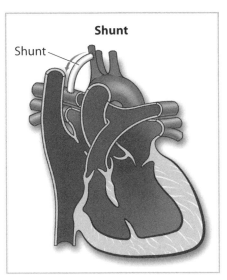

Shunt

Shunt

Can it be repaired?

Most children with tricuspid atresia can have surgery to allow their hearts to work more like normal. Connections are created between the body veins and the lung (pulmonary) arteries. This is usually done in two stages. First, the large vein from the upper half of the body (the superior vena cava) is connected to the lung arteries in a procedure called a Bidirectional Glenn Operation.

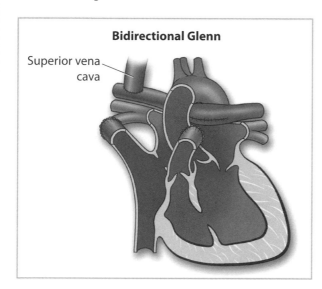

Bidirectional Glenn

Superior vena cava

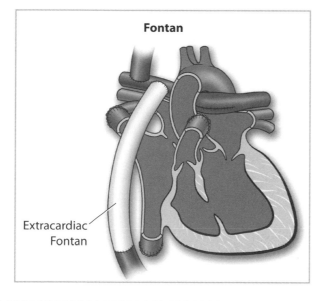

Fontan

Extracardiac Fontan

Later, the large vein from the lower half of the body (the inferior vena cava), as well as the veins from the liver, are connected to the lung arteries in a surgery called a Fontan Operation. Sometimes, at the time of the Fontan surgery, an opening is purposely left between the bluish (low-oxygen) and red (high-oxygen) sides of the blood flows. The Fontan operation may eliminate or greatly improve the cyanosis but, without a right ventricle that works normally, the heart doesn't work like a normal heart, which has two pumps. The Fontan procedure can be performed using a tube that goes around the heart as shown in the picture or with a path (baffle) that goes inside the heart. Both types of Fontan operations route the blue blood from the lower half of the body and liver to the lungs.

ᵃ Reprinted with permission. www.americanheart.org ©2009, American Heart Association, Inc. To review the information on normal heart function see www.americanheart.org/presenter.jhtml?identifier=770 and for endocarditis see www.americanheart.org/presenter.jhtml?identifier-11078.

What will my child need in the future?

Children with tricuspid atresia require lifelong follow-up by a cardiologist for repeated checks of how their heart is working.

What about preventing endocarditis?

Children with tricuspid atresia are at increased risk for developing endocarditis. Ask your pediatric cardiologist about your child's need to take antibiotics before certain dental procedures to help prevent endocarditis. See the section on Endocarditis for more information.

Truncus Arteriosus

(Note: before reading the specific defect information and the images that are associated with them, it will be helpful to review normal heart function.)

What is it?

Truncus arteriosus occurs when the two large arteries carrying blood away from the heart don't form properly and one large artery is present instead. This artery (the truncus) sits over a large opening or hole in the wall between the two pumping chambers (ventricular septal defect). This single great vessel carries blood both to the body and to the lungs.

Some children with Truncus Arteriosus have a condition called DiGeorge Syndrome.

Can it be repaired?

Surgery is necessary to close the ventricular septal defect and separate blood flow to the body from blood flow to the lungs. This is usually done early in infancy to prevent high blood pressure from damaging the lung arteries. A patch is used to close the ventricular defect. The pulmonary arteries are then disconnected from the single great vessel (the truncus) and a tube (a conduit or tunnel) is placed from the right ventricle to the pulmonary arteries. This is sometimes called a Rastelli repair.

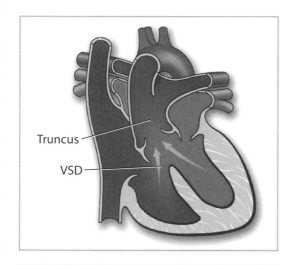

Truncus

VSD

Rastelli repair with patched septum and new pulmonary valve/artery

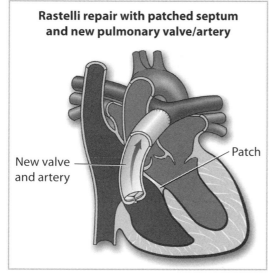

New valve and artery

Patch

Will my child need more surgery?

The conduit connecting the right ventricle to the pulmonary artery conduit may become narrowed and blocked (stenotic) over time, or the child may outgrow the conduit. It may have to be replaced from time to time. Timing of the replacement varies. The peripheral pulmonary arteries also may become narrowed and require treatment. Sometimes conduits and peripheral pulmonary artery narrowings may be dilated using a balloon-tipped catheter or an expandable stent in the cardiac catheterization laboratory. This procedure may help extend the time between operations for conduit changes. Sometimes surgery is required to enlarge the narrowed area. Your child's cardiologist will discuss whether a balloon/stent procedure or surgery is best.

The aortic valve is actually the large truncal valve from the single vessel, which arose over the ventricular septal defect before surgical repair. This valve sometimes becomes leaky over time and may need to be replaced.

What ongoing care will my child need?

Children with truncus arteriosus need regular follow-up with a pediatric cardiologist and they may need to take medicine after surgery. Your child's cardiologist will evaluate with a variety of tests including electrocardiograms and echocardiograms (see the Glossary) to determine when another procedure such as cardiac catheterization may be needed.

---

[a] Reprinted with permission. www.americanheart.org ©2009, American Heart Association, Inc. To review the information on normal heart function see www.americanheart.org/presenter.jhtml?identifier=770 and for endocarditis see www.americanheart.org/presenter.jhtml?identifier-11078.

What activities will my child be able to do?

If valve obstruction and leakage is mild and tests show good heart function and no abnormal heart rhythms, your child can usually participate in some sports. Your cardiologist may recommend avoiding certain intense competitive sports. Ask your child's cardiologist which activities are appropriate.

What about preventing endocarditis?

For patients with uncorrected or partially corrected truncus arteriosus, antibiotics are recommended before certain dental procedures to prevent endocarditis. See the section on Endocarditis for more information.

Ventricular Septal Defect (VSD)

(Note: before reading the specific defect information and the images that are associated with them, it will be helpful to review normal heart function.)

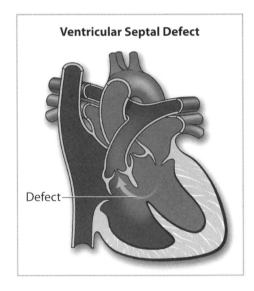

Ventricular Septal Defect

Defect

What is it?

A VSD is an opening or hole (defect) in the wall (septum) between the heart's two pumping chambers (ventricles).

What causes it?

In most children, the cause isn't known. It's a very common type of heart defect. Some children can have other heart defects along with VSD.

How does it affect the heart?

Normally, the left side of the heart only pumps blood to the body, and the heart's right side only pumps blood to the lungs.

In a child with VSD, blood can travel across the hole from the left pumping chamber (left ventricle) to the right pumping chamber (right ventricle) and out into the lung arteries. If the VSD is large, the extra blood being pumped into the lung arteries makes the heart and lungs work harder and the lungs can become congested.

---

[a] Reprinted with permission. www.americanheart.org ©2009, American Heart Association, Inc. To review the information on normal heart function see www.americanheart.org/presenter.jhtml?identifier=770 and for endocarditis see www.americanheart.org/presenter.jhtml?identifier-11078.

How does the VSD affect my child?

If the opening is small, it won't cause symptoms because the heart and lungs don't have to work harder. The only abnormal finding is a loud murmur (noise heard with a stethoscope).

If the opening is large, the child may breathe faster and harder than normal. Infants may have trouble feeding and growing at a normal rate. Symptoms may not occur until several weeks after birth. High pressure may occur in the blood vessels in the lungs because more blood than normal is being pumped there. Over time this may cause permanent damage to the lung blood vessels.

What can be done about the VSD?

If the opening is small, it won't make the heart and lungs work harder. Surgery and other treatments may not be needed. Small VSDs often close on their own. There isn't any medicine or other treatment that will make the VSD get smaller or close any faster than it might do naturally.

If the opening is large, open-heart surgery may be needed to close it and prevent serious problems. Babies with VSD may develop severe symptoms and early repair, within the first few months, is often necessary. The repair may be delayed in other babies. Medicines may be used temporarily to help with symptoms, but they don't cure the VSD or prevent permanent damage to the lung arteries.

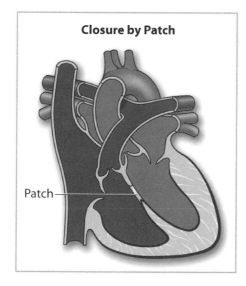

Closure by Patch

Patch

Closing a large VSD by open-heart surgery usually is done in infancy or childhood even in patients with few symptoms, to prevent complications later. Usually a patch of fabric or pericardium (the normal lining around the outside of the heart) is sewn over the VSD to close it completely. Later this patch is covered by the normal heart lining tissue and becomes a permanent part of the heart. Some defects can be sewn closed without a patch. It may be possible to close some VSDs in the cath lab.

ª Reprinted with permission. www.americanheart.org ©2009, American Heart Association, Inc. To review the information on normal heart function see www.americanheart.org/presenter.jhtml?identifier=770 and for endocarditis see www.americanheart.org/presenter.jhtml?identifier-11078.

If an infant is very ill, or has more than one VSD or a VSD in an unusual location, a temporary operation to relieve symptoms and high pressure in the lungs may be needed. This procedure (pulmonary artery banding) narrows the pulmonary artery to reduce the blood flow to the lungs. When the child is older, an operation is done to remove the band and fix the VSD with open-heart surgery.

What activities can my child do?

If the VSD is small, or if the VSD has been closed with surgery, your child may not need any special precautions regarding physical activity and can participate in normal activities without increased risk.

What will my child need in the future?

Depending on the location of the VSD, your child's pediatric cardiologist will examine your child periodically to look for uncommon problems, such as a leak in the aortic valve. Rarely, older children with small VSDs may require surgery if they develop a leak in this heart valve. After surgery to close a VSD, a pediatric cardiologist will examine your child regularly. The cardiologist will make sure that the heart is working normally. The long-term outlook is good and usually no medicines or additional surgery are needed.

What about preventing endocarditis?

Ask about your child's risk of endocarditis. Your child's cardiologist may recommend that your child receive antibiotics before certain dental procedures for a period of time after VSD repair. See the section on Endocarditis for more information.

ª Reprinted with permission. www.americanheart.org ©2009, American Heart Association, Inc. To review the information on normal heart function see www.americanheart.org/presenter.jhtml?identifier=770 and for endocarditis see www.americanheart.org/presenter.jhtml?identifier-11078.

Problems Affecting the Lungs

Many babies in an NICU have lung problems. Some of these problems are due to lung immaturity associated with preterm birth. Lung complications can result from problems with other body systems. This section explains some of the lung and breathing problems the medical team manage most often.

Transient Tachypnea of the Newborn

During development, the fetal lungs are filled with fluid, not air. During labor, hormones cause the lungs to begin absorbing fluid, and during vaginal birth much of the remaining fluid is squeezed out as the baby passes through the birth canal. The baby's circulatory system absorbs the remaining fluid in the first few hours after birth. Transient tachypnea of the newborn (TTN) or "wet lung" develops when there is a delay in reabsorption of this lung fluid after birth. Transient tachypnea of the newborn will improve over time and usually resolves in the first 2 to 5 days of life.

Babies Susceptible to Transient Tachypnea of the Newborn

Term or near-term newborns are most likely to get TTN. Babies born by cesarean section or rapid vaginal delivery are at increased risk for developing TTN.

Potential Problems Caused by Transient Tachypnea of the Newborn

Fluid in the lung traps air in the alveoli (small breathing sacs). This increases your baby's work of breathing and causes symptoms such as tachypnea (rapid breathing), cyanosis (bluish color of the lips or around the mouth and eyes), and moaning or grunting sounds with breathing. This increased work of breathing is tiring and makes it difficult to take in enough oxygen and get rid of carbon dioxide. Rapid breathing also makes sucking and swallowing difficult and may make it very difficult for your baby to eat.

Diagnosis and Treatment of Transient Tachypnea of the Newborn

A chest x-ray will show increased fluid in the lungs. Treatment includes giving your baby oxygen, fluids, and a warm environment. Some babies with TTN may require additional help with breathing. Nasal prongs (short tubes) may be placed in your baby's nose so that continuous positive airway pressure (CPAP) (see Chapter 9) can be used to provide extra oxygen and apply a small amount of pressure to your baby's lungs. This helps to push out the remaining fluid trapped in the alveoli. Usually TTN resolves in 24 to 72 hours. It should cause no further problems for your baby.

Meconium Aspiration Syndrome

Meconium is a sterile, dark-green substance produced in the fetal bowel before birth and is passed in the baby's first few stools (bowel movements). Sometimes meconium can be passed while the baby is still in the uterus, and it can be inhaled (aspirated) into the lungs.

At or after term, a decrease in the amount of oxygen reaching the baby in the uterus may cause the release of meconium from the baby's bowel into the amniotic fluid (fluid surrounding the baby). As the fetus "breathes" (makes breathing movements), the meconium can get into the mouth and airway. Babies who have inhaled a large amount of meconium into their lungs can have severe breathing problems after birth. This condition is called meconium aspiration syndrome (MAS). About 10% of all deliveries are complicated by meconium in the amniotic fluid, but only a small number of these babies experience breathing problems.

Birth Interventions for Newborns With Meconium-Stained Amniotic Fluid

Often meconium will be present in the amniotic fluid and on your baby's skin at birth, but it is not known if the baby has inhaled this material. The first goal in treating a baby with meconium-stained amniotic fluid is to ensure that meconium does not get into the baby's upper airway and inhaled with the first breaths. If the baby is vigorous and begins to cry immediately after birth, the health care team will wipe any visible meconium from your baby's face and then use suction to clear any meconium from the mouth and nose. If your baby is born limp, with a slow heart rate, and does not breathe on her own, an endotracheal tube (breathing tube) will be inserted into your baby's airway. Suction is applied, and any meconium present is removed from deep in the airway before the baby begins breathing.

Symptoms of Meconium Aspiration Syndrome

The presence of meconium in the amniotic fluid is the first sign that your baby may be at risk for MAS. After birth, you may notice that the dark-colored meconium has stained the baby's skin, fingernails, or umbilical cord a greenish color. Babies who have inhaled meconium into their lungs may be quite slow to breathe after birth, or they may have tachypnea (rapid breathing) or increased work of breathing (labored breathing) and cyanosis (blue color of the body and around the mouth).

Potential Complications of Meconium Aspiration Syndrome

The complications of meconium aspiration will depend on the degree of distress that occurred before your baby was born and the severity of the MAS. Meconium acts as a chemical irritant to the lungs, and although it is sterile, its presence may encourage the development of infection.

Mild meconium aspiration usually resolves with few complications. Babies with mild meconium aspiration may require extra oxygen and IV fluids for several hours to days following delivery. If your baby is breathing rapidly, feedings may be delayed or given by gavage (see Chapter 5). Sometimes administration of surfactant into the lungs may help to improve lung function (see page 225).

More severe cases of MAS can lead to complications requiring complex care. Some particles of meconium can be quite large and may block smaller airways. In some cases, a blockage traps air in the airway; in others, it keeps air from entering. This uneven inflation of the lung may lead to rupture of some air sacs and trapping of the air outside the lung (called a *pneumothorax*), discussed later in this chapter. Babies who have inhaled meconium into their lungs before delivery may become quite sick and need additional support such as mechanical ventilation and drug and fluid support. In combination with hypoxia (reduced oxygen to the tissues), severe meconium aspiration can lead to a serious complication called *persistent pulmonary hypertension of the newborn.*

Persistent Pulmonary Hypertension of the Newborn

Persistent pulmonary hypertension of the newborn (PPHN) occurs when a complex interaction of factors produces high blood pressure (hypertension) in the arteries supplying blood to the lungs. This forces blood away from the lungs where the blood is normally oxygenated. Without oxygenated blood from the lungs, the supply of oxygen to the body is decreased. Persistent pulmonary hypertension is a life-threatening problem for a newborn.

As the baby develops in the uterus, blood follows a path known as *fetal circulation.* This path allows oxygen-rich blood supplied by the placenta to circulate quickly to the baby's body. Much of this blood bypasses the baby's lungs, which do not function during fetal life. Two fetal shunts in the heart, the foramen ovale and the ductus arteriosus, produce the bypass. Because the lungs receive little blood flow and little oxygen, the vessels to the lungs are narrow (constricted). After birth, all blood must pass through the lungs to pick up oxygen for the body. The pressures in the heart change, and air with oxygen enters the lungs. The presence of oxygen relaxes the pulmonary blood vessels in the lungs. These 2 factors cause the closure of the fetal shunts and the change from fetal circulation to normal newborn circulation.

In term or near-term infants, several factors can interfere with this changeover from fetal to normal newborn circulation. These include abnormalities in the development of the lung, asphyxia, meconium aspiration, infection, hypothermia (low body temperature), and occasionally respiratory distress syndrome (RDS). These problems trigger hypoxia (lack of oxygen in the tissues), which keeps the pulmonary vessels constricted, forcing blood away from the lungs. That, in turn, changes the pressures within the heart, keeping the fetal shunts open in the heart. Poor circulation to the lungs results in less oxygen in the blood for body tissues, causing further hypoxia and a buildup of waste acid in the baby's body. This sets up a cycle of hypoxia and blood vessel constriction that is difficult to break.

Signs of Persistent Pulmonary Hypertension of the Newborn

The signs of PPHN are difficult to distinguish from those of other major illnesses. Your baby may be either slow to breathe at birth or tachypneic (breathing quickly), be cyanotic with a low arterial blood oxygen concentration (bluish color), be pale or mottled with low blood pressure, and have hands and feet that are cool to the touch or blue. As PPHN continues, your baby may become quite swollen because of low urine output and redistribution of body fluids.

Diagnosis of Persistent Pulmonary Hypertension of the Newborn

If your baby remains hypoxic (poorly oxygenated) despite good mechanical ventilation (with a respirator), PPHN is suspected. Additional tests can be done to show the presence of blood moving across the foramen ovale and ductus arteriosus in the heart. A cardiac ultrasound (echocardiogram) is often done to examine the functioning of the heart and rule out other cardiac problems. The echocardiogram is also used to measure the pressures in the heart and major blood vessels of the heart. These pressure measurements help to diagnose the severity of PPHN.

Treatment for Persistent Pulmonary Hypertension of the Newborn

The goals of treatment for PPHN are to improve oxygen levels in the blood, relax the blood vessels in the lungs, and maintain a normal blood pressure. Good ventilation will help increase the oxygen in your baby's system and relax the pulmonary vessels. In infants with problems affecting the lungs, good ventilation may be difficult to achieve, requiring high concentrations of oxygen and increased amounts of pressure. Ventilation may be improved with high-frequency ventilation or jet ventilation (see Chapter 12). Other possible treatments for severe, life-threatening PPHN include the use of nitric oxide and extracorporeal membrane oxygenation (ECMO) (see Chapter 12).

Normal blood sugar and blood pressure are maintained with IV fluid. Hypoxia may cause your baby's capillaries (tiny blood vessels) to leak fluid into the tissues. If that occurs, large amounts of IV fluid such as normal saline (salt and water) and different medications may be used to help stabilize the blood pressure.

Medications such as dopamine, dobutamine, or epinephrine may be given to help to raise your infant's blood pressure. Other medications, such as sodium bicarbonate, could be used to restore chemical balance in the blood if necessary. Antibiotics prevent or treat infection. Medications may be given to sedate your baby and alleviate any discomfort related to the ventilator. The medications will also help to decrease oxygen use. In some cases, medication will be necessary to paralyze your baby's muscles temporarily, to keep her from breathing against (fighting) the ventilator. Although unable to move her muscles, your baby can still hear your voice and knows that you are with her.

Your baby may be cared for on an open bed with a radiant heater to keep her warm. In addition, many babies with PPHN are very sensitive to noise, light, and handling. Your baby's nurse may use blankets and eye patches to protect her from light, and ear muffs to decrease noise. Those around your baby will be asked to be especially quiet. You should discuss your baby's care with the nurse so that she can help you find the best way to communicate with your baby at this difficult time.

Congenital Diaphragmatic Hernia

The diaphragm is the muscle that separates the chest cavity from the abdominal cavity and assists breathing. A congenital diaphragmatic hernia (CDH) is a birth defect in the diaphragm that occurs early in pregnancy, as the fetus is developing. There is normally a hole in the diaphragm during fetal development, but around the third month of gestation the hole should close. When the hole persists in the diaphragm, some of the organs normally found in the abdomen move up into the chest cavity. The abnormal opening can

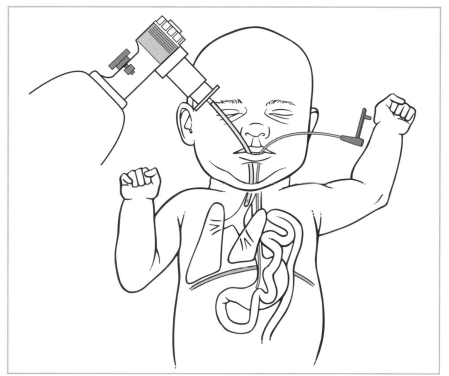

Diaphragmatic hernia.
A diaphragmatic hernia occurs when an opening in the diaphragm allows the bowel to push up into the chest cavity. As a result of the defect, the heart is pushed to the side by the bowel while the lung on the affected side is compressed and may fail to grow properly.

From: American Academy of Pediatrics, American Heart Association. Textbook of Neonatal Resuscitation. *5th ed. Kattwinkel J, ed. Elk Grove Village, IL: American Academy of Pediatrics; 2006: 7–8.*

either be on the right side or the left side. If the opening is on the right side, the liver and intestines will move into the chest cavity. If the opening is on the left side, the stomach and intestines will move into the chest. It is most common to have the defect on the baby's left side.

The lungs, digestive system, and diaphragm all develop at the same time during pregnancy. When the abdominal contents move into the chest cavity, there is not enough room for the lungs to develop properly. The condition of underdeveloped lungs is called *pulmonary hypoplasia* (see page 319). The intestines also may not develop properly because they are displaced into the chest cavity and may not get an adequate blood supply.

Signs and Symptoms of Congenital Diaphragmatic Hernia

When the defect is on the left side, the symptoms are observable soon after your baby is born. The most common symptoms include difficulty breathing, rapid heart rate (tachycardia), cyanosis (bluish color of the skin), and abnormal chest development with one side appearing larger than the other; the abdomen may appear caved in (concave). When the defect is on the right side, your baby may not have immediate or obvious symptoms.

Diagnosis of Congenital Diaphragmatic Hernia

In many cases, a prenatal ultrasound reveals the presence of a CDH, and the NICU team is ready to intervene immediately at birth. Your baby may not be able to breathe effectively because of the underdeveloped lungs. Often a baby will be intubated (have a breathing tube placed in the windpipe) immediately to keep air from entering the stomach and intestines. A chest x-ray is done to look for the presence of the abdominal contents in the chest cavity and to look at the abnormalities of the lungs. Because difficulty breathing is a common symptom, a blood gas will be performed to evaluate your baby's ability to maintain oxygen in the blood. Other tests often include an echocardiogram (ultrasound) of your baby's heart to look for any structural abnormality as well as coexisting PPHN.

Treatment of Congenital Diaphragmatic Hernia

Congenital diaphragmatic hernia is a life-threatening illness that requires neonatal intensive care and, unfortunately, is often fatal. Once your baby is intubated, a ventilator will be used to assist breathing. If breathing is very difficult and your baby is having difficulty maintaining a normal oxygen level in the blood, your baby may need nitric oxide therapy or placement on a temporary heart/lung bypass (ECMO) pump (see Chapter 12). The hole in the diaphragm is fixed when your baby is stable. The stomach, intestines, and other organs are moved from the chest cavity back to the abdominal cavity. The hole may be repaired with one surgery only, or there may be a need for subsequent operations.

Many babies will stay in the intensive care unit for a while following surgery. Although the abdominal organs are moved back to where they belong, the underdeveloped lungs may require prolonged treatment and breathing support for a while. When your baby no longer needs breathing support from the ventilator, she may still require oxygen and medications to help her breathe.

Follow-Up Care for Infants With Congenital Diaphragmatic Hernia

Babies born with CDH have long-term problems and need regular follow-up visits to the pediatrician. Continuing respiratory difficulty and the baby's inability to eat are 2 common problems that need close observation. Infants with the most serious lung problems are more likely to have problems with eating and are more likely to have difficulty growing. Your pediatrician will monitor your baby's progress and make recommendations for follow-up visits with other specialists.

Pulmonary Hypoplasia

Babies who have CDH may also develop pulmonary hypoplasia, a condition that limits full lung development. When the lungs do not develop properly during pregnancy, it may be difficult for your baby to breathe after birth. Healthy lungs have millions of small air sacs (alveoli) that look like a bunch of grapes. With pulmonary hypoplasia there are fewer air sacs than normal, the air sacs that are present are only able to fill partially with air, and the air sacs deflate easily due to a lack of surfactant (a soapy substance that keeps the air sacs from sticking together). When there is pulmonary hypoplasia, there is not enough blood flow to the lungs (pulmonary blood flow) to oxygenate the blood.

Babies Susceptible to Pulmonary Hypoplasia

Pulmonary hypoplasia has several causes and is often suspected based on maternal history or ultrasound findings. The most common risk factors for pulmonary hypoplasia include

- Inadequate space in the chest cavity, perhaps because of a CDH
- Inadequate amniotic fluid, perhaps from the amniotic membranes (bag of waters) leaking over a prolonged period
- Poor kidney development or lack of kidney development, leading to a decreased amount of amniotic fluid
- Other malformations or problems that cause a decrease in breathing movements that babies normally make before birth

Treatment of Pulmonary Hypoplasia

Treatment is dependent on the degree of lung hypoplasia, and management is based on the risk factor that caused the problem. Diaphragmatic hernia is the most common cause of pulmonary hypoplasia (see previous section on diaphragmatic hernia). If the hypoplasia is severe when your baby is born, breathing may be difficult and the medical care team will insert an endotracheal (breathing) tube. Your baby will then be moved to neonatal intensive care for continued support.

Outcome of Pulmonary Hypoplasia

The outcome for your baby is related mainly to the size of the lungs at birth and the presence of other problems. Most babies will have chronic lung problems that require close follow-up by your pediatrician and other specialists. Babies who develop pulmonary hypoplasia from lack of kidney development have a very poor prognosis.

Air Leaks

When a baby has trouble breathing, one possible complication is an air leak. This occurs when air ruptures one or several of the alveoli (breathing sacs) and then leaks into the spaces around the lung tissue. *Pulmonary interstitial emphysema* (PIE) is the term for this type of air leak. Air may collect in the space between the lung and the chest wall (producing a pneumothorax) or the space in the center of the chest containing the heart and major blood vessels (producing a pneumomediastinum). A pneumopericardium is a collection of air in the sac around the heart and is a life-threatening emergency.

Babies Susceptible to Air Leaks

Among healthy term babies, 0.5% to 1% may develop a spontaneous pneumothorax shortly after birth. These air leaks are associated with aspiration of fluid or meconium and usually do not require treatment. Term babies with severe meconium aspiration or PPHN may develop an air leak as a complication of ventilator treatment or positive pressure ventilation and usually will require intervention.

Preterm babies may develop air leaks because of the mechanical pressure needed to inflate lungs affected by RDS. The incidence of air leaks in babies with RDS is about 4%, but is decreasing as surfactant treatment increases.

Signs of an Air Leak

Some term babies with a pneumothorax show no symptoms. Other babies have mild signs of respiratory distress, such as tachypnea (rapid breathing). Premature or unstable infants with a pneumothorax show more signs of distress, such as cyanosis (blue coloring), hypotension (low blood pressure), uneven chest movement, and decreased oxygen saturation. If you were to listen to the lungs of these babies with a stethoscope, you'd hear softer breath sounds over the area of the leak.

Babies with PIE usually show general signs of worsening respiratory status, such as an increased need for oxygen and poor blood gases. A pneumomediastinum produces no specific symptoms. A pneumopericardium produces severe distress, including low blood pressure and heart rate, severe cyanosis, and shock.

Diagnosis of Air Leaks

A chest x-ray is used to diagnose air leaks. Sometimes a series of x-rays may be required to define the location and size of the air leak or follow its progress. If a baby has a sudden worsening of his respiratory condition, a bright light may be used on her chest to look for an abnormal "glow" that indicates a collection of air outside the lung. This procedure is call *transillumination*.

Treatment for Air Leaks

Infants with a small pneumothorax and mild symptoms may not require any treatment other than careful monitoring. If the pneumothorax is large or causing more significant symptoms, the air can be removed by inserting a needle attached to a syringe between the ribs into the space between the lung and the chest wall, removing the air through the syringe, and then removing the needle. This procedure is called *needle aspiration* or *needle thoracentesis*. If there is concern that the air may re-accumulate, a thin plastic tube (chest tube) attached to a suction device can be left in the space to drain the leaking air. In most cases, the ruptured alveoli repair themselves within several days and the chest tube can be removed.

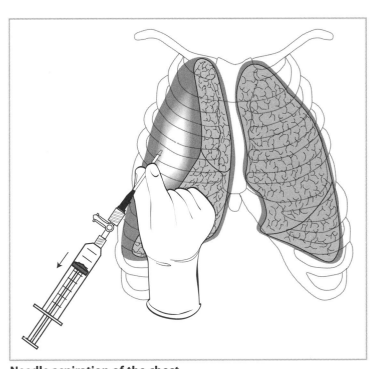

Needle aspiration of the chest.
To help treat a pneumothorax, a needle is inserted into the space between the lung and the chest wall. The air is drawn out through the needle.

From: American Academy of Pediatrics, American Heart Association. Textbook of Neonatal Resuscitation. 5th ed. Kattwinkel J, ed. Elk Grove Village, IL: American Academy of Pediatrics; 2006: 7–8.

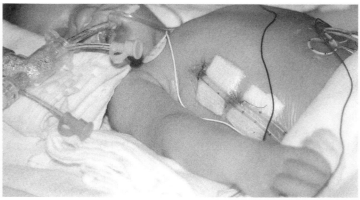

Chest tube.
A chest tube may be placed into the space between the lung and the chest wall to draw out and prevent re-accumulation of air. The chest tube is a clear plastic tube that is sutured to the chest and secured well with tape and sterile dressings. This baby's chest tube enters the skin between the right nipple and armpit area. A baby can have multiple chest tubes if needed.

Pulmonary interstitial emphysema is more difficult to treat because the air is trapped in many small spaces and cannot be removed. Babies with PIE are usually given gentle ventilator support until their lungs heal. The NICU team may allow the baby to have lower blood oxygen levels or higher carbon dioxide levels temporarily in order to decrease the ventilator pressure while the lungs are healing. In some cases, a special ventilator such as a high-frequency oscillator or jet ventilator may be used. Chapter 12 explains how these special ventilators work.

A pneumomediastinum does not need any treatment. The trapped air gradually reabsorbs.

A pneumopericardium must be treated quickly. A needle is inserted underneath the rib cage into the space around the heart, the air is drawn into the needle, and the needle is removed. If there is concern that the pneumopericardium will re-accumulate, a tube with suction attached may be inserted and left in place to drain the accumulated air.

Problems Related to Infection

Infection is a common problem in the NICU, especially among premature babies. Newborns are especially vulnerable to infection for several reasons.

- During the final few weeks of a term pregnancy, protective substances called *immunoglobulins* cross the placenta from mother to baby. Babies born early may not receive these substances.
- Other infection-fighting mechanisms are not fully developed at birth.
- Many of the diseases affecting babies require invasive treatment procedures involving IV lines, catheters, and endotracheal tubes. These devices may introduce infection to the body.

Chapter 9 explains how a baby's immune system functions and why infections are especially problematic for newborns.

Infection

An infection occurs when a bacterium, virus, or fungus enters a part of the body where it is not normally found and causes a reaction. You may also hear the term *sepsis,* which means that infection is present in the blood. The 2 terms, *sepsis* and *infection,* have slightly different meanings but may often be used to refer to the same thing.

Causes of Infection

Three types of organisms are responsible for most neonatal infections: bacteria, viruses, and fungi.

- **Bacteria** are living, single-cell organisms. In healthy humans, bacteria cover much of the outside of the body. They also live in the mouth, intestines, and vagina. Bacteria are found in the environment—on plants, in soil, and in water. Most are harmless; some may actually help protect us from other, harmful, bacteria. Problems occur when bacteria enter an area of the body where they are not normally found; then they may cause an infection. Bacterial infections are treated with medications called *antibiotics.*
- **Viruses** are tiny structures that can survive only by living inside other cells. Those cells (such as the cells in our body) protect the virus and make it difficult to detect and treat. We associate viruses with the common cold and the flu. Viruses are also responsible for illnesses such as measles, chickenpox, and herpes.
- **Fungi** are another type of living organism that can also cause infection. In infants, the most common fungal infection is yeast, caused by a group of fungi called *Candida.*

Some of these organisms are normally found in or on the body with no ill effects. They cause an infection only if they move to an area of the body where they are not normally found. Other organisms can be passed to the baby from the hands of parents, siblings, and caregivers. Still others live in the environment—in the water reservoirs of ventilators or incubators, for example.

Routes of Infection

Infections in the newborn fall into 1 of 3 categories, depending on how and when they occur: intrauterine (congenital), perinatal, and acquired.

Some organisms can cross the placenta and infect the baby while it is in the uterus. Called *intrauterine* or *congenital infections,* they are sometimes represented by the letters TORCH, which stand for toxoplasmosis, other, rubella virus, cytomegalovirus, and herpes simplex virus. Human immunodeficiency virus (HIV) may also be transmitted in this way. Babies born following an intrauterine infection may show a variety of symptoms, including growth restriction (small for gestational age), an unusually large or small head, a rash, an enlarged liver, and abnormal muscle tone and behavior. Intrauterine infections are relatively rare but can be quite serious. If infection occurs early in the pregnancy, it can result in brain, nervous system, or tissue abnormalities or even miscarriage.

The second route by which infants acquire infection is through the birth canal. These are called *perinatal infections.* Group B streptococcus (GBS) is an example of such an infection (see page 327). Organisms may move up the birth canal during the days before delivery and infect the baby in the womb, especially if the membranes rupture. A baby may also acquire an infection as she passes through the birth canal during delivery. Some organisms responsible for these perinatal infections may also cause illness in the mother. Others may live normally in the mother's vagina, causing no symptoms in the mother but producing significant illness in her baby. These types of infections are usually evident within a few days after birth.

The third type of infection in the newborn is an acquired infection, meaning that the infecting organism was passed to the baby after delivery. Organisms that cause acquired infections may be passed to babies from their parents or siblings, health care workers, or the hospital environment. Symptoms usually develop several days to weeks after delivery. Acquired infections are commonly spread through poor hand washing. Before you spend time with your baby, always wash your hands or use alcohol gel. When you are present at the baby's bedside, you can remind other members of the health care team to wash their hands before touching your baby if necessary.

Babies Susceptible to Infection

Newborns are especially susceptible to acquired infection because of an immature or weakened immune system. Other factors predisposing infants to infection are

- Prematurity
- Low birth weight
- Prolonged rupture of membranes
- Maternal fever or infection at delivery
- Fetal distress
- Multiple fetuses (twins, triplets, or more)
- Invasive procedures (IVs, intravascular lines, catheters, and so on)
- Birth defects

Signs of Infection

Babies who are developing an infection often show general signs of illness or signs that mimic other problems. Newborns with perinatal or acquired infections most frequently show signs associated with breathing, such as tachypnea (rapid respirations), retractions (pulling in of the chest muscles while inhaling), cyanosis (blue color of the body or mucous membranes), and grunting while exhaling. Other signs of infection are

- Lethargy (lack of energy) or irritability
- Temperature instability
- Abnormal muscle tone
- Seizures

- Apnea (pause in breathing of 20 seconds or longer) and/or bradycardia (low heart rate)
- Jitteriness
- Feeding problems (vomiting, diarrhea, increased amounts of the feeding remaining in the stomach)
- Unstable blood glucose levels
- Jaundice (different from the common kind of newborn jaundice)
- Poor perfusion (pale, mottled skin; cool hands and feet)

These signs may be subtle or quite dramatic, depending on the severity of the infection and the type of organism causing it. Also, none of these signs is specific for infection and may be caused by other problems or, in some cases, be of no particular significance.

Common Sites for Infection in Babies

Newborns may develop infections in many areas of the body. The most common location is the lungs—and the infection is called *pneumonia*. Other sites include the lining of the brain or spinal cord (meningitis); the blood (septicemia, bacteremia, or sepsis); the skin, especially around the umbilical cord; the bowel (gastroenteritis); and the bladder or kidneys (urinary tract infections).

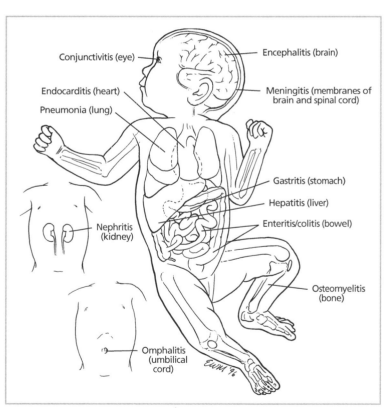

Diagnosis of Infection

To see if your baby has an infection, caregivers do a sepsis workup. They take samples of your baby's fluids (usually blood, urine, and spinal fluid). These samples go to the laboratory, where they grow in broth (cultures) or specialized tests are performed. If microorganisms (bacteria, viruses, or fungi) are present, the culture or special test is positive, indicating an infection.

Sites of infection.
Babies may develop infections in many areas of the body. The most common location for a neonatal infection is the lungs. Other sites include the skin, bowel, bladder, kidneys, heart, and bone. Infection may also occur in the lining of the brain or spinal cord, or as a generalized infection in the blood.

Cultures usually take 24 to 48 hours to develop before a result can be read, and the special tests may take hours or days to get the result. Sometimes bacteria on the skin will get in the culture (a "contaminant") so the antibiotics may need to be continued until this is confirmed.

Samples will be taken from other areas of your baby's body—such as chest secretions or wound swabs—to check for specific types of infections. X-rays of the chest or abdomen may also be done. Less common infections require additional tests.

Treatment for Infection

The first treatment for infants suspected of having an infection is antibiotics—medications that are effective against bacteria. Initially, your baby receives antibiotics that are effective against many different types of bacteria. As caregivers learn more about the type of organism causing your baby's infection, they may give a more specific antibiotic.

Supportive care is also provided to increase your baby's ability to fight the infection. A warm environment, IV fluids, adequate nutrition (oral or IV), and oxygen or ventilation as needed are examples of supportive care.

Specific infections may require additional treatment. Pneumonia sometimes requires intubation of the trachea and use of a ventilator until your baby's lung function begins to improve. Sedatives or anticonvulsant drugs, such as phenobarbital, may be used in the treatment of meningitis or encephalitis.

Short- and Long-Term Complications of Infection

The problems resulting from infection depend on the severity of the infection, the type of organism causing it, and your baby's condition. Some organisms are aggressive, causing significant problems; others have only minor effects. Very low birth weight babies are more likely to be seriously ill with an infection than larger, healthier babies.

Significant infections cause several short-term problems. Some organisms release substances (toxins) into the bloodstream that can interfere with the blood's ability to clot. As a result, your baby may bleed excessively—a condition called *disseminated intravascular coagulation (DIC)*. Shock may accompany infection if the organism interferes with your baby's blood pressure or heart function. Shock occurs when the blood circulation doesn't deliver enough oxygen and fuel to the body for its needs. This can occur for a variety of reasons.

- Hypovolemia (decreased blood volume)—caused by bleeding, vomiting, or diarrhea or because fluid has left the blood vessels and leaked into the body tissues
- Heart failure—caused by infection of the heart cells, or inadequate oxygen to the heart's blood vessels

Any critically ill baby may show signs of shock. These signs may be seen immediately after birth or because of other medical problems.

- Increased heart rate
- Low blood pressure
- Pale, mottled skin
- Decreased oxygen levels in the blood
- Low urine output
- Chemical imbalance in the blood (especially too much acid)

Shock is treated by

- Supporting the baby's blood pressure with fluids and medications
- Keeping the baby warm and well-nourished
- Ventilating the baby to improve oxygenation
- Treating the cause of the shock where possible (for example, giving antibiotics to fight an infection)
- Correcting chemical imbalances
- Sedating the baby to decrease oxygen use

Long-term complications of infection depend on the infecting organism and the site of infection. Treatment with antibiotics usually clears a bacterial infection from the body. Some types of infection may cause damage that takes longer to heal. Severe pneumonia requiring ventilator support may contribute to lung problems, such as bronchopulmonary dysplasia (see Chapter 9).

Meningitis results in brain and nervous system complications, such as motor or mental disabilities, in 2% to 50% of cases. Infections of the kidney or bladder require follow-up investigations to rule out structural abnormalities that may have led to the infection. Blood, skin, and bowel infections usually do not cause long-term complications unless they are accompanied by severe illness.

Group B Streptococcus

"Group B strep," which stands for group B beta-hemolytic streptococcus (GBS), is a type of bacteria found in the birth canal in about 20% of healthy women. This organism does not usually cause any symptoms in the mother, but in some cases may be responsible for urinary tract infection or chorioamnionitis (infection of the amniotic membranes that surround the baby before birth).

The presence of GBS can be detected before the onset of labor if the birth canal and rectum are swabbed (cultured). This GBS screening is usually done at about 36 to 37 weeks of pregnancy. If you carry this organism, you will receive antibiotics during labor to help prevent transmission of the organism to your baby after rupture of the membranes or during delivery through the birth canal. Group B strep can cause sepsis (bacteria in the blood), pneumonia, and/or meningitis in newborns. Risk factors for infection include prolonged rupture of membranes (more than 12 hours), maternal fever, and low birth weight. Approximately 60% of babies born to mothers with GBS have the organism on their skin, but only a small number (1%–2%) of those babies develop GBS sepsis and pneumonia. Those who do become infected can become seriously ill. Often infants with GBS sepsis and pneumonia show respiratory symptoms that mimic those of other respiratory problems, such as RDS. The infection can progress rapidly, with development of shock, apnea, and PPHN (see page 315).

Treatment of sepsis and pneumonia consists of antibiotics and supportive care (temperature control, ventilation, nutrition). In severe cases, your baby may receive immunoglobulins—substances found in the blood that fight infection—or a stimulant of the baby's bone marrow to make more infection-fighting cells.

Birth Defects

At birth, some babies show distinctive physical abnormalities. Others may have hidden abnormalities of the internal organs or organ systems. The medical term for these abnormalities is *congenital* (existing at birth) *anomalies*. The common name for them is *birth defects*.

Causes of Birth Defects

Abnormalities are generally identified as having 1 of 4 basic causes: genetic, environmental, a mixture of the 2, or unknown.

Genetic Defects

As humans, we each have a genetic code that determines who we are: whether we are tall or short, blond or brunette. No 2 people share the same genetic makeup except identical twins.

The information that makes each of us unique is carried on genes found in the 46 chromosomes that are carried in every cell in our body. All cells in the body contain identical genes. When a new life is formed, 23 of the 46 chromosomes come from the mother and 23 from the father.

Problems at the time of fertilization can prevent the chromosome pairs from joining properly. This results in a chromosome, or genetic, defect. How severe the defect is depends on the type of problem it causes. In most cases, chromosome defects are so serious that the fetus cannot survive, and a miscarriage occurs. Sometimes babies with chromosome abnormalities are born alive with birth defects in one or more organs, sometimes severe and sometimes mild.

Down Syndrome

The most common chromosome abnormality is Down syndrome—also called *trisomy 21*. (The word trisomy means 3 chromosomes, and babies with Down syndrome have an extra 21st chromosome.) A child with Down syndrome has 47 chromosomes instead

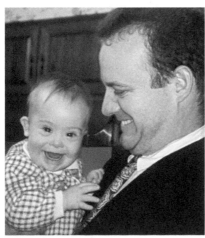

Down syndrome.
A baby with Down syndrome, showing some facial features typical of the syndrome: slanted eyes and broad, flat nose.

of the normal 46. The extra chromosome affects the development of the body, causing the features of Down syndrome, which may include short, wide hands; a crease across the palm of the hand; slanted eyes; a broad, flat nose; low-placed ears; and decreased muscle tone. In addition to producing these visible features, the extra chromosome found in Down syndrome interferes with mental development and may affect structures such as the heart and/or bowel. The risk of Down syndrome is higher when a woman becomes pregnant after age 35, but most children with this condition are born to mothers younger than 35. Extra chromosomes also occur from time to time in other chromosome pairs, such as trisomy 13 and 18; these syndromes are less common than Down syndrome but have much worse outcomes.

Environmental Agents

Much has been written about the influence of the environment on the developing fetus. Although there is a great deal that we don't know, we have identified some specific drugs, chemicals, and toxins that can cause birth defects. These agents—called *teratogens*—can cause problems for the fetus if exposure occurs during a critical period of development, usually the first trimester (the first 13 weeks of pregnancy). Remember that these agents do not always cause problems and that the benefits of some drugs must be weighed against the harm of untreated illness in the mother. Women attempting pregnancy and pregnant women should discuss any use of prescription and nonprescription drugs (including alcohol and recreational drugs) with their medical provider.

Mixed or Unknown Causes

Unfortunately, for most birth defects the cause is either not known or thought to be a combination of genes and the environment. Some of these problems may be detected before delivery, but many will not be diagnosed until after the baby is born. Two birth defects of unknown or mixed origin are described here.

Cleft Lip and Cleft Palate

Problems in the development of the lip and palate may occur alone or as part of a pattern of defects, called a *syndrome*. A cleft lip is a defect that involves an opening from the upper lip to one or both nostrils. A cleft lip may be accompanied by a cleft palate, an opening on the roof of the mouth that connects the oral and nasal cavities. The hole in the palate may cause feeding problems and may need procedures or therapy for dental and speech problems.

If your baby's cleft lip or palate is discovered by ultrasound before birth, you may have referrals to specialists even before she is born. By the time your baby arrives, you will already have received some education and guidance, and specialists will be ready to help with your baby's care. In any case, early treatment involves the use of special feeding devices to reduce feeding problems. Surgery to correct cleft lip and palate will be done later in infancy.

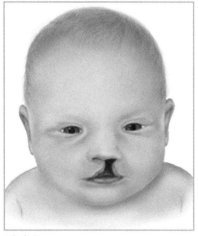

Cleft lip.
A cleft lip is a defect that involves an opening from the upper lip to one or both nostrils. This baby's defect involves one nostril.

From: Centers for Disease Control and Prevention, National Center on Birth Defects and Developmental Disabilities.

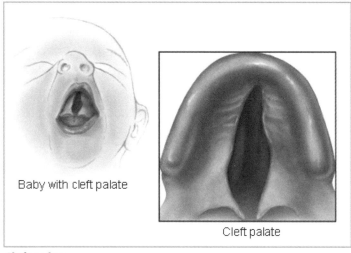

Baby with cleft palate

Cleft palate

Cleft palate.
A cleft palate is an opening on the roof of the mouth that connects the oral and nasal cavities.

From: Centers for Disease Control and Prevention, National Center on Birth Defects and Developmental Disabilities.

Gastrointestinal

Some of the more common birth defects of the gastrointestinal tract are explained below.

Omphalocele

An omphalocele occurs when some of the contents of the abdomen (usually bowel) are in a membranous sac in the base of the umbilical cord. The presence of an omphalocele is sometimes associated with other birth defects of the heart, kidneys, intestine, or brain. After delivery, a baby with an omphalocele will be taken to surgery, where the surgeon

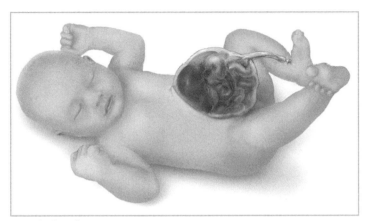

Omphalocele.

An omphalocele occurs when abdominal contents push out into the base of the umbilical cord. The abdominal contents are contained in a membranous sac; however, the sac may rupture at or before delivery.

From: Centers for Disease Control and Prevention, National Center on Birth Defects and Developmental Disabilities.

will try to place the bowel back into the abdomen and close the defect. If the defect is large, the surgeon may place a plastic bag over the bowel and gradually ease it back into the abdomen in stages. If it is very large (a "giant" omphalocele), it may be covered with creams to fight infection and to promote growth of skin from the edges of the sac. Over several weeks, the skin will completely cover it, and then the corrective surgery can be delayed to several months or even years, when it is safer.

Gastroschisis

Similar in appearance to an omphalocele, a gastroschisis occurs in a different way. In this defect, the contents of the abdomen (bowel, stomach, and liver) are pushed outside the abdomen through an opening in the abdominal wall. Because no membrane covers the exposed bowel or other abdominal contents, they are exposed to the amniotic fluid in the uterus and become swollen and matted.

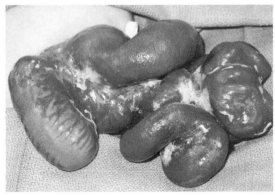

Gastroschisis.

A gastroschisis occurs when the contents of the abdomen (bowel, stomach, liver) are pushed outside the abdomen through an opening in the abdominal wall. Because there is no membranous sac to protect the organs from amniotic fluid, they can become swollen and matted.

Courtesy of Kenneth Gow, MD, Seattle Children's Hospital, Seattle, WA.

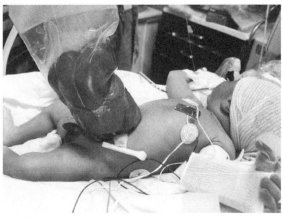

Gastroschisis repair.

A pouch or "silo" may be placed over the bowel in the operating room. Over the next several days, gravity gradually pushes the bowel back into the abdomen, and then the defect in the abdominal wall can be closed surgically.

Courtesy of Kenneth Gow, MD, Seattle Children's Hospital, Seattle, WA.

Gastroschisis is usually not associated with other anomalies except for blockages of the intestines. It requires immediate coverage with a bag to prevent infection and large fluid losses. Putting the bowel back into the abdomen in one step is often difficult because of the amount of swelling present. Instead, a pouch or "silo" may be placed over the bowel in the operating room. Over the next several days, gravity gradually pushes the bowel back into the abdomen, and then the defect in the abdominal wall can be closed surgically.

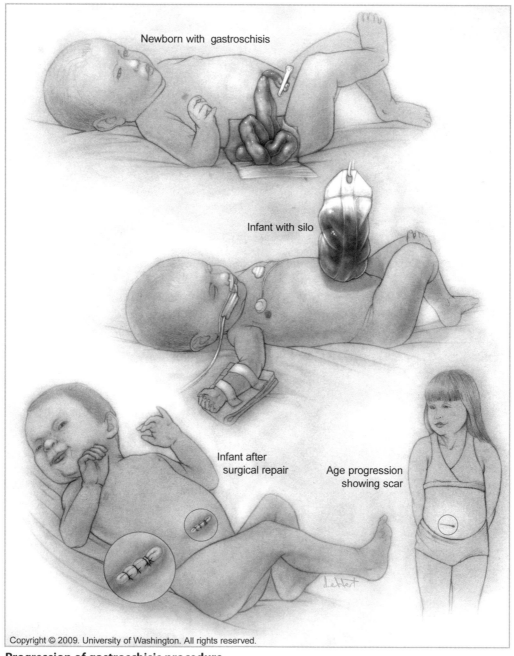

Newborn with gastroschisis

Infant with silo

Infant after surgical repair

Age progression showing scar

Progression of gastroschisis procedure.

©2009. University of Washington. All rights reserved. Used with permission.

Tracheoesophageal Fistula With Esophageal Atresia

A tracheoesophageal fistula (T-E fistula) is an abnormal connection (or "fistula") between the trachea (windpipe) and the esophagus (food pipe); it occurs during fetal development. Of babies with fistulas, 30% to 40% also have other types of anomalies. The J-type fistula, the most common type of T-E defect, has a pouch where the upper part of the esophagus ends. This pouch collects saliva that cannot be swallowed.

Before birth, polyhydramnios (a greater than normal amount of amniotic fluid) is often the first sign of a fistula. Signs in the newborn include increased saliva, respiratory distress, and choking or blue spells during feeding. A fistula can be diagnosed with x-rays.

If your baby has a T-E fistula, she will be kept NPO (not fed by mouth), and a special suction catheter will be used to drain the saliva and prevent choking. Surgery will be scheduled to repair the defect. If the parts of the esophagus are close together, the surgeon will reattach them in one step. If they are too far apart, a 2-step repair will be done. In the first step, a tube will be inserted into your baby's stomach to allow feeding. (See Chapter 16 for information about gastrostomy tubes.) Four to 6 weeks later, a second operation will be done to reconnect the ends of the esophagus. Strictures (narrowing) of the esophagus at the site of reattachment may develop. Reflux (food moving up the esophagus from the stomach) is another possible complication.

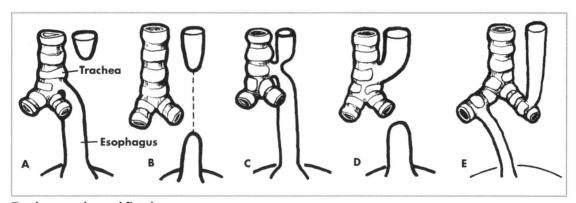

Tracheoesophageal fistula.
Possible variations of a tracheoesophageal fistula include

A: Atresia (blockage) of the esophagus with fistula from the lower esophageal segment. This is a J-type fistula, the most common type of fistula.
B: Absence of the middle third of the esophagus.
C: Atresia of the esophagus with fistulae from both upper and lower segments.
D: Fistula from the upper esophageal segment.
E: Fistula from both upper and lower segments.

From: Gray SW, Skandalakis JE. Embryology for Surgeons: The Embryological Basis for the Treatment of Congenital Defects. *Philadelphia, PA: WB Saunders; 1994:72. Reprinted by permission.*

Duodenal Atresia

A duodenal atresia is a blockage of the duodenum (upper portion) of the small bowel. The reason blockages occur is unknown. Up to 70% of infants with duodenal atresia have associated defects.

Duodenal atresia causes abdominal distention (bloating) and vomiting. The blockage can be diagnosed on x-ray and is treated with surgery. Complications usually occur only if there are associated defects.

Staying Informed

This chapter has explained many of the serious medical problems that bring an infant to the NICU. No more than a few will apply to your baby. This information is intended to give parents a basic understanding of each problem, but it is not intended to replace detailed discussions with your baby's caregivers. Write down your questions, and discuss them with your baby's care team. Keep in mind that just as each baby is unique, so is each NICU. There are different approaches to treating many of these problems. New discoveries are helping to improve the care of tiny and sick infants every day. Some of those discoveries may have an impact on the information in this chapter even before you read it. In medicine, as in many other areas of life today, things change quickly. The best approach is to keep asking questions.

Chapter 11
Neonatal Surgery

Everybody was doing something to help.

Piglet, wide awake suddenly, was jumping

up and down and making "Oo, I say" noises;

Owl was explaining that in a case of Sudden and

Temporary Immersion the Important Thing

was to keep the Head Above Water....

Diane B. Longobucco, RNC-NIC, MSN, APRN, NNP-BC

Surgery on newborns—called *neonatal surgery*—is not an unusual event. Seriously ill infants may have surgery soon after birth to ensure their survival.

Neonates may need one or more surgeries during their hospital stay because of complications of prematurity, serious illness, or other factors. Other babies may be in the well-baby nursery or even discharged home when they develop life-threatening emergencies. And some parents may know far ahead of time that their baby will need to return to the hospital for a planned surgical treatment.

This chapter looks at common aspects of neonatal surgery including informed consent for the procedure, preparations for the surgery, anesthesia and pain relief, and care immediately following surgery. This information is intended as a general guide for parents of infants undergoing all types of surgery. Specific questions about your baby's procedure and care should be addressed to your neonatal intensive care unit (NICU) team and your pediatric surgeons.

Getting the Information You Need

When you first hear the words "Your baby needs surgery," you may be overwhelmed by questions. For most parents, these questions fall into 3 basic categories: Who will be involved? What will the surgery involve and will my baby be alright? What is surgical informed consent?

The Surgeon

General pediatric surgeons are trained to perform surgery on infants and children. They perform a variety of surgeries involving the gastrointestinal tract and the chest region, as well as other procedures. They have experience with many of the surgically correctable congenital anomalies mentioned in Chapter 10. Surgery to treat disorders of specific body systems—such as the brain, heart, kidneys, and bones—is performed by surgeons who specialize in that particular body area. Surgeons with specialized expertise may operate on adults as well as children and infants.

Not all hospitals treat enough critical congenital problems to be expert. If your baby needs a special type of surgery, such as cardiac surgery, he may be transferred to a large university medical center or a children's hospital. The neonatology staff at your hospital will help transfer your baby to a center that specializes in the care required. Transfer to another hospital, especially if it is far from your home, may present more challenges, such as transportation, more time off from work, and child care. It may help to know that babies with unusual or complicated problems need surgical expertise as well as an experienced team of physicians, nurses, nutritionists, and others who know how to manage care after surgery and provide follow-up after the hospital stay. This usually requires the many resources available at a large medical center or children's hospital.

If your baby has a complex problem that requires surgery, you may want to explore treatment options by talking with the surgeon. Resources/support groups may also be available on the Internet to provide you with information on a condition and questions you may need to consider; however, Internet information varies in its accuracy and currency. (See Appendix D for information about how to use the Internet wisely.) If the surgery is not an emergency, it's often advisable to request a second opinion, as you would for any surgical procedure for yourself. This may involve meeting with different surgeons in different hospitals and bringing your baby's x-rays and lab information with you. This process may give you peace of mind about your baby's treatment.

Many neonatal problems are treated in basically the same way by most medical teams. However, some surgeons develop their own styles and may perform single-stage corrective procedures—that is, they correct the problem in one operation. Others perform multiple-stage corrective procedures. Depending on where your infant is treated, who the surgeon is, and the extent of the problem, he may undergo several surgeries, but another infant with a similar problem may have the correction made in one surgery. Keep in mind that your baby's condition may not be identical to another infant's, so you may not be able to compare. Sometimes the condition of the baby dictates how a surgery will be performed. If a baby is very sick and on the ventilator, he may not tolerate a long procedure under anesthesia and the surgery may have to be done in stages.

What You Should Know About the Surgery

Before you agree to a surgical procedure for your baby, you'll want the answers to questions similar to those listed below.

About the Procedure

1. Why does my baby need surgery? What will happen if he doesn't have this surgery?
2. What type of procedure will be done?
3. Are there alternatives to surgery or to a specific surgical procedure?
4. How long will the surgery take?
5. Who will perform the surgery?
6. How many times has the surgeon done this procedure?
7. Will my baby need more than one surgery?
8. When will I meet the surgeon?

About the Anesthesia

1. What type of anesthesia will my baby receive?
2. Will my baby be intubated (on a ventilator) during and/or after the surgery?
3. How long will the anesthesia last?
4. When will my baby wake up?
5. Who is the anesthesiologist?
6. When will I meet the anesthesiologist?

About the Postoperative Course

1. How soon will I see my baby after surgery?
2. Will my baby recover in the NICU or in a different unit?
3. How will my baby look after surgery (for example, will he have an incision, tubes, bandages, or swelling)?
4. Will my baby be given pain medication? If so, what type?
5. Will my baby be given any other medications, such as antibiotics?
6. How long will the stitches (drains, tubes, and other medical equipment) stay in place?
7. How long will my baby need to stay in the hospital following the surgery?
8. When will we see the surgeon again for follow-up care?
9. Who covers for this surgeon if the surgeon is needed and not immediately available (a surgeon who is part of the same group practice or a surgeon from another practice)?

Surgical Consent

Before any surgical procedure, the medical team must get the patient's agreement to the surgery—called *consent*. Because you are the legal guardian for your baby and your baby can't speak for himself, you will be asked to sign the consent form.

In a teaching hospital, surgical residents may perform all or part of your baby's surgery, although the attending surgeon will be present in the operating room (OR). The physicians performing the surgery are usually the ones who obtain the consent. Therefore, the attending surgeon or a surgical resident, rather than the neonatologist, will present the consent form to you. For simple, straightforward procedures, such as central venous line placement or circumcision, a physician from the NICU may obtain your consent. The hospital's policies dictate who obtains consent and what the form includes.

Consent forms vary from hospital to hospital, but all of them should include certain basic points.

1. The name(s) of the attending physician(s) (the surgeon[s] who will perform or oversee the procedure)
2. The name of the procedure that is to be performed
3. The fact that potential risks and complications have been explained to you

When you sign the consent, you are agreeing that the named physician(s) will perform the named procedure and that you understand the procedure, as well as the possible risks and complications. When you sign a surgery consent, consent for anesthesia is implied so a separate consent for anesthesia may not be necessary. However, in many institutions hospital policy dictates that an anesthesia consent also be obtained.

Consent forms can be relatively simple and specific to the particular procedure, while others are complex and difficult to read. Some consents are all-inclusive. This means they include consent for other actions that might be needed along with the surgery, such as a blood transfusion or additional medical tubes or drains. Some hospitals obtain separate consents for blood transfusions.

Take as much time as you need to read and understand the form. Don't be intimidated by someone who may be in a rush. If your baby is having a procedure on one side of the body (for example, eye surgery), make sure that the consent states the correct side of the body (for example, left eye). If the form contains abbreviations you don't understand, have them spelled out clearly. Before you sign the consent, be sure that you understand every word, especially the words that have been written in by the person obtaining your consent.

Read the entire consent form before you sign it. There may be a lot of fine print, but you need to read that too so that you understand exactly what you are signing. Most consents list all of the potential complications of the surgery, including such things as death and loss of a limb. You should not be overly concerned about these potential complications, but you should ask the surgeon about the chances of serious complications. The phrase "informed consent" means that you understand what you are agreeing to and that all of your questions have been answered. If you have any questions about anything to do with the surgery, get your questions answered before you sign the consent.

Preparations for Surgery

"The day of our baby's surgery was almost as stressful as our first day in the NICU. We asked many questions, sometimes more than once. Information helped us to calm down and feel a little more in control."

Neonatal surgery is not always an emergency. You may know weeks ahead of time that your baby will need surgery and you will need to wait for your baby to grow large enough for the procedure. In most cases, some preparation is required before surgery. The extent of this preparation depends somewhat on the complexity of the surgery. Here are some basic steps that may be done before surgery.

Common Neonatal Surgical Procedures

Central line placement: A thin, flexible catheter is placed into a larger vein to deliver fluids, nutrients, and medications to the body. *Broviac catheters* are placed through an incision under the skin, into a vessel, and enter the vena cava, a large vessel that carries blood to the heart. A *PICC line* (peripherally inserted central catheter) is threaded through a needle into a vein, into the vena cava.

Circumcision: Removal of the foreskin of the penis. (See Chapter 15.)

Colostomy: A surgically placed opening on the baby's abdomen into the colon that allows stool (feces) to drain from the bowel into a collecting bag. A colostomy is most commonly placed after surgical removal of a portion of the large (lower) intestine. (See Chapters 10 and 16.)

Exploratory laparotomy: Surgery used to examine the abdominal organs and to aid diagnosis. Depending on what is discovered during exploratory surgery, major surgery may be needed.

Fundoplication: A procedure used to treat severe gastroesophageal reflux. A procedure (most commonly known as *Nissen fundoplication)* in which the top of the stomach is sewn around the lower end of the esophagus (food pipe) to prevent stomach contents from flowing back into the baby's esophagus (reflux).

Gastrostomy tube: A tube used for feeding, which is inserted through a surgically created opening in the abdominal wall into the stomach. (See Chapter 16.)

Hernia repair: A procedure performed in the inguinal area (pelvic region) to repair a weakness or gap in the muscle wall after contents of hernia (usually intestines) are pushed into an adjacent body cavity.

Ileostomy: A surgically placed opening on the baby's abdomen that allows stool (feces) to drain from the bowel into a collecting bag. An ileostomy is most commonly placed after surgical removal of a portion of the small (upper) intestine. (See Chapter 16.)

Laser photocoagulation: Laser is used to produce heat that causes tissue destruction in the retina and stops the progress of ROP.

Patent ductus arteriosus ligation: Surgical closure of the ductus arteriosus. The ductus is an open blood vessel (patent ductus arteriosus) in the heart that allows blood to bypass the lungs in utero and normally closes after birth. When this fails to close after birth it is sometimes necessary to surgically close it by cutting it or tying it off. (See Chapter 9.)

Thoracotomy: A surgical incision of the chest, necessary for placement of a chest tube. A chest tube drains air or fluid from the space surrounding the lungs.

Tracheostomy: A surgical opening made in the neck and into the trachea (windpipe). The baby breathes through a tube placed in this opening instead of through his nose or mouth.

Ventriculoperitoneal shunt: A device used to drain excess fluid from the brain; used in treatment of hydrocephalus. (See Chapter 10.) A thin tube, called a *shunt,* is inserted into the ventricle of the brain, passes underneath the skin, and drains the excess cerebrospinal fluid into the abdominal cavity where the fluid is reabsorbed.

Anesthesia Support

If your baby requires anesthesia, you will meet the anesthesiologist and perhaps members of the anesthesia team. An anesthesiologist is a physician specially trained to administer medications that provide anesthesia (partial or complete loss of feeling and consciousness) and analgesia (pain relief). An anesthesiology resident may be working with the attending anesthesiologist. Some institutions use certified registered nurse anesthetists, who are specially trained to administer anesthesia in collaboration with the attending anesthesiologist. The visit from the anesthesia team is your chance to ask questions regarding your baby's anesthesia. Sometimes your baby will need to be intubated (tube in the windpipe) for anesthesia and may be on a ventilator (breathing machine) after surgery. You should ask about the type of anesthesia planned and potential complications.

Laboratory Support

Depending on the type of anesthesia and surgery your baby will require, tests may be needed before surgery. Complete blood counts, measurement of blood electrolytes (such as sodium and potassium), and a chest x-ray or ultrasounds are frequently performed on infants who will have general anesthesia (put to "sleep" for the surgery).

Respiratory Support

Even if your baby is breathing on his own, a tube may be placed in your baby's throat (intubation), and he may be attached to a ventilator before surgery. This makes it possible for the anesthesiologist to control your baby's breathing in the event that anesthesia or pain medications affect the baby's ability to breathe on his own.

Intravenous Support

Your baby may be kept NPO (no food given by mouth) for a time before surgery because medications for anesthesia and pain relief can cause nausea and vomiting. If your baby vomits during or after surgery, the empty stomach helps prevent the possibility of choking and aspiration (fluid entering the lungs). Your baby will have an intravenous (IV) line to provide fluids and glucose until the surgeon determines that he can begin to eat again. The length of time before feeding resumes depends on many factors, including the type of procedure and the medications used for anesthesia and pain control, but mostly on the return of bowel function after the use of anesthetics.

Temperature Support

Your baby must be kept warm during the ride to and from the OR and in the OR itself, which is usually cooler than the NICU. Your baby may wear a hat, and his arms and legs may be wrapped in a soft material to retain warmth. Your baby may go to the OR covered in warm blankets in the NICU incubator, on a radiant warmer, or in a warm battery-powered transport incubator. Whatever the transport method, most surgeons use a radiant warmer during surgery to keep the baby warm. In some cases, the surgery will be done in the NICU or a room adjacent to the NICU to avoid the problems of transport to and from the OR.

Parent Support

The NICU staff are aware that this event is very stressful for parents and will support you by providing information about your baby's condition. A NICU nurse, the NICU clinical nurse specialist, or a clinical nurse specialist who works for the surgical team will usually educate and inform parents before the surgery. Some parents also find it helpful to speak to other parents whose infants have had a similar procedure.

Another source of support may be your own clergy or the chaplaincy service at the hospital. If you have not yet done so, you may wish to have your baby baptized or blessed before surgery. Your NICU nurse or social worker can help you make arrangements.

Time Out

All hospitals follow The Joint Commission Universal Protocol for Preventing Wrong Site, Wrong Procedure, Wrong Person Surgery. This is called a *time out*. This means that people involved in your infant's surgery will ask you over and over again what surgery is being done, and perhaps what side of the body the surgery is on. Someone may mark the site (if it will be done on the right or left side) and recheck your baby's identification several times. This repetitive checking and questioning does not mean that the surgical team does not know what type of surgery they are performing on your infant. Time out is a safety procedure in place to minimize medical errors.

Waiting for the Outcome

On the day of the surgery, you may wish to stay with your baby until he goes to the OR. Some hospitals even allow parents to accompany their baby to the OR. Others allow you only as far as the elevator or doors to the OR. Ask the nurse who provides your preoperative information about specific policies.

Your baby is probably on the OR "schedule" for a certain time. Remember that the schedule may change, depending on other surgeries and activities in the OR. The NICU or OR staff should let you know about major changes in the day's schedule so that you can adjust your expectations for receiving information and seeing your baby after the operation.

On the day of the surgery, make sure that you know where you can wait to be kept informed of the surgical progress and when you will be able to speak to the surgeon

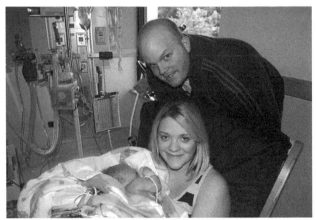

Preoperative preparation.
These parents spend a few quiet moments with their baby before his complex heart surgery. See his postoperative photos on pages 348 and 351.

afterward. Some physicians have nurses (usually the clinical nurse specialists) who will keep you informed during the course of the operation. If not, remember that emergencies and delays in other areas of the OR may delay your child's surgery. Also, procedures sometimes take longer than expected.

Try to find a comfortable place to wait during surgery (some hospitals have special waiting areas for families), and bring a book or magazine to read or something else to do. Make sure you eat something the day of surgery, especially if the procedure is a lengthy one. You don't want to feel faint when you are finally able to reunite with your baby.

Surgical Anesthesia

Only a couple of decades ago, newborns were subjected to major surgery and painful procedures without anesthesia. It was believed that babies did not need anesthesia during surgery because they did not "feel" pain. This belief began to change in the 1970s, as research in this area increased. As a result, pediatricians, surgeons, and anesthesiologists started to explore methods of safe anesthesia for infants. Even through the 1980s, giving babies anesthesia, even for complex surgeries, remained controversial.

Research in 2 major areas has made neonatal surgery without anesthesia rare today. First, researchers have studied how newborns perceive pain and how their bodies metabolize (break down) medications. Second, safer medications have been developed for anesthesia and pain relief in children and adults. In the 1980s, the American Academy of Pediatrics began to support the use of local or general anesthesia in all newborns undergoing surgical procedures and today consider it unethical to perform surgery without anesthesia. Even circumcisions are performed today with topical and/or local anesthesia.

The type of anesthesia is determined by several factors including the surgical needs, the age of the infant, whether the infant will be extubated (taken off of the ventilator and allowed to breathe on his own) at the end of the surgery or shortly after, the need to control blood pressure, and the need for pain control in the postoperative period. The numerous techniques available include inhalational gas techniques, IV drug administration, regional anesthetic techniques, muscle relaxants, and narcotics such as fentanyl. If extubation is planned at the end of surgery or shortly after, the anesthetic medication must be adjusted so most of the anesthetic effects have worn off by the time the baby needs to breathe on his own. The anesthesiologist, in conjunction with the neonatologist and the surgeon, will decide what type of anesthetic is best for your baby. The anesthesiologist must explain all of the possible risks and side effects, which may sound like a frightening list of complications. However, your baby is unlikely to experience many of the risks and side effects the anesthesiologist names for you. Every baby reacts differently to anesthesia, and the surgical team is prepared to deal with complications that may occur as a result of your baby receiving anesthesia.

Types of Anesthesia

Anesthesia types used in neonatal surgery include topical, local, regional (nerve blocks), and general. Each has its own special uses.

Topical Anesthesia

Topical anesthetics are those that are applied to the skin. When applied prior to a procedure, the medicine enters the underlying skin and the area becomes numb (loses the ability to feel touch and pain). Although topical anesthesia is not effective for major surgery, it is reliable and successful and used in many minor procedures.

Nerve Blocks

When used in an awake or sedated patient, a nerve block eliminates the patient's ability to feel pain in a specific area. There are 2 types of nerve blocks: local anesthesia (in which a small, specific body area loses sensation or becomes numb) and regional anesthesia (in which a larger area of the body is unable to feel sensation or pain). Anesthetics used for dental procedures are classified as nerve blocks.

Local Anesthesia

Local anesthesia is used when a small, specific area of the body is numbed for a procedure or surgery. Many adults have had local anesthesia for dental procedures. In the newborn, local anesthesia is commonly used during circumcision. Before surgery begins, the baby receives an injection of medication in the area of the procedure. An effective block numbs the area, and the baby does not feel pain during surgery.

Regional Anesthesia

"When the doctor said Tyler would have an epidural, I felt better about the surgery. I had an epidural in labor and knew it had worked well for me."

Regional anesthesia results in the inability to feel pain while the patient remains awake. Two types of regional anesthesia used for neonatal surgery include caudal epidural and spinal anesthesia. For newborn, preterm, or maturing preterm infants undergoing surgical procedures, regional anesthesia has become more popular than general anesthesia because it does not have many of the undesirable side effects of general anesthesia. Regional anesthesia is often combined with general anesthesia to assist with early extubation and postoperative pain relief. Regional anesthesia can be used when the operation is elective (planned), the site of the surgery is below the level of the umbilicus (navel), and the procedure is expected to take less than 2 hours in preterm and former preterm infants. Regional anesthesia is frequently used during inguinal hernia repair as infants undergoing this procedure often fit these criteria.

Regional anesthetics such as epidural blocks can be administered by a single injection or through a catheter, a tiny tube placed in the epidural space around the spinal column. Multiple doses of the medication can be administered through the catheter. At the end of the operation, the catheter can also be used to deliver medication for postoperative pain. The infant may be awake during regional anesthesia but is usually given a sedative. The benefit of regional anesthesia is that your infant does not need general anesthesia and ventilator support. After surgery, your baby may be groggy, but this effect decreases as the medication wears off.

General Anesthesia

General anesthesia is most often used for the larger, more complex operations within the body cavities. This type of anesthesia is sometimes said to "make the baby sleep," but in reality, the baby has loss of consciousness and loses the ability to feel pain. Medications that produce general anesthesia are given through an IV line or inhaled. Other medications, such as sedatives or muscle relaxants, may be used with the anesthetics to help reduce the amount of the anesthetic medications needed.

Administration Through Intravenous Line

The IV approach to inducing general anesthesia may include a combination of various drugs, including muscle relaxants, barbiturates, propofol, narcotics, and ketamine, because these drugs produce sedation, analgesia, and amnesia. The IV method commonly uses a drug called *fentanyl*, a narcotic frequently used for pain relief in the NICU. Given at higher doses than those used for pain relief, fentanyl is an effective anesthetic for infants undergoing major surgery. Narcotics such as morphine sulfate and others may also be used as a neonatal anesthetic. A major side effect of all narcotics is respiratory depression (slowing of breathing). Therefore, infants who receive narcotics for anesthesia require intubation and monitoring in case of breathing difficulties.

Administration by Inhalation

General anesthesia may also be induced by using inhaled anesthetics. In this approach, the baby breathes in a gas form of an anesthetizing medication. This type of anesthesia works well, is easy to administer to a patient of any size, and is rapidly metabolized by the body. Dosages can be adjusted throughout the surgical procedure so that the baby can be extubated after the procedure and will wake up shortly. If the baby will not be extubated for a day or two, extra anesthetic may be given toward the end of the operation to provide sedation and pain relief. Before the procedure, ask what the anesthesiologist and surgeon plan to do in the OR and after the procedure. You will then be prepared if your baby is groggy or unresponsive when you see him after surgery.

Side Effects

Although useful, effective, and easy to administer, general anesthesia has the most side effects of all anesthetics used for newborns. The most common side effects are apnea (a cessation of breathing for 15–20 seconds), periodic breathing, low oxygen levels, heart or circulation problems, and a slow heart rate. It is unclear exactly why postoperative apnea occurs, although it may have the same causes as apnea of prematurity (see Chapter 9) or may be due to leftover sedation effects of the anesthetic or muscle relaxant. Apnea that occurs after surgery usually resolves within 24 hours.

To reduce the chances of postoperative apnea, elective surgery is usually postponed until the infant is at least 44 weeks' postconceptional age (about 1 month after the expected due date). If this is not possible, infants who are already home should be admitted and monitored for at least 24 hours after surgery. Some physicians prescribe caffeine before surgery because it can regulate the respiratory center and reduce the occurrence of apnea. Frequently, if a formerly preterm infant requires surgery such as a hernia repair, the procedure is performed a few days before discharge. The infant can be monitored for a day or two after the procedure without prolonging the hospital stay.

One study showed that those infants most likely to develop apnea had lower (less than 30%) hematocrits. As a result of this study, some physicians place infants on iron supplements before surgery and delay surgery if the baby's hematocrit is low. Rarely are infants transfused right before surgery unless the hematocrit is very low or the procedure is an emergency. It is impossible to predict exactly which infants will develop postoperative apnea, but adhering to guidelines about age and hematocrit seems to reduce risks.

When the Surgery Is Over

Most babies return immediately to the NICU after surgery, bypassing the recovery room or post-anesthesia care unit. In some hospitals, your baby may go to a specialized postoperative intensive care unit, such as a neurologic or cardiothoracic unit. If that is the case, your baby may be transferred back to the NICU after a few days or may remain in the specialized unit until discharge.

What to Expect Right After Surgery

Immediately after surgery, the recovery nurse will be very busy assessing your baby's overall condition, recording frequent vital signs, and obtaining lab specimens and x-rays. A baby who has undergone a simple surgical procedure, such as central venous line placement or hernia repair, usually requires less intervention postoperatively than does a baby who has undergone complex surgery. Again, these are general guidelines. Your baby's situation will be unique, and policies vary from unit to unit. Once the immediate postoperative tasks are completed, and as long as your baby is stable, you'll be encouraged to spend time with your baby. The time you spend with your infant in the initial postoperative period may be brief, but will increase as your baby's condition improves and he is able to interact with you.

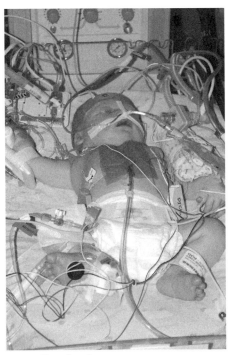

Immediately after surgery.
After his cardiac surgery, this newborn is covered in tubes and wires. The dressing on his chest covers a large open incision.

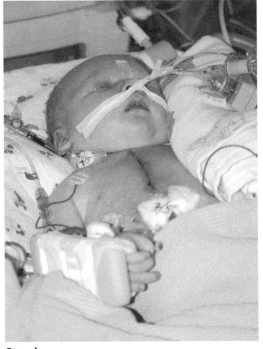

Steady progress.
The baby makes steady progress in the days following surgery and requires less intensive support.

You will soon feel relieved when your baby comes through surgery, things settle down a bit, and you can concentrate on his recovery. You will want assurances that your baby's pain is being controlled and that your role as a parent is valued. Your knowledge of your baby's unique cues for demonstrating pain and indicating other needs will be valuable to the medical team during this time. Ask questions about your baby's condition and participate in your baby's care as he stabilizes.

Pain Relief After Surgery

"After surgery, the nurse showed me how to cup my warms hands around Brian's feet. He seemed to like that, and it made me feel better to be doing something for him."

The nurses and medical team caring for your baby will assess your baby's pain by monitoring his vital signs and activity level and will decide which medications or techniques will provide the best relief. Pain perception seems to be different from infant to infant, and a combination of medication and comfort measures may be necessary.

Acetaminophen

Most infants experience discomfort after surgery, but not all infants require a lot of pain medication. For simple procedures, a dose or two of acetaminophen (Tylenol or Tempra) may be all that is required. Acetaminophen is given by mouth or as a rectal suppository. It relieves mild to moderate pain and may be combined with a narcotic if your baby requires more pain relief.

Narcotics

If your baby has undergone major surgery (cardiovascular, urogenital, gastrointestinal, or neurologic), narcotic pain relief may be used. These drugs are often administered through an IV, eliminating the need for a needlestick. They can be administered as a single dose, or continuously as an IV infusion if your baby requires pain relief for a few days.

Morphine sulfate and/or fentanyl are 2 of the most common narcotics given, although there are several that may be used. The risks and benefits of each drug are considered before they are prescribed for your infant.

Two side effects of both morphine and fentanyl are tolerance and dependence. Tolerance to a drug means that progressively higher doses are required to achieve the same therapeutic effect. Dependence means that the patient becomes used to the effects of the drug and stopping it abruptly can cause withdrawal symptoms. If these drugs are administered at high doses or for more than a few days, your baby may be weaned from the drug (the dosage slowly decreased over time) rather than having it abruptly discontinued.

Sedatives and Hypnotics

In addition to pain medications, sedative drugs may also be given to your infant during the postoperative period. These drugs produce sedation, hypnosis, and amnesic effects but have no effect on pain. They produce a generalized calming effect and a sleeplike state in which there is no memory of the event. Common drugs in this category include benzodiazepines (midazolam and lorazepam) and chloral hydrate.

Non-Pharmacologic Techniques

Many interventions, in addition to medications, can help relieve pain. These may include facilitated tucking or containment, touching, stroking, holding, swaddling, and speaking softly to the baby. Some babies respond to a few drops of a high concentration of sugar water (sucrose) given through a nipple. This method works in the brain, similar to a narcotic, by reducing the perception of pain.

These interventions help some babies, but others may become more agitated. If you have used a particular type of touch that has relieved your baby's discomfort in other circumstances, it may now help soothe him after surgery. Talk to your nurse about your baby's pain cues and techniques of containment or positive touch you can use with your baby.

Be sure to ask what medications and techniques will be or are being used to control your baby's pain. Not all units manage postoperative pain relief in the same way, but understanding what is being done to relieve your baby's pain will help reduce your anxiety as well.

The Postoperative Period

As your baby stabilizes and makes progress, you'll be able to participate more in his care for longer periods. The amount of equipment attached to your baby may determine when you can hold him. Until then, remember that your voice and touch are an important part of your baby's care and recovery. Babies generally recover more quickly than older children, and your baby may rapidly shed the extra tubes and equipment.

As your baby heals, usual care patterns will resume. Vital signs will be needed less frequently, and your baby's sleep will be interrupted less often. Depending on the type of surgery, your baby's surgeon or neonatologist will decide when your baby can start eating. Sutures or staples used to hold the skin together while it heals are generally removed 1 week after surgery, so if your baby is discharged before then, you'll need to return to the surgeon's office to have them removed. Many sutures are made from natural materials that the body will absorb and do not require removal.

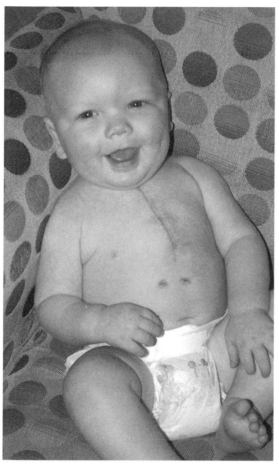

Happy at home.
This baby continues his recovery at home with involved parents who support his development and advocate for his health care needs.

It's not always possible to determine immediately if a surgical procedure is successful. You may need to wait while your baby undergoes some tests (x-rays, scans, and so on) to evaluate the adequacy of the surgery. Often, gastrointestinal surgery requires a waiting period. Then your baby may have a test called a *barium swallow*. For this test, your baby is fed a small amount of oral contrast and is then x-rayed. The contrast material shows up on x-ray and clearly defines the gastrointestinal tract for evaluation.

If your baby was cared for in a specialty unit postoperatively, he may be transferred back to the NICU when special postoperative care is no longer necessary. For some babies, surgery is the last hurdle before discharge. For others, it may be a step along the course of continued hospitalization.

The usual discharge criteria (such as adequate age, adequate weight, and ability to feed) apply postoperatively. Your baby's discharge plan and follow-up care will include any special needs or technological assistance required at home.

Your baby's postoperative condition and whether or not your baby requires more surgery will determine how much follow-up you will have with the surgeon. If your baby has had a hernia repair, he will probably need to be seen only once after discharge to assess proper healing. If your infant has undergone complex surgery, however, you and your child may develop a long-term relationship with the surgeon.

The Parent's Role in a Baby's Recovery

Surgery, even on very small babies, is commonplace in most NICUs. Understanding your baby's condition and the procedures involved helps reduce anxiety. Be sure you understand what the surgery is supposed to accomplish, and ask as many questions as you can think of before and after the procedure. Seek support from your baby's nurses, your social worker, and friends and family who can be there for you during this stressful time.

Surgery may be the last major barrier to discharge—and for some, it can be the most difficult and frustrating. Your baby may have been almost ready to go home—taking most or all feedings from the breast or bottle and off of most medications. Immediately after the surgery your baby may be very sick, not eating, and on all monitors again, but most babies heal quickly and this period will be short-lived. You are a very important part of your baby's recovery. Your voice and touch can do much to comfort your sick baby and help make this difficult time pass quickly for both of you.

Chapter 12
Diagnostic and Therapeutic Techniques: Progress and Promise

"Pooh!" cried Piglet, and now it was his turn

to be the admiring one. "You've saved us!"

"Have I?" said Pooh, not feeling quite sure.

Ellen Tappero, DNP, RN, NNP-BC

The complexity of your baby's care in the neonatal intensive care unit (NICU) presents challenges to nurses and physicians. It also presents opportunities to use state-of-the-art technology.

Since the 1960s, rapid advances in the computer industry have brought about an explosion of technology in the NICU. This technology has changed not only the way the health care team works with high-risk babies, but also the appearance of the NICU. Although the NICU may seem cluttered with a lot of high-tech equipment, that "clutter" allows older, time-tested treatments to be monitored more closely and applied more effectively, with less risk of complications.

Like other specialty areas, neonatology has its own language and alphabet-soup shorthand. RDS, SGA, and ABG—abbreviations for respiratory distress syndrome, small for gestational age, and arterial blood gas—may become part of your everyday conversation after only a day or two in the NICU. Extracorporeal membrane oxygenation, therapeutic cooling, and magnetic resonance spectroscopy—3 of the treatments and diagnostic approaches explained in this chapter—may seem more intimidating because you'll hear them less often. This chapter highlights and explains some of the technical advances and procedures that are being used in many NICUs across the United States and Canada. If your baby's care involves any of these technologies, you'll be better prepared to understand the health care team's explanations after you've learned a bit about them.

This chapter focuses on 4 treatment approaches and 4 diagnostic imaging advances.

- High-frequency ventilation (HFV)
- Extracorporeal membrane oxygenation (ECMO)
- Inhaled nitric oxide (iNO) therapy
- Therapeutic hypothermia
- Computed tomography (CT) scans
- Ultrasonography
- Magnetic resonance imaging (MRI)
- Magnetic resonance spectroscopy (MRS)

Not all of these complex therapies and diagnostic tools will be used for your infant. In fact, not every NICU will use or have all of them available. To keep things simple, focus on those therapies or tools that play a part in your baby's care. These explanations are somewhat general, and you may need to ask your baby's health care team for more information.

Therapeutic Treatments

Some of the most common problems NICU infants experience are associated with breathing and with getting enough oxygen to the body systems, tissues, and the brain. The 4 treatments discussed in this section have had dramatic effects on seriously ill infants in many NICUs. It will take more time for the newest treatment, therapeutic hypothermia for the prevention of brain injury, to prove its safety and efficacy, but clinical studies with term newborns show a great deal of promise, and this therapy is quickly becoming the standard for eligible infants.

High-Frequency Ventilation

Chronic lung disease (CLD) remains a leading cause of extended hospital stays as well as significant respiratory problems for infants. As a result, many efforts in modern neonatal care have focused on methods that might reduce the incidence of this complication. Over the last 20 years, a great deal of laboratory and clinical research has focused

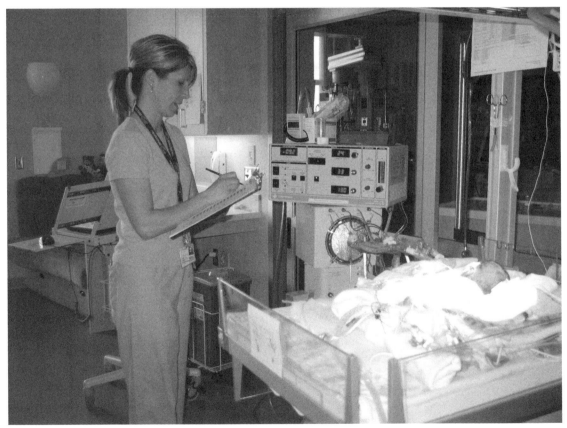

HFV.
A baby on HFV rests on a radiant warmer, closely monitored by the NICU nurse.

Courtesy of Providence Sacred Heart Medical Center & Children's Hospital, Spokane, WA.

on HFV, and it has become an important tool in the neonatal provider's arsenal for providing breathing support to infants in severe lung failure.

Conventional ventilators require high pressures to deliver the volume of gas necessary to inflate a "stiff" (noncompliant) lung. But medical professionals believe that the high pressures and high concentrations of oxygen required by conventional ventilators may cause injury to the lungs and airways, including such conditions as air leaks in the lungs (called *pulmonary air leaks)* and bronchopulmonary dysplasia (BPD), which lead to CLD. High-frequency ventilation is a form of mechanical ventilation that delivers small tidal volumes (amount of air inhaled and exhaled with each normal breath) at rapid rates in an attempt to avoid those complications. High-frequency ventilation is not always the preferred choice, and your baby's medical providers will determine which ventilator therapy seems best for her unique situation. Some studies show no advantage for HFV over conventional mechanical ventilation in the prevention of BPD; therefore, they are not recommended as initial therapy in the treatment of RDS for preterm infants.

When first introduced in the early 1990s, HFV was used as a "rescue" therapy for infants with severe lung disease who appeared to be "flunking" or who were not improving with conventional ventilation. Many studies have demonstrated that HFV is an effective method of providing both oxygenation (supplying oxygen) and ventilation (removing carbon dioxide from the blood). It has been used most successfully on infants with pulmonary air leaks, such as pulmonary interstitial emphysema (PIE), pneumothorax, and pneumopericardium. (See Chapter 10 for a discussion of pulmonary air leaks.) Originally used only before an infant was placed on ECMO or to enhance the delivery of nitric oxide therapy, HFV has gained popularity as a more conventional means of ventilation as more clinical studies have been completed. High-frequency ventilation has also been used with limited success on infants diagnosed with RDS (see Chapter 9), diaphragmatic hernia, persistent pulmonary hypertension of the newborn (PPHN), and meconium aspiration. (See Chapter 10 for information on these conditions.)

With conventional ventilators, the machine rate is measured in breaths per minute. When an infant is on HFV, the machine rate is so fast that counting the number of breaths per minute is virtually impossible. Instead, the health care team will use the term *hertz* to state the HFV rate. One hertz (Hz) is equal to 60 cycles of the ventilator. For example, a high-frequency ventilator set to run at 15 hertz delivers 900 cycles (or "breaths") per minute. For premature infants, between 10 and 15 hertz is a typical setting for a high-frequency oscillatory ventilator. Term infants will usually start with 7 to 10 hertz. A ventilator set to operate at 7 hertz would deliver 420 cycles or "breaths" per minute. This is a typical operational setting for a high-frequency jet ventilator.

The health care team's evaluation of the baby on HFV is different than when the baby is on conventional ventilation. Infants can breathe on their own during HFV, but it may be hard to tell at times because of the vibrating "breaths." The team must observe or feel the vibrations or wiggling of the chest rather than listen with a stethoscope.

Two techniques are commonly used for producing HFV.

High-frequency jet ventilation (HFJV) is produced by delivering short bursts (high-speed pulses) of gas directly into the trachea (windpipe) and down the airways to the alveoli at a rate of 240 to 600 cycles or "breaths" per minute. The nursing staff and other members of the health care team refer to this type of ventilator as the *jet*. This type of HFV was the first to be approved by the US Food and Drug Administration (FDA) for use in infants with RDS complicated by pulmonary air leaks and is still being used for this type of respiratory problem in NICUs today. It seems to be most effective for respiratory problems in larger infants in whom carbon dioxide elimination is the biggest problem.

During normal breathing, you actively bring air into your lungs by expanding your chest wall and thus inflating your lungs. In exhalation, you relax the respiratory muscles of your chest wall and diaphragm, passively deflating your lungs. To allow your baby to have sighs (deep breaths) and continued expansion of the alveoli at the end of expiration, HFJV is used in conjunction with a conventional ventilator. It is similar to conventional mechanical ventilation in that the expiration phase is passive; air is exhaled by the "automatic" recoil (bounce-back) of the chest wall and lung.

High-frequency oscillatory ventilation (HFOV) is quite different from HFJV. High-frequency oscillatory ventilation actually vibrates the air; it opens the lungs with a sustained breath and then vibrates (oscillates) around that pressure using a vibrating diaphragm or piston that alternates between pushing and pulling small volumes of gas within the airway. It operates at rates ranging from 600 to 900 cycles ("breaths") per minute. In HFJV, passive recoil of the lungs and chest wall expels gas from the lung. In HFOV, the gas is actively pulled out of the lung during exhalation. This method of HFV is therefore classified as active expiration. High-frequency oscillatory ventilation has been compared with conventional ventilation in a number of studies and it is in widespread use in many neonatal centers. At present, it is most often used to treat preterm infants with RDS and pulmonary air leaks, such as PIE, as well as for term infants who are approaching ECMO criteria. Studies using animal models have shown that the combined use of surfactant replacement therapy and HFOV may have a synergistic effect in reducing lung injury and improving outcomes. High-frequency oscillatory ventilators have been available only since 1990, however, and were not FDA approved until March 1991. The health care team may also refer to this type of ventilator as the *oscillator*. Research continues to be conducted to evaluate the long-term effects of this technique.

Once HFV is started (it doesn't matter which technique is used), you'll notice that your baby begins to shake. Shaking of the chest and abdomen is the most obvious, but in very small infants, the whole body may appear to tremble. Don't be alarmed. This is a normal result of HFV therapy. The amount of vibration produced during HFV depends on the rate and pressure being used as well as on the size of the infant. When HFV is used in adults, patients describe the vibration as "soothing." The continuous motion appears to relax infants as well; as a result, fewer sedatives are needed to keep infants on HFV from fighting the ventilator. Infants are eventually weaned from HFV and placed on a conventional ventilator, nasal continuous positive airway pressure (CPAP), or a nasal cannula, where they remain until they no longer require any breathing or oxygen assistance. (See Chapter 9 for information about nasal CPAP and the nasal cannula.)

"The NICU equipment is amazing. It's absolutely magic."

Extracorporeal Membrane Oxygenation

The machine used for ECMO (pronounced "EK-mo") is a modification of a heart-lung bypass machine that allows for a longer period of therapy than the one used in

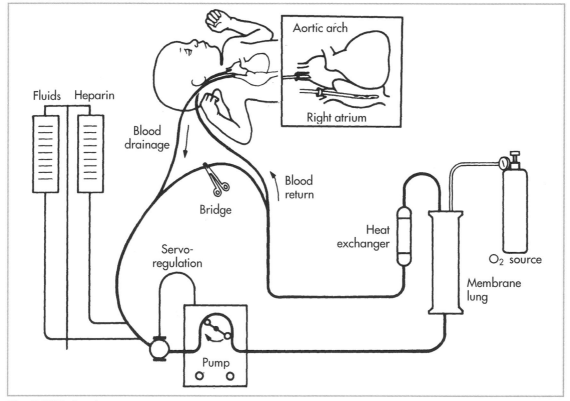

The ECMO circuit.
ECMO acts as an artificial heart and lung for critically ill late preterm and full-term infants who do not improve with conventional ventilation or medications.

From: Nugent J. Extracorporeal membrane oxygenation (ECMO) in the neonate. In: Beachy P, Deacon J, eds. Core Curriculum for Neonatal Intensive Care Nursing. *Philadelphia, PA. WB Saunders; 1993:180. Reprinted by permission.*

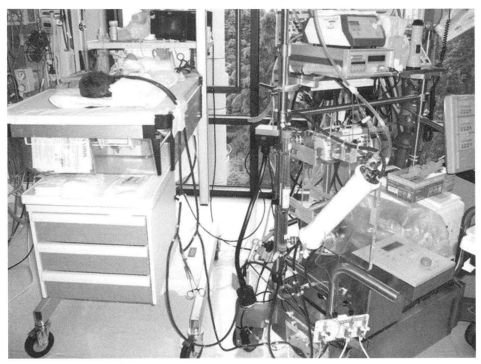

Extracorporeal membrane oxygenation.
Each baby on ECMO is staffed by a nurse and an ECMO specialist (usually a nurse, a respiratory care practitioner, or a perfusionist) who has received hours of special training on both the equipment and the physiologic process.

the operating room for open heart surgery. Extracorporeal membrane oxygenation provides cardiac (heart) and respiratory (lung) support to the 2% to 5% of critically ill late preterm infants (gestational age 34–36 weeks) or term infants with severe lung failure who do not respond to the usual therapy of maximum conventional ventilation or medications. Extracorporeal membrane oxygenation is surgically and technically complex and is not available at every NICU; therefore, if your baby requires ECMO treatment she may be transferred to another hospital. At present, infants are considered for ECMO when other therapies have failed and the baby continues to deteriorate. Extracorporeal membrane oxygenation is usually only offered in circumstances when the problem is reversible or temporary. These infants usually have one of the following problems: lung infection such as pneumonia, meconium aspiration syndrome, RDS, PPHN, or a congenital diaphragmatic hernia.

Large tubes (catheters) need to be placed in the baby's blood vessels; therefore, only babies weighing more than 4 pounds are candidates for ECMO. Babies who have large bleeds in their brains and babies who have chronic lung changes from being on the ventilator for more than 2 weeks are generally not considered good candidates for this procedure.

Because ECMO is an invasive procedure, physicians will explain the process, the possible complications, and how they expect your baby to respond to the treatment. You will need to sign a consent form (see Chapter 11) giving them permission to insert the catheters and begin the therapy.

Types of Extracorporeal Membrane Oxygenation

There are 2 types of ECMO: venoarterial (VA) bypass and venovenous (VV) bypass. The method selected depends on whether the infant needs both heart and lung support or mainly lung support.

Venoarterial Bypass

If both heart and lung support is needed, ECMO is started by placing the infant on VA bypass. The surgical procedure required to place the ECMO catheters—called *cannulation*—is usually performed by a surgeon with the operating room staff in attendance. Cannulation is commonly done at the infant's bedside to avoid the risks involved in moving a critically ill infant to and from an operating room. The ECMO machine is brought to the baby. Before the catheters are placed, the infant is given medications for pain, for sedation, and to briefly paralyze her (stop all muscle movement) to prevent the formation of an air embolus (bubble) in the bloodstream.

For VA ECMO, 2 tubes (catheters) are used. The first tube (catheter) is placed in a large neck vein on the baby's right side and is then gently threaded (pushed or advanced) into the right atrium of the heart. A second catheter is placed next to the first one, but it is inserted into the carotid artery (a large artery in the neck that carries blood from the heart to the brain) and advanced to the infant's aortic arch (vessel through which the body is supplied with oxygenated blood). After the catheters are inserted, an x-ray is taken to confirm that they are in the correct positions. The catheters are then connected to the ECMO circuit, which has been primed (filled) with heparinized adult donor blood. The heparin keeps the blood from clotting when it is exposed to the surfaces of the catheters and ECMO circuit tubing.

Venoarterial ECMO therapy—in which a catheter is placed in both a vein (veno) and an artery (arterial), as just described, is used for infants with heart or blood pressure problems. The advantage of VA bypass is that it supports not only the lungs, but also the heart. Therefore, if heart function is a concern, VA ECMO will be used. A disadvantage of VA ECMO is that the carotid artery is usually tied off after decannulation (removal of the catheter). However, many units are now repairing the carotid artery if the ECMO run has been less than 7 days, which returns circulation to its normal pathway through the carotid artery.

Venovenous Bypass

The second method for initiating ECMO is a VV bypass. A double lumen catheter (a catheter with 2 canals inside) is placed in a vein in the neck. This approach is used in infants who do not have problems with blood pressure or heart function. The advantage to this method is that once the ECMO therapy is completed, the carotid artery does not need to be tied off, as it must be in a VA bypass. Infants who are started on VV ECMO and later develop blood pressure problems or continue to have low oxygen levels can be changed over to VA ECMO if necessary.

In VA ECMO, dark blood (blood containing little oxygen—deoxygenated blood) is drained by gravity from the infant through the catheter that was advanced into the right atrium of the heart. The ECMO pump (which acts as an artificial heart) pushes this blood through the rest of the ECMO circuit. As the drained blood passes through the membrane oxygenator (which acts as an artificial lung), carbon dioxide is removed and oxygen is picked up. The blood enters the oxygenator dark (deoxygenated) and comes out bright red in color (oxygenated). When the blood leaves the oxygenator, it is warmed in the heat exchanger and returned to the infant through the arterial catheter.

The procedure for VV ECMO is the same as in VA bypass except that the blood is drained and returned through the same catheter, the one in the right atrium. This catheter has 2 lumens (openings). One-half of the catheter drains the dark blood and the other half returns the oxygenated (red) blood to the infant.

Extracorporeal Membrane Oxygenation Therapy

Extracorporeal membrane oxygenation saves lives, but it does require more staff and equipment than conventional management of respiratory failure. Each baby on ECMO is staffed by a nurse and an ECMO specialist (usually a nurse, a respiratory care practitioner, or a perfusionist) who has received hours of special training on both the equipment and the physiologic process. The staff is required to monitor and maintain a trouble-free ECMO circuit 24 hours a day, both providing routine maintenance of the circuit and taking emergency actions when unexpected, potentially catastrophic events occur. The baby's regular care is often the responsibility of another nurse while the baby is on ECMO. A physician familiar with ECMO and the infant's plan of care must be available 24 hours a day; this may or may not be the infant's primary physician. The costs of the equipment and the staffing needed to run the circuit add up to a high daily ECMO charge. These charges are usually reimbursed by insurance companies, however, and should not play a part in your decision to use ECMO as a treatment for your infant.

Even though your infant is supported by ECMO and is not using her lungs to breathe, she will remain on the ventilator. Very low settings (low pressures and low oxygen concentrations) are used to "rest" your baby's lungs. The tube in the infant's trachea (windpipe) allows secretions to be suctioned out, and the light breaths from the ventilator help keep the baby's lungs inflated.

When ECMO is started, the pump is at first set at a low flow rate to check for leaks in the system and to ensure that the gravity flow of blood from the venous catheter is adequate. The flow rate of the pump is gradually increased until about 80% of the blood your infant's heart pumps out (cardiac output) is diverted through the ECMO circuit. This usually requires flow rates of 90 to 120 milliliters per kilogram (of infant weight) per minute (mL/kg/minute). At maximum flow rates, your infant's arterial blood gases should be normal. This high flow rate means that ECMO is doing most of the work of providing oxygen to your baby's blood. While on high flow rates, infants usually remain quiet and may receive pain medications as well as a sedative to ensure comfort. Babies on ECMO may open their eyes, breathe on their own, and occasionally move their arms and legs in response to stimulation, such as your voice or a soft touch.

As your infant improves, the ECMO flow rate is decreased and more blood goes to her lungs for the exchange of oxygen and carbon dioxide. A decrease in the amount of ECMO support (or a decrease in the percentage of bypass) over a period of several days is an important sign that your baby is improving. Eventually, she will no longer need ECMO support to maintain adequate gas exchange at low ventilator settings.

When the ECMO flow rate is decreased to 30 to 50 mL/kg/minute it is called "idling." If your baby's improved lung function remains stable at low ventilator settings during idling, the catheters are clamped, and a trial period off ECMO is attempted. If your baby's arterial blood gases deteriorate, the catheters are unclamped, and ECMO support is resumed. If blood gas values remain good while your infant is off ECMO, the catheters are removed from your baby's neck (decannulation). After decannulation, your infant will be weaned from the ventilator as tolerated and routine NICU care will be resumed.

How long an infant remains on ECMO varies depending on her condition and on the recovery of both heart and lung function. Most newborns average 5 to 7 days on ECMO. Length of treatment depends on the age of the infant, the original illness, the amount of damage to the lungs before ECMO was started, and any complications that may have occurred during ECMO.

Risks and Complications of ECMO

Although ECMO therapy has improved the outcome of infants with severe lung failure, there are risks associated with this procedure.

Bleeding: Heparin is added to the blood in the ECMO circuit to prevent it from clotting when it comes in contact with the surfaces of the catheters and circuit tubing. The amount of heparin needed is monitored closely, and the infant's bleeding times (amount of time it takes for a small quantity of blood to clot) are tested frequently to minimize risks. Bleeding may occur anywhere in the body, including the brain. If bleeding does occur and cannot be stopped, ECMO therapy may be discontinued.

Infection: Any time a catheter is introduced into the body, there is always a risk of infection. Infants on ECMO may be given antibiotics (drugs to prevent or fight infections) throughout the ECMO run and are watched closely for signs of infection.

Blood transfusion reactions/complications and/or infections: Infants on ECMO usually require several transfusions of blood products. As with all blood transfusions, there is a risk of hepatitis, AIDS, and/or a blood transfusion reaction. All blood from the hospital's blood bank is screened for these and other viruses, but a small risk of acquiring a disease is always present.

Mechanical failure: A mechanical failure can occur at any time. Although safety precautions are used, the circuit tubing could break, the oxygenator could fail, and the neck catheter could accidently be pulled out, to name only a few of the possibilities. The ECMO specialist watching the circuit is trained to handle just such emergencies. Should one occur, the infant will be placed on increased ventilator settings until the problem is resolved and ECMO can be resumed.

Emboli: Air emboli (bubbles) and tiny clots can move from the ECMO circuit into the infant's bloodstream, leading to complications and possibly death. Safety precautions are taken, and the ECMO specialist monitors the circuit continuously for both air and blood clots.

Of the total number of babies that have been placed on ECMO for respiratory problems, 76% have survived. This figure is lower than in the early 1990s, when the survival rate was reported at 80%. However, with newer technology and treatment modalities, babies who eventually require ECMO are sicker than in the past. For these sick babies, ECMO is indeed a lifesaver. Babies are offered ECMO treatment only if there is a high likelihood of not surviving without it. According to the 2009 Extracorporeal Life Support Organization Registry Report, survival rates for infants on ECMO to treat each of these causes of lung failure are as follows:

- Meconium aspiration: 94%
- PPHN: 78%
- RDS: 84%
- Infection/pneumonia: 58%
- Congenital diaphragmatic hernia: 51%
- Sepsis: 75%
- Pulmonary air leak syndrome: 74%

Overall, studies show a strong benefit for using ECMO related to survival at the time of discharge.

Neurodevelopmental Outcome

Because infants who are treated with ECMO are critically ill at birth, it is difficult to determine whether their neurodevelopmental outcome is a result of the original illness (when there was a low oxygen concentration in the blood) or strictly related to ECMO therapy. Several follow-up studies have been conducted to assess both medical and developmental outcomes of infants treated with ECMO. Studies show that the neurodevelopmental outcome among infants treated with ECMO is consistent with the developmental outcome of infants who had severe respiratory failure and were treated with conventional therapy.

The long-term effects of ECMO during later childhood and adult life remain unclear. Further studies are needed, but it seems that ECMO is safe and that normal development is possible depending on the infant's diagnosis prior to treatment.

"My own mother had a premature baby 30 years ago. When she visited Janis, I know she was thinking 'if only we had known about this back then.' But at the same time, she was glad that her grandchild was going to live."

Nitric Oxide Therapy

Approval of iNO by the FDA in December 1999 brought another therapeutic advance to neonatal medicine. As recently as the mid-1980s, nitric oxide (NO) had a bad reputation as a common air pollutant found in cigarette smoke and smog. It was blamed for acid rain and the depletion of the ozone layer and was suspected of causing cancer. Nitric oxide is a small, light molecule that investigators have only recently discovered is a crucial part of the body's neurochemical system. It is essential for activities ranging from digestion to blood pressure regulation. It is not to be confused with laughing gas, or nitrous oxide, which you may have received at the dentist's office or in the operating room.

In the early 1990s, much attention was focused on the role of NO as a blood pressure regulator. Cells that line the inner walls of both veins and arteries release NO; from there, it migrates to nearby muscle cells and relaxes them. This dilates (enlarges) the blood vessels allowing more blood flow and lowering blood pressure. Keeping this discovery in mind, neonatal physicians looked more closely at infants who had persistent pulmonary hypertension, a condition in which the arteries in the lung are constricted.

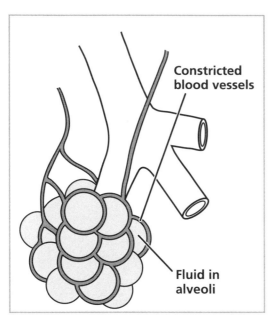

The fetal lung.
The fetal lung has diminished blood flow because of constricted blood vessels.

From: American Academy of Pediatrics, American Heart Association. Textbook of Neonatal Resuscitation. *5th ed. Kattwinkel J, ed. Elk Grove Village, IL: American Academy of Pediatrics; 2006:1–4.*

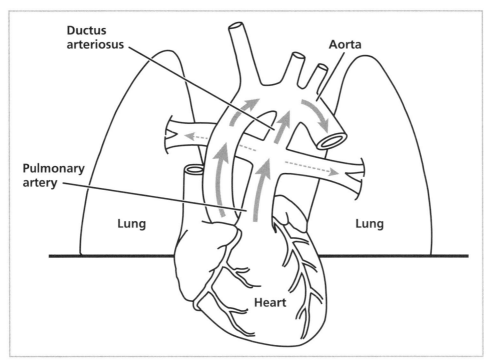

Patent ductus arteriosus.
The open ductus arteriosus allows blood to flow past the lungs of the fetus.

From: American Academy of Pediatrics, American Heart Association. Textbook of Neonatal Resuscitation. *5th ed. Kattwinkel J, ed. Elk Grove Village, IL: American Academy of Pediatrics; 2006:1–4.*

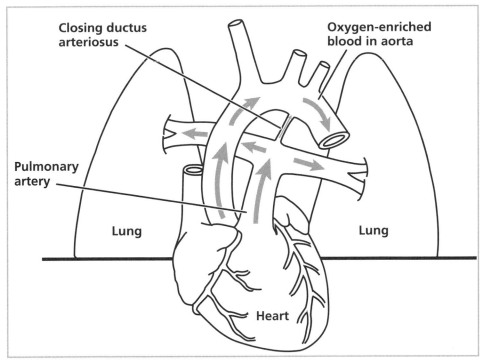

The ductus arteriosus beginning to close.
At birth, the ductus arteriosus closes off and allows more blood to flow to the lungs. The increased blood flow through the lungs supplies body tissues with oxygen as the baby breathes.

From: American Academy of Pediatrics, American Heart Association. Textbook of Neonatal Resuscitation. 5th ed. Kattwinkel J, ed. Elk Grove Village, IL: American Academy of Pediatrics; 2006:1–6.

In the uterus, fetal lungs serve no respiratory purpose; the placenta supplies the fetus with oxygen. The alveoli of the lungs are filled with fluid rather than air. Therefore, the blood that flows through the lungs is unable to pick up oxygen and carry it to other parts of the body. The blood flow through the fetus's lungs is much less than what is needed after birth. This diminished blood flow is the result of the partial closure of the arterioles (vessels in the lung) located next to the alveoli (see page 366). The constriction (closure) of the arterioles results in a large amount of blood being diverted through the ductus arteriosus. The ductus arteriosus is a small blood vessel near the heart that connects the vessel that supplies blood to the lungs (the pulmonary artery) to the vessel that supplies blood to the body (the aorta) (see page 366).

At birth, when a newborn takes her first few breaths and expands her lungs, the arterioles (blood vessels in the lungs) open up and let more blood flow through the lungs. Blood that was previously diverted through the ductus arteriosus (while the baby was in the uterus) now flows to the lungs, where it picks up oxygen and carries it to the body. The ductus no longer serves a purpose, and it eventually closes (see page 367).

In preterm infants with RDS or term infants with conditions such as meconium aspiration, infection/pneumonia, or congenital diaphragmatic hernia, the respiratory compromise may be complicated by PPHN (see Chapter 10) caused by low blood oxygen levels. In these infants, the non-oxygenated blood that would normally go to the lungs is forced away from the closed arterioles and is channeled through the ductus arteriosus (which never closed or may have reopened after birth) to the aorta, leaving the blood unoxygenated. This creates a vicious cycle of unoxygenated blood in the body, leading to further pulmonary arteriole constriction.

In the past, vasodilators (drugs used to open or widen the blood vessels) and ECMO have been used to treat PPHN. Vasodilators have had limited success because they performed inadequately. They either produced too little vasodilation or they produced too much, widening the blood vessels to the point where the blood pressure in the whole body became too low. Extracorporeal membrane oxygenation has been effective in supporting these infants, but the therapy is invasive and can have major complications.

Nitric oxide was first described as an endothelial-derived relaxing factor, which is a vasodilator produced by the body. This relaxing factor has been shown to contribute to the normal opening of the pulmonary vessels after birth. Any alteration in the body's production of this molecule may result in failure of the pulmonary vessels to relax. Investigators have found that inhalation of NO (delivery of NO to the infant through a tube in the windpipe) allows the gas to diffuse directly into the smooth muscle of the pulmonary vessels, producing vasodilation. Giving NO by inhalation is thought to be most effective in dilating pulmonary (lung) vessels, but not the systemic (rest of the body) blood vessels, therefore avoiding the problem of a low blood pressure in the body.

Several studies have shown that in term and late preterm infants with respiratory failure unresponsive to the usual methods of support, inhaled NO increased the level of oxygen in the baby's blood and reduced the need for ECMO. Another study demonstrated that newborn survival without CLD was increased in the patients treated with inhaled NO.

Premature newborns with underdeveloped lungs and severe oxygenation problems that do not respond to conventional ventilator support and surfactant therapy have also been successfully treated with inhaled NO. Inhaled NO continues to be investigated for its use on premature infants. One study concluded that inhaled NO did not decrease the rates of death or bronchopulmonary dysplasia in infants born weighing less than 1,500 grams. Another study showed inhaled NO seems to benefit the larger preterm infant (birth weight at least 1,000 grams), showing a substantial decrease in death and bronchopulmonary dysplasia. No short-term negative outcomes were identified in preterm infants weighing 1,000 to 1,200 grams.

Recent studies have shown that the neurodevelopmental outcome of term and preterm infants treated with iNO does not seem different from that of infants treated conventionally and with ECMO. However, the initial improved pulmonary outcome has not changed the need for outpatient treatment of lung disease or translated into a decrease in rehospitalization rates. Despite the positive findings, the risks and benefits of inhaled NO are still being carefully considered because long-term outcomes remain unclear.

Although treating newborns earlier in their disease progression may not improve the mortality statistics, earlier treatment may prevent the disease from progressing, and long-term outcomes may be affected by preventing more severe disease. Inhaled NO has the potential to change the management of severe neonatal respiratory failure, but there are still questions to be answered. Does pretreatment with surfactant improve the response to inhaled NO? Can it be used in infants without PPHN? What is the optimal dose? Does HFV augment the response to inhaled NO? Will earlier treatments with more conventional therapies such as surfactant and HFV be as effective as inhaled NO? Future studies will need to answer some of these questions and continue the investigation to prove NO to be both safe and effective at decreasing pulmonary hypertension.

Therapeutic Hypothermia for Hypoxic-Ischemic Encephalopathy

Hypoxic-ischemic encephalopathy (HIE) is a common cause of brain damage in the term newborn. (HIE is also discussed in Chapter 10). It is a term that is used to describe abnormal neurologic behavior in the newborn period that is the result of a hypoxic-ischemic event. These events occur before or during birth and are the result of hypoxia (the lack of or a decreased amount of oxygen in the blood) and ischemia (a reduction or cessation of blood flow to the brain). The hypoxia and ischemia may occur at the same time or one after the other. Before birth, hypoxia is the result of an improperly functioning or detached placenta (abruption) or an obstruction to blood flowing through the umbilical cord, which can eventually lead to respiratory and cardiac problems. Some risk factors of hypoxia in the fetus before birth include placental abruption, placenta previa, umbilical cord compression, umbilical cord prolapse, abnormalities in placental circulation, rapid or prolonged labor, maternal hypertension, maternal cardiac arrest, uterine rupture, fetal heart rhythm irregularities (cardiac arrhythmias), and fetal to maternal transfusion (blood loss from the fetus to the mother's circulation). Hypoxic-ischemic events lead to asphyxia (a progressive buildup of acid with a decrease in oxygen and an increase in carbon dioxide in the blood) and are caused by a compromise or cessation of placental or pulmonary gas exchange. Ultimately, these events cause a dysfunction of the baby's brain (encephalopathy). This type of damage can occur in both term and preterm infants. The site of the brain injury depends on the gestational age of the newborn and the maturity of the blood vessels as well as the metabolic activity of the brain. (See Chapter 10 for more information on asphyxia.)

Hypoxic-ischemic encephalopathy is often divided into 3 categories or stages: mild, moderate, and severe. Mild HIE almost always has a good outcome, and treatment is usually only supportive in the newborn period. Moderate to severe HIE continues to be an important cause of acute brain injury for term infants. In technically developed countries, asphyxia during labor or birth affects 3 to 5 per 1,000 live births, and subsequent moderate to severe HIE occurs in 0.5 to 1 per 1,000 live births. Worldwide, HIE is a major problem affecting infants. Death occurs in 10% to 60% of these infants in the newborn period, and 25% of survivors have long-term neurologic disabilities. There has been no significant improvement in the treatment of this tragic event over recent decades, and only supportive care has been available.

In recent years, we have begun to understand the processes that lead to neuronal (nerve cell) death with hypoxic-ischemic brain damage. Experimental studies have indicated that neuronal death occurs in 2 phases. The first phase is early (primary) neuronal damage seen with the initial injury. During this phase there is exhaustion of the cell's high energy stores, which leads to cell rupture and death of the cell. This is also known as *primary energy failure*.

Recovery and reperfusion, that happens during resuscitation, may lead to complete recovery or to a secondary phase of late neuronal damage or reperfusion injury. Whether the cell injury can be reversed depends on several factors, which include the severity of the initial injury, the baby's body temperature, and the other disease processes that are occurring at the same time. The late or delayed neuronal death occurs approximately 6 to 15 hours after the initial injury and can last for hours to days. In this second phase, the cells shrink with retention of the cell membrane rather than rupture, as is seen with early neuronal damage. This secondary phase is associated with encephalopathy, increased seizure activity, and a worsening neurologic exam. The secondary phase of energy failure accounts for a significant proportion of the final cell loss after severe hypoxic-ischemic insults.

Recent studies indicate that induced hypothermia (cooling), started before the second phase of energy failure, protects the brain from injury. The precise mechanism by which hypothermic neuroprotection occurs is unknown, but it is believed to modify the cells that would have died during the secondary phase of energy failure, leading to their survival. Hypothermia may also protect neurons (cells that transmit brain messages) by reducing the brain's metabolic rate, which reduces energy use and therefore reduces neuronal loss.

The possibility that mild cooling might be beneficial has been known to clinicians for almost 300 years. Hypothermia as a strategy for protecting the brain has been used since the 1950s by cardiologists to maintain brain function when the heart is purposefully stopped during open heart surgery. Over the past few years, several studies and multiple systematic reviews of therapeutic hypothermia in the newborn have been published and evaluated. An important outcome of these reviews is that in term infants with moderate to severe encephalopathy, cooling decreases mortality (the death rate) without increasing major neurodevelopmental disability in survivors. There is also some evidence of harm from therapeutic hypothermia, such as decreased platelet counts and low blood pressure, but the benefits of therapeutic cooling on survival and neurodevelopment outweigh these short-term problems.

The 2 methods currently being studied to provide hypothermia as a neuroprotective intervention are selective head cooling and whole body cooling. With either method, the baby is cooled with a goal of keeping the rectal temperature at approximately 34.5°C (94°F). The heart rate of the baby falls, but as long as the blood pressure and oxygen saturations are stable, no intervention is needed. The baby requires therapeutic hypothermia for a period of 24 to 72 hours. At the end of the cooling period, rewarming will begin over a 4- to 24-hour period.

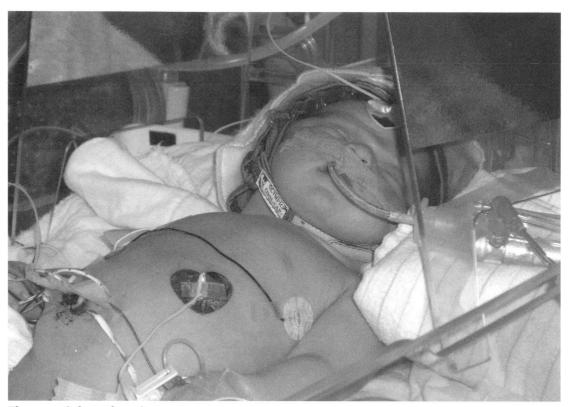

Therapeutic hypothermia.
This infant is wearing a head cooling device in an attempt to prevent brain injury following birth asphyxia.

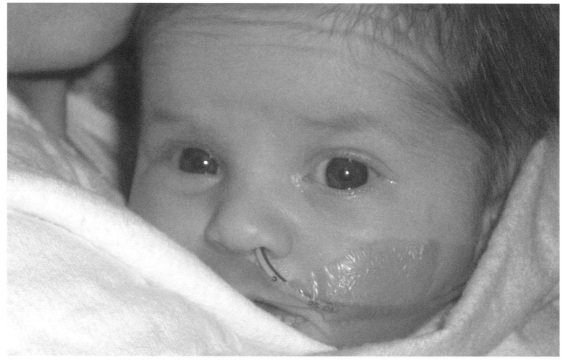

On the road to recovery.
This baby is now convalescing and will require neurodevelopmental follow-up to ensure her best possible outcome.

It is difficult to make a distinction whether head cooling is superior to whole body cooling because study results using both methods were similar. Selective head cooling can be achieved using a cooling cap over the scalp while the body is warmed by an overhead warmer to limit the degree of systemic hypothermia. Whole body cooling involves the baby lying on a cooling mattress. The long-term effects of hypothermia as a neuroprotective therapy for HIE at school age and later are not yet known.

Hypoxic-ischemic encephalopathy remains a challenging problem for the health care team. Selection of babies to receive this treatment include being term or near term in gestation, meeting the criteria of moderate to severe HIE, and starting the procedure prior to 6 hours of age. Currently, therapeutic hypothermia is the only intervention that shows promise in improving neurologic outcomes in full-term newborns with HIE. One in 6 babies, especially those with milder degrees of encephalopathy, will see some benefit from the therapy. However, for those babies with severe HIE, the outcome is not as promising.

As the mysteries of brain injury continue to be unraveled, a variety of neuroprotective strategies will emerge, targeting the pathways that lead to cell death. Extensive experimental data from adult and neonatal animal research strongly support a combination of pharmacologic agents (drugs) with therapeutic hypothermia to improve the outcomes of babies with brain injury. Future studies should evaluate simpler methods of cooling, earlier or later initiation of cooling, the most appropriate method of rewarming, the duration of rewarming, and the effect of hypothermia combined with pharmacologic agents. Future studies will also need to address long-term follow-up focusing on cognitive abilities such as learning and thinking, and neuromotor abilities such as walking and talking.

Diagnostic Imaging Techniques

"I'm a computer engineer. For me, it was easier to understand what the nurses told me about the equipment than what they told me about our baby."

Imaging techniques are simply methods for "seeing" inside something without opening it up. These techniques play a vital role in helping to identify (diagnose) the cause of medical problems. Important diagnostic imaging techniques developed since the early 1980s have revolutionized the field of diagnostic radiology by giving health care providers a better look at the internal structure and function of a baby's organs. Diagnostic imaging methods have gone from invasive examinations (tests in which catheters needed to be inserted or dyes had to be injected) to noninvasive and painless examinations, such as real-time ultrasonography and CT scanning. These techniques offer the health care team a tremendous amount of insight into such neonatal problems as congenital malformations, hydrocephalus, and intracranial hemorrhages (sometimes referred to as *bleeds)*. (See Chapters 9 and 10 for an explanation of these problems.)

More recently, MRI and MRS have extended the health care team's ability to detect physical abnormalities in specific areas of the body. The potential diagnostic value of MRI and MRS for the newborn is just beginning to be appreciated. In many cases, only one imaging technique may be used; however, they may often be used in combination to give a clearer picture of the problem. Each of these diagnostic imaging methods has its advantages and inconveniences, as the explanations that follow indicate.

Computed Tomography

The procedure called computed tomography—CT or CAT scan for short—became recognized as a diagnostic imaging tool in 1973. It involves aiming a very narrow beam of radiation at a specific layer of tissue and getting a computer-assisted reconstruction of the x-ray slices to provide a 2-dimensional picture of internal structures. Just as in a conventional x-ray, on a CT scan, bone absorbs the largest amount of x-rays and appears white; air absorbs the least and appears black. Because soft tissue is neither as dense as bone nor as thin as air, it appears as shades of gray. A CT scan is much more sensitive to tissue densities (thicknesses) than is a conventional x-ray. It can also detect changes in much smaller areas of tissue than a conventional x-ray can.

A CT scan is used to help determine the extent of a malformation or disease. It provides precise detail of the anatomy despite bone covering the area or overlapping of nearby body structures. In newborns, it is used most frequently to detect brain injury (cerebral lesions). It is not very useful in detecting chest (thoracic) defects because heart and lung movements distort the image. Injecting the infant with a contrast material through an IV site (known as *contrast enhancement)* can help measure blood flow to an area or define an abnormality. For most lesions in newborns, however, contrast enhancement for a detailed view of the blood vessels is not necessary.

Computed tomography scans are more reliable than ultrasonography or MRI in diagnosing or excluding certain kinds of brain and spinal cord hemorrhages, such as subarachnoid (below the innermost membrane covering the brain), subdural (below the outermost membrane covering the brain), and intraparenchymal (within the tissue of the brain). These small lesions may not be seen on ultrasound, and they may not be as easy to distinguish on MRI. (See Chapter 9 for information on intraventricular hemorrhage and the grading of these lesions.)

Because motion distorts the CT scan image, newborns usually need to be restrained and sometimes sedated for the study. However, new generation CT scanners are much faster than older models, and the need for sedation has markedly decreased. Computed tomography scanning is also unsuitable for repeated use because of the cumulative radiation dosages and the hazards of moving the infant from the NICU to the hospital's radiology department. For these reasons, real-time ultrasound at the baby's bedside has become the preferred method for diagnosing brain hemorrhages in newborns.

Ultrasonography

Ultrasonography uses high-frequency sound waves to evaluate internal anatomic structures, tissue movement, and blood flow. This diagnostic technique was first introduced into obstetric practice in 1966, but wasn't used routinely with newborns until 1979. It is now common obstetric practice to have a prenatal ultrasound done early in pregnancy to evaluate the fetus.

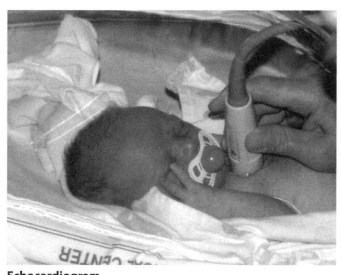

Echocardiogram.
The ultrasound machine can be used to scan the baby's heart.

Ultrasound imaging is based on mapping variations in reflected sound waves (echoes) within a specific region of the body. Using electronic mechanisms, a transducer in contact with the infant's skin sends brief ultrasound pulses through the tissue. These pulses are reflected by tissue interfaces (boundaries between 2 surfaces) and returned to the transducer as an echo. The transducer both sends (emits) the initial impulse and receives the reflected impulse. A computer constructs a 2-dimensional image from the reflected sound energy. Only tissues that are reflective enough to send back echoes are recorded and displayed on the scanner. Whether tissue is reflective depends on its density. The differences in the strength of the returning signals (echoes) are displayed on the scanner as various shades of gray. The stronger the reflection (the denser the tissue), the brighter (more echogenic) the image will appear on the scanner. Ultrasound cannot be used to scan bone, the lungs, or the bowel because the interfaces between soft tissues and bone and between soft tissues and air do not produce echoes. This method is used frequently in the NICU to scan the infant's brain to rule out intraventricular hemorrhages. If bleeding has occurred, its progression and the reabsorption of the blood will be followed with repeated ultrasounds.

The following are advantages of ultrasonography as a neonatal diagnostic tool:

- No ionizing radiation is necessary. Therefore, ultrasonography can be used frequently to evaluate the brain or to monitor the progression of bleeding inside the brain.
- No sedation is required. Injection of contrast material is not necessary.
- Ultrasound can be performed at the infant's bedside with portable equipment.
- Ultrasonography is less costly than CT scanning or MRI.
- The procedure is noninvasive and therefore considered mandatory in evaluating infants suspected of having heart disease.

Ultrasonography has the following disadvantages:

- Bone, excessive fat, and gas act as barriers, totally blocking or distorting images. Certain parts of the body must be scanned through a "window"—in the case of the brain, through the anterior fontanel (soft spot). The usefulness of echocardiography (ultrasound scan of the heart) is limited when overinflated lungs or chest wall deformities prevent adequate imaging.
- The usefulness of the scan depends on the operator's ability and the type of equipment used.

Ultrasound scans cannot differentiate tissues with similar structural composition. The interface (boundary) between the 2 tissue types is not well displayed on ultrasound. Computed tomography scanning is a superior method for imaging of tissues with similar structural compositions because it detects different densities. For example, a CT scan can differentiate the white and gray matter in the neonatal brain because the 2 have different densities (white matter regions have more water). Ultrasonography cannot.

A technique called *Doppler ultrasound* can be used along with regular ultrasonography by simply "flicking" a switch on the machine. Doppler complements 2-dimensional ultrasound because it detects disturbances in blood flow resulting from abnormal anatomic structure. Doppler-derived calculations are useful in estimating blood flow and the severity of stenotic (narrowing) lesions. From Doppler ultrasound, estimates can be made about blood velocity (speed) and the direction of blood flow. These estimates are based on changes in sound wave frequencies reflected from moving structures, such as circulating red blood cells. Doppler ultrasound is most often used in echocardiography of the heart and in determining blood flow in the brain. Despite the availability of new imaging techniques, ultrasonography and Doppler ultrasound remain the first choice in NICUs because they make a quick bedside diagnosis possible and lack side effects.

Magnetic Resonance Imaging

The theoretic basis of MRI is complex. The technique is based on interactions between the field of a large magnet in the imaging equipment and the atoms in the body. The magnetic field aligns the nucleus of a cell in the general direction of the magnetic field.

Once aligned, these nuclei can be shifted out of alignment by using short bursts of radio waves. The atoms send out a signal that a specifically designed computer converts into thousands of mathematical calculations and then displays in the form of images. These images provide the health care team with a wealth of information for use in diagnosis and treatment planning.

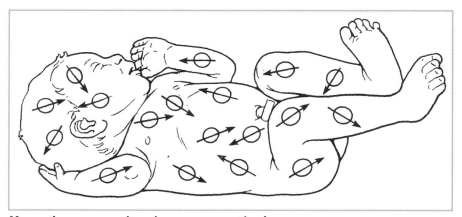

Magnetic resonance imaging—unmagnetized.
The body has randomly arranged spinning atoms.

From: Theorell C. Diagnostic imaging. In: Kenner C, Brueggemeyer A, Gunderson L, eds. Neonatal Nursing. Philadelphia, PA: WB Saunders; 1998: 752. Reprinted by permission of Elsevier.

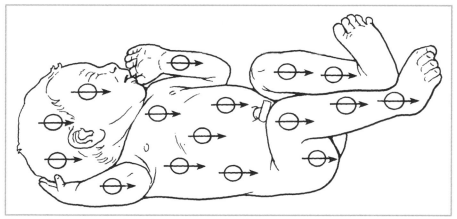

Magnetic resonance imaging—magnetized.
Once magnetized, the spinning atoms of the body are aligned in one direction. Short bursts of radio waves then shift the nuclei out of alignment. The resulting signal creates images that provide the health care team with information for use in diagnosis.

From: Theorell C. Diagnostic imaging. In: Kenner C, Brueggemeyer A, Gunderson L, eds. Neonatal Nursing. Philadelphia, PA: WB Saunders; 1998: 752. Reprinted by permission of Elsevier.

Particularly appealing for use in newborns, MRI is noninvasive, does not use ionizing radiation, and has no known adverse effects. It differs from CT scanning in that dense bone or fatty tissue does not affect the images produced. Magnetic resonance imaging produces better images of soft tissue than either CT scanning or ultrasound. It can show the degree of brain maturity in a premature infant, as well as allow earlier and more precise assessment of bleeding in both the gray and the white matter of the brain.

The disadvantages of MRI are its non-portability, its substantial equipment and operational costs, the length of time required to collect the necessary data, and the fact that access to the critically ill infant is limited during the procedure. The quality of the images produced by MRI is excellent, however. Magnetic resonance imaging holds great promise for future applications in the care of newborns.

Magnetic Resonance Spectroscopy

Magnetic resonance spectroscopy has also entered the clinical arena of magnetic resonance techniques routinely used for the evaluation of the brain and, like MRI, permits noninvasive study of the newborn. Magnetic resonance spectroscopy provides a biochemical assessment to the structural features seen on the MRI. It extracts information about the chemical composition of tissues. Rather than mapping out an image, as seen with an MRI, a plot graph representing the chemical composition of a region of tissue is generated. Magnetic resonance spectroscopy can be used throughout the body, but it has proved to be of particular importance in the evaluation of the baby with hypoxic-ischemic brain injury. As brain cells damaged by the hypoxic-ischemic event begin to deteriorate and die, the chemicals released by the cells vary in concentration depending on the phase of destruction (see the section on HIE for more information). The sequence of biochemical concentration levels seems to follow the sequence of delayed energy failure seen in HIE. The MRS assessments can be done sequentially, and studies have shown that the elevations and declines in certain chemicals (such as lactate) correlate with the severity of the brain injury and subsequent neurologic problems. Magnetic resonance spectroscopy may therefore be useful in identifying infants who would benefit from early therapeutic interventions.

Magnetic resonance spectroscopy complements conventional MRI, and they should be used together to formulate care plans. The information gathered improves diagnostic capabilities, improves the development of appropriate management plans, and helps to formulate a realistic plan as to what parents can expect in the future related to neurologic outcomes.

The Importance of Parenting

The NICU you enter today is very different from the NICU of even a few years ago. Advances in respiratory care as well as in noninvasive monitoring and diagnostic techniques have been incredible. Both nursing and medical research are constantly changing the way sick babies are treated.

Understanding the basics of NICU technology prepares you to ask questions about your baby's treatment. The NICU team understands that this technology can be overwhelming for parents and that it may contribute to your feelings of powerlessness and frustration. Keep asking questions, and stay involved in your baby's care. The NICU in which your baby is a patient may not have access to some of this technology. Discuss with your baby's medical provider whether such technology would be beneficial and whether it is worth the risk of transport to a facility that has the desired equipment. The technology in the NICU is important to your baby's survival and holds promise for better neonatal outcomes, but it cannot replace the importance of your voice, your touch, and your long-term commitment as an involved parent.

Chapter 13
When a Perfect Baby Is No More

"Pooh, promise you won't forget about me, ever.

Not even when I'm a hundred."

—Christopher Robin

Denise Maguire, PhD, RN-BC, CNL

There are few struggles in life as difficult as the heartbreaking loss of a perfect baby, whether from severe disability or death.

Not only must you face your own shattered dreams, you might have to manage the practical details of the situation and support those around you who are also trying to cope with this tragic loss. This experience will change who you are and how you live. It may be difficult to find anything positive in these events. But as this experience unfolds, please remember that *you* are your baby's parent. Although the opportunities to "parent" your baby may be limited or very different from what you hoped, you will participate in the important decisions that affect you and your baby. Everything you do will help create the memory you will have for the rest of your life.

Many health care providers may not be familiar with your culture or family customs, but they very much want to respect them. They will count on you to tell them what is important for you and your family at this time, and how decisions are normally made. Things can happen very quickly in the neonatal intensive care unit (NICU), often with little notice. There might be a special ceremony you performed with your previous children that might be done a little differently to keep the tradition alive. Many traditions are symbolic representations of welcoming a new baby into the family. The nurses often have suggestions that they know have been helpful for other families if you are unable to think clearly. Your baby should be welcomed, even if it must be just before you say goodbye.

This chapter will cover several difficult, but different situations. Scan the headings for the topics that will help you most.

Difficult Choices for a Severely Disabled Infant

A child may be born with a congenital condition that is not compatible with life, or develop severe complications after birth. In either case, the perfect child that parents hope for is lost. Having a severely disabled child will greatly affect your life, and recognizing this is important. You will be faced with very hard decisions that must be made, and there is not a single right answer. Each child and each family is different. Talking with social workers, clergy, physicians, nurses, family members, and friends can give you all the information they have, but ultimately you must make the decision regarding your child's future. This chapter will help you learn about some of the options available to you.

Alternatives to NICU Care

The kind of care provided in a NICU is usually acute care. The NICU is a fast-paced environment that focuses on complex procedures designed to support infant recovery for a relatively short period. Because of this, it is not always the best place for some infants, particularly those who have a chronic (long-term) or fatal condition. Infants born with acute problems (congenital heart defects, kidney disorders, and seizure disorders, for example) may be stabilized but not cured in the NICU. Other infants develop severe complications and have physical or mental disabilities because of their prematurity or illness. Infants born with chronic syndromes may require long-term care after initial diagnosis and stabilization in the NICU. From the first day of NICU admission, the goal of the care team is to discharge all infants. Infants may be discharged to their homes or to other facilities that can provide specialized care. When an infant develops major chronic problems, a facility other than the NICU may be the best option for providing specialized care. This may be a difficult decision for you, but one that needs to be made.

If a decision for long-term care needs to be made, the medical team will give you a clear explanation of your infant's condition and what they believe is the prognosis (long-term outcome). Unfortunately, the prognosis for many problems is not certain, and the information you may want the most might not be available. As frustrating as it may seem, time might be the only thing that may clearly reveal your child's physical and mental abilities. At this point, your baby will benefit from a change to a health care team in a different environment that focuses on individualized physical and developmental therapies of infants with long-term problems. The NICU is not able to provide that kind of care.

The options for long-term care clearly depend on your baby's medical condition. Some of the common options available include

- Home care
- Transitional care facilities
- Long-term care facilities
- Palliative and hospice care
- Foster care or adoption

Your baby's social worker can be a valuable source of information and support as you learn about the various care options available to you. The social worker will know about suitable care facilities in the region where you live. If you live far from the NICU, the social worker will coordinate your baby's discharge with a social worker near your home. Financial assistance and regulations vary from state to state, and a social worker can describe the options available to you based on your baby's condition and your family's situation. Your baby's nurse or social worker may also suggest that you speak to a parent whose child has similar care requirements. Many parents find conversations of this sort helpful in some aspects of decision-making. Appendix D lists parent organizations that may be able to provide support and answer your questions, should you like to take advantage of it.

Home Care

Taking home a baby who is very ill or seriously disabled can place tremendous hardships on the family, but it doesn't mean it should not be done. It is often a good decision for some families of an infant who is not expected to live very long. Bringing such a child home affects all members, and parents should especially recognize the impact that home care may have on the baby's siblings. Some children who have grown to adulthood with disabled siblings view it as the best experience of their childhood. Other children raised with disabled siblings grow up resenting the loss of parental attention and lack of financial resources. If you are considering caring for a seriously ill or disabled infant at home, read Chapter 16. This chapter provides details about what to expect about your infant's needs at home and the kinds of things you should plan for. This should be a joint decision of both parents because the stress it brings could be a potential source of conflict.

Transitional Care Facilities

A transitional care facility is a place that infants can go for care after the NICU and before going home. A transitional facility can be a rehabilitation hospital, and its patients often include older children and adults. Transitional facilities prepare patients for discharge home, and only those who have a possibility for discharge are admitted. Infants may be admitted to transitional or rehabilitative facilities to be weaned off a ventilator, for administration of or weaning off total parenteral nutrition, or to manage specific developmental issues. A team from the transitional care facility often comes to the NICU to meet you and your baby, evaluate your infant's medical condition, and determine if their facility can meet your infant's needs.

Once your infant is admitted to a rehabilitation facility, a new plan of care is developed, which is shared with you and everyone involved in your infant's care. This ensures that everyone caring for your baby knows the outcome goals. Parents gradually assume more of their infant's care at transitional care facilities, and visiting policies are usually quite liberal. Most facilities allow the entire family to visit and really get to know the baby. The atmosphere in such facilities is more relaxed than in a NICU, and the care given and the decisions made are not emergent. Change happens at a slower pace than in the NICU, and the atmosphere is more conducive to learning about your baby's needs. The goal of the rehabilitation facility is to discharge your baby home. Rehabilitation facilities that encourage active parent participation can greatly ease the transition between hospital and home.

Long-Term Care Facilities

"The decision to use a chronic care facility for our baby was the right decision for us. She gets loving care, and we are still very much her parents."

If your baby has a poor prognosis, such as severe physical or mental disabilities or a condition that is ultimately fatal, a long-term care facility (also called a *chronic-care facility*) may be the best option after the NICU. Infants who are not expected to improve may be admitted to a long-term care facility rather than a transitional facility or going home. Factors that will help you decide if a long-term care facility is best for your family are your financial resources and the feasibility of home care. Not every region provides long-term care, or it might be very far from your home. Although the usual goal of long-term care facilities is not discharge, it may still be a possibility for your infant. Home care does not work for every family, and a long-term care facility may offer options that best meet the needs of your child and family.

Palliative and Hospice Care

"Palliative care does not mean you've given up hope. It redirects your efforts toward making sure your baby is comfortable and has the best possible quality of life."

Palliative care is a service for people who are debilitated with incurable conditions and may be another option for families who choose to take their infant home, if it is available in your region. The goal of palliative care is to help families make choices in the best interest of their baby that are based on their personal and religious beliefs. A team of professionals work together to provide the best pain management (if necessary), social support, and access to needed resources such as respite care. Nurses and/or social workers make regular home visits to assess infant and family needs, discuss changes with the physician, and provide psychosocial support to family members as needed. Palliative care may help enable a smooth transition to home for the family bringing home a severely disabled infant.

Palliative care is sometimes confused with hospice care, which is directed at the end of life. Hospice also uses a team of professionals who work together to ensure a comfortable and peaceful death. Hospice may also be available in an inpatient setting. Sometimes both services can be found in the same organization. The unit social worker will tell you about these options, and if there are any in your region. Sometimes they are limited to adult patients and are unable to accept infants.

Foster Care or Adoption

Foster care or adoption is sometimes an option when the NICU is no longer the best place for your baby and you are unable to parent your baby. Although a difficult choice, it may be the best one for your family. This is a conscious choice you should make only after obtaining all of the facts about your child's illness and prognosis from the medical team. You should also receive counseling from an adoption social worker, who can help you with decision-making, facilitate the process, and provide resources for follow-up care for you and your family. Some states have a medical foster care program that provides medically based care for children with complex medical needs.

All parents who place a child in foster care or for adoption should see the child before doing so. If you have been told that your baby has some severe deformities or abnormalities, this is especially important. Descriptions often make these defects sound worse than they actually are. Most parents only see their baby, and don't focus on the deformity.

A very important part of the adoption or foster care process is saying good-bye to your baby. Even though your baby has not died, you will grieve the loss of your child and your role as parent and primary caretaker. You will never forget your baby and always remember this important part of your life. Saying good-bye is a concrete act that begins your healing process and establishes a last memory of your child.

The Hardest Choice of All—Letting Go

In the delivery room, doctors and nurses cannot always identify which babies might have a fatal condition. When they don't know, they usually do everything they can to save the baby's life. They are not always successful, and some babies die despite vigorous treatment. Other babies stabilize, are admitted to the NICU, and are then found to have conditions incompatible with life. Sometimes an infant may develop a condition that no longer responds to treatment. When a baby has a condition that is incompatible with life or is no longer responding to treatment, you may be asked to participate in making the most difficult decision of all—that of allowing your baby to die.

Family Presence at Resuscitation

When an infant is very unstable, there is always the possibility that the baby might "arrest." When nurses and doctors talk about arrest, they are referring to a condition in which the heart stops beating or beats ineffectively (cardiac arrest), or the baby stops breathing (respiratory arrest). Respiratory arrest can be a frequent event in the NICU, and is usually treated first by "bagging" the baby with a bag and face mask, followed by insertion of a tube down the baby's airway (intubation). The tube is then connected to a respirator, which takes over or helps the baby to breathe. Cardiac arrest is less frequent, but is a very serious event that requires resuscitation. Cardiac arrest can happen during a respiratory arrest, or any time depending on the baby's condition and diagnosis. Resuscitation usually involves someone manually giving the breaths with an airway bag, administering medications to help the heart start going again, and manually pumping the heart on the outside of the chest. Sometimes a unit alarm will be called to bring more help from NICU staff to your baby's bedside. Invasive procedures may be required to help resuscitate an infant, such as inserting chest tubes (a surgical procedure) and intravenous or central lines for fluids and medications. Sometimes blood or blood products are given emergently. Everything that can be done to save a baby's life is done as quickly as possible. It may appear chaotic, but everyone has an assigned duty and has practiced it many times.

If your baby is so unstable that there is a real possibility that he or she may have an arrest, you may want to ask about the unit policy on family presence during resuscitation. It is not recommended that other children witness resuscitation, because it is unlikely they would understand what is going on; however, some units let parents stay with their baby during a resuscitation. If you can and want to stay, they will call a chaplain, social worker, or other health care team member to stay with you. That person will be able to explain what is happening. They can also leave the room with you if you don't want to stay any longer. The doctor or neonatal nurse practitioner in charge of the resuscitation can also ask you to leave at any time if it is thought to be in your best interest. Parents whose emotions make it difficult for doctors and nurses to concentrate on the resuscitation may also be asked to leave.

Please know that many parents do not want to stay, and that is OK. Deciding not to stay does not reflect on you as a parent in any way; it is regarded as a matter of personal choice. Only you know what is best for you. If you think you might want to stay, it is best to know ahead of time if it is possible.

Ethical and Legal Considerations

Most health care professionals believe that parents should participate in decisions about the future of their child. The courts decided in 1986 that parents should be the primary decision-makers for their child, as long as the decisions made were in the child's best interests. In addition, the US Supreme Court stated that child protection is a responsibility of the individual states and that each state, through its own child abuse and neglect laws, can intervene if it believes that parents are not acting in the best interests of their child. The rulings provide guidance for parental input and a multidisciplinary hospital committee to review both medical and ethical aspects when critical decisions about disabled and gravely ill infants are being made.

The Role of the Ethics Committee

An ethics committee is made up of a variety of different people, and often includes doctors (neonatologists, pediatricians, or subspecialists), nurses, social workers, chaplains, ethicists, and laypeople (someone from the community who is not a hospital employee). The members usually have a special interest in medical ethics, and may have studied ethical decision-making in school. The ethics committee is asked to give an opinion to help resolve issues when there does not seem to be a right answer. Cases involving complicated, difficult treatment decisions are presented to the committee. The committee provides an important opinion because it is based on principles of biomedical ethics.

Not all decisions regarding whether to continue or stop treatment are difficult to make. Some may be straightforward; after a thorough assessment, it may be clear that the infant has a condition clearly incompatible with life, and futile medical therapies can be discontinued. Ethics committees exist for decisions that are not straightforward. They allow a forum for those involved with the baby to offer facts, information, and opinions about the child and prognosis.

In some hospitals, parents may attend the ethics committee meeting or parts of it. In other hospitals, a nurse or a social worker acts as the parents' advocate. If you are excluded from meetings, it is to allow the committee to discuss the case freely and form a unified opinion. If you and the committee can reach a mutually agreeable decision, you will work with the health care team directly involved in your baby's care to formulate a plan to implement the decision.

It is unusual that the ethics committee, the health care team, and parents are unable to agree on a plan of action. Doctors and nurses prefer to do everything they can to respect your wishes and honor your beliefs. In the rare event that agreement cannot be reached, referral to a court of law may be the next step. A child welfare agency may seek guardianship of your child if the hospital does not believe you are acting in your baby's best interests. This is usually a last resort, after everything has been tried to resolve the problem, including getting a second medical opinion. In a court of law, when one side presents the case for life, the judge(s) will usually rule that the life of the infant be continued.

Communication Strategies for Negotiating Difficult Decisions

Parents are not solely responsible for making decisions about continuing or withholding medical treatment for their baby. These decisions are negotiated with the medical team, bearing in mind that parents are valuable partners in the medical care of their baby. When faced with a difficult decision, the goal is for parents and medical providers to agree on an action plan.

Every family is different and there is no one right answer. The best answer is the one that meets the needs of your baby and your family. These suggestions may help enhance communication between you and your health care providers.

1. Do not get critical information about your baby over the telephone or by e-mail. Your baby's medical provider should set up an appointment in person to be held in a quiet and private place.

2. If your infant's condition has a name, ask the medical care provider to write it down for you. What caused the problem? Sometimes it is not any one specific condition that has led to the baby's critical situation, but rather a series of complications resulting from the original illness or series of illnesses.

3. Ask for the medical facts about your baby's condition. What are the choices for treatment? Can the outcome of each choice be predicted?

4. If necessary, remind care providers to use language you can understand and at a pace that allows you to consider the information and ask questions.

5. Tell your baby's medical provider if there are cultural aspects that influence your decision-making process. Should a particular person in your family receive this information? Who is in charge of negotiating decisions with medical staff? Are there topics that should not be discussed with a family group? What cultural, dietary, or religious practices are important to your family in this situation?

6. Take your time. Let the medical care provider know when you are overwhelmed with information and need a break. This also gives you time to think of questions and write them down.

7. Repeat the information in your own words to make sure you understand what you have been told.

8. If English is not your native language, or if other members of your family do not speak and/or understand English well, ask for a medical translator. Do not use a family member, a friend, or a child to translate.

9. This is not solely a medical decision. There are emotional implications and perhaps even financial consequences of your decision. You are encouraged to discuss your feelings and fears and questions with other medical providers, a social worker, a spiritual counselor, family members, and anyone else whom you trust to listen to you and support your decision-making.

10. If possible, your medical provider should connect you to families who have faced this decision to withhold treatment or raise a disabled child. These families may offer more information and perspective for decision-making.

11. Well-intentioned health care providers may want to protect you from seeing your baby if he has birth defects. Be with your baby, touch and hold him if you want to do so. Most parents are grateful for this opportunity to spend time with their baby.

12. If your hospital bioethics committee will review your case, ask if you may attend. You may be invited to share your preferences. Take a support person to the meeting with you if possible.

13. Read all informed consent documents carefully. Ask questions if you don't understand what you are being asked to agree to. You have a right to get information in words you can understand.

14. What is the follow-up plan for decision-making and future discussion?

The Decision-Making Process

As a parent of a child with an incurable condition, you may be asked to help plan the timing and circumstances of your child's inevitable death. You have the right to continue your baby's care, to add no further treatment, or to stop treatment and make sure your infant has a comfortable death. When faced with these difficult decisions, the doctors, nurses, and other health care team members will provide you with as much information as possible about your child's condition and prognosis. The recommendation to allow a baby to die is not made by a single person, or by the parents alone. Like you, the team wants what is best for your baby, and your input is essential.

Your baby's doctor or nurse practitioner will let you know if they think the best thing to do is to stop treatment and allow your baby to die. They will also tell you why they think that is the best option. Generally, the neonatologists and other medical team members have reached their recommendation together, based on your baby's test results and discussion in team meetings.

The decision to stop treatment for your baby is very complicated. Unlike the members of the ethics committee and the NICU staff, you will have to live with your loss every day. Although the doctors and nurses make their recommendations very thoughtfully, they know it is very different for you. Sometimes parents want to know what the doctors and nurses would do in this situation—but that doesn't matter.

The decision to stop treatment is made only when you are ready, and after thoughtful consideration of everyone involved. When the medical team makes a recommendation, you may not be ready. You may even be shocked that they asked. It may seem unimaginable what they are asking you to consider. After the shock wears off, you might begin to hear what they have to say. When facing this situation, ask as many questions as you need to, and then ask again to make sure you understand the answers. Some questions do not have answers, but the team will answer everything they can. See page 390 for communication strategies for treatment decision-making. You can also ask for a second opinion.

Once a decision is made to remove life support, care of you and your baby will shift to providing as much support and comfort as possible. Parents often feel a great sense of relief when they are involved in a decision that has been so difficult. You might still second-guess yourself and have some doubts, but these are normal feelings that will take time, and sometimes professional help, to resolve. This may be the hardest experience you will ever have, but your participation ensures that you are a parent who only wants the best for your baby. When treatment becomes futile and your baby is not going to get better, making the decision for a peaceful and comfortable death is a parental right you can assert and will never regret.

"Do Not Resuscitate" Orders

If the decision is made to let your infant die or to withdraw life-sustaining equipment, the doctor, neonatal nurse practitioner, or physician assistant caring for your child will talk with you about how this will be done. Most often, babies on ventilators have their breathing tubes removed, or the medications to maintain circulation are stopped. When mechanical support is withdrawn, babies are often sedated to prevent pain and suffering. If you have any questions or concerns about the procedure or pain relief, ask before anyone takes any action.

If a decision has been made to remove your baby from life support, the medical provider will write a "do not resuscitate" (DNR) order. The DNR order prevents vigorous lifesaving measures from being carried out. If your baby is being supported with complex medical technology and you have made a decision that further treatment is futile, a DNR order allows the withdrawal of that technology so that the baby can die peacefully. Sometimes a DNR order is needed before a baby with a lethal condition is sent home or transferred to hospice care. Some states require a DNR order before a patient is transferred to hospice care.

Bringing the Baby Home to Die

Not all infants with fatal anomalies or diseases require a lot of technological support, and you may wish to take your baby home to die. If you decide to take your baby home, the NICU team will help you develop a home care plan, teach you what to expect as your baby's condition worsens, provide a contact person who will be available at all times to answer questions and give support, and provide an alternate plan in case home care becomes too difficult. If necessary, your baby can be readmitted to the hospital for supportive care (with a DNR order). Find out before discharge whether your baby would be readmitted to the NICU or to another unit.

Sending a baby home to die is unusual, and some units may have little or no experience with these circumstances. Speak with the nurse manager about what you would like to do and how you would like to do it. Some requests take time, so try to plan in advance and be flexible. Nurse managers and social workers can help you decipher rules and regulations, allow you to maintain control of the situation, and arrange events to your satisfaction.

Preparing to Say Farewell

"The doctors and nurses understand if you want to cry. I know this because they cried with me."

You may feel very alone during this time, but you are probably surrounded by others who are also experiencing this loss. Grandparents, your older children, and close friends and relatives will grieve with you. Shielding them from the reality of the situation does not make the loss easier for you or them.

Family Participation

Most NICU staff encourage family members, including older siblings, to be together as a family when a baby dies. Spending time with the infant gives family members the opportunity to "know" the baby and have their own memories. This is also the opportunity to incorporate your family traditions into your baby's life. If there is time to plan a traditional ritual, let your baby's nurses know what you want to do. Most traditions can be accommodated, but individual situations vary. It's best to check with the nurses first. Sometimes a private room may not be available, although the death of a baby is a high priority. If there is very little time to plan a traditional ritual, ask the nurses how you can achieve the spirit of the tradition given the situation. Some parents may not have had a tradition in the past but would like to create one for this baby. Talk with nurses, grandparents, and others who might be able to suggest something special for your baby. Rituals such as baptism are often accommodated. Most people don't think of death as an "event," but it is certainly a significant event in your baby's short life. It should be marked by something meaningful to you.

Events may occur quickly. Birth, death, and funeral may occupy only a few days. Experiencing this tragedy together as a family will help everyone get through it. In addition, when the family talks about the baby in the future, all of the family members who participated will be able to share their memories and support.

Reuniting Mother and Baby

If the baby was transported to another hospital, both parents may not be with him when difficult decisions are made or when the infant is near death. Find out what can be done to get mother and baby together. Laws, rules, and regulations vary widely, so ask the social worker and nurses for help when considering your options.

If you are the mother and you are medically stable, an early hospital discharge may be arranged to allow you to go to your baby. A mother may also be medically transferred to the hospital where her baby is receiving care (health care coverage may influence this option). If hospital discharge is not an option, ask for a "pass" that allows you to leave the hospital but to return at a prearranged time for continued hospital care. In some cases, the hospital caring for your baby may authorize a back transport of the baby to the original hospital. Before agreeing to back transport, find out if your insurance carrier will cover the cost of the baby's transport and continued care at the mother's hospital.

Organ Donation

"I felt lucky because we could donate our baby's organs to save another baby. At least there was some comfort in knowing our baby's death brought hope to someone else."

In 1984 Loma Linda University Medical Center in California began performing heart transplants in newborns with a fatal congenital heart defect called *hypoplastic left heart syndrome*. Before transplantation became an option, a series of complex surgeries was the only hope for these children. These surgeries were high risk and had a high mortality rate. Without some type of surgical intervention, this defect is always fatal. Heart transplants have increased the number of infants with hypoplastic left heart syndrome who survive and thrive.

Hearts are not the only organs transplanted; livers, kidneys, blood vessels, and corneas have all been successfully transplanted to infants and small children. Medications that reduce rejection of transplanted organs have been greatly improved and have increased the success rate of transplants.

Infants who die in the NICU, however, are rarely eligible to become organ donors. The criteria for brain death are very strict, and newborns rarely meet it. The criteria for organ donation are also strict: The infant must be brain dead and infection-free, and the organs that will be taken must be functioning normally. Specific tests—such as various blood tests, sonograms, and radiologic studies—are performed to evaluate each organ.

You may ask about the possibility of organ donation, someone from the hospital may ask (such as a chaplain), or someone you have never before met may ask (such as a trained professional from the organ donation center). If your infant is dying and you would like to donate his organs, talk to the medical provider in charge of your baby's care. All hospitals that participate in Medicaid and Medicare programs are required to refer all potential organ donors to their local organ procurement organization to be evaluated as possible organ donors. If the patient meets the criteria, a hospital representative or a transplant coordinator will talk with the family.

Neonatal organ donation is a very personal and emotional decision. Organ donation is not a choice between life and death; only infants who are brain dead can be organ donors. The infant will die whether he is an organ donor or not. Ask as many questions as you have. Transplant recipients or their families may also work or volunteer for these programs, providing support, comfort, and information to families. The counselors who work with the transplant team are highly trained. They talk regularly with families wrestling with unexpected death and the decisions surrounding these tragic circumstances. You may want to speak with family members and clergy. It may not be an option at all if not allowed by your religious beliefs. If your infant becomes an organ donor, organ donation will not delay a funeral. Your baby will not be disfigured, so an open casket service will still be possible. The surgeons, nurses, and staff who perform these procedures are sensitive and caring individuals who respect your infant as a person and who recognize your sorrow.

Organ donation may be a way of having something good come out of this terrible experience. Although it will not bring your child back to you, it may allow someone else's child to live. This is a very giving attitude—one you may have difficulty feeling fully at the time of your baby's death. Looking back, however, parents who have donated their infant's organs have not regretted it. Again, this is a personal decision that parents should make as a team. But knowing that someone else was given a second chance at life may ease your sadness and grief at a later time.

Naming the Baby

If you have not yet done so, name your child. Naming your baby will help you and others recognize that your baby was born and died, although that life was brief. It's up to you whether to use one of the names you may have selected before your baby's birth or to save those names for another child. Naming your child also establishes a memory that you will be able to reflect on later. Referring to a child by name, even after death, gives dignity to that life. Everyone deserves a name.

Baptism and Other Rituals

Talk to your baby's nurses about the need for baptism or other important spiritual customs you wish to observe. Religious clergy are welcome in the NICU at your request, or ask for chaplaincy services if you wish clergy of a specific denomination. Nurses who know about your customs and religious preferences will respect your wishes. If you are not present at the time of death, you might consider performing rituals important to your family even after death, if appropriate.

NICU Staff Behaviors

Education and personal coping strategies for managing death and dying influence how NICU staff members behave around the family of a dying baby. Most staff members are knowledgeable about the process and are wonderfully supportive. Some team members, however, may seem to withdraw emotionally. Although they know that further treatment of your baby is futile, some doctors and nurses feel a great sense of failure when they realize there is nothing left "to do." If a staff member withdraws from you emotionally, do not interpret it as a criticism of your decision. The withdrawal probably reflects the staff member's own difficulty dealing with the many issues surrounding death in the NICU.

At the Time of Death

When your infant is dying, the main priority is the baby's comfort and companionship. If you are in the NICU, the staff will make arrangements for you to hold your baby, preferably in a private, quiet area. Your baby may still be attached to equipment or may be freed from most tubes and wires. After your infant has died, you will have all the time you need to say good-bye to your child. If you are not in the unit when your infant is dying, your baby's nurse may hold and comfort your baby. When you arrive, the nurse can make arrangements for you to see and hold your baby one last time.

This may be the only time you are able to "parent" your baby, and it may be the only time you have been able to hold and care for your baby without wires and tubes getting in the way. You may hold your baby at any time during or following death. Some NICUs allow families to gather in a private hospital room to hold the baby and say good-bye. You may ask the nurse to stay with you or just to be available if you call. Feel free to unwrap your baby's blanket and examine every inch. Even if your baby has a birth defect, be sure to focus on the wonderful things that may be perfect, such as fingers and toes. This is important parenting time, so do not feel pressured or hurried.

In some cases, a physician may prescribe medications that will dull the emotions of a grieving mother. Taking a sedative at this time may make it difficult to fully participate in the last moments of your baby's life, or even to remember the details of it. Although it may seem like a good idea, avoiding such a painful part of life may cause regrets later. If sedative medications are offered to you, be sure to fully discuss the pros and cons with your medical provider.

Remembering Your Baby

"A year after Jessica's death, I was ready to see the pictures the nurses had taken the day she died. I called the NICU and her primary nurse sent them along with a lovely note about Jessie. Now I treasure these things."

Most units have a camera and will offer to take pictures of your baby. There is an art to photographing a critically ill or deceased baby, and to some extent, the expertise of the photographer will determine the quality of the photo. You may suggest that your baby be dressed or wrapped in a blanket and that your baby's arms and legs be supported with blanket rolls or your hands. You may wish to hold your baby for a family portrait. Some parents find these photos comforting; others are uncomfortable with them. If you do not want the photos, the staff will store them for you. If they don't take them home right away, many parents request them some time after their baby's death.

Some parents want to videotape their last moments with their baby. Most hospitals do not allow videotaping of critical events, but you might be able to if your baby's death is anticipated in a controlled setting—for example, when you are holding the baby in a private room. Pictures and videotapes are something you may put away and review on important dates, such as your baby's birthday, death date, and special family holidays. Be sure to ask if you think you might like to videotape, because it needs to be planned.

You may also take home all of the baby's belongings, such as blankets, clothing, footprints, tape measure, crib card, and even a lock of hair if you would like it. You may find all of this comforting, but if you do not, at least hold onto these items. You may be glad to have them later on.

After your baby dies, the nurse bathes the baby before taking him to the morgue. The nurses usually do this task, but you are welcome to assist or give the bath yourself. Doing something like this for your baby may help you say good-bye. After the bath, you may want to rock and hold your baby again. After you have said good-bye, your baby will receive identification tags and be carried to the morgue.

Seeing Your Baby Again

If you wish to see your baby again, or if you were not present when your baby died, you may call the NICU and make arrangements to spend time with your baby. Most NICUs will provide a private place, wrap the baby in a warm blanket, and allow you to spend more time with your baby. Ask how the hospital arranges a viewing and holding time after the baby has left the NICU.

Taking the Next Step

After your baby has died, you will be asked to consider an autopsy. You will also need to make decisions about a funeral and burial or cremation, notify family and close friends about your baby's death, arrange for transport if your baby did not die at a hospital near your home, and perhaps deal with nursery furnishings and baby gifts. Again, take as much time as you need to sort out your choices. If you are having trouble, call on those who have helped and supported you up to now—your nurses, doctors, family, friends, social workers, and clergy.

Obtaining an Autopsy

Unless the cause of your baby's death is crystal clear, an autopsy may be one of the best things you can do. It may answer questions and provide explanations for what happened. There is no guarantee that it will answer all your questions, but an autopsy may be the best way to figure out what happened. Sometimes the results have implications for future pregnancies not only for the mother, but for her blood relatives as well.

An autopsy will not significantly delay any funeral arrangements you may wish to make, so timing should not be a consideration in your decision. If other family members would like to see the baby before the autopsy, let everyone know when you give autopsy consent. In addition, an autopsy will not influence the type of wake or funeral you wish to have. An open casket is still possible because pathologists are able to perform autopsies without disturbing the baby's face or hands.

The doctor caring for your baby is usually the person who will ask you for the autopsy consent. If your baby died in a community hospital or smaller medical center, ask the doctor if it would be advantageous to have the autopsy at a larger medical center with a regional NICU or at your regional children's hospital. Sometimes pathologists at large centers or children's hospitals have more expertise with infant autopsies and access to more resources than a community hospital.

If you agree to an autopsy, make an appointment with your social worker and your baby's doctor to review the results. The early results may be known in a few days, but the detailed results can take 6 weeks or more. It's up to you when you want to learn the results. One month to 6 weeks after the death seems to be the time many parents are ready for this appointment; life has settled into a new routine, and you may be ready to hear the results. Usually, the doctor and social worker who cared for your baby will meet with you and explain the results and, if you wish, give you a copy of the report.

Any questions you may have can be answered at the meeting, but if you want more information at a later date, the doctor should be a resource to you.

An autopsy will probably not provide all of the information you hope to have. The cause of death sometimes remains unknown, and this can be frustrating. Although the autopsy may not identify the exact reason for your baby's death, it may reassure you that a number of possibilities—for example, genetic problems or suspected malformations—were not the cause. It will also provide information that might be useful when thinking about future pregnancies.

Funeral Arrangements and Transport

A funeral will let you, your family, and close friends say good-bye to your baby in a public way as a celebration of your baby's short life. It also allows public recognition that this was a person who lived and had a profound influence on the lives he touched.

Parents or family members are financially responsible for funeral arrangements. Depending on the state in which you live, financial support may be available. If you are unclear about how to arrange a funeral, ask your nurse, social worker, or clergy about resources available to assist you. Your social worker should be able to provide a list of reputable funeral homes and other available resources. Funeral homes sometimes help defray the cost of a funeral for an infant, and churches sometimes have special burial areas for infants and children.

Your beliefs may clearly define the type of funeral you will have, and a clergy member can assist you with the arrangements. Parents whose religious affiliation does not strictly prescribe funeral arrangements must make decisions about a traditional funeral and burial, a cremation and funeral service, or a simple memorial service (sometimes called a *celebration of life),* which may involve a simple gathering of close friends and family members at a location of your choice, with separate arrangements for the body.

If you have some definite ideas about how the wake and funeral should be handled, explain them to the funeral director. If you are having difficulty expressing your needs to a stranger, enlist the support of a resource person from the NICU (such as your nurse, social worker, or chaplain) who can make phone calls with you. The funeral director is providing a service for you and should be able to meet your needs or, if something is absolutely impossible, to offer you acceptable alternatives. Do not feel shy or embarrassed about asking questions. Request an itemized list of the funeral home's charges and then consider cost-effective alternatives. For example, you may save a significant amount of money by dressing your baby yourself before he is taken to the funeral home.

If your baby dies far from where you wish to bury him, the funeral home can arrange transport or, if local laws allow, you may be able to transport the baby yourself. A knowledgeable funeral director or the hospital's grief counselor, social worker, or chaplain can help. Most are familiar with infants' and children's funerals. If you don't know how to proceed, ask someone to assist you.

Talking With Friends

"Most of our friends were there for us, helping out whenever they could, or just listening to us talk about our baby. But I was surprised and disappointed that some of my friends didn't call me after Joshua died. Really, what's so hard about saying, 'I'm so sorry this happened. Can I do anything to help?' "

As painful as it may be, you'll need to tell your close friends what happened. If your baby's life was very short, friends may not be aware of the events surrounding the birth, and this may be your first chance to speak with them about your baby. Calling close friends helps mobilize support, validates your feelings of loss as they express their shock and grief, and helps you find a way to live with this loss. If you wish, ask a few close friends to pass the news to other friends. This relieves you of endless phone calls. It may also prevent uncomfortable situations in which unknowing friends congratulate you on your baby's birth or bring gifts for the baby.

The Nursery and Baby Gifts

How you put away the baby's nursery is personal. You may wish to do it a bit at a time or all at once. You may wish to do it all yourself, with your partner, or with other family members. Some parents request that family members or close friends put away the nursery for them. As grieving parents, you may need to clearly tell your family members how you want to handle it. They may think they should "protect" you from this painful task. Putting away the nursery may be a form of healing closure, or you may decide that it would be better for others to do it for you. Both ways are fine, because it is entirely up to you. You must do what is best for you.

There are no rules of etiquette for returning baby gifts. You may choose to save some gifts in remembrance of your baby or for a special baby in your future. No one expects you to give back their gift . If you don't want them, consider donating them to a shelter or other volunteer organization. Those who have given gifts are probably also those from whom you have or will receive sympathy. When you thank them for their support, let them know what happened to their gift.

If someone lent you furniture or other baby items, or made a major investment, however, offer to return the item. Make all of these decisions at your own pace. You'll know when it's time.

Understanding Grief

Grief is an emotional response that occurs when someone close to you dies or when something else you value (such as a "perfect" birth experience) is lost. Grief is not an intellectual or rational response. Grief reactions differ from person to person, just as the depth and range of other emotions do. Grief is a very strong emotion. Because of its emotional nature, grief is very unsettling. A grieving person may feel loss of control, overwhelmed, and irritable. Some physical and behavioral signs of grief are given on page 402.

It's important to recognize that no 2 people grieve the same way. Not everyone experiences all of the stages of the grief process, and individuals experiencing the same loss may not experience the stages at the same time or in the same way (see below). Partners may also grieve differently because their level of attachment to the lost child or the lost outcome is different. Mothers grieve differently from fathers, and children grieve differently, depending on their age.

Loss of a Twin or Other Multiple

Multiple births can be a special event, but parents who lose one child from a set of twins or other multiple births face a unique situation. The loss of one child is not compensated by the survival of another. The child who is lost is always missed, always mourned, even if only privately.

Caring for the surviving twin may continually be a source of both sadness and joy. Your emotions are on a roller-coaster ride as you both celebrate the birth and life of a healthy

Stages of Grief[a]

> **Shock:** The first reaction is often numbing disbelief and shock. You may not want to believe that your baby is dying or has a lethal condition. It's almost impossible to understand that such a thing has happened. Physical symptoms may include weakness, crying, and aimless activity. This stage can last from a couple of hours to weeks.
>
> **Suffering:** Once the shock wears off, it is followed by intense emotional pain. You may not be able to imagine your life without your baby, which causes great sadness. Some people wonder if there was something they might have done to prevent this tragedy. You may be angry with yourself, others, or both. You may question, "Why me?", or bargain with a higher being ("I will never swear again if you bring him back."). You will need a lot of emotional support during this time. Later in this stage, you will move into a period of depression and loneliness. The full impact of your loss is felt in this stage. Much of the strong emotions have drained, leaving an empty hole in your heart. Many friends and relatives are living normal lives, and sometimes forget about what you live with every day. Although most days are spent doing "normal" activities, the loss is still palpable, just under the surface. This stage can last from months to years.
>
> **Recovery:** After a long time, the depression and loneliness start to fade, and you become able to live your life fairly normally. Of course you still miss your baby, but you can plan for the future. Your pain begins to recede into the background of your life.

[a]Adapted from © Jennie Wright, 2008. Available at: http://www.recover-from-grief.com. Reprinted by permission.

child and grieve for what has been lost. Because of the turmoil around the death of one infant, parents may feel like they are ignoring the needs of the other. They may feel guilty that they can only provide the basic needs of their other infant, such as feeding and diapering, but cannot attend to their emotional needs.

It is not unusual for grieving parents to wish that all their babies had died. Some parents may feel it would be easier just to grieve rather than to grieve while continuing to deal with ongoing NICU problems. These are perfectly normal feelings. With time, a balance

Signs and Symptoms of Grief[a]

Physical Signs	
Gastrointestinal System	**Cardiovascular System**
Anorexia and weight loss	Cardiac palpitations ("fluttering" in chest)
Overeating	"Heavy" feeling in chest
Nausea and vomiting	**Neuromuscular System**
Abdominal pain or feeling of emptiness	Headaches
Diarrhea and constipation	Vertigo (dizziness)
Respiratory System	Syncope (fainting)
Sighing respiration	Brissaud disease (tics)
Choking or coughing	Muscular weakness or loss of strength
Shortness of breath	
Hyperventilation	

Behavioral Signs	
Feelings of	**Disturbed Interpersonal Relationships**
Guilt	Increased irritability and restlessness
Sadness	Decreased sexual interest and drive
Anger and hostility	Withdrawal
Emptiness and apathy	Crying
Helplessness	
Pain, desperation, and pessimism	**Inability to Return to Normal Activities**
Shame	Fatigue and exhaustion or aimless overactivity
Loneliness	Insomnia or oversleeping
Preoccupation With the Image of the Lost Infant	Short attention span
	Slow speech, movement, and thought processes
Daydreams and fantasies	Loss of concentration and motivation
Nightmares	
Longing	

[a]From Gardner SL, Hauser MM, Merenstein GB. Grief and perinatal loss. In: Merenstein GB, Gardner SL, eds. *Handbook of Neonatal Intensive Care.* 6th ed. St. Louis, MO: Mosby-Elsevier; 2006:921. (Modified from Lindemann E. *Am J Psychiatry.* 1944;101:144–146.; Marris P. *Loss and Change.* New York, NY: Pantheon; 1974; and Colgrove M. *How to Survive the Loss of a Love.* New York, NY: Lion Publishing; 1976.) Reprinted by permission.

can be found. With time, you can learn to be happy for the surviving baby and develop the ability to deal with that child's problems while grieving for the baby who has died. If one or both of the parents cannot find joy in the life of the surviving child, additional professional help may be needed to provide a warm, nurturing environment as that child grows. Each parent reacts to the death of a multiple birth differently. The only way to get through the experience is to talk about it and respect each other's feelings.

Differences in How Men and Women Grieve

"Losing your baby changes your marriage. You both have to make an effort to stay close, and stay strong. It takes time and a whole lot of patience."

Expression of grief varies between men and women. This is partly because societal expectations of behaviors for each gender sometimes determine appropriate masculine and appropriate feminine behavior. Society expects men to be strong and unemotional in a crisis, while women are allowed to cry and "fall apart." Women may feel as though they have to take care of their mate, both physically and emotionally. Men may become distant and uncommunicative, unable to show emotions because it makes them too vulnerable. They may be too ashamed to show their partner how lost and sad they feel, believing that they have to be strong. A man may not want his partner to see him in this lost, vulnerable state. Fathers have been ignored during the grieving process because of the erroneous belief that they do not experience the same loss as mothers. Fortunately, popular culture has become far more accepting of masculine displays of emotion. Greater freedom to display their emotions and grieve openly may let men resolve their grief in a healthier manner.

Sometimes men return to work rapidly after the death of a baby. When they focus on their work, it may appear that they are either not grieving or have moved beyond their grief. Neither may be true. The difference may be that they are not alone all day long focusing on their grief. When they come home, they may need to set their own grief aside to provide support to a grieving mother. Men often find themselves in a different situation than a woman does, and that alone may influence how they grieve.

Lack of communication between partners has been cited as one of the reasons for the high divorce rate among couples who have lost an infant to death, congenital anomalies, or intellectual disability (sometimes referred to as *mental retardation*). The loss of a child may be the first major crisis a couple faces together. It can be frightening to see your partner lose control, and it may be difficult to deal with a crisis if both of you are lost, overwhelmed, and unable to support each other. The stress is great, and the potential for misunderstanding each other is high. Couples who communicate well are often able to deal with small misunderstandings before they become insurmountable problems.

Coping With Grief

At this point in your life it may seem that nothing will ever make you feel good again. No one can tell you exactly how to get through this experience, but you may find some of the following suggestions helpful.

If you have previously experienced a loss or have survived crises before, try to recall what helped you most in that situation. Was it spending time with a friend? Or attending a group session? Also, try to maintain your usual daily habits, even if you are unable to sleep. A sense of "routine" may help you feel more normal and less "lost."

During this time, you may find relief by expressing yourself artistically. This serves 2 purposes. First, it can help you sort through your emotions day by day. Second, when everything is over and for many years to come, your work will provide you with remembrances and memories of a bittersweet time. It is entirely up to you whether you share these outlets or keep them private. Some parents have developed their journals into published books after their NICU experience has ended. Some creative coping strategies include writing (a letter to your baby, poetry, a journal, blogging), scrapbooking, drawing, painting, creating pottery, or sculpting.

Others have found solace in activities such as exercising, taking long walks, and talking to supportive friends and family. There are many local chapters of other parents who have lost children. Sometimes talking to others who have experienced the same or similar event is very helpful. The NICU social worker can give you some contacts, or you may be able to find them on the Internet.

When they feel ready, many parents find it helps to plant a tree as a memorial to their baby, donate time or money to a children's charity, become a parent volunteer and lend support to other NICU parents, or become politically active for a children's cause.

Helping Others Cope With Grief

Coping with your own feelings may seem like all you can do right now, but as you move through your grief, you may find yourself supporting those around you.

Grandparents

Your baby's grandparents will grieve in their own ways for their own reasons. Like parents, they grieve the loss of the future. Grandparents develop their own fantasies about their grandchild—what the baby will look like, what they will do together, what they hope the child will become. When a grandchild dies or is severely disabled, grandparents also mourn the loss of that future.

In addition, grandparents hurt for you, their own children. They never stop being parents, and your pain compounds their grief. But don't overlook the support your parents offer. They may be separated from the situation enough to help you make plans and decisions.

Your Baby's Siblings

Sibling grief reactions vary, depending on the age of the sibling. Although younger children may not fully comprehend what has occurred, even the youngest child will sense the emotional turmoil surrounding the loss of the baby. The table below describes how children of different ages understand the meaning of death.

Unlike adults, children do not grieve continuously; rather, they grieve sporadically. Much to your surprise, your children may be able to continue their daily routine and play and eat as usual. Then, when you least expect it, one of them may remember something about the baby and become very sad.

A Child's Developing Concept of Death[a]

Age	Cognitive Understanding	How Experienced
Infant (to 12 mo)	None	Indirectly through parental grief expressed in emotional withdrawal, inability to provide concern and continuity in caregiving behaviors, overconcern because of fear of recurrent loss
Toddler (1–3 yr)	Little understanding of cause and effect Death may be confused with sleeping or being away	React to changes in behavior of grieving parents and reflect their feelings and anxiety
Preschooler (3–6 yr)	View death as a temporary state and not an inevitable occurrence Believe that they are the center of the universe and can do anything, and that thinking is doing (thoughts have the power of actions)	Expect the dead to return—ask questions about "when" Fear (and feel guilty) that negative thoughts or actual death wishes caused the death
School age (6–12 yr)	Understand that death is inevitable and irreversible 6- to 9-year-olds personify death as a separate person (skeleton, bogey man) About 8 years old: "death phobia," a normal developmental stage characterized by preoccupation with thoughts of own death or that of a loved one Reasons concretely with ability to see cause-and-effect relationships	Realize death occurs in adults like parents and even in children; realize death is permanent, not temporary, state May show interest in biological aspects of death and details of funeral
Adolescent (12 yr)	Able to think abstractly about death like the adult; philosophical reasoning	Similar to that in adult

[a]From Gardner SL, Hauser MM, Merenstein GB. Grief and perinatal loss. In: Merenstein GB, Gardner SL, eds. *Handbook of Neonatal Intensive Care.* 6th ed. St. Louis, MO: Mosby-Elsevier; 2006:943. Reprinted by permission.

Some predictable grief reactions occur in children. They may feel guilty because they believe that they caused their sibling's death or disability by wishful thinking. They may have resented the baby and feel secretly relieved when the baby does not come home. They may misbehave as an attention-getting ploy and may regress in their behavior (go back to thumb-sucking or bed-wetting, for example). They may experience frightening thoughts that others are going to die. They may also be frightened at the strong emotions they see from you for the first time.

Children are as unique as adults and may grieve in unique ways. An unconcerned attitude that continues without any change, however, may be a signal that your child is denying the situation or is unable to express his or her emotions. Your child may benefit from professional counseling in dealing with the feelings; no child should be totally non-reactive to the loss of a sibling.

Even though it can be difficult while you are grieving, remember that your surviving children need you. Be as honest as possible with your children without going into too much detail. Answer questions concisely with as much explanation as you feel is appropriate. It's all right to admit that you don't have all the answers. Resources are available to assist you, but remember: You know your children best. Trust your instincts as you struggle with what to say.

When explaining death to children, use real words and express the problems honestly. Children may need reassurance that the same thing will not happen to them. Avoid talking about death as going to sleep; that may result in sleeping problems. Be honest: "The baby was born too early and she was too small," "The baby's heart didn't work right and he couldn't make it," "The baby was born very sick and she died," and especially, "The baby's problems are nobody's fault."

If you decide not to let your child see the baby in the NICU, do not withhold knowledge of the infant. Even children as young as 2 or 3 years can sense a parent's turmoil and know that something very sad is occurring. Parents should honestly acknowledge what is happening and how they feel. Young children (generally those older than 6 to 8 years) can participate in a funeral or memorial service and may benefit from saying good-bye to their infant sibling.

A unique problem sometimes faces the sibling survivor(s) of a multiple pregnancy in which one or more of the babies have died. Survivors often feel a sense of missing something; they shared a womb with their sibling(s) yet do not share their lives. As soon as your child begins to ask questions about his birth, tell your surviving child or children their birth story, and address any fears and questions. You may develop unique ways of celebrating events for the survivor(s) while remembering your lost infant(s). Your family will decide the best way to celebrate and mourn simultaneously.

Friends

Friends may respond to your loss in a number of ways. Some who are sad and scared for you may withdraw simply because they do not know what to do or say. Others may be more comfortable with your grief, stay close, and support you through this difficult time. Many people have difficulty speaking to mourning parents and say nothing or the wrong thing. You will probably encounter many well-intentioned people with a knack for saying the wrong thing: "You're young; you can have others" and "This happened for the best." You will probably also have dear, close friends who realize that "I'm sorry," "We're thinking of you," or just their presence is a great comfort to you.

Duration of Grief

Your life has now changed forever. Things are never the same after a child dies. But you will eventually find a new place of emotional peace where you feel comfortable and belong.

An Individual Timetable

In general, the grief process can take several years and depend on 4 individual influences.

1. The nature of your loss
2. The level of significance of your loss
3. Your willingness to experience the intensity of your feelings about your loss
4. The quality of the support system available to you

People grieve at their own pace, depending on the variables just listed and on their personality. The first year is usually one of experiencing all of the "firsts," living a full year of special dates (birthdays and holidays) and feeling the acute pain of your loss as these dates occur. Even though your baby's death may not affect how your family celebrates a particular event, you may feel your loss most at family gatherings.

The second year is usually spent looking toward the future, reorganizing your life without your baby in it. As time passes, your loss will feel less physically painful, and you'll learn to laugh again. Expect to experience occasional "blue" days, when some date or event causes you to reexperience your grief. If you feel you are too sad for too long, consider a support group or private therapy.

Chronic Sorrow

Grief may never completely resolve in the case of a disabled or chronically ill child. This may result in an ongoing process known as chronic sorrow. Having a child with a severe, long-term disability reminds parents everyday of something they have lost. It is not expected that you "accept" the situation and "get over" your grief. It is a natural response to a tragic situation. Chronic sorrow is influenced by many factors and its intensity changes from time to time. Chronic sorrow doesn't feel the same all the time. Sometimes the sorrow is strongly felt, such as when an important milestone is missed. There might not be any first steps or Little League. At other times, it is barely perceived or mixed with moments of joy. It is not a sorrow that can be cured, nor is it abnormal. It is an unresolved sorrow because caring for or giving up a physically or mentally impaired child is an unresolvable situation.

Accepting help from others can help you conserve your strength, especially when your situation is ongoing. Respite care (time away) for you and your partner can help you recharge. Especially if your child is difficult to care for, you need to take breaks to avoid exhaustion. Don't be embarrassed to ask for help. Others, even close friends and relatives, may not realize how difficult your situation is every day. Community resources may also provide respite care and/or sponsor support groups. A social worker may be able to help you locate such resources. Support groups have been formed for almost every illness and disease (see Appendix D). Most parents find them helpful as a source of information, if not emotionally.

At some point, you will learn how to live with your situation and be able to function and grow, albeit much differently than you may ever have imagined.

What Is "Normal"?

Throughout the grief process, both for a child who has died or a chronically ill child, you may wonder if you are normal. "Is feeling this emotion normal?" "Have I been feeling sad, angry, or confused for too long?" Most people are able to work through their grief with help from their partner, family members, friends, and coworkers. However, you may want to obtain help from a therapist, family counselor, social worker, or other professional if you feel you need it or if any of the following occur:

- You are afraid you may physically harm yourself or someone else; you have thoughts of suicide.
- You are participating in activities that may damage your health (drugs, alcohol abuse or overeating).
- The support of friends and family members is not enough.
- You sustain repeated losses.
- You think very poorly of yourself and feel out of control, depressed, or "stressed out" all the time.

A Bittersweet Time

Few things in life are more difficult than making decisions for a disabled, chronically ill, or dying baby. Drawing on the love and support of family, friends, and the health care team will help you make the choices that will ultimately be best for you and your child. It may take time for your decisions to feel completely right. The choices facing you are complex and will awaken many new emotions. As time goes by, though, you'll be thankful that you were empowered to make these choices for your baby and grateful that you were able to control some aspects of this very overwhelming time in your life.

Chapter 14

One Step Closer to Home: The Intermediate Care Experience

"All right," said Eeyore. "We're going.

Only Don't Blame Me."

Karin Menghini, RN, MSN, NNP-BC

One day when you call to check on your baby, the nurse will tell you, "It's graduation day! Your baby will be leaving the NICU and moving to the step-down (or intermediate care) unit."

Graduation sounds like progress (and it is!), but what else changes? Being a neonatal intensive care unit (NICU) parent has meant dealing with daily changes, but by now you have developed a comfort level with the NICU staff, equipment, routines, and visiting procedures. Things may be different in the new unit. This change means another period of adjustment.

This chapter explains what intermediate care is and what happens if this change in care means your baby must move to a new space within the unit or to a new hospital. It also looks at ways in which you'll continue to build a more active role in your baby's care.

The Intermediate Care Experience

Some babies go home directly from the NICU, but most NICU babies are eventually transferred to a step-down unit for less intensive care before discharge. The step-down unit may be within the NICU itself or very nearby. Some NICUs transfer babies to a community hospital, possibly closer to your home, for continued convalescence. Knowing what to expect in the way of routines, staff members, and your role during this period of hospitalization will help alleviate your stress and enable you to participate in your baby's care more fully.

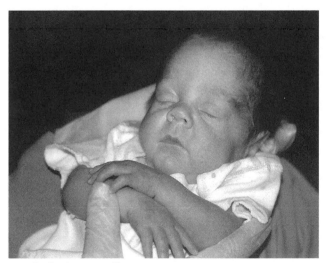

Ready for intermediate care.
With most of his medical crises behind him, this baby is now a "gainer and grower."

Intermediate Care Defined

The name of the step-down unit and the babies who qualify for admission vary from hospital to hospital. The unit may be called *intermediate care, NICU step-down, special care, growing preemie unit, Level II unit,* or something else. Whatever the unit is called, your baby's transfer means that she has matured beyond the need for intensive life support. With a few rare exceptions, your baby is past the life-and-death crises and is on the road home. Parameters for intermediate care vary widely among nurseries but, in general, your baby is off the ventilator and now needs less intense nursing care and observation.

As your NICU nurse prepares you for your baby's transition to this new phase of care, she may describe the intermediate care nursery as a quieter place, more able to work with your baby's sleep-wake cycles and abilities to interact with her less hectic surroundings. Because growing babies need a lot of undisturbed rest, feeding time is usually the best time for interaction; therefore, your nurse may suggest that you begin to spend this time with your baby, learning about her emerging personality, cues, and behaviors. Your baby no longer requires frequent intensive nursing care, so expect her nurse to have 3 to 4 other babies under her care. Some intermediate care settings keep the same nursing staff (your baby may even keep the same primary nurse) for the entire hospitalization. Or the nurse in the intermediate care unit may supervise specially trained nursing assistants who help with feeding, vital signs, and other care tasks. Occupational or physical therapy personnel may be more visible in intermediate care as they work with you and your baby on feeding skills, positioning, comforting, and other behavioral and physical tasks. In intermediate care, there is generally a greater focus on parent involvement. Learning to care for your baby becomes the focal point of your visits.

When you call to check on your baby in intermediate care, there will most likely be a different focus on what is reported. Unless some complication occurs, your baby's condition will change much less often than in the NICU. Lab work, x-rays, and other tests are less frequent in intermediate care, and monitor alarms are heard less often. The staff focus on your baby's progress and your plans for actively participating in care and discharge planning.

Emotional Changes

In the NICU, you probably developed trusting relationships with members of the NICU staff—usually those staff who always discussed your baby's case openly and honestly and were willing to listen to your feelings and concerns. If your move to the intermediate care nursery means a change of personnel, you'll probably miss the comfortable working relationships you shared. You and your baby will need some time to get acquainted with a new team and to learn how to communicate well with that team. Eventually, you will develop good communication and trusting relationships with staff members in the intermediate care nursery, just as you did with those in the NICU.

As things slow down, you may find that emotions from the past weeks are catching up with you. Your baby's major crises are over, but as you start to relax, you may also begin to feel the emotions that you've been too numb to acknowledge until now. You may have been too frightened or overwhelmed to express some of those feelings, but now they seem to come tumbling out at your partner, the nursery staff, and anyone else who is willing to listen. This outpouring will slow down eventually.

There are ways to gain control over these emotions. Think about what you are feeling. See your behavior as an expression of overwhelming emotion. Talk to a friend, your partner, or a counselor. Write in a journal or talk into a tape recorder. The length of time this process takes depends on the length of time your child was in the NICU, how early in your pregnancy your infant was born, how many life-and-death crises your baby experienced in the NICU, your support system, and your personal coping style. Ask your baby's nurse if the hospital has a support group, social worker, clinical nurse specialist, chaplain, or other person who supports the emotional needs of parents. Ask if they have "graduate" NICU parents who volunteer to talk with families about their similar NICU experiences. Do not be afraid to share your feelings with the doctor, nurse practitioner, physician assistant, or bedside nurse caring for your baby. Everyone is available to help. These emotions and feelings are normal. Keep in mind that what you have been going through would be very stressful for any parent. Find coping skills that work for you.

By now you've observed and learned so much about NICU practices, your biggest challenge in adjusting to this new unit will be accepting that *different* is not necessarily *wrong*. Adjusting to new faces and new routines will take time. Your communication techniques (see Chapter 3) may need review and fine-tuning as you negotiate a new plan of care for your baby. If you're not given an orientation list for the intermediate care unit, review your original NICU orientation list (see Chapter 4) and ask about the plan for the remainder of your baby's hospital stay. This effort will communicate to staff that you're interested in how this new unit works. Most importantly, it will help you get comfortable so you can focus on learning to care for your baby before she is discharged. In addition to learning about the new unit routines, communicate your baby's likes and dislikes, including her typical behavior patterns, with the staff. They will be most appreciative of the information during this period of adjustment for both you and your baby.

Transport Back to the Community Hospital

"It was great to bring James back to our birth hospital. Some of those nurses had helped care for him the day he was born so sick, and we knew they would take good care of him now."

If your baby was transferred to the NICU from a community hospital, the doctor, nurse practitioner, or physician assistant may discuss transporting her back to your community hospital for continued convalescence and preparation for discharge. Back transport—also called *return transport*—is common in hospitals where NICU beds are used for the sickest infants and less intensive care is done in community hospitals in the area. The community hospital is often closer to your home and may allow you to spend more time with your baby.

Anxieties About Transfer

Feelings of anxiety as you face yet another change are normal. A tour of the community hospital special care nursery can help allay many concerns about a transfer. Ask your social worker or primary nurse to call the nurse manager or clinical nurse specialist at the community hospital nursery and make an appointment for you to tour the nursery. Also check the financial aspects of back transport with a financial counselor or your insurance company to ensure that your coverage provides for back transport and transfer of hospital care.

Community hospitals with special care nurseries are pleased and excited to care for your baby. Because basic care of a growing preterm or convalescing infant does not require the high level of vigilance and technology found in major medical centers, you may discover that you can learn to care for your baby in a more relaxed atmosphere and also receive more individual attention at the intermediate care nursery.

If your baby requires complex care—for a colostomy or a shunt, for example—you may need reassurance that the specialists involved in her care will still be available through the intermediate care nursery. Ask what access the community nursery has to specialty staff— such as neurologists, ophthalmologists, and pulmonologists—for consultations. Ask the nurse at the community hospital at what point it might be necessary to transport a baby with unanticipated difficulties back to the NICU and how this would be accomplished.

Your community hospital may be closer to home than the regional NICU and more convenient for visiting your baby. People who can help you and your baby make the transition to home are available at the community hospital and are very familiar with local support sources, such as medical equipment supply companies and community home health services.

With your questions answered, you should feel more secure about your baby's transfer to a community hospital intermediate care nursery. Most parents find this more peaceful atmosphere a welcome relief after the NICU.

If, however, you have serious reservations about the ability of the community hospital nursery to meet your baby's complicated care requirements or about follow-up services, make your concerns heard immediately to your discharge planner or neonatologist. You may not be able to make the ultimate decision, but a compromise may be reached that meets the needs of both your baby and the NICU. A delay in transfer or transfer to a different community hospital may be possible, but this will no doubt be a collaborative decision. Even though your feelings are running high, it's important to maintain some objectivity and present your case calmly and in a spirit of cooperation. You and the NICU staff have invested a lot to get your baby to the point where intermediate care is possible. Everyone shares your goal of a healthy baby at discharge.

Adjusting to This Change

As the transport incubator carrying your baby rolls into the intermediate care nursery at your community hospital, you may ask yourself just how you'll survive the stress of another adjustment. This may be a difficult transition. Many parents suffer separation anxiety and even feelings of abandonment as they leave the security of the NICU. Sometimes they transfer those angry feelings to the new nursery staff, delaying the development of good communication. But as you allow yourself to become comfortable with these new faces and routines, the sense of partnership will return.

Transport is stressful for babies too. Yours may be sleepier or more irritable than usual or may not tolerate feedings well for the first 24 hours in the new environment. Some babies require a slight increase in supplemental oxygen following a transport or lose weight for the first few days. These temporary setbacks rarely reflect poor caregiving by the new nursery staff. Given an opportunity for quiet rest, your baby will quickly recover and adapt to this new environment. This is not the time to introduce new stressors, however, such as stepping up the bottle or breastfeeding schedule or quickly weaning your baby out of the incubator to a crib. Use this interim period to acquaint yourself with the staff and new routines.

Unlike the parent whose baby convalesces in and is discharged from the same unit in the same hospital, you face the additional challenges of adjusting to and working with 2 hospital routines during this experience. It may help to know that the basic principles of intermediate care are the same in almost all step-down nurseries. The remainder of this chapter focuses on the intermediate care experience and what you may expect during this period of hospitalization.

Your Expanding Role in Care

"First, I bargained with God to let my baby live. Then I worried about whether he'd be normal. Now I'm worried that I won't be able to take care of him at home. It helps to talk to the nurses about your biggest worry of the moment."

Except in the unlikely case of complications, the intermediate care nursery is the gateway to home. In this environment suited for instruction and supervised practice, you and your baby will master the skills necessary for discharge. This is the time to take a more active role in your baby's care.

Negotiating the Schedule

You'll need to know your baby's schedule of activities to participate in care. Ask about the feeding schedule, bath time, and special treatments such as respiratory therapy or physical therapy. Let the nurses know what you already feel comfortable doing (for example, changing a diaper) and what skills you're ready to tackle (such as giving vitamins). Nurses will gladly save a feeding or bath for parents or rearrange your baby's schedule to fit your schedule if this is discussed ahead of time. The intermediate care nursery also provides an excellent opportunity to begin or continue kangaroo care (see Chapter 5). Holding your baby in this special way gives you a chance to get to know her before homecoming.

Working With Your Baby's Cues Now

As a NICU parent, you've learned about infant states and cues and are beginning to recognize your baby's individual behaviors (see Chapter 4). As your baby becomes more stable and mature, she will develop distinct patterns of sleep and wakefulness. This will make it easier for you to communicate with her and meet her needs.

Your baby may take a few minutes to wake to the quiet alert state before feeding, for example. If you find your baby already awake or crying, you can use comforting techniques to reestablish a quiet alert state. If your baby is quietly looking at you, she is telling you to proceed. Remember to introduce only one type of stimulation at a time. If your baby can look at your face, try speaking gently. Once your baby can handle both looking and listening, try rocking. Watch for new ways your baby has learned to cope with stimulation, such as finger sucking, and encourage use of those coping tools. If the room is noisy or the lights are bright, your baby may become overstimulated. Be alert for signs of stress, and provide time-out periods when necessary. Because feeding time can be especially stressful for babies still perfecting their skills, ask the staff to help you control the environment as much as possible. Developing a communication tool, such

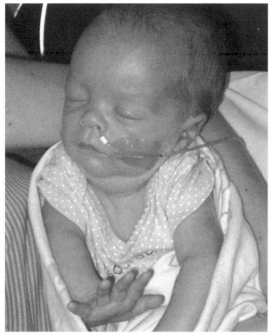

Disengagement cues.
This baby is signaling a need for a break by closing her eyes, turning her head away, and splaying her fingers.

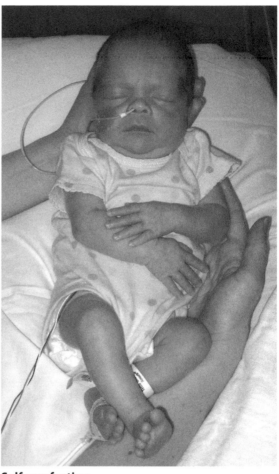

Self-comforting.
This same baby shows increasing skill at self-comforting by flexing her arms to her midline and bracing her feet.

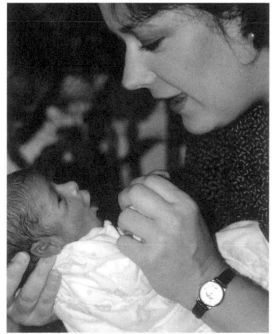

Clear invitation cues.
As your baby convalesces and matures, his periods of alertness are more sustained. This results in clear invitation cues from your baby.

as a bedside care plan or communication sheet about what your baby likes and dislikes, is a helpful, easy way for all staff to get to know your baby's preferences and behaviors.

Positioning Your Baby

When holding your baby, position her so her arms, shoulders, and back flex forward. Preterm infants tend to extend backward because they did not have as much time in the flexed position while in the uterus as term babies did. Unless corrected, this backward extension can cause movement difficulties and delays in meeting developmental milestones. Sometimes a referral to a physical or occupational therapist is necessary and may help during the hospitalization as well as for follow-up after discharge.

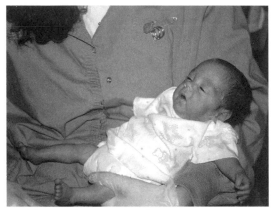

Positioning for organization.
Your baby may still need help with positioning in order to organize herself. This baby is sprawled in the nurse's arms and has difficulty focusing on the nurse's voice.

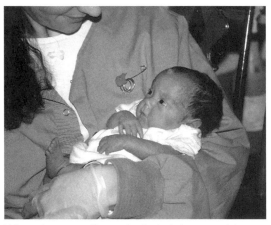

When the nurse flexes the baby's legs, positions his arms in midline, and holds him close, the baby can concentrate and learn about his surroundings.

The bigger your baby becomes, the more she will move around in bed. You have probably noticed positions she seems to prefer. Most babies prefer flexed positions and like boundaries around their bodies. You can help your baby get comfortable by making boundaries or nesting her with rolled blankets while she is in an incubator. The head of the bed may be tilted up if your baby tends to spit up after feeding.

When homecoming approaches and your baby transitions to an open crib (see page 437), the boundaries and extra nesting materials will be removed from her bed so that safe sleep practices can be followed. This includes putting her to sleep on her back. A sleep sack may also be introduced when in a crib to help with positioning and comfort yet discourage overheating from the use of multiple blankets. Become familiar with recommendations to reduce the risk of sudden infant death syndrome (SIDS), also known as *crib death,* and start incorporating them into your baby's routine while in the hospital. These are covered in Chapter 16.

A baby's head movement must sometimes be limited to keep respiratory equipment in place. This can leave the baby's head temporarily flattened on the sides. The look of this "preemie head" concerns most families. Fortunately, head shape corrects with time, usually after your infant can hold her head up independently. More tips for helping to "round out" your baby's head are on page 489.

Diapering Your Baby

You probably changed your baby's diaper for the first time in the NICU. The diaper may simply have been lying under your baby, or you may have had to work with adhesive tabs or a diaper cover. Your baby's nurse showed you how to gently lift your baby's legs, clean the diaper area, and replace the diaper. This once daunting task may have become routine by now; if not, it soon will. As you diaper your baby, be sure to examine the diaper area for rashes or redness and to note the consistency and color of the stool. You'll learn to recognize what amount is normal; the amount will increase as your baby grows.

You should notify your baby's nurse of any change in skin condition and then find out how to treat the problem. If the diaper area is red, a thin coat of clear ointment (such as A+D) will protect the area and help it heal. If a diaper rash develops, a zinc-based ointment (such as Desitin) may be applied, the skin may be left open to the air, or a heat lamp may be used to speed healing. A moist, bright red, solid-looking rash may indicate a yeast infection, which usually requires prescribed medication.

Performing Cord Care

Because many NICU babies stay in the hospital for more than 2 weeks, parents rarely need to concern themselves with caring for the umbilical cord site. The remainder of the umbilical cord dries up and falls off within 2 weeks. The cord site should be kept open to air, clean, and dry. The nurses will teach you any other care required. In most units, the baby is not given a tub bath until the cord has dried and fallen off.

Dressing Your Baby

Your first experience dressing your baby will probably involve putting on a hat or a pair of booties. Dressing your infant in real baby clothes may be scary at first. Those little arms and legs look very fragile. The staff are used to handling these little ones, and their confident movements may look harsh when you're still a bit afraid even to move your baby. But those little arms do fit in sleeves, and the legs go in the leg holes just like other children's. All parents are nervous at first, and your baby has been through a lot. Watch the nurses, and ask questions as they demonstrate dressing your baby. Take your time until you're comfortable. Before long, you'll be able to dress your baby completely without a second thought.

Feeding Your Baby

"When Maria got to intermediate nursery and really started eating well, I couldn't pump enough breast milk to keep up. That's when the lactation specialist helped me most. Her encouragement kept me going, and in a few weeks, my milk supply caught up with Maria's appetite."

Feeding is quality time for you and your baby. You can participate in feeding even before your baby is ready to tackle a complete breastfeeding or bottle feeding. Ask if you can hold your baby during gavage feeding.

Care providers base their feeding decisions on your baby's weight, gestational age, and general condition. The health care provider determines the plan for introducing what feeding, in what concentration and volume, and by what route. Protocols often guide the nurse in advancing your baby's feeding to more volume or more breastfeeding or bottle feeding. The earlier in gestation a baby is born, the slower feeding progresses. Chapter 5 explains infant feeding in detail.

You may be able to hold your baby during gavage feedings, but when your baby begins breastfeeding or bottle feeding, you may certainly hold her while feeding her. The nurse will stay nearby until you're comfortable and will offer help as needed. You might feel nervous at first, but you'll come to look forward to this special time with your baby.

Infants usually begin the transition from tube feedings to breastfeeding or bottle feeding by trying the breast or bottle once per shift or per day. At the same time, a plan is prepared for increasing the frequency of nipple (breast or bottle) feedings. As your infant is able, she will progress from one or more breastfeedings or bottle feedings per day to finally all nipple feedings.

Another approach to feeding is determined by infant feeding cues. Being awake and ready to feed as feeding time approaches, bringing her hands to her mouth or rooting (moving about searching for something to suck on), readily taking her pacifier, and having good muscle tone at feeding times are all cues that she is ready to breastfeed or bottle feed. If she has a number of readiness cues (this will happen more on some days than others), she is offered an opportunity to breastfeed or bottle feed. Ask your nurse what approach your hospital uses.

When bottle or breastfeeding frequency is increased, your baby may not gain weight for a time. In fact, some babies lose a little weight during this transition. After a few days, weight gain begins again. See Chapter 5 for more information on weight gain and growth.

Every NICU approaches the transition from gavage feeding to breastfeeding differently, so discuss your baby's feeding plan with your medical team. If your premature baby is now 32 to 34 weeks' gestation and you notice feeding cues, be assertive in your desire to introduce breastfeeding or bottle feeding.

If you are breastfeeding, it may be necessary to supplement the feedings with gavage feedings to ensure adequate nutrition at each feeding. When your baby is able to get milk from the breast, bottles will be introduced until your baby can breastfeed every time and gain weight from breastfeeding alone. Other units introduce the breast and bottle simultaneously. Each unit practices feeding advancement differently, so communicate your ideas clearly and prepare to be flexible.

Some mothers worry that once introduced to bottle feeding, their baby will find breastfeeding more difficult. Breastfeeding and bottle feeding are different skills, but most babies are adaptable. Recent studies indicate that nipple preference is more apt to occur when a baby is fed only from a bottle for weeks before breastfeeding is attempted. If the 2 are introduced together or within days of each other, the baby rarely has problems switching to the breast from the bottle. Chapter 5 has more information about this concern on page 134.

Using the Bulb Syringe

A bulb syringe is used to remove secretions from a baby's mouth and nose. Until your baby can effectively clear her nose, the syringe will be used when she seems bothered by nasal stuffiness or discharge. To use a bulb syringe, first squeeze the bulb; then place the tip of the syringe gently into the baby's nostril (don't push it in). Releasing the bulb suctions the secretions. Don't hold the opposite nostril closed; this could cause painful pressure in the ear. Don't push the tip of the syringe too far into the nostril, because the tissue is easily damaged. Swelling as a result of tissue damage only complicates nasal stuffiness. If her nose congestion doesn't bother her (only you), she probably doesn't need to be suctioned. To clean the bulb after use, force hot water through the bulb syringe, adding infant bath soap to the water if desired. Be sure to rinse any soap thoroughly from the bulb.

Massaging Your Baby

You may be able to massage your baby as part of caregiving in the intermediate care unit. If you want to try massage, it's important to remember all of the things you know about your baby's tolerance for stimulation. Vimala McClure's book *Infant Massage: A Handbook for Loving Parents* (2000) is written for parents of term infants but contains a helpful chapter on massaging premature babies.

When you begin massage, the first step may simply be to "contain" your baby by putting a firm hand on her head or chest or by holding her arms and legs in a flexed position. Light massage tends to irritate very young preterm babies, but these infants enjoy small amounts of firm, gentle stroking. The unit may have a nurse or occupational therapist who is a licensed massage instructor and who can teach you the skills.

Bathing Your Baby

Each hospital has different criteria and routines for tub bathing infants, and even sponge bathing may be postponed until the staff feel your baby is medically stable. You should be able to bathe your baby several times before discharge, however, so you can practice this care task with supervision.

Most babies do not require a bath more than 2 or 3 times per week. Cleansing the diaper area and washing the baby's hands and face are all she will need on most days. When your baby's umbilical cord (and circumcision site if your baby boy has been circumcised) are healed, you may be taught tub bathing.

Just as dressing your baby can be frightening at first, giving your baby that first bath can be overwhelming. Your baby's nurse will teach you the components of a special care bath—among them, removing electrode patches and protecting intravenous (IV) sites from water. When your baby can tolerate a tub bath, the nurse will provide a working surface, a warming light, a bathtub or basin, and the necessary linen and bath supplies. At first, you'll probably serve as an assistant while the nurse gives most of the bath and demonstrates important points. As your confidence grows, you'll do more of the work, using the nurse as your resource.

Remember to celebrate these special moments and consider taking photographs or journaling about your experiences. They will be lifelong memories.

Gaining independence.
The nurse in intermediate care stands by to offer assistance but allows you to do as much caregiving as possible.

Taking Your Baby's Temperature

Use of a thermometer is an important skill that every parent or caregiver should be comfortable with before the baby's discharge. A baby's "normal" temperature depends in part on age, weight, metabolism, and other health factors, but most NICU experts agree that a baby's normal axillary (armpit) temperature is in the range of 97.5°F to 99°F (36.4°C–37.2°C). Your baby's rectal temperature should be in the range of 98°F to 100°F (36.7°C–37.8°C). A rectal temperature of 100.4°F (38°C) or greater usually indicates fever in a baby. The most common methods for taking your baby's temperature are axillary (armpit), tympanic (ear), skin (with a fever strip), and rectal (in the baby's bottom). While your baby is still in the hospital, an axillary temperature will be used most often. If illness is suspected, the nurse may check a rectal temperature. The tympanic method and fever strips are less reliable methods for infants and are further discussed in Chapter 16.

An axillary temperature—one taken in the armpit—is easy, usually more pleasant for you and your baby than a rectal temperature, and it's a perfectly acceptable way to assess temperature. This is probably the method the nurses will teach you. It's important to place the tip of the thermometer against skin in the center of the underarm. Hold the arm firmly while the temperature is registering—this takes about 2 minutes. With a digital thermometer, this method is quick and accurate.

A rectal temperature is most accurate but can cause injury and may be unpleasant for your baby. After your baby is home and if you suspect that your baby has a fever, your baby's care provider will probably ask you to take a rectal temperature. Therefore, learn how to take a rectal temperature before your baby goes home (see page 493).

A rectal thermometer should be well lubricated (with petroleum jelly or a lubricating jelly like K-Y) before insertion. Depending on your baby's size, the thermometer should be inserted 1/2 to 1 inch into the rectum. Never force a rectal thermometer. If you can't insert it gently, pull it back toward the rectum and gently probe in another direction. The recommended position for your baby is lying on her tummy over your legs or on a firm surface such as a changing table. This lets you control your baby's movements and prevents her from rolling onto the thermometer, which could cause an injury.

Whether you take an axillary or rectal temperature, it's important to use the same method each time when monitoring your baby's temperature. Readings vary by as much as 2°F between axillary and rectal, so alternating methods makes it difficult to compare results. When reporting your baby's temperature to your health care provider, be sure you mention whether you used the axillary or the rectal method.

Giving Medications

If your baby will go home on medications, the nurses will teach you how to draw up the dose and give it to your baby. They should also teach you about the common side effects of any drugs your baby will be taking. Appendix B offers detailed information on many of the medications commonly given to babies. Chapter 16 gives tips on how to manage problems you may encounter with medicines at home.

Practice drawing up and administering your baby's medications before your baby comes home. For many medications, you'll need to learn how to use a syringe to accurately measure the dose. Some medications should be mixed in a small amount of formula or breast milk to prevent stomach upset. Others need to be given directly into your baby's mouth. Breastfeeding mothers may be taught to give all medications directly into their baby's mouth just before nursing or halfway into the feeding. An alternative method is to express some breast milk into a bottle to be used for medication administration. Ask your nurse which method the hospital recommends. Your health care provider or specialist is usually responsible for adjusting dosages as your baby grows.

Ask why your baby is on each medication and how long she will need to take it. Babies are often weaned from medications prior to discharge. Drug levels or other tests may be needed at certain intervals to assess the medication's effectiveness. In some cases (for example, with theophylline, caffeine, or phenobarbital), the baby may be allowed to outgrow the dose. The drug dose will be increased only if the baby shows the need—if, for example, apnea or seizures continue or recur. Ask the intermediate care nurses and the physicians as many questions as needed until you are comfortable with this part of your baby's plan. You need to know enough about your baby's medications to be a partner in her care after discharge. Once your baby is discharged, your health care provider is your resource, and you will be your child's primary case manager and advocate.

Learning Infant CPR

Every parent should know how to perform infant CPR. You can learn CPR in a couple of different ways. You can find a class through your local Red Cross or fire department. Many hospitals offer infant CPR classes as part of their parent education programs. Consider purchasing a self-directed learning kit such as the *Infant CPR Anytime* program. Using the kit allows you and your family to learn infant CPR in the comfort of your own home and practice the skills of CPR over and over again. Attend a class or purchase a kit and learn this important skill now, well before going home. Don't wait until the mad rush just before discharge. (See Appendix E for CPR information.)

Learning Special Care Tasks

If your baby will be going home with special equipment for care, get involved in learning how to manage the equipment and do these tasks as soon as possible. Special care tasks include gavage feeding; gastrostomy, colostomy, and tracheostomy care; and oxygen use for emergencies, during feedings, or by nasal cannula or ventilator. Chapter 16 contains more information on caring for babies with these special needs at home.

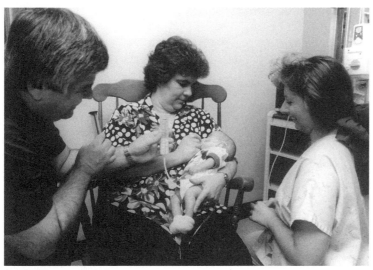

Special care skills.
Now is the time to learn special skills you will need for your baby's care at home. This father gives the gastrostomy feeding while the mother offers the baby a pacifier. The nurse provides teaching and reassurance to the family. This father and son appear again on page 506.

Have the nurses explain what they are doing as you watch. After a few times watching, do the task while a nurse talks you through it. Don't expect to perform the task as easily as the nurse does. The nurse has had a lot more practice! Gradually, the nurse will do less coaching as you gain confidence. Don't wait until your baby's last week in the hospital to learn these skills. Give yourself plenty of time to practice and get help if you need it.

Networking

Contact with the parents of other NICU graduates can be helpful—both before and after your baby's hospital discharge. Your baby's move to the intermediate care nursery is a good time to begin making contacts. When available, support groups may be helpful. There may also be a support network of parents with previous NICU experience who can give you valuable insights and information. Call or meet with 2 or 3 other families. They can provide priceless guidance as you face decisions about a pediatrician or other health care provider and all of the other choices you'll need to make as your baby's discharge date approaches.

Watching for Complications

"In the beginning, you expect complications and scary moments. In intermediate care, setbacks are more surprising, more disappointing, because you think those times are behind you."

When your baby is stable enough to graduate to intermediate care, she is generally considered past the real dangers that may have been present while she was critically ill. A few medical conditions can affect progress, but most cause only a temporary setback. Rarely, these conditions can mean readmission to the NICU.

Apnea and Bradycardia

Apnea, bradycardia, and desaturation (see Chapter 9) often occur in babies born at less than 32 weeks' gestation, and episodes may continue in the intermediate care nursery. The staff will monitor the frequency, intensity, and duration of the episodes.

If your baby was not having apnea or bradycardia in the NICU or if the frequency or intensity of the episodes increases now, this may be a sign of illness. If this happens, the physician, neonatal nurse practitioner, or physician assistant will order tests to find the cause. If the apnea and bradycardia are because of immaturity, your baby may receive medication (theophylline or caffeine) to decrease the episodes. If your baby is put on medication, drug levels in the blood may be checked periodically. As your infant grows, the doctor adjusts the dosage or allows your baby to outgrow the dose if apnea and bradycardia resolve.

Unless they are a side effect of another illness, apnea and bradycardia often resolve around your baby's original due date. If your baby is ready to go home before that date, mild apnea and bradycardia may need to be managed before discharge. Management of the situation depends on the philosophy of your baby's neonatologists. Your baby may require continued monitoring in the hospital, may require testing with a pneumogram before discharge (see page 442), or may be a candidate for home monitoring and/or medication. If your baby goes home with a monitor, you'll be instructed in monitor use and infant CPR.

Infection

Your recovering baby is prone to many kinds of infection. Despite the best precautions of staff and visitors, infections do occur. Some infections, such as thrush, are minor and respond to treatment rapidly. Others can be more serious.

Thrush

Your baby might get a yeast infection—called *thrush*—in her mouth. It looks like thick white patches on the tongue or gums. You cannot wipe these patches off. Infants with thrush often have feeding problems because of tenderness in the affected area. Thrush is usually treated with oral medication. Page 138 has more information about thrush.

Other Infections

Signs of other infections may include feeding difficulties (intolerance, vomiting, abdominal swelling, or poor feeding), decreased activity, increased frequency of apnea and bradycardia, unstable temperature, and increased work of breathing. When the health care team becomes aware of these signs, your baby may have blood work, a spinal tap, a urine culture, or x-rays to identify the cause of infection. Intravenous antibiotics may be started, and your baby may be made NPO (no nutrition by mouth) as a precaution. Rarely, your baby may be transferred back to the NICU for respiratory support, for increased monitoring, or simply for IV medications. It is also rare that a baby overwhelmed by an infection will die. Most infections respond well to treatment, and your infant will be back to normal in 2 or 3 days. Chapters 9 and 10 provide more information about infections in newborns.

Hernias

Preterm infants are at risk for hernias—protrusion of a body part (such as a loop of intestine) through a muscle weakness or unusual opening inside the body. If your baby develops a hernia, most eventually require surgical repair.

Inguinal Hernia

The most common hernia is called an *inguinal hernia*. This condition occurs most often in males and usually presents as a bulge in the groin, especially after crying or straining during a bowel movement. Sometimes girls get inguinal hernias, which cause a bulge, or swelling, above or along the labia.

Usually a boy's testicles stay in the inguinal canal (high in the groin, not down in the scrotal sac) until about 32 weeks' gestation. At that time, the testicles descend into the scrotum. But in preterm babies, part of the intestine may push through a remaining gap in the muscle wall into the scrotum. This may affect one or both sides and appears as a swelling above or in the scrotum.

As long as the hernia is reducible (the intestine can be easily and gently pushed back through the opening), immediate surgical correction is not necessary. Surgery to repair the hernia may occur before discharge or around the time your baby weighs around 2 kilograms (or 4½ pounds). Surgery can also be postponed until the child is older or requires other surgery. If the hernia becomes incarcerated (trapped in the scrotum), the scrotum will become blue and painful, and immediate surgery is necessary.

Umbilical Hernia

Another area where the muscle may not close properly is around the umbilical cord. An umbilical hernia causes the umbilical area, or belly button, to push outward when the baby cries. As long as there is no redness or discoloration, there is no cause for concern. This condition usually corrects itself as your baby grows and the abdominal muscles strengthen and thicken. In general, surgical correction is not recommended before the age of 3 to 5 years.

Gastroesophageal Reflux

A condition known as *gastroesophageal reflux* (GER) occurs when the opening at the entrance of the stomach has not matured and allows food to move back up the esophagus. A baby with GER might vomit 3 or 4 times per day and loses a significant amount of her feedings. She may have episodes of apnea, bradycardia and desaturation during feeding, signs of discomfort during feeding, difficulty advancing volume, poor digestion, and poor weight gain. Many preterm babies show symptoms of GER and most outgrow it as they reach term age (their original due date).

A variety of factors may contribute to the dysfunction of the junction at the esophagus and stomach. Reflux may be caused by respiratory distress that causes the diaphragm and abdominal muscles to work harder than they should, positioning an infant on her back, bearing down with abdominal muscles during movement, and large volumes of food causing pressure on the junction at the esophagus and stomach. Feeding small amounts more frequently, feeding continuously by pump (although gavage tubes are associated with increased reflux symptoms), raising the head of the bed, or placing the baby on her tummy after feeding may help alleviate this condition. If tummy positioning is used, continuous cardiorespiratory monitoring must be used and the baby must be transitioned to back sleeping prior to discharge to reduce SIDS risk. If the condition is severe, treatment may include medication or surgery. The surgery to correct reflux is called *fundoplication* (see page 516).

Anemia

While your baby is in intermediate care, blood counts (hematocrit or hemoglobin) will be checked weekly or as the baby's situation requires. Preterm NICU babies are at risk for anemia (low red blood cell count) because their NICU stay required drawing of blood for testing and evaluation of treatment, and the body system that makes red blood cells (RBCs) is immature. (See Chapter 9 for more information.) Rapid growth also causes a decrease in blood counts. Babies often cannot replenish their blood supply fast enough to keep up with the necessary blood tests in the NICU; therefore, blood transfusions may be given to correct anemia. In some institutions, the medication Epogen (EPO) is given to help stimulate RBC production.

Anemia can cause low oxygen and glucose levels in the blood, which can cause the tissues and organs to function improperly. Infants with anemia may appear pale and lethargic, have an increase in apnea and/or bradycardia, and not eat well. Infants on respiratory support may have regular transfusions. Keeping the blood count normal is important for keeping oxygen levels normal and allowing timely weaning from oxygen.

Most babies who have graduated to intermediate care are able to maintain their oxygen levels without help, so they shouldn't require many transfusions. In intermediate care, blood counts are allowed to drop lower than in the NICU to stimulate the baby's own RBC production system. When an infant receives transfusions, the production of RBCs in the bone marrow is not stimulated. A low RBC count is the necessary stimulus to trigger production. As with all immature systems, full functioning takes time.

When the hemoglobin and hematocrit drop, the body system that produces RBCs is stimulated to replenish the lost supply. A blood test called a *reticulocyte count* (retic) shows the amount of developing RBCs produced. If the retic count is within normal limits, transfusion will be postponed in the hope that the baby's system will do its job. In most infants, the process corrects itself without complication. Occasionally a baby may be transfused in the week before discharge. In that case, your health care provider's office may schedule follow-up lab work after discharge.

Moving Closer to Home

Your baby's graduation to the intermediate care unit is an exciting time. It is one step closer to home! As an emerging expert of your baby's behavior and special needs, you know you have more to learn. You'll begin to feel more like a parent as you assume most, if not all, of your baby's caregiving before discharge. The more time you have to learn and practice your parenting skills in this more relaxed setting, the easier things will be in the long run. Go slowly, but don't procrastinate. Your baby will soon be homeward bound.

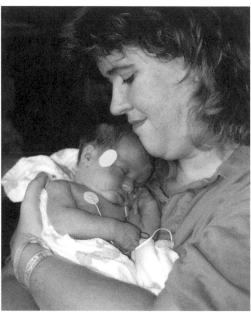

Being together.
Your feelings of belonging to each other can take a while to develop, but time and patience result in a strong bond.

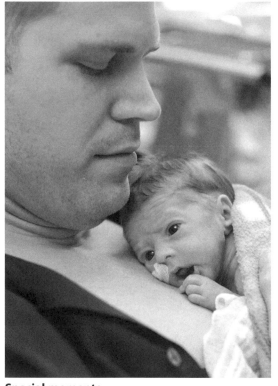

Special moments.
The intermediate care setting is usually quieter than intensive care and offers more moments for just being together. This dad and baby are enjoying skin-to-skin care.

Courtesy of Gigi O'Dea.

Chapter 15
Homeward Bound

"Think of all the possibilities, Piglet,
before you settle down to enjoy yourselves."
—Eeyore

Karin Menghini, RN, MSN, NNP-BC

By the time your baby is eating well, gaining weight, and in an open crib, you should be very familiar with the process of discharge planning.

When your preterm baby's weight nears 4 pounds (1,700–1,800 grams), or your sick baby's special needs are stabilized or resolved, he may be almost ready for discharge. But discharge planning for all neonatal intensive care unit (NICU) babies begins long before these milestones are achieved. Soon after your baby was stabilized in the NICU or was transferred to intermediate care, the health care team began work on a final discharge plan. Your baby's primary nurse, his nurse practitioner, a case manager, or a clinical nurse specialist may have been assigned to coordinate all aspects of the plan. The plan details teaching for parents, referrals that will need to be made to specialists or community services, and equipment if it is needed for home care. If your baby's care will be complex following discharge, you may attend a meeting with representatives from all of the departments that have helped care for your baby. Representatives from community agencies—such as public health, home health agencies, and equipment supply companies—may also attend the meeting. Ask your baby's nurse about your hospital's process for discharge planning so that you can work with the staff to prepare your baby, yourself, your home, and your family and friends for this long-awaited event.

Signs of Progress

Once your baby is in the intermediate care unit, the signs of progress change. Even though your baby may go to intermediate care while still on oxygen or intravenous fluids, the primary focus now becomes your baby's ability to feed by bottle or breast, grow and gain weight, regulate body temperature, and organize behavior into meaningful patterns.

Because discharge depends on the interaction of many factors, your baby's caregiver may not be able to pinpoint an exact date far ahead of time. When the physician or nurse practitioner finally sets a date, it may be right around the corner. That's why it's important to begin learning care skills and preparing your home when you first notice signs of progress.

Less Frequent Measurement of Vital Signs

Your baby's vital signs (temperature, heart rate, and breathing rate) will probably be taken only before feeding and then, eventually, only before every other feeding. Some units will discontinue the cardiorespiratory monitors and pulse oximetry when your baby has had no apnea, bradycardia, or desaturation for a specific period. Routine measurements used to assess your baby's well-being—such as measurement of abdominal girth and daily urine dipstick screening—will be discontinued. Unless your baby has an ongoing cardiac or respiratory condition, frequent measurement of blood pressure and accurate measurement of intake and output may also be discontinued.

More Demands for Attention

Your baby is growing up and may begin demanding more attention. He may awaken before feeding time and move around or fuss. He may quietly watch a mobile or just enjoy the surrounding activity. Older babies may even enjoy sitting up in an infant seat or swing for short periods.

Your baby may also seem irritable and inconsolable at times. The transition from an incubator to a crib, from tube feeding to breastfeeding and/or bottle feeding, and from sick to well requires a lot of energy. Some babies get overwhelmed by all of the activity. Others simply seem to be bored with hospitalization and ready to move on. In any case, this is a wonderful time to pay careful attention to your baby's cues and to consider snuggling, rocking, talking, and increasing or decreasing activity to find out how your baby responds to these actions.

Gaining and Growing

Your baby will gradually take more of his feedings in larger amounts from the breast or bottle and fewer feedings by gavage. This transition to the breast or bottle can be a slow process. (See Chapter 5 for more information.) Weight gain will usually average about 1/2 to 1 ounce (15–30 grams) per day. Don't worry if your baby doesn't gain weight every single day. After a day or two of little or no weight gain, he will probably gain well for the next few days. Look at the average weight gain over several days to a week and you should see a good overall gaining trend. (See Chapter 5 for more information on weight gain and growth.)

Measurements of length and head circumference are also good indicators of overall growth. Many units measure these 2 parameters weekly; however, the baby's gestational age, degree of illness, ability to absorb nutrition, and hereditary factors must be considered. Depending on a baby's gestational age, head circumference increases about 1/2 to 1 centimeter per week on average during the first weeks after birth. A growing baby's length increases about 1/2 to 1 centimeter per week, with an average length increase of about 10 to 12 inches (25–30 centimeters) in the first year.

Moving to a Crib

Maintaining body temperature involves calories and oxygen. The more energy your baby uses to keep warm, the less he will have for growing and healing. Your baby will progress from the incubator or radiant warmer to an open crib based on his ability to regulate body temperature. This ability depends, in part, on gestational age and weight. The transition is usually gradual, but your baby may be returned to the warmer environment at the first sign of inability to maintain temperature. It's not unusual for a baby's weight gain to slow, or even for weight to drop, for a day or so during the weaning process to an open crib.

Giving Care Independently

As discharge nears, you're likely to need the unit staff less often for routine care procedures. Your baby's nurse may still talk you through the more complex tasks, but by now you should be fairly comfortable taking a temperature or changing a diaper. Use your nurse as a resource whenever you have questions or need assistance during this learning period.

Learning What's Normal for Your Baby

"Our nurse said she would not only wean Matthew's oxygen, but wean us from total dependence on the NICU."

As nurses check vital signs, change diapers, and do other tasks, they constantly assess your baby. Assessment is noticing the baby's general condition and what might be different from the baby's typical condition. An important part of learning to care for your baby is learning what is normal and understanding how to recognize a change. A parent is often the first and best person to point out a change in their baby's general condition, including both positive changes and potential concerns or changes in behavior.

Corrected Age

If your baby was born early, he really has 2 birthdays. The day your baby was born is the official date of birth, but your original due date is also an important milestone for your baby.

When you measure your baby's development—that is, when you look at what is appropriate behavior for an infant of your baby's age—consider both of those dates. You'll need to determine your baby's corrected age, or postmenstrual age, to know where he should be developmentally.

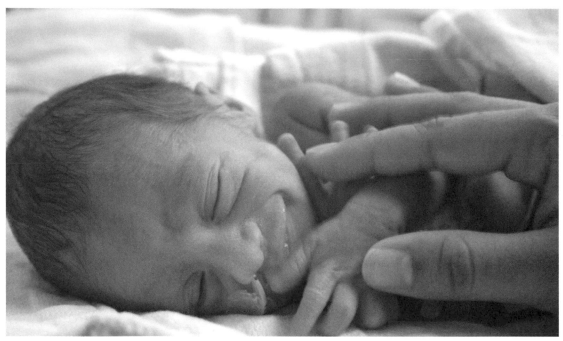

Connecting.
As your baby matures, he will become increasingly responsive to your touch and voice.

Courtesy of University of Washington Medical Center, Seattle, WA.

Calculating corrected age isn't difficult. Begin with your baby's actual age in weeks (number of weeks since the date of birth) and then subtract the number of weeks your baby was preterm. This is your baby's corrected age. A term pregnancy is 40 weeks' gestation. To determine the number of weeks premature your baby was at birth, subtract his gestational age at birth from 40. For example, if your son was born at 28 weeks' gestation, he was 12 weeks (3 months) premature. If he is now 6 months old (24 weeks since birth), his corrected age is

Actual age in weeks minus	Weeks premature	=	Corrected age
24 weeks -	12 weeks	=	12 weeks (3 months)

In this case, even if your son is 6 months old, you should expect him to be at or near the developmental level of a 3-month-old term baby. It would be unrealistic to expect your son to be physically ready to sit up with very little support or on his own—a skill that is frequently emerging in term babies around the age of 6 months. Your baby may just be beginning to roll over, which is developmentally normal for a term baby of 3 months and, therefore, for a baby whose age is 3 months corrected. Pages 542 through 544 include a useful table listing developmental milestones for infants and children of various ages.

Parents are often frustrated by well-meaning family and friends who express concerns about their baby's development. People may think your son is delayed for a 6-month-old, for example, when in fact he is performing ahead of his corrected age of 3 months.

Explaining corrected age and why your baby is so small can get tiresome after a while, and many people continue to be confused. Don't worry—you'll only need to correct for prematurity until your child reaches the age of 2 to 2 1/2 years. Most will catch up developmentally by this age.

Temperature

The nurses have probably already taught you how to take your baby's temperature. (If not, review the instructions in Chapter 14 and get help from your nurse.) Taking a temperature is an important skill for parents to master before the baby comes home.

Check with your baby's caregivers to find out what temperature they consider normal for your baby. Most experts recommend that a baby's normal axillary (armpit) temperature is in the range of 97.5°F to 99°F (36.4°C–37.2°C). The range for a rectal temperature is 98°F to 100°F (36.7°C–37.8°C). A rectal temperature of 100.4°F (38°C) or greater usually indicates a fever. The range of acceptable temperatures varies slightly among medical providers in different parts of the country.

Heart Rate

By watching your baby's cardiac monitor in the NICU, you probably became familiar with your baby's normal heart rate—and also with the fact that heart rate increases when a baby is active and awake and decreases during deep sleep. The resting heart rate for an infant is usually 120 to 160 beats per minute, but the normal range is broad—from 80 beats per minute during deep sleep for older infants to more than 200 beats per minute during crying. Unless your baby has a heart condition, you will probably not routinely check heart rate.

Breathing Rate

A healthy baby's respiratory rate ranges from 40 to 60 breaths per minute. If your baby is working hard to breathe, the outline of the ribs is more visible, the respiratory rate may have increased, and your baby tires quickly when eating. If your baby will go home with a chronic respiratory condition, discuss with your nurses what is normal for your baby and what should be reported to your health care provider.

Color

By now, you probably know your baby's "normal" color. A change in color from a central pink (of lips, tongue, and gums) to pale, dusky, or yellow may indicate infection or a breathing or heart problem. Color changes also occur with desaturations associated with apnea and bradycardia. If your baby has apneic and/or bradycardic episodes, it helps to know what kind of color changes your infant shows just before or when these episodes begin so that you can intervene quickly. Color is a primary indicator of your baby's health status. Learn what is normal for your baby and what changes should be reported to your care provider.

Cry

When your baby's breathing tube was removed, you probably heard him cry, perhaps for the first time. Over time, that first hoarse cry changed to what is now your baby's normal cry. Sometimes when a baby is sick, the cry becomes weaker or higher pitched. As your baby grows, you'll be able to tell the difference among hunger cries, tired cries, and sick cries.

Urine

Most babies have a wet diaper at least 6 times a day. If your baby has a chronic respiratory or cardiac condition, you'll want to note the number of diapers he wets in an average day. (If you switch to super-absorbent diapers at home, it may be difficult to tell if the diaper is actually wet.) Ask your nurse or health care provider at what point you should report an increase or decrease in wet diapers. You may also wish to note the color and odor of your baby's urine, especially if he will take medications at home. Your baby's nurse or health care provider should tell you if his medications will affect how often he will have a wet diaper or if his urine will have an odor or a different appearance.

Stools

You'll also want to be aware of your baby's normal bowel patterns before he is discharged. As your baby progresses to full feedings, bowel movements will change in consistency and color. A healthy baby has softly formed or mushy bowel movements without much odor. A constipated baby strains hard or cries during a bowel movement and produces small, hard, pellet-like poop. Notice how flat or round your baby's tummy is and whether it is soft or hard. If your baby does not have a bowel movement for several days, his tummy may become firm and distended. Notify your baby's nurse or doctor if you have concerns about changes from normal patterns.

Diarrhea is watery and foul smelling and demands immediate attention. Babies with diarrhea become dehydrated easily, and this can be life-threatening. Notify your baby's health care provider immediately any time your infant has more than one diarrhea stool.

Spit-up or Vomit

Spitting up is a common occurrence for most babies. Air bubbles from the stomach bring up a small amount of milk, which runs out of the baby's mouth. Different from spitting up, vomit is ejected from the stomach with force and comes flying out of the baby's mouth. If your baby vomits more than one feeding or consistently spits up more than a tablespoon, let your baby's health care provider know. Also, if the vomit is green or looks different than normal spit-up, notify your health care provider immediately.

Predischarge Testing

While you're learning all you can about your baby's care, the discharge coordinator or case manager is planning your baby's final tests and making preparations for discharge. Common discharge tests are explained here, but not all NICU babies require all of the tests discussed. Ask your baby's nurse what to expect as discharge draws near.

Eye Exam

If your baby was 30 weeks' gestation or less or weighed less than 1,500 grams (3 pounds, 5 ounces) at birth, he will have an eye examination at between 4 and 7 weeks of age. Babies born after 30 weeks' gestation and weighing between 1,500 and 2,000 grams may also have this type of eye examination if they had an especially difficult NICU course. Follow-up exams will be scheduled if the findings of the first exam warrant them. The exam is to identify any changes in the eye tissue caused by retinopathy of prematurity (see page 255).

Hearing Test

Hearing tests—also called *audiology screenings*—are done in most nurseries before discharge. Electronic sound and response monitoring determine if your baby can hear. Environmental conditions, such as surrounding noise or a crying baby, can cause inconclusive results, however. If this happens, a retest should be scheduled in a more controlled environment. If your baby responds to your voice or to noise-making toys held where he can't see them, there is usually no reason for concern. After discharge, your child's hearing should be monitored by your health care provider at periodic health exams. If you are concerned about your baby's hearing, never hesitate to insist on a more extensive hearing exam. These are available at a pediatric audiologist's office or in pediatric outpatient rehabilitation centers.

Newborn Metabolic Screening

Every baby is tested soon after birth to identify some rare but potentially serious or life-threatening conditions. The number of tests varies by state. Newborn metabolic testing can yield inconclusive results if the baby is very premature, is critically ill, or required a blood transfusion prior to metabolic testing. If the screening test suggests a problem, your baby's doctor will speak directly with you and will order follow-up testing. Become aware of the screening test results prior to discharge from the NICU and communicate the findings with your community pediatrician. (Chapter 9 also discusses metabolic screening related to premature infants.)

Blood Count

A final hematocrit or hemoglobin and reticulocyte level are usually done the week of discharge. Although it's unlikely, your baby might be anemic and either need a transfusion at this time or be placed on iron medication to assist his bones in making new red blood cells. (Chapter 9 has information about anemia.) If so, follow-up lab tests will usually be done in the pediatrician's office or an outpatient clinic.

Sleep Study (Pneumogram)

Infants with continuing apnea and bradycardia may have a special test to help determine the cause of these episodes. Depending on your region of the country, the test is called a *sleep study,* a *pneumocardiogram,* or a *pneumogram.* Philosophies vary regarding the use of pneumograms, and not all NICUs use them. A pneumogram does not answer every question about the baby's apnea and bradycardia, and interpretations of the test vary regionally. The American Academy of Pediatrics (AAP) states that "pneumograms are of no value in predicting sudden infant death syndrome (SIDS) and are not helpful in identifying patients who should be discharged with home monitors." Chapter 16 discusses pros and cons of home monitors.

Cranial Ultrasound

If your baby was born younger than 30 weeks' gestation, she has probably had several ultrasounds of her head to detect intraventricular hemorrhage (Chapter 9). Some NICUs will perform a cranial ultrasound or other brain imaging study near the time of hospital discharge for babies weighing less than 1,000 grams at birth. Your neonatologist may also suggest magnetic resonance imaging near your baby's original due date to help predict the need for early intervention services and ensure the best possible developmental outcome. Sometimes a different brain imaging technique may show abnormalities that a screening ultrasound will not. This does not mean that the initial ultrasounds were misinterpreted, but merely that each test has limitations.

Getting What Your Baby Will Need

While your baby is growing stronger and getting ready to go home, it's time to pull out all of the baby care books that you hid away because they seemed so irrelevant to your NICU experience. Look over the baby supply and home preparation lists and start accumulating what you'll need. Now is also the time to cue eager friends or family members who have been waiting for the right moment to give you a baby shower.

Your baby will need many of the items on a basic newborn layette list (page 443). But as a NICU graduate, he may have some special needs as well. The information that follows should help answer many of your questions about baby supplies.

Sample Layette

Clothing
4–6 shirts
6–8 stretch suits
6 one-piece T-shirts with snaps at waist or crotch
4–6 gowns or kimonos
2 or 3 sweatshirts or sweaters
1 or 2 dressy outfits for special occasions
6 pairs booties or socks
12 fabric diaper covers if using cloth diapers
5-dozen cloth diapers (may also be used as burp
    cloths) or disposable diapers

Seasonal
Snowsuit
Warm hat
Warm booties
Cotton hat or bonnet
Cotton booties
Sunsuit or romper

Bedtime
2–3 sleep sacks
6 receiving blankets
2 crib blankets
2–4 crib sheets
6–12 lap pads
2 waterproof pads
Baby intercom
Nightlight

Bath Time
2–4 bath towels
6–8 washcloths
Plastic bathtub
Foam bathtub liner (foam bath pillow)
Brush and comb set
Baby shampoo
Baby scissors

Health Care Supplies
Cool-mist humidifier
Thermometer and lubricant
Infant acetaminophen as recommended by your
    baby's health care provider
Medicine spoon
Plastic rolling cart or trays for special care supplies
Bulletin board and calendar

Furniture
Bassinet or cradle
Crib and mattress or portable crib
Chest of drawers
Laundry hamper
Diaper pail for cloth diapers
Rocking chair or recliner
Toy box

Outings
Diaper bag
Car safety seat
Stroller

Breastfeeding
2 or 3 nursing bras
Nursing pads
Hospital-grade electric breast pump
Containers for breast milk storage

Bottle Feeding
Disposable nurser kit
8 four-ounce or eight-ounce bottles
Baby formula recommended by your
    baby's health care provider

Miscellaneous
2 or 3 pacifiers
Baby toys
Baby record book
Baby care books
Baby laundry soap

For Later
Front carrier and/or backpack
Baby swing
High chair
Play yard
Bibs
Feeding spoons and cups
Childproofing supplies

Clothing and Diapers

By the time they are ready for discharge, many preterm babies fit into newborn-sized clothes. You may decide to purchase a few "going out" items in preemie size for special occasions, but keep in mind that your baby will quickly outgrow them and seldom use them.

Newborn diapers generally work fine for most preterm babies at discharge. Some hospitals send home a small supply of preemie diapers at discharge. You might ask the nurse if your hospital does this. If not, consider getting a few weeks' supply before your baby's discharge.

Diapers will be part of your life for a long time, and your baby will use about 3,000 diapers in his first year, so give some thought to your choices. Choices include cloth or disposable diapers. Both choices impact the environment: disposable diapers are not biodegradable and will add to the 18 billion disposable diapers a year already going to the landfill. Cloth diapers use a lot of water and detergent, and the diaper service delivery trucks use fuel and pollute the environment by being on the road.

Disposable diapers are very absorbent and decrease the amount of contact between your baby's skin and urine. However, it makes it more difficult to monitor how much urine your baby is producing. To decrease the environmental impact, check to see if your community has started recycling or composting used disposable diapers—this is a new trend worth investigating.

Cloth diapers are not as absorbent as disposables and require a plastic, cotton, or terry cloth cover. If you choose cloth diapers, either you or your diaper service must wash and dry them. Washing diapers requires a considerable amount of time and effort, and doorstep pick-up and delivery of diapers may not be available in your community or may be outside your budget.

You may begin with a preference for cloth or disposables and then change your mind as your baby grows, or you may decide to use a combination of cloth and disposable supplies.

Breastfeeding Aids

If you have been breastfeeding your baby, you will have the basic supplies already. You need 2 or 3 well-fitting nursing bras, containers for expressed milk, and perhaps a few bottles and nipples if your baby needs a supplemental bottle. Most breastfeeding mothers of NICU graduates also need to continue to use an electric breast pump at home for a while after their baby's hospital discharge. If your health care provider has recommended test weighing your baby before and after feeding to see how much milk he is getting at the breast, obtain a baby scale designed for this purpose by the time your baby comes home. (See Chapter 5 for information about breast pumps and baby scales.)

Bottles and Formula

Your baby may require special formula. Your local pharmacy should be able to order it for you, or the hospital can give you information on other sources. Ask your social worker or nurse about the expense of special formula and if you should be aware of any other information. For example, is special formula considered a medication and therefore tax deductible or covered by insurance or the government-funded WIC program (Special Supplemental Nutrition Program for Women, Infants, and Children)? Does the formula manufacturer provide formula for families under special circumstances? Investigate these possibilities and talk with the families of other NICU graduates. Special formula can be a major expense. Get all of the cost-saving advice you can.

If your baby will be discharged on regular or premature discharge baby formula, he will no doubt make this transition before discharge. Find out which baby formula your care-giver recommends and why. Find out if the recommended brand is interchangeable with another brand. Differences in formula content may affect your infant's digestion. Figure out which retailer in your local area carries the formula you will need before discharge. Some premature discharge formulas may need to be ordered ahead of time for smaller stores, but larger retailers may stock them routinely.

Most hospitals use ready-to-feed (premixed) formula. At home, you may wish to buy a less expensive form of the recommended formula. You'll find ready-to-feed, concentrated-liquid, and powder formulas on your grocery store's shelves. The powder type is usually the least expensive. Compare costs, and read the preparation instructions to decide which is most time- and cost-effective for you. Follow the instructions carefully, making sure you add the correct amount of powder or concentrated formula and water to the mixture. Ready-to-feed is a convenient option for traveling and to have in your diaper bag to use in case of emergency.

Water from most public water systems is acceptable for infant use. To be sure, however, ask your baby's health care provider about the necessity of boiling supplies when pre-paring formula, including the water used to dilute concentrate or powder formula. Most physicians are comfortable with a thorough washing of all supplies with hot soapy water and a bottle brush. Dishwashers are also efficient for bottle washing. If you have an alter-nate water source, such as a well, or if lead or high fluoride levels in the water are a con-cern, check with your baby's caregiver or the public health department for their recommendations.

Once your baby comes home, he will soon be eating regular baby portions, so special little bottles are rarely necessary. Many parents prefer the nursing systems that use plastic bags, feeling that their infant takes in less air during feeding. Other parents feel that washable plastic bottles are more environmentally responsible. You may need to try a few different options in terms of nipples and bottle types before you find one that your baby prefers.

Thermometer and Acetaminophen

In case of illness, you'll need a reliable, easy-to-use thermometer. You may choose a digital model that can be used safely in your baby's armpit (a rectal or oral model works), or buy a rectal model for rectal use only. Glass mercury thermometers are not recommended because they break easily, putting a hazardous substance (mercury) in your home. Forehead strip thermometers (fever strips) are not as accurate as a true thermometer and not recommended for routine use.

Acetaminophen may be given for fevers and for possible discomfort of immunizations. Acetaminophen drops (such as Tylenol and Tempra) are the easiest form of this medication to give to infants. Always keep a bottle available, remembering to store it in a locked cabinet. You may need it for fevers and later for teething discomfort. Check with your health care provider for the proper dosage.

Car Safety Seat

It's very important to place your baby in an approved car safety seat when you take him anywhere in a vehicle. In all 50 states, car safety seat use is mandated by law. Your lap is never a safe place for your baby in a moving vehicle. If your baby needs your attention and can't wait until you reach your destination, stop the car in a safe place to help him. After all that you and your baby have been through to get to this point, why take a chance with your baby's life by ignoring this basic safety rule of the road?

Many NICUs perform a car safety seat "trial" prior to discharge of premature babies. If this is the case, bring the car safety seat you intend to use to the unit for the trial. During this time, your baby's heart rate, breathing, and oxygen saturation will be monitored to see if the baby's upright position in the car safety seat causes any problems. If there are any concerns with the test results, the staff may recommend different options for car safety seat use. The AAP publishes many brochures describing various car safety seat models and options. See Appendix C for car safety seat information and resources.

Stroller

First-time parents are usually amazed by all of the baby paraphernalia necessary for a simple trip to the store. Strollers are invaluable for carrying not only your baby, but all of the supplies and equipment your baby needs. If your baby requires a cardiac monitor or oxygen, purchase the best-manufactured stroller you can afford. Compare brands, and talk to other parents of special care babies before deciding. Look for safety features, sturdiness, compartments and storage space, and ease in collapsing and setting up. Umbrella strollers and most baby backpacks and carriers do not give adequate head and back support for young babies.

Nursery Monitor

Different from a cardiac monitor, a nursery monitor is an intercom (and sometimes a video camera) that helps you hear your baby wherever you are in the house. When selecting a monitor, check range, power requirements, and ease of use. Remember that your baby monitor may pick up signals from other baby monitors in your neighborhood, and your neighbors' baby monitors may be able to pick up everything happening in your baby's room. Purchase one with more than one channel to decrease the risk of interference with your other electronic devices, and keep your receipt in case you need to return it to the store.

To keep your baby safe from accidental injury—for example, strangulation by the monitor cord or electrical shock from putting parts in his mouth—be sure to place the base of the monitor and other accessories out of your baby's reach, and never take this equipment near water such as in the bathroom.

Humidifier

Ask your care provider about the likelihood that your baby will need a humidifier. A humidifier combats dryness in home air and may be recommended to keep respiratory secretions liquid and mobile and to help prevent infection.

Shop carefully for a humidifier. The most popular models are ultrasonic, which turn cold water into mist through high-frequency vibrations. You may wish to investigate demineralization filters or to use only distilled water in this unit. Another option is a warm-mist humidifier, which increases air humidity by boiling water like the old-fashioned steam vaporizers. Bear in mind that a humidifier containing hot water is hazardous around small children, tends to be noisy, and may overheat a small room.

Any humidifier must be kept scrupulously clean to prevent molds and bacteria from growing in the water reservoir. Check the manufacturer's recommendations for the best way to clean your model. As with any electrical equipment, the humidifier and its cord should be placed out of your baby's reach.

Bulletin Board and Calendar

A bulletin board and a calendar are not on most baby supply lists, but many parents of NICU graduates have a multitude of people and medical appointments to coordinate. Use the bulletin board to post each person's business card, or write each person's name, identification (pediatrician, lactation specialist, health insurance agent, and so on), telephone numbers, address, and other important information on a 3-by-5–inch card and put those on your board. Next to that health care team list, post a calendar on which to keep track of your baby's appointments, developmental milestones, and visitors; you may even post your bill payment schedule here. Some parents also post their baby's medication schedule and other information they refer to frequently, such as instructions from the physical therapist. This bulletin board will become your "communication station"— especially if your baby's care needs are complex. You may eventually outgrow the need for this organizational tool, but most parents find it helpful during the first few months at home. Some parents use a notebook or personal digital assistant (PDA), which can be taken to medical appointments, to keep track of this information.

Arranging for Medical and Other Care After Discharge

Your baby is making good progress toward a homecoming date. You've purchased supplies and equipment, and you're comfortable with most of your baby's care tasks. Before your baby is discharged from the hospital, you need to arrange for his continuing medical care.

Choosing Your Baby's Health Care Provider

Parents are sometimes caught the week before their baby's discharge without a clue as to who will provide their baby's care. As soon as you're able, begin the interviewing process and choose a health care provider. Finding a new caregiver can be an unsettling experience, especially after you've come to know and trust the hospital staff. Don't delay your search. As with any new relationship, expect a time of adjustment, uncertainty, and nervousness until trust is established. You need time to get acquainted.

Most neonatologists do not see infants outside the NICU or intermediate care unit, but depending on where you live, they may be able to recommend various health care professionals in your area. Get recommendations weeks before discharge. Your insurance program may have a list of health care providers; bring the list to the NICU for help in choosing a provider. Nurses, close friends, or parents of NICU graduates are other possible sources of recommendations. If you do not have access to a pediatrician where you live, a healthy NICU graduate may be cared for by a family physician or qualified pediatric nurse practitioner. After you have a few names in hand, call and schedule a "meet the provider" visit. Ask if this visit is free of charge or covered by your insurance, because some offices will charge for this time. As you interview potential candidates, keep in mind that personality type and coping styles—both yours and the provider's—play a large part in the decision. Health care professionals run the gamut from telling parents everything and involving them in all decisions to telling them as little as necessary and making most decisions themselves. Other questions to ask include

- Where do you have hospital privileges? If our baby requires readmission to the hospital, will you be the primary provider or will you refer to a specialist?
- Is this your primary office location? Do you have other "satellite" offices near my home?
- What are your office hours?
- Do you do some lab testing in your office? What types of tests do you perform?
- Can we review our child's medical record during the course of care?
- How would I schedule an appointment?
- Who is available to answer baby care questions during the day? After hours?
- How far in advance do I need to call for a routine checkup?
- How is billing handled?
- Do you care for other babies with histories similar to my baby? What is your training and experience with a baby like my baby?
- Will other providers in your practice see my baby? May I meet them today?
- What procedure do we follow if we need you on a weekend or at night?
- How do we handle emergencies—should we call you first or go directly to the emergency department?
- Do you offer parent education classes?
- What is your philosophy about vaccinations? Breastfeeding or bottle feeding? Circumcision?

Babies with special needs should have one doctor who is able to follow their progress. Choosing a pediatrician before your baby is discharged allows the neonatologist or primary physician caring for your baby to speak directly with the pediatrician or to send the doctor a written discharge summary of your baby's hospital course. If at all possible, your baby should be seen by a consistent caregiver rather than at a general health unit or clinic, where medical personnel change often. Many pediatricians accept patients on public assistance if you are without private insurance. In some states, Medicaid will also provide transportation for you to take your baby to the doctor.

Your pediatrician will become an important resource person as your special care baby continues to grow and develop. The pediatrician you choose should be trained in the care of infants and children with special conditions, such as prematurity, or special needs, such as technology dependence.

Establishing a Medical Home

A medical home is not a building. A medical home is a concept of care that means families and care providers work together to coordinate all of a child's care. It means having a "home base" for health care focused on the whole child, not just one part. In a medical home, you are valued as the expert in your child's care and treated as an important member of your child's health care team.

Your baby may go home with ongoing special health care needs. You may need help locating resources, getting referrals, making appointments, and coordinating your baby's care with several health care providers. Your primary health care provider in your baby's medical home will be your guide during this process—helping to identify, access, and coordinate all of the medical and nonmedical services your baby needs. This ongoing relationship will serve as a home base, a *medical home,* to look at the needs of not only your baby, but your family needs too. The provider in your medical home cares for your baby in partnership with you. Ask your primary care provider about establishing a medical home for your baby.

Understanding Referrals

Certain specialists may continue to follow your baby after discharge. To help you, hospital staff will refer you to the appropriate health care agencies. Your baby's health care provider will be notified of the impending discharge. The neonatologist may call the physician and discuss your baby's hospital course or may arrange for a copy of the discharge summary to be sent to the office. Some health care professionals may prefer to see your baby in the hospital before discharge. Some neonatologists give parents a copy of the discharge summary. This is helpful in case you change doctors or have to see other specialists. When you receive this summary, make copies to distribute, and be sure to keep one for yourself. Keep one in your diaper bag at all times so that you have the information handy in case of emergency. If you have questions about anything you read in the summary, ask your baby's nurse, or make an appointment with the neonatologist.

The special care nursery staff should give you the names of specialists who have served as consultants during hospitalization. If your baby had an intraventricular hemorrhage, for example, a neurologist may have been monitoring your baby's progress and will continue follow-up care after discharge. Some neonatal units have a developmental pediatrician who specializes in treating babies with deficits common to preterm birth or prolonged hospitalization. Consulting physicians will usually meet with you or talk with you on the phone. They will indicate when and where follow-up exams should occur. Part of the work of parenting a NICU graduate is coordinating your baby's medical appointments.

To comply with legislation (Individuals with Disabilities Education Act, formerly Public Law [PL 99-457]), all states must have some mechanism for tracking preterm infants or those who are at risk for developmental delays or health problems. (See Chapter 17 for more information on this law.) After discharge, affiliated service providers may contact you at regular intervals to assess your baby and refer you to community resources as needed. These programs operate through the public health department. Some hospitals also have their own NICU follow-up clinic for developmental screening or appointments with specialists. Ask your discharge coordinator how this works in your region.

Decisions to Make as Discharge Nears

If many miles have separated you from your baby, now is the time to use any available resources to spend as much time as possible with him before discharge. Ask your discharge planner for help with this very important aspect of parent education. But whether you're close to your baby's hospital or far away, you still need to make more decisions and preparations before your baby comes home. Ask your NICU social worker about facilities such as the Ronald McDonald House or rooming-in facilities at the hospital.

Rooming-In

For various reasons, you may find the prospect of taking your baby home frightening. To decrease this anxiety, some hospitals offer rooming-in, an arrangement that allows parents to stay overnight at the hospital to care for their baby independently. Nursery staff are immediately available if needed during this time. Rooming-in validates parent learning and lets parents see for themselves what baby care will be like at home. Most parents feel that rooming-in builds their confidence and eases the transition to home.

Timing of the rooming-in experience is important. Ideally, rooming-in should take place as close to discharge as possible. To simulate the home environment, try to have any home monitoring equipment in place during rooming-in.

Rooming-in for parents who must learn about oxygen and other devices might be necessary for as long as 4 or 5 days. You may wish to complete your rooming-in experience a day or two before your baby's discharge date. A good night's sleep the night before discharge may help ease some of the inevitable anxiety of your baby's homecoming.

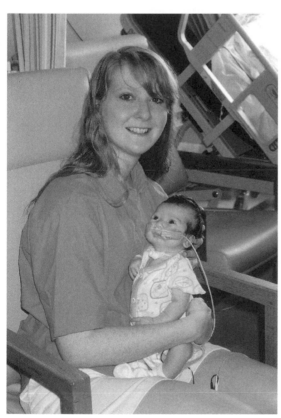

Rooming-in.
Spending a night or two in the hospital with your baby allows you to care for your baby as if you were at home. The nursery staff are immediately available if needed. Rooming-in is especially helpful if your baby's care is complex, as for this baby who is going home with a feeding tube and a tracheostomy.

Investigating Professional Services

Parents of babies who will require special care at home have additional preparations to make. Chapter 16 explains how to manage the equipment and special treatments your baby may need after discharge. It may be helpful to read that chapter before you investigate home health agencies and equipment supply firms. There may be many companies providing equipment or nursing care in your area, or there may be very few.

If your health care coverage gives you options for choosing a home health agency, you have many things to consider (see pages 453–454). First, check with your insurance carrier to find out exactly what is and what is not covered. Consider that some companies that provide nursing care may also provide equipment; others do not. You'll need to weigh the convenience of dealing with one company against the cost. Talking with other parents of NICU graduates can help. The hospital staff may also recommend companies (staff may call them "vendors"), but feel free to shop around.

Insurance companies acknowledge the cost-effectiveness of home care instead of prolonged hospitalization. They see the wisdom and cost savings of discharging a baby home as soon as possible. The ultimate goal of most insurers, however, is for parents to learn to assume the care of their infant themselves and to rely on the local pediatrician, emergency medical service (EMS) system, and hospital services when the child experiences illnesses or emergencies. Parents must therefore realize that home care nurses will usually not become permanent caretakers. The length of time they will be in your home will depend on your insurance company's policies and the perceived need of your baby. When an infant's care requires it, these policies may be challenged. In most instances, however, your child's condition will improve over time, and he will need less care. In more serious cases, exceptions will be made. But it's important that you understand the insurer's goal—for you to assume the care of your infant as quickly as possible.

Choosing a Home Care Provider[a]

Congratulations! Your baby will soon be discharged from the hospital. This is an exciting time; there is much to learn and do.

Target Discharge Date: _____

You have been asked to choose a home care company to provide special equipment and nursing care for your baby. You may be given a list to choose from. This is an important decision. Here are some things to ask.

Step 1. Ask your doctors and nurses what equipment your baby will need. They will need to order the supplies and nursing care.

- Heart and breathing monitors
- Oxygen, including flow rate (liters per minute)
- Feeding equipment
- Intravenous equipment
- Other special equipment

Step 2. Ask if a home care nurse is needed.

- How often can the nurse visit?
- What will the visits be like?
- Will the nurse know about NICU babies?
- How long will the nurse be needed?

Step 3. Work with the social worker and your insurance company to see how this special care will be paid for.

- Set up an appointment to talk with your social worker.
- Ask if your baby is eligible for supplemental social security or any other special funds.
- Identify who you should speak to at the insurance company:
  Name:_____Phone:_____
- If possible, request one person to handle your case (sometimes called a case manager).
- Find out what services and equipment are covered by your insurance policy or by Medicaid.
- What are my benefits for home care?
- Are nursing visits covered?
- If so, how many visits are covered per year?
- Do I pay for home therapies, such as physical therapy, occupational therapy, and speech therapy?
- What out-of-pocket expenses will I have?

Choosing a Home Care Provider, continued

Step 4. Look for a good home care provider.

To be sure that you find a good provider, ask more about the company.

- Has your company passed state credentialing or accreditation evaluations?
- Do you meet all state licensing requirements?
- Do you share patient satisfaction scores?
- Can you provide a reference?
- Then talk with another family and ask if they are happy with the company.

To check on the services the company provides ask

- Do you provide home nursing care visits?
- Can the nurse visit as often as I need?
- Do you have enough nurses available?
- Do the nurses know how to work with the equipment my baby has and his/her care needs?
- Do you have a backup plan for nursing care in case of illness or emergency?
- Will the home care nurses and therapists come to the hospital and get to know my baby before discharge?
- If needed, do you have nurses that speak my language?
- Do you provide medical equipment (monitors, oxygen, feeding tubes, etc)?
- Do you provide other therapies (nutrition, physical, occupational, speech, developmental)?
- Do you work with a pharmacy for medications and intravenous nutrition needs?
- How do the home care nurses and therapists communicate with my baby's primary health care providers?

Step 5. Work with the durable medical equipment company to get all of the needed supplies.

- Do you take payment from my insurance company?
- Has your company passed state credentialing or accreditation evaluations?
- Do you have the equipment my baby needs?
- Do you provide special formulas or medications?
- Do you have respiratory therapists that work with babies?
- Will you provide equipment training?
- Will you set up the equipment in my home at a time when I can be there?
- Do you have someone on call 24 hours a day for emergencies or questions?

Planning ahead for all of your baby's discharge needs will help make the process much smoother for everyone involved in your baby's care.

Step 6. Explore resources and develop connections with other families who have experienced caring for a special baby.

ªAdapted with permission from Gracey K, Hummel P, Cronin J. Choosing a home care provider. *Adv Neonatal Care.* 2004;4(6):365–366. (http://lww.com).

Immunizations

The first immunization your child received was most likely the hepatitis B vaccine. The first dose of hepatitis B vaccine is given at birth to newborns weighing 2 kilograms (4 pounds, 6 ounces) or more. If your newborn weighed less than 2 kilograms, the first dose of hepatitis B vaccine is given at 30 days of age if your infant is still in the hospital or at time of hospital discharge if this occurs before 30 days. In some situations, the first hepatitis B vaccine dose will need to be administered within 12 hours of birth regardless of the infant's birth weight.

If your infant is in the hospital for 60 days or more, your baby's care provider will talk to you about the immunizations routinely given at that time. (See the immunization schedule on page 456.) These are the same vaccines your infant would receive in the doctor's office at a 2-month checkup. With exception of the hepatitis B vaccine, the immunization schedule for preterm infants is the same as that for term babies. You don't have to correct for how early the baby was born. These routine immunizations include diphtheria, tetanus, and pertussis (DTaP) vaccines; the inactivated polio (IPV) vaccine; *Haemophilus influenzae* type b conjugate (Hib) vaccine; pneumococcal conjugate (PCV7) vaccine; the second dose of hepatitis B (Hep B) vaccine; and rotavirus vaccine. If your baby is still in the hospital when 2 months old, the rotavirus vaccine will not be given until your baby is ready to go home or right after discharge from the hospital. Acetaminophen may be given to your baby to decrease the chance of fever after immunization.

If your infant was very preterm, has experienced respiratory problems requiring treatment in the nursery, or has significant heart disease, your baby may be at increased risk of rehospitalization due to respiratory syncytial virus (RSV) infection. Palivizumab (Synagis) is an intramuscular injection given monthly for 1 to 5 doses during the RSV season to lower the risk of severe RSV infection in certain premature infants born before 35 weeks of gestation or certain infants with congenital heart disease. Your neonatologist or pediatrician will determine if your baby should receive this medication. Some hospitals administer the first dose before the baby is discharged while other babies are given the first dose after they leave the hospital.

Immunizing your baby is an important investment in his health and protects him from rehospitalization. But your new baby is not the only one who needs immunizations. Be sure that your other children and the adults in your home are up to date on all of their immunizations. Ask whether you need a booster dose of tetanus and diphtheria vaccines (due every 10 years) and whether you and the people who will be in contact with your baby need a booster dose of the vaccine, which also gives protection against pertussis (whooping cough). Everyone older than 6 months in your family and everyone who will take care of your baby should also receive the influenza vaccine before flu season starts each year. By immunizing yourself, your children, and your baby's caregivers, you are protecting your baby until he is old enough to receive all of his own immunizations.

Recommended Immunization Schedule for Persons Aged 0-6 Years—UNITED STATES 2009

For those who fall behind or start late, see the catch-up schedule

Vaccine ▼ Age ▶	Birth	1 month	2 months	4 months	6 months	12 months	15 months	18 months	19–23 months	2–3 years	4–6 years
Hepatitis B[1]	HepB	HepB		see footnote 1		HepB					
Rotavirus[2]			RV	RV	RV[2]						
Diphtheria, Tetanus, Pertussis[3]			DTaP	DTaP	DTaP	see footnote 3	DTaP	DTaP			DTaP
Haemophilus influenzae type b[4]			Hib	Hib	Hib[4]	Hib	Hib				
Pneumococcal[5]			PCV	PCV	PCV	PCV	PCV			PPSV	
Inactivated Poliovirus			IPV	IPV	IPV	IPV	IPV				IPV
Influenza[6]					Influenza (Yearly)						
Measles, Mumps, Rubella[7]						MMR	MMR		see footnote 7		MMR
Varicella[8]						Varicella	Varicella		see footnote 8		Varicella
Hepatitis A[9]						HepA (2 doses)				HepA Series	
Meningococcal[10]										MCV	MCV

Legend:
- Range of recommended ages
- Certain high-risk groups

This schedule indicates the recommended ages for routine administration of currently licensed vaccines, as of December 1, 2008, for children aged 0 through 6 years. Any dose not administered at the recommended age should be administered at a subsequent visit, when indicated and feasible. Licensed combination vaccines may be used whenever any component of the combination is indicated and other components are not contraindicated and if approved by the Food and Drug Administration for that dose of the series. Providers should consult the relevant Advisory Committee on Immunization Practices statement for detailed recommendations, including **high-risk conditions:** http://www.cdc.gov/vaccines/pubs/acip-list.htm. Clinically significant adverse events that follow immunization should be reported to the Vaccine Adverse Event Reporting System (VAERS). Guidance about how to obtain and complete a VAERS form is available at http://www.vaers.hhs.gov or by telephone, 800-822-7967.

IS0084

(For necessary footnotes and important information, see reverse side.)

1. **Hepatitis B vaccine (HepB). (Minimum age: birth)**
   At birth:
   - Administer monovalent HepB to all newborns before hospital discharge.
   - If mother is hepatitis B surface antigen (HBsAg)-positive, administer HepB and 0.5 mL of hepatitis B immune globulin (HBIG) within 12 hours of birth.
   - If mother's HBsAg status is unknown, administer HepB within 12 hours of birth. Determine mother's HBsAg status as soon as possible and, if HBsAg-positive, administer HBIG (no later than age 1 week).
   After the birth dose:
   - The HepB series should be completed with either monovalent HepB or a combination vaccine containing HepB. The second dose should be administered at age 1 or 2 months. The final dose should be administered no earlier than age 24 weeks.
   - Infants born to HBsAg-positive mothers should be tested for HBsAg and antibody to HBsAg (anti-HBs) after completion of at least 3 doses of the HepB series, at age 9 through 18 months (generally at the next well-child visit).
   4-month dose:
   - Administration of 4 doses of HepB to infants is permissible when combination vaccines containing HepB are administered after the birth dose.

2. **Rotavirus vaccine (RV). (Minimum age: 6 weeks)**
   - Administer the first dose at age 6 through 14 weeks (maximum age: 14 weeks 6 days). Vaccination should not be initiated for infants aged 15 weeks or older (i.e., 15 weeks, 0 days or older).
   - Administer the final dose in the series by age 8 months 0 days.
   - If Rotarix® is administered at ages 2 and 4 months, a dose at 6 months is not indicated.

3. **Diphtheria and tetanus toxoids and acellular pertussis vaccine (DTaP). (Minimum age: 6 weeks)**
   - The fourth dose may be administered as early as age 12 months, provided at least 6 months have elapsed since the third dose.
   - Administer the final dose in the series at age 4 through 6 years.

4. **Haemophilus influenzae type b conjugate vaccine (Hib). (Minimum age: 6 weeks)**
   - If PRP-OMP (PedvaxHIB® or Comvax® [HepB-Hib]) is administered at ages 2 and 4 months, a dose at age 6 months is not indicated.
   - TriHiBit® (DTaP/Hib) should not be used for doses at ages 2, 4, or 6 months but can be used as the final dose in children aged 12 months or older.

5. **Pneumococcal vaccine. (Minimum age: 6 weeks for pneumococcal conjugate vaccine [PCV]; 2 years for pneumococcal polysaccharide vaccine [PPSV])**
   - PCV is recommended for all children aged younger than 5 years. Administer 1 dose of PCV to all healthy children aged 24 through 59 months who are not completely vaccinated for their age.
   - Administer PPSV to children aged 2 years or older with certain underlying medical conditions (see MMWR 2000;49[No. RR-9]), including a cochlear implant.

6. **Influenza vaccine. (Minimum age: 6 months for trivalent inactivated influenza vaccine [TIV]; 2 years for live, attenuated influenza vaccine [LAIV])**
   - Administer annually to children aged 6 months through 18 years.
   - For healthy nonpregnant persons (i.e., those who do not have underlying medical conditions that predispose them to influenza complications) aged 2 through 49 years, either LAIV or TIV may be used.
   - Children receiving TIV should receive 0.25 mL if aged 6 through 35 months or 0.5 mL if aged 3 years or older.
   - Administer 2 doses (separated by at least 4 weeks) to children aged younger than 9 years who are receiving influenza vaccine for the first time or who were vaccinated for the first time during the previous influenza season but only received 1 dose.

7. **Measles, mumps, and rubella vaccine (MMR). (Minimum age: 12 months)**
   - Administer the second dose at age 4 through 6 years. However, the second dose may be administered before age 4, provided at least 28 days have elapsed since the first dose.

8. **Varicella vaccine. (Minimum age: 12 months)**
   - Administer the second dose at age 4 through 6 years. However, the second dose may be administered before age 4, provided at least 3 months have elapsed since the first dose.
   - For children aged 12 months through 12 years the minimum interval between doses is 3 months. However, if the second dose was administered at least 28 days after the first dose, it can be accepted as valid.

9. **Hepatitis A vaccine (HepA). (Minimum age: 12 months)**
   - Administer to all children aged 1 year (i.e., aged 12 through 23 months). Administer 2 doses at least 6 months apart.
   - Children not fully vaccinated by age 2 years can be vaccinated at subsequent visits.
   - HepA also is recommended for children older than 1 year who live in areas where vaccination programs target older children or who are at increased risk of infection. See MMWR 2006;55(No. RR-7).

10. **Meningococcal vaccine. (Minimum age: 2 years for meningococcal conjugate vaccine [MCV] and for meningococcal polysaccharide vaccine [MPSV])**
    - Administer MCV to children aged 2 through 10 years with terminal complement component deficiency, anatomic or functional asplenia, and certain other highrisk groups. See MMWR 2005;54(No. RR-7).
    - Persons who received MPSV 3 or more years previously and who remain at increased risk for meningococcal disease should be revaccinated with MCV.

Additional information about vaccines, including precautions and contraindications for vaccination and vaccine shortages, is available at http://www.cdc.gov/nip or from the CDC telephone hotline, 800/232-4636 (English and Spanish). Approved by the Advisory Committee on Immunization Practices (http://www.cdc.gov/nip/acip), the American Academy of Pediatrics (http://www.aap.org), and the American Academy of Family Physicians (http://www.aafp.org).

Immunization Protects Children

Regular checkups at your pediatrician's office or local health clinic are an important way to keep children healthy.

By making sure that your child gets immunized on time, you can provide the best available defense against many dangerous childhood diseases. Immunizations protect children against hepatitis B, polio, measles, mumps, rubella (German measles), pertussis (whooping cough), diphtheria, tetanus (lockjaw), Haemophilus influenzae type b, pneumococcal infections, and chickenpox. All of these immunizations need to be given before children are 2 years old in order for them to be protected during their most vulnerable period. Are your child's immunizations up to date?

The chart on the other side of this fact sheet includes immunization recommendations from the American Academy of Pediatrics. Remember to keep track of your child's immunizations—it's the only way you can be sure your child is up to date. Also, check with your pediatrician or health clinic at each visit to find out if your child needs any booster shots or if any new vaccines have been recommended since this schedule was prepared.

If you don't have a pediatrician, call your local health department. Public health clinics usually have supplies of vaccine and may give shots free.

American Academy of Pediatrics

DEDICATED TO THE HEALTH OF ALL CHILDREN™

The information contained in this publication should not be used as a substitute for the medical care and advice of your pediatrician. There may be variations in treatment that your pediatrician may recommend based on individual facts and circumstances.

3-4E3

Deciding About Circumcision

Opinions vary regarding the necessity of circumcision (removal of the skin covering the tip of the penis). For some, circumcision is a religious requirement. For others, this decision is often more emotional than intellectual. You might want to visit credible Web sites and read some articles explaining the benefits and risks of circumcision. (See Appendix D for how to use the Internet wisely.) Information is available on the AAP Web site. Ask the nurses in the newborn nursery about the percentage of parents in your region who opt for circumcision. As your son grows up, he will no doubt see a mix of circumcised and uncircumcised males. This is not an easy decision for many parents. Make sure you have enough information before you sign a consent.

The AAP states that routine circumcision of babies is not medically necessary. Complications of circumcision are rare but include bleeding, pain, and infection. If you do decide to circumcise your son, it will usually be done right before discharge. If your baby requires other surgery (hernia repair or ostomy closure, for example), the procedure may also be done at that time.

Some physicians prefer to perform circumcision in their office after your baby is older and larger. Check with your insurance carrier to see if your insurance covers circumcision. Your health insurance or Medicaid may not cover circumcision, and an office visit may be less expensive than a hospital procedure. If you decide to circumcise your baby, ask the doctor performing the circumcision about regional anesthesia and pain relief before and after circumcision.

Your baby's nurse or physician will instruct you in circumcision care. You'll be told to call the doctor if you notice bleeding, swelling, or drainage. In most cases, you will be instructed not to give your baby a tub bath until the circumcision is healed.

Preparing Yourself, Your Home, and Your Family

"On the day our baby came home from the hospital, we showered most of the attention on his big sister. She wore her "big sister" shirt to day care and took cupcakes to celebrate. She had her dinner on a special new plate just for big sisters. She felt very important, and that helped her adjust to having a new baby in the house."

As your baby grows and heals in the intermediate care nursery, you will have a lot to do. It can be overwhelming at times. Go slowly, but don't procrastinate. Preparation gives you a chance to mobilize some of your anxious energy to make a difference in your child's future.

Preparing for an Emergency

Graduates of NICUs have a higher rate of rehospitalization than the average newborn population. Common reasons for unexpected readmission are dehydration because of vomiting or diarrhea, upper respiratory infections, hernia complications, persistent or increased apnea, or shunt repair.

Now is the time to prepare for an emergency, before one arises. Before your baby is discharged, go to the hospital where your baby is most likely to be readmitted. Know the fastest route from your house, and an alternate route, as well as the locations of the hospital's emergency entrance, parking, and admitting office. Be prepared to call the EMS system for an ambulance if you believe your baby's condition is critical, however. Post 911 or your community's EMS number on all of your phones and program your baby's care providers' numbers in your cell phones as well. Being ready will prevent panic in case of an emergency.

If you know your baby will come home with a cardiac monitor, a ventilator, or oxygen, you also need to contact public services to ensure that you will receive priority help in community emergencies. The EMS system (or nearest fire station) and your utility providers (water, electric, and gas) should all be aware that you have a baby with special needs in your home. Ask your baby's nurse, case manager, or discharge planner for this letter to send to your utility companies. Be sure to notify them when your child is no longer technology dependent or if you move.

Housecleaning

Many parents feel they must "sterilize" their home with industrial-type cleaning products to eliminate germs and dust before their baby's homecoming. The family pet may be permanently banished outdoors or given to a new owner. Although the intent behind these precautions is admirable, they often are not necessary and generally are impossible to keep up. Few families can maintain such high standards of cleanliness while giving baby care and normal living the priorities they must have.

Rely on common sense as you prepare—and maintain—your home. A thorough cleaning is enough. Harsh cleaning solutions and insecticidal sprays can leave residual odors that may irritate or even harm your baby.

Tobacco Smoke

Babies—especially those who have had or are having breathing difficulties—are at risk for a number of problems from exposure to tobacco smoke. No one should smoke in the home, around your baby, or anyplace where your baby spends time, such as in the car. The AAP Committee on Environmental Health has identified these problems with secondhand smoke exposure: decreased lung growth, decreased lung function, and increased frequency of lower respiratory tract infections and respiratory symptoms. Research also clearly shows that exposure to smoke can cause ear infections and related hearing problems, increased incidence of hospitalization related to bronchitis or pneumonia, and increased risk for SIDS. If you need more information or literature—for example, to convince family or close friends of the dangers of secondhand smoke to your baby—contact the American Lung Association or the AAP (see Appendix D).

Pets

Pets are important members of the family. Banishing a beloved companion may cause resentment. Instead, prepare your pet for your baby's arrival. Bring home clothing or a blanket with your baby's scent on it before your baby is discharged. Siblings can help by spending extra time with the pet. Be alert for signs of aggression or jealousy when your baby comes home, and never leave your dog or cat unsupervised near your new baby. Extra attention and discipline will solve most problems.

Keeping your pet out of your baby's sleeping area may help reduce the risk of fur or dander irritating the baby's breathing passages. When your baby is developmentally mature enough to lie outside the crib, place a clean blanket or mat under the baby to keep fur, dander, dust, and carpet fibers from irritating the baby's airway during playtime.

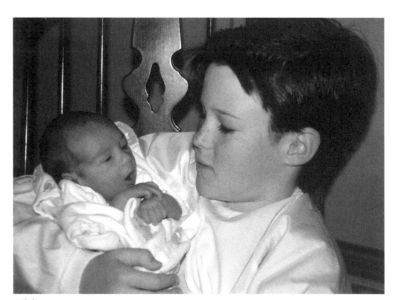

Sibling concerns.
As discharge day nears, your other children may have concerns about how life will change with a new baby at home.

Carefully assess all of the factors involved in having a pet, and talk with your health care provider as you decide on a reasonable approach.

Siblings

Prepare your older children for what life may be like when their baby brother or sister comes home. Plan to spend special time alone with each of your other children a short time after your baby comes home and repeat this daily. Encourage and allow them to talk about their feelings. This should reduce episodes of acting out. Most parenting books include information on helping siblings adjust to a new baby.

Visitors

You'll need a traffic control plan for visitors. Start thinking about this before your baby's discharge, and set up a visiting schedule. Don't turn down offers of help, but use your calendar to keep track of who is planning to visit. Place limits on the number of visitors to your home. Your needs deserve top priority, and entertaining others is probably not at the top of your list right now. Let friends and extended family know that you'll need some time to adjust to this new baby at home and that you'll let them know when you're ready for visitors. Caring family and friends will respect your need for privacy and give you the time you need to make this adjustment. (Chapter 16 provides some suggestions for visitor control.)

Thinking About Child Care

If you intend to use child care within 2 or 3 months of your infant's discharge, this is a good time to start your search. The early months at home will fly by. You'll be absorbed in your baby and in your family's adjustment to this new addition. While your baby is still hospitalized, you'll have more time to explore the possibilities.

During your baby's first year, you may want to limit the number of children he is exposed to because exposure increases the risk of illness. Not everyone can afford home care, and some families find it too invasive. Child care in someone's home offers a controlled environment with a low caretaker-to-child ratio. Look for a referral service, which can tell you ahead of time about age ranges, pets, smoking, training, years of experience, and hours. Personal referrals generally provide information from a parent's perspective on the personality of the care provider and the type of care given. Both large and small child care settings should offer informal visitation. See Chapter 16 for more information about important considerations when choosing an out-of-home child care.

Babies who will need complex care require special consideration. Quality child care for special needs infants is often hard to find, and you may face long waiting lists. For mothers who plan to return to work quickly (paid maternity leave may be used up during the NICU stay), the search for child care should begin as early as possible.

Emotional Readiness

You're probably overwhelmed reading all of this, but believe it or not, in time you'll adjust. Start now by making sure that your expectations are realistic. When your baby comes home, you will experience times of great stress, nights when you'll be tempted to return your baby to the hospital, and moments when you'll wonder what you ever saw in your partner. Know that these feelings will pass. Before your baby comes home, think about your personal arsenal of coping mechanisms, focus on the positive, and enjoy your many good experiences with your baby.

Everyone develops individual coping mechanisms, but some general principles apply.

- Without an outlet, emotions take a toll on your body. Exercise; cry in the shower; scrub floors; talk to a counselor, pastor, or friend; or keep a journal—but do not lock in your feelings. If you are increasingly ill, accident prone, fatigued, or depressed, try something different, or get help. These are red flags of emotions that need expression.

- You deserve an occasional break from the full-time responsibilities of caring for a special needs baby. Even parents of healthy term infants need a break periodically to sleep, to have some adult interaction, to exercise, or just to have a change of scenery. Couples need time alone together. Siblings need time alone with their parents. People cannot just "make do" indefinitely. Communication breakdowns and acting-out behavior should be clear signs of a need for attention. Have at least one support person trained to babysit. If you have home nurses, take an hour or so for yourself occasionally. Have an "at-home date" while someone else is responsible for the baby's care. Do not wait for spontaneous breaks in the chaos, or you will be too exhausted to enjoy them.

- Pay attention to how you manage your own anxiety about your infant and his care. It is easy to become crisis prone. Hypervigilance (a constant high level of worrying and watching) is a method of trying to decrease anxiety, but it is counterproductive. This behavior is a sure course to burnout. Your disappointment when illnesses arise or developmental milestones are not met will be as dramatic as your expectations are unrealistic. Be observant of changes in your baby's behavior, and develop methods of getting feedback (from a pediatrician, nurses, and friends) to help you assess without panic. All in all, be realistically optimistic.

- Develop a positive parenting image. If you have other children, draw from your experience. If not, give yourself a series of pats on the back for getting this far. Have confidence in your present level of competence and in your willingness and ability to continue to learn. Learn to trust your instincts as a parent.

- Feeling overwhelmed is a sure sign that you need help, a break, or a new plan. When you are overly stressed, break things down into small steps.

- Make lists to feel in control and enjoy the satisfaction of checking things off when complete.

- Make a list of things others could help you do. Asking for help is sometimes difficult, but this is certainly the time to do so. When people ask, "Is there anything I can do?" do not politely insist, "We'll be OK." Share your list with them and let them choose something that suits them. Suggestions might include providing meals (freezable), shopping or running errands, doing laundry, cleaning or doing things with your other children, doing yard work, and calling people with progress reports so you can rest (or play).

Celebrating

Last but not least, celebrate your baby's arrival home. Consider ways to bring a sense of celebration to your baby's homecoming. When your baby's health care team finally sets a discharge date, consider planning a celebration dinner with your partner a few days before your baby is discharged. Once your baby comes home, it may be a few weeks or more before you can find much quality "couple time" in your schedules.

Discharge Day at Last!

Discharge day is a collage of excitement, fear, jangling nerves, and uncertainty. In spite of all of the preparations—learning your baby's care needs and perhaps spending a night or two rooming-in—even the most competent parent feels nervous about assuming total responsibility for a baby at home.

Miscommunication often causes delays on discharge day. You may arrive first thing in the morning to be told that you'll have to wait for one more test, for the results of a previous test, or for a doctor or nurse practitioner to examine your baby or write an order. You may find this frustrating—or, if you are especially anxious, you may appreciate this short reprieve.

When everything is finally in order, make sure you get a copy of the baby's discharge summary. Dress your baby in the special going-home clothes you've brought with you, and take a tour through the unit so that the nurses can say good-bye and celebrate with you.

Some parents want to do something special for the staff. Thank-you cards, a letter to the hospital administrator expressing appreciation of the NICU and nursery staff, and letters and pictures from home are the most valuable gifts you can give the staff. They enjoy seeing the progress your special baby makes.

Now you're on your way out the door with reams of discharge instructions and bags of supplies, toys, and baby clothes. Don't forget your baby!

On Your Own

Your baby's homecoming is a big event. Homecoming is also an adjustment—a time of shifting values, expectations, and priorities. Parents of NICU graduates have all of the concerns of parents of healthy term infants, and then some. Don't isolate yourself and try to handle everything alone. You know people who can and will support you. Lean on the counsel of others, your own spiritual resources, and any other support you're offered. Take a moment to appreciate those who have helped you get to this point, and be proud of all you have learned about caring for your new baby.

Chapter 16
Home at Last

"Pooh!" he whispered. "Yes, Piglet?"

"Nothing," said Piglet, taking Pooh's paw.

"I just wanted to be sure of you."

TrezMarie T. Zotkiewicz, RNC-NIC, MN, APRN

Welcome home! Your telephone is ringing, your baby is crying, your children are screaming, your dog is barking, your dishes and laundry are piling up—it all seems to be too much to handle.

Bringing your baby home (finally) can be quite overwhelming. All of the other demands of everyday life will be waiting for you, along with your new baby and her special needs.

While your baby was in the hospital, your primary focus was on learning about her special care needs and, by discharge, you had probably become quite competent in your baby's care. Now that you're home, though, everything seems to have turned into chaos. Relax! This is normal for anyone with a new baby in the house, even for experienced parents. It's especially true for parents of preterm babies or other infants with special needs.

Parenting any baby, especially one born at risk, demands an enormous amount of physical and psychological adjustment. Most parents eagerly anticipate their baby's homecoming, but even the most experienced and prepared parents find the first few weeks an incredible challenge. This chapter offers practical suggestions and guidance for parents of preterm infants or of babies with special needs who are finally at home.

How Homecoming Affects You and Your Family

"When I spent time with Adam at the hospital, he was always so quiet. The second I brought him home, he started crying. Finally, I called his nurse and learned that he cried a lot for her too. Adam kept crying, but at least I didn't take it so personally."

The transition from hospital to home is marked by moments of excitement, joy, anxiety, fear, uncertainty, and even depression. Parents who have spent time learning about their baby's care before discharge tend to feel less apprehensive about caring for their baby at home, but they, too, may experience a flood of new fears and face overwhelming responsibilities.

Even though you're relieved that your baby is home, you may find that you miss the attention and support of the hospital staff. You may feel alone and abandoned as you make the adjustment to independent parenting. This is particularly true if family and other support is limited. For some parents, the first days at home with their neonatal intensive care unit (NICU) graduate are as stressful as were the first days in the NICU.

Feelings of Panic

You may feel panicked now that you have total responsibility for your baby's care. Until you're suddenly "cut off" at discharge, you may not realize just how much you have come to depend on the hospital staff for support. You may suddenly realize how much your baby's illness, the hustle-bustle of the NICU, and your continued concerns in intermediate care distracted your attention. You may feel as though you don't remember a single thing you were taught about caring for your baby.

It may help to realize that these feelings are common among most parents who bring home a new baby. In spite of all of your preparations, expect this to be a stormy period as you and your family make the necessary adjustments. It may be of some consolation to know that you now share something with parents of healthy term babies: feelings of uncertainty and clumsiness with baby care at home. Although much of your anxiety may come from your baby's fragile beginnings and potential for future complications, you may be able to relate to the feelings expressed by this mother of a healthy term baby girl: "I finally had my baby home with me. I couldn't believe how tiny she was. She needed me for everything—she had to learn about me, about our family, and our home. After all our planning and expectation, I felt totally unprepared as her parent. That first week at home I checked on her every few hours to make sure she was breathing. I tried to prevent her from crying—yet she seemed to cry all the time. She fed every couple of hours at first, and we both had to learn how to breastfeed. I had so many questions about what to do with and for my baby. I felt constantly exhausted, worried, and nervous. But she was mine…and I felt so happy and proud."

Your feelings of panic should diminish as you find that you are indeed surviving. You may do things differently than they were done in the hospital, but as long as the decisions you make keep your baby safe and thriving, you can have confidence in them. Take advantage of any support you are offered because of your baby's NICU stay. Depending on where you live and your health care coverage (private insurance vs government program), a home health nurse, or a NICU home visit nurse can reinforce your discharge teaching, validate your feelings, and help you anticipate upcoming questions and concerns. If your NICU or intermediate care nursery does not provide a home visit, don't hesitate to call the unit for help during the first weeks at home.

Feelings of Grief and Guilt

When you first reunited with your baby in the NICU, you were probably assured that your baby's problems were not your fault and were, in fact, outside your control. Yet you may have felt guilty anyway and said to yourself many times, "If only I had…." Soon, though, the daily challenges of NICU survival overshadowed those feelings.

Now that your baby is home, feelings of sadness and guilt may resurface. Your NICU graduate may not be the baby you envisioned during your pregnancy. Your NICU experience was probably very different from your fantasy of an uncomplicated birth, a short hospital stay, and an exciting homecoming for a healthy newborn baby. Parents also feel guilty when they continue to grieve for what might have been instead of feeling grateful for or accepting of the child they have.

This cycle of grief and guilt usually passes as you gain confidence caring for your baby and adjust to your role as a parent. Support from your family, friends, and health care providers is important as you resolve these feelings and develop healthy parenting attitudes.

If your depression persists or if you continue to have upsetting memories of the NICU experience, seek help from a health care professional. Postpartum depression is a very real risk for NICU moms, so seek advice if you think you have been feeling too sad or anxious for more than a few weeks (see Chapter 6). Review your experience and feelings with someone familiar with your NICU experience; this may help you manage your feelings of loss and put them into proper perspective. Your focus has been on meeting the physical and emotional needs of your baby. Keep in mind that your own mental health goes hand in hand with your baby's healthy growth and development.

Feelings of Attachment

The bonds you established with your baby during hospitalization are very real. But development of true intimacy may have been difficult because of the lack of privacy and the distractions of hospital technology. Now that your baby is home, she may suddenly seem like a little stranger. You may worry if you do not have strong feelings of love toward your baby.

Give yourself some time to get to know your baby—and to let your baby get to know you. At first, your baby will make incredible demands on your time and attention and seem to give back little. But as you gain confidence in meeting your baby's needs, she will begin to respond to your efforts with quiet alertness, more frequent eye contact, and that first amazing smile. All relationships take time to grow, and ultimately you will feel attached to and loving toward your baby.

Feeling Overwhelmed

It's a fact that NICU graduates are more at risk for abuse and neglect than are healthy term infants. Some parents purposefully keep an emotional distance between themselves and their baby as protection in case the baby dies. Preterm, chronically ill, and technology-dependent infants tend to be more irritable than term infants. The additional stress parents feel because of these behavioral differences and their infant's special care requirements may contribute to the alarming rate of child abuse and neglect in the population of NICU graduates.

Recognize when you have reached your limit and need a break from your baby. There is nothing bad or abnormal about feeling as though you are going to "lose it" with your baby. Walk away, calm down, and get help before you act on your out-of-control feelings. Call a family member, a friend, your pediatrician, your local social services department, your home health agency, or a parent support hotline. Talk about your feelings, and plan ahead so that someone can relieve you on very stressful days.

Impact on Your Older Children

The introduction of a new family member is traumatic for siblings—even when the baby is healthy. A baby who has had and may still have special needs causes repeated turmoil for your older children.

The NICU experience likely disrupted your family's routine, and in spite of your best efforts, older siblings may feel left out and less loved. During the NICU experience, your other children were probably aware of your tension and knew that the goal was to bring their new brother or sister home. Siblings who were involved in the baby's progress and who visited the baby in the hospital seem to make the homecoming adjustment more quickly than those who never interacted with the baby. But the reality of homecoming is still stressful for most siblings.

Once the baby is home, your other children may be surprised that your attention is still focused so intensely on the baby. You can help children adjust to their new role as older brothers and sisters

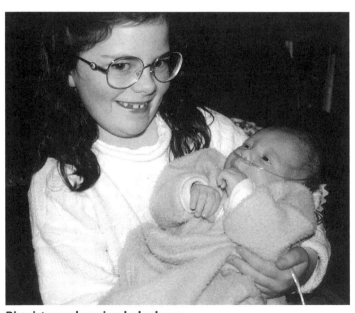

Big sister welcoming baby home.
Older children face many adjustments when your baby comes home. This is the time to involve them in the baby's care if they are interested.

by suggesting activities appropriate to their age level. Before discharge day, arrange a special dinner or dessert just to celebrate this new status as an older sibling. Involve your children's teachers—perhaps by sending cookies to school along with a picture of the baby. One family's baby announcement gave the focus to the older sibling: "I'M A BIG SISTER!" was printed on the front of the card, and the baby's statistics were displayed in one column, with the sibling's age, weight, and height in the facing column. Another parent sent a balloon bouquet to her daughter at home and signed the card with the new baby's name. And a father showed sensitivity to both his partner's and his older child's feelings by setting up a surprise baby shower with the "secret" help of the older child—and including a few special gifts for the older sibling(s). Certainly, plan a small gift for each older sibling the day you bring your NICU graduate home.

As your children now watch the baby take even more of your time, attention, and love, their reactions may be similar to those shown during your baby's NICU stay. You may notice that they seem angry at you or the baby, regress to thumb-sucking or bed-wetting, act out to get your attention, anger easily, or have difficulty concentrating in school.

If older children are interested, involve them in the care of the new baby as much as possible, even though this may sometimes mean more work for you. Try not to criticize any "help" you receive, and praise a job well done. The more you can include older children in caregiving, the sooner they will adjust to the new baby's presence and be less frightened of any illness or disability.

Spend some special time alone with each child, even if just for a few minutes of snuggling, reading a book, or taking a walk together. The addition of a new baby changes your relationship with your other children, and working through this adjustment together is an important part of your growth as a parent and as a family.

Coping as a Family

"We not only learned to recognize Casey's cues, but each other's stress cues as well. My husband knew I needed a break when I started talking to myself. And I knew he was struggling when he started singing his old high school fight song. It may sound strange, but it worked for us."

Your baby's homecoming will have an impact on the entire family. The stressors, as well as the solutions, will be unique to each family. A lot depends on how much special care your baby requires at home. Here are several recommendations from parents and professionals.

- Talk honestly and openly with one another, share ideas, and listen to one another.
- Trust your instincts and your ability to adequately care for your baby.
- Acknowledge the fact that life will be different now that your baby is home, and talk about what this means to you and your family.
- Openly discuss feelings of isolation or lack of privacy and ways to actively cope with or change these stresses.
- Take time out for yourself, as a couple, or with other children and family, away from your baby—even if these periods are short.

Managing Visitors

When your baby comes home, your friends and neighbors may assume that the crisis is over and be less available for support. On the other hand, friends who were nowhere to be found during your NICU crisis may now knock on your door to see your new baby and expect to be treated as visitors.

Each family handles this transition differently, but most health care providers and parents of NICU graduates will tell you to limit visitors. Your priority is to care for your baby and yourself. That may mean ignoring the doorbell at times and screening phone calls with caller ID or an answering machine. Hang a sign on your door indicating your readiness (or unreadiness) for visitors: "Mom and Baby Are Sleeping Now." Or try a direct but humorous approach: "Welcome! Our Favorite Visitors Bring Snacks and Stay 30 Minutes or Less!"

The more people your baby comes in contact with, the greater the risk of infection. Healthy visitors may be welcome, but anyone with a cold, cough, open sore (such as a fever blister), or communicable illness should not be allowed near the baby. Most people understand when you explain that a common illness picked up from an older child or adult can develop into a serious setback for a NICU graduate.

Try to limit how much visitors handle your baby. Remember, good hand washing is the best prevention against illness. Also, keep your baby from becoming overstimulated, which can occur from too much handling. A polite way to discourage holding is to secure your baby in an infant seat and see that she stays there.

You probably won't want to discourage all visitors, however, because you'll need help once your baby is home. Those friends who have seen you through your crisis will want you to be honest about your needs now that your baby is home. Now more than ever, you may need to make a list of things people can do to help you, such as running errands, helping with laundry, or watching your children while you nap. Now is not the time to be Super Parent—ask for and accept help! For these first stressful weeks at home, allow yourself to put your family's needs first.

Financial Stress and Career Changes

Financial burdens may place added stress on your family. You may need to take an extended absence from work or even leave your job to care for your baby at home. If you did not do so before your baby's discharge, you may need to check with your social worker regarding your rights to a family leave of absence (see Chapter 7). Even under the best of circumstances, a loss of income may have far-reaching consequences on your family's future.

Maintaining your medical coverage often means a lack of freedom to move or change jobs—for fear that the baby will not be covered by a new insurance policy. On the other hand, some parents may relocate so as to have access to medical care for their baby that would otherwise be unavailable or too far from home. Help is available for families of NICU graduates under financial stress. Work closely with your social worker and your hospital financial counselor to devise a plan (see Chapter 7).

Most NICU parents experience some degree of crisis as they adjust in the first 4 to 6 weeks after homecoming. Be patient. Give yourself some time to get off the emotional roller-coaster before expecting to settle into some semblance of a normal life.

What to Expect From Your Baby—The Unexpected

Babies are unique in the way they react to their surroundings and signal their needs. A large part of gaining confidence as a parent is feeling that you are adequately meeting your baby's needs. Parenting a NICU graduate can be challenging at first, especially if your baby does not signal those needs clearly or does not act predictably.

Behavioral Differences Between Preterm and Term Babies

Compared with term infants of a similar chronological age, many NICU graduates are challenging, difficult, and often frustrating for the first 3 to 6 months after arriving home. See the box on page 474 for a summary of these differences. Preterm infants tend to be more irritable, less responsive, and less predictable than healthy term infants. These patterns of behavioral disorganization are most noticeable in the areas of sleep, activity, and feeding. Term infants with chronic illnesses requiring NICU time may exhibit some of these behaviors as well. Try to be patient. Recognize that your baby needs time to learn about your home environment, just as you need time to develop your routine. Most infants outgrow these differences within the first year of life and grow into typical toddlers. Until that time, however, your baby may try your patience. By understanding her behavior and helping her to become more organized, you'll find it easier to get into a routine.

Behavioral Differences Between Preterm Infants and Term Infants in Their First Months at Home[a]

Preterm infants are often different from healthy term infants. Preterm infants usually
• Are less predictable and harder to read
• Spend less time awake
• Are less alert and responsive when awake
• Are less active but fussier
• Are more difficult to soothe, and more withdrawn
• Have shorter, more disorganized, sleep-wake cycles
• Arouse with fussing more frequently at night
• Have a weaker suck, so demand to be fed more often
• Are less adaptive to new people and situations
• Show delayed development of motor self-help skills, such as sitting without support

[a]Adapted from Gorski PA. Fostering family development after preterm hospitalization. In: Ballard RA, ed. *Pediatric Care of the ICN Graduate*. Philadelphia, PA: WB Saunders; 1988:27, 29. Reprinted by permission.

Sleep Patterns

Don't expect your preterm baby to sleep through the night for many months. Unlike a term baby, who might sleep a full 6 to 8 hours at night by 4 months of age, your baby may not accomplish this task until 6 to 8 months or later. During this transition period, play with your baby during daytime awake periods. Keep night feedings as quiet and as businesslike as possible, with minimal or soft lighting. This will help your baby learn the difference between day and night and may help you get much-needed sleep at appropriate hours. But remember, it may take several weeks before your baby gets her days and nights straight!

Babies vary in how easily they settle down to sleep. Follow the same steps each time you put your baby down to sleep to help her learn a personal going-to-sleep routine. At first, you'll probably jump up and go to your baby at the first crying sound. But as you get to know each other and as you notice your baby's self-comforting skills, you need to allow your baby to console herself and go back to sleep on her own. Self-comforting is an important skill for your baby. Beginning early to teach your baby to fall asleep on her own will ease you through the later developmental stage (at 6–9 months corrected age) when sleep problems may emerge once again.

To help your baby rest, try playing the radio softly or placing a ticking clock in the room for those first few weeks at home. In addition, a soft night-light may be reassuring to you both. Let your baby suck on her fist or a pacifier if this seems calming.

Fussing

"The medications, the breathing treatments, the special formula—
it takes a lot out of you. Sometimes I would wonder how I could keep
going, and then Rachel would look right at me and smile. That gorgeous
toothless smile would revive me. She's worth every bit of hard work."

Although your baby will sleep up to 16 hours a day at first, her actual sleep intervals may be short. She may awaken and fuss every 2 to 3 hours until 3 to 4 months' corrected age. These fussy periods may or may not coincide with hunger.

Your baby communicates some needs by fussing and crying. You'll learn to recognize the different cries your baby makes. If she is fed, is not too hot or too cold, has a clean and dry diaper, and is not uncomfortable or ill—but will not calm down with gentle holding, talking, or rocking—she may simply be tired or overstimulated. Put her down in a quiet place and let her try to pull herself together or go to sleep.

But what if your baby doesn't settle down and just keeps crying? You can try a variety of consoling techniques until you find what works best for your baby. Try rocking her, either in a rocking chair or in your arms. Some babies prefer an up-and-down motion to side-to-side movement, which may actually be stimulating. This is why some babies find a rocking swing comforting. (Use a swing only if your baby passed the car safety seat test and has no respiratory problems in a sitting position.) Other babies like to be sung to or to hear music. Still others enjoy being gently stroked or patted, massaged, held skin-to-skin on your chest, or swaddled snugly (but not too tightly). Make sure your baby can get at her hand or pacifier if sucking is comforting. Your baby may prefer a walk, either in your arms or in a stroller or a carriage. A warm bath has a calming effect on most babies, but not all.

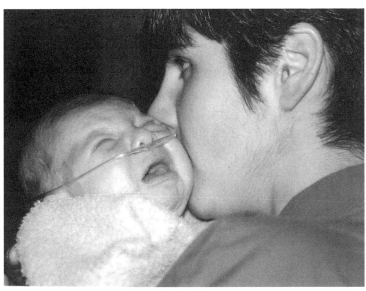

Crying.
Crying is stressful for babies and parents alike. Give yourself some time to figure out why your baby cries and what works best to calm him.

As concerning as these crying episodes may be, it is important to know that many babies go through a fussy or "colicky" period that begins anywhere from 2 to 4 weeks' corrected age, peaks around 6 weeks' corrected age, and usually resolves by 3 months' corrected age, but can last until 6 months' corrected age. (See pages 437–438 for how to calculate corrected age.) For some babies, this fussy period occurs at the same time every day (usually late afternoon or early evening). For others, it appears to be related to feedings, but experts now know that it is also a time when your baby is developmentally becoming more alert and aware of her environment and may have difficulty handling all of the new sensory stimulation she is receiving. Without your knowing, your baby may be swallowing more air as she feeds and looks around the room in excitement to the noise of the television, people talking, or dog barking. This may result in more gas or stomach upset along with overstimulation of her maturing brain. In other words, your baby becomes overwhelmed by the end of the day and needs a good cry to help her relax! But getting her to calm down may be a challenge. Colic does seem to be more pronounced and tends to last longer in premature infants and NICU graduates, which may require very inventive calming strategies. Try the strategies stated previously, and try the sound of a vacuum cleaner or a fan, the smell of an article of your clothing in the crib, or a drive in the car.

During your baby's first months at home, you'll be learning what she likes and doesn't like. The most frustrating thing for parents is that the same comfort measure doesn't work every time—and may not work 2 times in a row. When you find something that works, stick with it until it doesn't work any longer. Babies like consistency and rituals, especially as they get older.

Baby care experts Sears and Sears recommend "baby-wearing," not just as a response to crying, but to prevent crying and promote parent-infant attachment and the baby's development. You could place your baby in a front pouch and "wear" her around the house while you cook, clean, or even pay bills, for example. If you're doing active chores, be sure to keep safety in mind. This technique may make your baby cry less and enhance her learning. Check with your baby's care provider before using a baby pack or pouch—sometimes NICU graduates do not have enough muscle strength to keep their airways open in an unsupported position.

Some parents worry about spoiling their infant with too much holding. Don't worry. Experts agree that holding a baby in the early months meets the infant's basic need to feel safe. In fact, babies who are picked up as soon as they begin to cry tend to cry less often and for shorter periods than do babies whose parents don't respond quickly.

This doesn't mean you have to pick your baby up with every peep you hear. As your baby grows, let her learn about and explore personal ways to self-comfort. She will discover that sucking her fist, holding her blanket, or clasping her hands together will help her feel better for a few moments.

How long to let your baby cry remains controversial. Some baby care experts feel that you should never let your baby cry it out alone. They recommend a quick response to your baby's cry to satisfy the need for security and to let your baby know that she is important. These experts argue that by meeting your baby's dependence needs, you foster a more independent child. Well-known pediatrician Dr T. Berry Brazelton is in this group, arguing that letting your baby cry it out only teaches her that you've deserted her in this time of need, but that doesn't mean you must jump at the first whimper.

Others feel that as long as your baby is in a safe place and her basic needs for safety, nourishment, and comfort are met, a few minutes of crying will not hurt her. Some babies seem to need to cry themselves to sleep—possibly because of fatigue or overstimulation or as a stress release—and will not be comforted by standard measures. If your baby is particularly demanding every day, make a plan for someone to relieve you periodically, even if only for an hour or so. You will need a break so that you can return to your baby in a more relaxed state of mind.

If your baby has special medical needs or turns blue with crying, you may not be able to let her cry even for a few minutes. And if your baby has a tracheostomy tube, you won't be able to hear her cry. You may need to purchase a bell to tie around an ankle (the bell is sewn inside the cloth bracelet for safety) to alert you that your baby is upset.

You'll probably find that as you adjust to your baby, you'll be less upset by her crying. This is not to say that you should become so desensitized to your baby's crying that you don't respond to basic needs. Whether you decide to respond to your baby's cry immediately or wait a moment, the important thing is to do what you feel is right. Trust your instincts. Try a combination of approaches before you decide which one is right for you and your baby. It's important to balance a baby's need for your love and attention with the developmental need to learn self-consolation.

Concerns About Feeding

Now that your baby is home, you'll be making more independent decisions about when and how much your baby eats. Most parents discover things they didn't learn about their baby's eating habits while the baby was in the hospital and wonder if they are "doing it right" at home. Learning about feeding your baby takes time. But as you see your baby gaining and growing every day, you'll begin to feel more confident in your decisions.

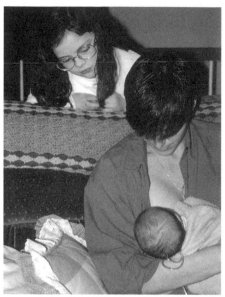

Breastfeeding at home.
Making the transition to breastfeeding at home can be challenging. Your older child may feel left out of this part of baby care, and you may miss the support of the hospital staff. Call on all available community resources to help ensure your success.

Helping Your Baby Eat Well

Minimizing distractions during feeding time is important for all babies, but especially for those who are easily overwhelmed and become stressed from too much stimulation. Monitor your baby's behavioral cues throughout the feeding. Does she frequently yawn, sneeze, hiccup, get frantic, or lose interest and fall asleep in the middle of feeding? Talking to and looking at your baby while she nipples or having the television on may be too much stimulation for your baby to handle.

If your baby seems unusually stressed during feedings when there is a lot of activity around, you may want to turn her feeding period into a "quiet time" for the whole family. If you're lucky, younger children may imitate older ones who are relaxing with quiet activities while the baby eats. Sometimes another family member can keep siblings occupied while you feed the baby in a quieter area of the house.

Here are some suggestions for a successful feeding experience.

- If you're bottle feeding, prepare the formula in advance. Do not heat the bottle in the microwave because microwaves heat bottles unevenly and you could scald your baby's mouth. Place the bottle in hot water or a bottle warmer instead and check the temperature of the milk against your wrist to make sure it is lukewarm.
- Minimize distractions in the room. Dim the lights, turn down the television or radio, and so on.
- Support your baby's head, neck, and hips, flexing them slightly.
- To help your baby anticipate the feeding, place your finger or a few drops of breast milk or formula in her mouth.
- If necessary, gently support your baby's jaw with your finger to keep the milk in her mouth.
- Identify the appropriate nipple for your baby. This should be established prior to discharge, but if you need to change nipples, remember that preemie nipples (supplied by the NICU) allow the milk to come out quickly—as your baby gets older, she may gag or choke from a flow rate that is too fast. Conversely, nipples used to complement breastfeeding tend to have slower flow rates, which may frustrate your baby.
- While making eye contact, talk softly or not at all. Watch for signs of overstimulation.

- Monitor your baby's behavior for signs of stress, and give her a break when necessary.
- Allow for frequent rest breaks and burps.
- Give your baby time to recover after the feeding is over.
- Never put your baby to sleep with a bottle propped or allow her to sleep with a bottle once she is old enough to hold her own. This is a bad habit that will ultimately lead to tooth decay and possibly ear infections.

How Much and How Often to Feed

Before your baby's discharge, her health care provider probably gave you written guidelines for how much and how often to feed her. Special high-calorie formulas (also called *enriched formulas*) designed specifically for premature infants are often continued at discharge to maintain optimal weight gain during this transition to home. Some babies need to continue a specific feeding schedule and fluid restrictions after discharge. Your health care provider may adjust that schedule only after weighing and examining your baby in the office. Other infants may be able to feed on demand—meaning that the baby determines how much and how often to eat, according to her feeding readiness cues.

The doctor or nurse practitioner should have told you before discharge whether to feed your baby on demand or to follow a feeding schedule (for example, 2 ounces or 60 cc every 3 hours) for the first few weeks to ensure continued weight gain. Allowing your baby to feed when she indicates readiness encourages behavioral development, which may produce better weight gain and encourage establishment of sleep patterns. Until she is more mature, she may not have a predictable sleeping or feeding schedule. She may wake up hungry every 2 to 3 hours, may sleep for 4 hours, or may wake up hungry and then fall asleep halfway through a feeding.

If you'll be feeding your baby on demand at home, you should begin to feed her this way before discharge. This will give you an opportunity to learn the behavioral cues your infant uses to signal readiness to eat. In the first few weeks after discharge, a breastfed baby needs 8 to 10 and possibly more feedings per day. A bottle-fed baby may need at least 6 feedings per day.

Your health care provider may suggest that you consider a modified demand schedule for breastfeeding a preterm infant who is 35 to 36 weeks' gestation at the time of discharge. This is because a preterm infant's need for sleep may override the desire to feed, resulting in poor weight gain or dehydration. Your health care provider may suggest feeding your baby every 2 to 5 hours, with a minimum of 6 feedings per day. You may need to continue to use a breast pump with this approach to ensure an adequate milk supply. Still other health care providers may recommend breastfeeding at least 8 times per day. Clearly, feeding schedules need to be individualized depending on your baby's weight gain. A visit from a home health nurse or lactation specialist during the first week or two after discharge can help to resolve breastfeeding issues. However, the bottom line is weight gain. Your health care provider should give you some weight gain goals to check on every week or two.

As your baby grows, so should her appetite. If your baby takes less than what she needs at a feeding, she may wake up earlier or take more at the next feeding. If she takes in too much or eats too quickly, she may spit up. Once she is able to take in more at each feeding, the time between feedings may lengthen. It's particularly nice when your baby starts lengthening the time between feedings at night, letting you get more sleep.

If you are breastfeeding and your baby is working hard to nurse, or if it is unclear how much milk your baby is getting, you may be instructed to supplement the amount your baby takes at the breast. Your health care provider will ask you to provide either breast milk or formula by using a bottle, a supplemental nursing device, finger feeding, or cup feeding so your baby will receive enough calories for growth (see Chapter 5). If a bottle is used, Dad or another caregiver may at times give the supplement so you can get some rest. Usually, once your baby is sucking and swallowing for at least 15 minutes at the breast and is growing and gaining weight, the health care provider will discontinue supplementation. Whenever you are supplementing your baby's meals (with breast milk or formula) you must continue to pump/express your milk in order to maintain your milk supply. Supplementation without pumping will allow your baby to be fed, but you will receive less stimulation, which you need to make milk. If you do not keep up your supply, then supplementing will result in less and less breast milk production over time. Not understanding this concept is the most common mistake mothers make after taking a NICU graduate home.

Some health care providers recommend test weighing the baby on a scale designed especially for this purpose. (See Chapter 5 for more information about test weighing.) By weighing your baby before and after breastfeeding, you can accurately calculate how much milk she is receiving at each feeding. This ends the guessing and insecurity about how much your baby is eating and may increase your confidence in your ability to breastfeed.

How Long to Feed

Feeding length varies, depending on how frequently your baby wants to eat and how easily she tires while feeding. Breastfed infants may begin nursing only a few minutes on each side and may require more frequent feedings. You should hear sucking and swallowing, along with some pauses. Gradually, your baby may work up to nursing 20 minutes or more on each side. The usual length of time it takes a breastfed infant to complete a feeding is 20 to 40 minutes. Breastfed infants tend to take twice as long as bottle-fed infants to eat. But as long as your baby seems content after feeding and is gaining weight (weight checks may need to be done at home or in the doctor's office), there's no reason to limit feeding time. In fact, your baby may become frustrated if you end the feeding too soon. Babies nurse not only to satisfy hunger, but also to satisfy their need for sucking, security, and comfort. Falling asleep or ceasing to suck are the usual indicators that a feeding is over.

In general, a feeding for a bottle-fed baby should not last longer than 20 to 30 minutes. Most babies will finish much sooner than that (in 10–20 minutes). If your baby is unable to take everything by nipple and requires supplementation by gavage (a feeding tube), you should still try to limit the total feeding time to 30 minutes. Your baby will have more difficulty gaining weight if she uses all of her calories to get through long, perhaps stressful, feeding periods.

Weight Gain

As you settle into a feeding routine, you may wonder whether your baby is gaining enough weight. Optimal weight gain is 15 grams (1/2 ounce) per day before your baby's due date and 20 to 30 grams (a little more than 1/2 ounce to 1 ounce) per day for the first 6 months. It is important to note the rate of weight gain and not the percentile placement on the growth chart. An easy to remember rule of thumb for weight gain is a goal of 1 pound per month minimum. Your baby's care provider will plot measurements of weight, length, and head circumference on the growth chart by corrected age. There are special growth curves for premature infants that allow your doctor to follow her growth by her corrected age. The smallest preterm infants will appear not to thrive when their growth is plotted on charts designed for full-term babies.

Your health care provider may recommend weekly weight checks at the office to check for adequate weight gain or by the home health nurse for the first few weeks after discharge or longer. It's important that your baby be weighed naked on the same scale each time to accurately assess weight gain. Once your baby demonstrates good growth at home, everyone (including you) will relax a bit.

Feeding Challenges

"It helps if you are confident with your baby's care before you leave the hospital so you can go home and train other people to help you. You need two or three people, whether they be family or friends, to help."

Some babies are more challenging to feed than others. Before your baby was discharged from the hospital, your nurse probably talked with you about her feeding style and helped you practice feeding your baby. The nurse, the lactation consultant, or an occupational therapist may have worked with you on specific feeding and positioning techniques that work best for your baby. If you roomed-in before discharge, you had the chance to feed your baby several times in a row. Now you'll put all of that practice to good use at home.

A bottle-feeding infant who gulps rapidly and then spits everything up may need a nipple that delivers the formula more slowly. You might need to try a few different types of standard bottle nipples before you find the one that works best. You may need to regulate the length of time the nipple is in your baby's mouth as well. Frequent burping and feeding the baby in a more upright position may also help prevent spitting up. Use of a bottle with a collapsing bag inside also helps.

Breastfeeding babies are usually able to adjust to the fast flow of milk that accompanies the mother's let-down reflex (also called the *milk-ejection reflex)*. Sometimes babies who are just learning to breastfeed have difficulty with a moment of faster milk flow and may stop breathing, choke, or spit up. One solution to this problem is to pump for a few minutes before the baby begins to nurse. This will decrease the surge of milk entering your baby's mouth as your milk lets down. Another technique is to get the baby latched on well and then slowly recline (in a reclining chair or against pillows behind you) so that the baby is positioned nearly on top of your breast. Then when the milk lets down, your reclining position lessens the force of the milk spray into the baby's mouth, and any overflowing breast milk can easily dribble forward out of the baby's mouth.

Your baby may have been discharged with an apnea monitor (discussed later in this chapter) to alert you to severe episodes of apnea (pauses in breathing) or bradycardia (slowing of the heart rate). If your baby tends to hold her breath (common also with gulpers), watch her breathing pattern and color during feedings. If you notice breath holding or a color change (to pale, dusky, or blue) at any time during a feeding, take the nipple out of your baby's mouth. Try gentle stimulation—rubbing or patting your baby's back, for example—to wake your baby up and remind her to breathe. The rubbing or patting may also bring up a burp. If you find you need frequent vigorous stimulation to keep your baby breathing during feedings, call your health care provider at once.

Some babies work hard to suck. Whether it's because their oral-motor development is still immature for their corrected age or because of unresolved breathing problems, they may need a special nipple made for premature infants, which is softer and allows more milk to come out with less effort. Take care when feeding with this nipple to keep your baby from choking if the milk comes out too rapidly. These nipples are not sold commercially and should be used at home only on recommendation of your health care provider. Because the nipples can be washed in hot, soapy water and reused, you don't need too many of them. If your baby needs this type of nipple, the nursery may have provided you with a supply at discharge, or you may have to special order them.

Babies typically outgrow the need for a preemie nipple within the first month after they're home. By that time, they are usually approaching the weight of a term newborn and are able to make the switch to a commercial nipple. If your baby begins to cough and sputter on the milk as her suck gets stronger, she may be ready for a standard nipple. You may need to try several nipples before you find the one that works best for your baby.

If you have difficulty feeding your baby after discharge, contact your health care professional. Frequently, all you need is a phone call to the NICU or intermediate care nursery for some advice and reassurance from a nurse who is familiar with your baby's eating habits. If not, an outpatient referral to a lactation specialist or an occupational therapist may be in order.

As your baby gets older, it is important to remember that transitioning to semisolid food and from breast or bottle to cup should be based on your baby's corrected and developmental readiness and not on chronological age. For example, if your baby was born at 24 weeks and is now 6 months old, she is not developmentally ready for spoon feedings because her corrected age would only be 2 months (24 weeks old now minus 16 weeks premature = 8 weeks old corrected age). Resist family pressures to feed your baby semisolids too early. Studies have shown that this may increase your baby's risk of food allergies. Your baby will let you know when she is developmentally ready for solid foods when she has good head control in an upright position and when she begins reaching for other family members' food.

A Feeding Log

Whether your baby is breastfeeding or bottle feeding, you may want to keep a log of each feeding for the first few weeks or month at home. Use a notebook to document

1. Feeding times
2. Feedings missed (for example, when your baby begins to sleep longer at night)
3. Time at breast or amount per bottle
4. Any spitting up and approximately how much
5. Wet and dirty diapers
6. Special comments (for example, is your baby satisfied after a feeding, or does she cry a lot; does your baby fall asleep in the middle of the feeding, or does your baby need to be awakened for feedings?)

All of these observations are worth noting. Bring this information with you when you take your baby to your health care provider. It will help your health care provider decide if your baby is taking in enough calories to grow. You may be concerned that your baby frequently spits up 1 to 2 teaspoons after each feeding, for example. As long as your baby is gaining weight adequately, your health care provider may advise you just to continue monitoring the amounts and to practice reflux precautions, such as holding the baby more upright during feedings, burping frequently, and elevating the head of the bed.

On the other hand, you may report that your baby is irritable, cries all the time, and needs to be bundled or dressed warmly to maintain her temperature. This history will help your health care provider determine why your infant isn't gaining weight despite a healthy appetite. Your baby is most likely burning up calories crying, working to breathe, or keeping warm. An increase in the amount and/or frequency of feedings is usually all that your baby needs. Occasionally, special additives to breast milk or formula or specially prepared high-calorie formula may be necessary to promote adequate growth and development if your baby was not initially discharged home on these. Because most babies today are already sent home with specially prepared high-calorie enriched or premature formulas or supplements to breast milk, more adjustments may need to be made by your health care provider in order to increase the caloric concentration of the breast milk or formula or increase the amount or frequency of the feedings.

Keeping a log is a simple and valuable way to work in partnership with your baby's health care team. Appointments at the health care provider's office are often only 15 to 30 minutes long, giving you little time to organize your questions. If you come prepared with your written questions and information log, you will be able to make the most of your office visit. Once your baby has established a consistent pattern of feeding and gaining weight for you at home, you can comfortably retire your feeding log as part of your baby book.

Other Common Homecoming Concerns

It may have seemed like an eternity until you were able to take your baby home. Now, at last, you have control over your baby and your family life—or do you? The normal elements of baby care may not be so routine for you. The first few days, weeks, and even months at home may in fact be unsettling. This section addresses some common concerns, with the goal of helping you to organize your family life once again.

Sudden Infant Death Syndrome

Many parents worry about their baby's chances of death from sudden infant death syndrome (SIDS), often called *crib death*. This syndrome is the third-leading cause of death in the first year of life in the United States, exceeded only by congenital malformations and disorders related to prematurity and low birth weight. However, the actual incidence of SIDS in this country and Canada is actually low, at less than 0.6 SIDS-related deaths per 1,000 live births.

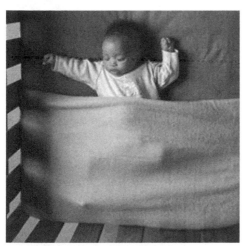

Safer use of a crib blanket.
If you use a blanket, place the baby's feet at the end of the crib. Place the blanket no higher than the baby's chest. Tuck the edges of the blanket under the crib mattress.

Courtesy of National Institute of Child Health and Human Development.

The media have played an important role in keeping parents informed of the latest scientific theories about SIDS. But at this time, no one theory explains these infant deaths. A panel from the National Institute of Child Health and Human Development (NICHD) modified the definition of SIDS in 1992, saying that it is "the sudden death of an infant under 1 year of age which remains unexplained after a thorough case investigation, including performance of a complete autopsy, examination of the death scene, and review of the clinical history." Although there is ongoing discussion about changing this definition, it is still used today.

In 1992 the American Academy of Pediatrics (AAP) recommended that infants be positioned for sleep on their side or back instead of prone (tummy down). At that time, a nationwide campaign called Back to Sleep was launched and promoted positioning all babies on their back (or side-lying, as second choice) for sleep instead of on their tummy. As a result of this simple change in sleeping position, the SIDS rate in the United States dropped by more than 50% and from the second-leading to the third-leading cause of death in infants. Since the AAP published its last statement on SIDS in 2005, it no longer recognizes the side-lying position as a reasonable alternative to back sleeping. Studies showed that side-lying infants were often found tummy down due to the unstable nature of the position; therefore, side-lying is no longer advised.

Sudden Infant Death Syndrome Risk Factors

Many countries have been involved in the study of SIDS. Several factors seem to be associated with an increased relative risk for SIDS. They include

- Low birth weight. The risk of SIDS is higher among infants born weighing less than 5 pounds, 8 ounces (2,500 grams), and higher still if birth weight is less than 3 pounds, 5 ounces (1,500 grams).
- Prematurity and intrauterine growth restriction/small for gestational age. These factors contribute significantly to an increased risk of SIDS, but apnea of prematurity does not. Up to 18% of all SIDS cases occur in preterm infants. But preterm infants diagnosed with apnea of prematurity do not have a higher incidence of SIDS than do other premature infants. Further, there is little evidence to support that home cardiorespiratory monitoring has any impact on SIDS prevention, including in the preterm population.

- Gender. Male infants have a 50% higher incidence of SIDS than do female infants.
- Race and ethnicity. The highest SIDS rates have been found in African American and Native American Indian/Alaska Native populations—more than 2 to 3 times the national average for Asians, whites, and Hispanics.
- Geography. Rates of SIDS declined all over the world as most developed countries also adopted a Back to Sleep policy. Australia, New Zealand, Northern Ireland, and Italy generally have the highest incidence of SIDS (1–1.5 per 1,000 live births); whereas Hong Kong, The Netherlands, Denmark, and Japan have the lowest rates (0.1–0.3 per 1,000 live births). The United States and Canada, along with several other countries, fall in between (0.4–0.6 per 1,000 live births).
- Season and climate. Some studies have identified an increased incidence of SIDS during cold months, but other factors may also contribute to this increased risk. They include infection (colds and flu are more common in winter months), temperature of the baby's room (too warm), nutrition or metabolic processes, infant care practices, and lifestyle.
- Cigarette smoking during pregnancy increases the SIDS risk 3 to 4 times. Smoking in the household is another separate risk factor.
- Substance abuse by the mother.
- Lack of prenatal care.
- Low socioeconomic status.
- An unmarried mother.
- Young maternal age (teenage).
- Short interval between pregnancies.
- Prior SIDS death. There is a 1% increase in the risk of SIDS above the baseline for subsequent babies when an older sibling has died of SIDS.
- History of illness preceding death.

Other factors related to SIDS are also being investigated at this time. These include

- **Age.** Sudden infant death syndrome generally occurs in infants younger than 6 months. The peak incidence of SIDS occurs between 2 and 4 months of age, and SIDS does not appear to occur before the age of 1 month in full-term infants. In the preterm population, the peak incidence of SIDS is between 43 and 46 weeks postconceptional age (3–6 weeks after the baby's original due date) regardless of gestational age.
- **Breastfeeding.** Studies on breastfeeding having a protective effect against SIDS have not been conclusive. Many of these studies, however, suggest that factors associated with breastfeeding, rather than the breastfeeding itself, are protective. Therefore, breastfeeding is encouraged for many beneficial reasons, but the evidence is insufficient to recommend breastfeeding as a strategy to reduce SIDS. In other words, no one could blame a SIDS death on failure to breastfeed.

- **Immunizations.** The combination diphtheria-tetanus-pertussis (DTaP) vaccine has *not* been associated with a higher risk of SIDS.

Reducing the Risk of Sudden Infant Death Syndrome

Unless you have received special sleep position instructions from your baby's care provider, remember that all babies, including premature and low birth weight infants, should be placed on their back to sleep. For premature infants with respiratory distress (bronchopulmonary dysplasia or chronic lung disease) and for infants or premature babies with certain upper airway malformations (such as Robin Syndrome), gastro-esophageal reflux disease, or other medical problems, sleep studies may be required prior to discharge from the hospital in order to determine the safest sleep position. Any alteration from the Back to Sleep recommendation must be discussed with your health care provider.

You may have seen your baby nested on her stomach in the NICU, on top of a soft pad and surrounded by rolled blankets (or commercial positioning cushion) in order to promote flexion. This positioning was done at an earlier time in your baby's life to decrease gastrointestinal reflux, improve developmental tone, or decrease other symptoms such as apnea, and while under close medical supervision and cardiorespiratory monitoring. Do not position your baby on her tummy or her side to sleep at home. Place your baby on her back to sleep.

The following are things you can do to reduce the risk of SIDS:

- Don't overdress or overbundle your baby or overheat your baby's room. Your baby should be lightly clothed for sleep, and the bedroom temperature should feel comfortable to a lightly clothed adult. Your baby should not feel hot to the touch and should not be moist or sweating. Be aware that continuing to use the knit hat at home may result in overheating your baby and is therefore not recommended. Your baby should be able to maintain her body temperature without the knit hat by the time she goes home.
- Some studies suggest running a ceiling fan or turning on a small fan in your baby's room for better circulation—which may help decrease the risk of SIDS (not proven at this time).
- Place your baby on a firm mattress covered only with a sheet. Avoid soft sleep surfaces, such as fluffy bedding, pillows, beanbags, or water beds, which may increase your baby's risk of suffocation.
- Avoid maternal and household smoking. Maternal smoking during pregnancy has been identified as a major risk factor in almost every SIDS study. Household smoking has emerged as a separate risk factor for SIDS. Avoiding an infant's exposure to secondhand smoke is advisable for numerous health reasons (discussed later on page 500) in addition to the SIDS risk.

- Consider offering a pacifier at naptime and bedtime throughout the first year of life. Although the reason is unknown, pacifiers have been shown to decrease the risk of SIDS. If your baby doesn't want it or if it falls out of her mouth, do not force it or prop the pacifier in place.
- Avoid commercial devices marketed to reduce SIDS or developmental tools used in the NICU to foster flexion and containment. None have been tested sufficiently to show efficacy or safety.
- Do not use home cardiorespiratory monitors in an effort to reduce the risk of SIDS— they do not.

Concerns About Back Sleeping

Most new parents are aware of the recommendations for positioning babies on their back for sleep. Your own parents or grandparents, however, raised "tummy sleepers," and may have the following concerns about back sleeping:

- **Choking.** The most common fear about the back sleeping position is that the baby will spit up and choke while asleep. If your NICU graduate has special issues that put her at risk, you will know this prior to discharge and receive special sleep positioning instructions. Healthy NICU graduates are able to turn their heads or protect their airways if they spit up.

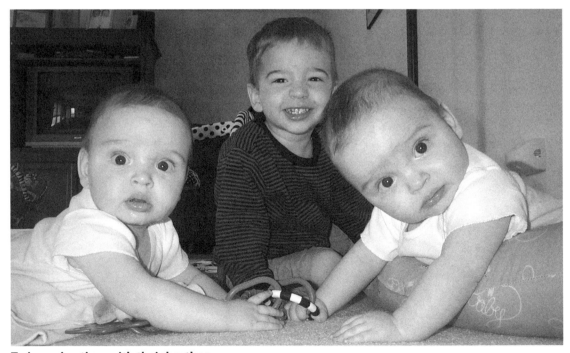

Twins enjoy time with their brother.
Tummy time builds neck and shoulder muscles needed for rolling over and helps a "flattened" head to round out.

- **Flat head.** Technically called *positional plagiocephaly,* your baby's head may be flat in the back and narrow on the sides. The head usually rounds out as the baby matures, holds her head up independently, and spends less time on her back. In the meantime, encourage plenty of supervised tummy time when your baby is awake, and avoid placing your baby in car safety seat carriers or "bouncers" for excessive lengths of time. Change the position your baby faces in the crib every few weeks or change the crib to the other side of the room (the baby's attention will be drawn to the center of the room rather than the wall) so that she is not always lying on the same side of her head. These strategies should help take the pressure off of the back of the head. If plagiocephaly occurs despite these preventive measures, talk with your health care provider about a referral to an occupational or physical therapist.
- **Delayed motor development.** Some worry that because the baby spends so much time on her back, it will take a long time to master the skill of rolling over. Allowing the baby plenty of supervised time on her tummy while she's awake will build the necessary neck and shoulder muscles she needs to roll over.

Be sure that everyone who cares for your baby knows the importance of positioning her on her back for sleep. Babies who are accustomed to a back sleeping position who are then placed on their tummy for sleep (for example, at naptime) have a very high risk of SIDS.

Family Bed: Not Recommended

Before you can establish a sleep routine with your baby, there are some important facts and controversies you need to know about sleeping arrangements. Our culture has traditionally frowned on parents sleeping with their infants and children, because we emphasize the development of independence and the importance of privacy. But behavioral specialists began promoting sharing a bed with your infant as a personal and individual decision. Some of your friends may have shared their bed with their newborn and/or young children. As current research emerged on SIDS risk factors (stated previously), the AAP determined that the safest place for your baby to sleep is in the room where you sleep, but not in your bed.

Your baby should sleep in her own safety-approved crib or bassinet, on a firm mattress with a fitted sheet. Never put your baby in your bed or on a chair, sofa, or waterbed to sleep. If bumper pads are used, they should be thin, firm, and well-secured. They should not be soft like pillows. If blankets are used, they should be tucked in and around the crib mattress and they should not reach any higher than your baby's chest. It is safer to use sleep clothing or sleep sacks instead of a blanket to avoid overheating. Blankets should not be used for "nesting" or to provide boundaries for your baby. The AAP does not recommend this practice at home because extra padding and blankets may increase your baby's risk of SIDS. Finally, it is important to keep all pillows, quilts, comforters, sheepskin, and stuffed toys out of your baby's crib. They can cover your baby's face and suffocate her—even if she is positioned on her back.

Placing your baby's crib or bassinet near your bed (within arm's reach) will make breast-feeding easier and allow you to better watch over your baby. This is especially true for parents of infants who require frequent nighttime feedings or who have special needs, such as medical treatments around the clock. These babies should also sleep in the same room with their parents. Sudden infant death syndrome prevention studies out of Europe recommend that infants should sleep in their parents' room for the first 6 months of life. Once your baby does transition to her own room, the purchase of a nursery monitor (see Chapter 15) enables you to hear your baby from a different room in the house. This should help give you peace of mind and allow you (and your baby) to sleep better. However, no study has ever shown that such monitors reduce the risk of SIDS or any other adverse event.

Co-bedding (sleeping in the same bed) of twins and other multiples in the hospital setting is another practice that remains controversial. Although many behavioral specialists consider co-bedding developmentally beneficial to twins and multiples, the potential increased risk of SIDS and other health problems has not been well studied or documented. There are not enough data to support that co-bedding of twins and other multiples is safe and therefore it is not recommended in the home setting.

Bathing

You can bathe your baby any time it's convenient for you. Don't feel you must stay with the hospital schedule, although knowing the logic behind that schedule is helpful.

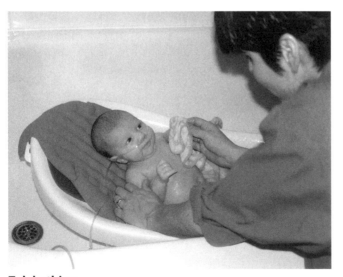

Typically, it's better to bathe before feeding, because a bath involves a lot of handling, which may cause spitting up if your baby has a full stomach. On the other hand, a bath followed immediately by a feeding may exhaust your baby. If your baby feeds poorly after a bath, you may need to allow time for a rest before feeding.

Tub bathing.
Bath time will become play time as your baby grows older. A sponge insert helps support this slippery baby and allows him to feel more secure.

As long as you keep your baby's face, neck, skin folds, and diaper area clean, you don't have to bathe her every day. A sponge bath will suffice until your baby can tolerate a tub bath without undue stress. On the other hand, a tub bath can be a relaxing and rewarding time for both you and your baby. For many babies, it may be less stressful than a sponge bath. Some parents get into the tub with their baby to hold and snuggle as they wash. This provides skin-to-skin contact for you and your baby. Remember to hold your baby securely and be sure the bath water isn't too hot for your baby.

With practice, you'll find the tub-bathing method that works best for you. There are only a few rules for tub bathing your baby: Don't let your baby get cold, and keep your baby safe. Never leave your baby unattended in the tub. If the phone or doorbell rings and you must answer it, wrap the baby in a towel and take her with you. If you must reach for something or turn away, keep one hand securely on your baby.

Bathe your baby in the warmest area of the house—preferably one free from drafts. You'll need only a few inches of water that feels comfortably warm to your wrist or elbow. Your baby will be slippery when wet; try placing a soft towel in the bottom of the tub, or buy a preformed sponge insert for the tub. Use a mild soap (ask your health care provider for a recommendation) to wash your baby's body. No soap is needed on your baby's face. Avoid using lotions; they may irritate your baby's skin. Most health care providers also advise against powder, which can irritate your baby's breathing passages.

If your son was circumcised shortly before discharge, you were probably instructed not to tub bathe him until the circumcision is healed. If you chose not to have your baby circumcised, you simply need to wash the penis at bath time. Don't try to pull back the foreskin. It will naturally separate from the penis over several years, and as your son grows you'll teach him to wash carefully as part of his daily routine.

Keeping Your Baby Warm Enough

Before discharge, you learned how to take your baby's temperature. Unless you've been instructed to check your baby's temperature routinely, you'll probably take it only when you suspect illness. But how can you tell if your baby is maintaining a comfortable body temperature?

It's not necessary (and not recommended) to turn your heat up to a sweltering level to keep your baby warm. This is a very common mistake parents make when bringing a new baby home—even when the baby is not premature. A normal household temperature that is comfortable for an adult in light clothing is recommended and is fine for most babies. If you have special concerns, ask your health care provider for advice. In the first few days at home, you may wish to check your baby's axillary (armpit) temperature randomly to see how she is adjusting to the temperature of your home.

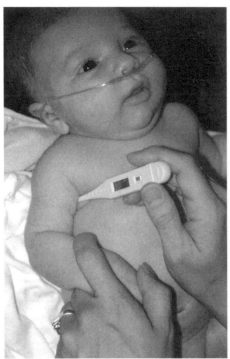

Taking a temperature.
Taking an axillary temperature is safer, easier, and less stressful than taking a rectal temperature. Remember to tell your health care professional what method you have used when you report your baby's temperature.

Because most of your baby's heat loss occurs from the surface of her head, your baby may have worn a soft cotton knit hat, day and night, while in the NICU. Prior to discharge, however, your baby should be able to maintain a normal axillary temperature in the range of 97.5°F to 99°F (36.4°C–37.2°C). The range for a rectal temperature is 98°F to 100°F (36.7°C–37.8°C) in an open crib, wearing light clothing, and no knit hat, especially if she was born term. The knit hat your baby wore in the hospital is usually not recommended at the time of discharge because of its potential to overheat your baby, especially as she gets closer to term or 5 pounds (2,268 grams). Ask your health care provider for recommendations on this matter if your baby is having trouble maintaining a normal temperature. If your baby was premature, it is especially important to determine prior to discharge if she can maintain a normal axillary temperature in an open crib while wearing light clothing and no knit hat.

Remember that the AAP cautions against overdressing your baby because overheating is a known risk factor for SIDS. The AAP recommends dressing your baby in the same layers of clothing that you would wear to be comfortable. If you're comfortable in a T-shirt and shorts, for example, your baby probably needs a footed jumper suit. On a cooler day, when you need a shirt and a pullover sweater, dress your baby in a jumper suit and a sweater. Avoid the temptation to overdress your baby. The most reliable way to determine temperature is to take your baby's temperature with a thermometer. The AAP recommends using the rectal measurement (in the baby's bottom) for newborns up to 3 months of age. However, this route is generally not recommended for very small or premature infants—the axillary method (under the armpit) is preferred unless you suspect illness. Ask your health care provider which method he or she prefers. Digital/electronic thermometers are inexpensive, safe, and accurate. Do not use a mercury thermometer (the glass kind with silver liquid inside). Mercury is a hazardous substance and these thermometers are dangerous if they break.

When you don't suspect illness, your baby's appearance or behavior may give clues to her temperature status. Usually, a baby who is dressed too warmly will fuss, turn red, and possibly sweat. A rectal temperature of 100.4°F (38°C) or greater usually indicates a fever. A cool baby may also fuss but will not turn red and may have cool, pale, or marbled-looking hands and/or feet. The temperature of a baby's hands or feet may not be reliable, but if her tummy feels cool, add a layer of clothing and check her temperature in an hour or so. If your baby seems consistently cool or isn't gaining weight despite eating well and being otherwise healthy, call your health care provider.

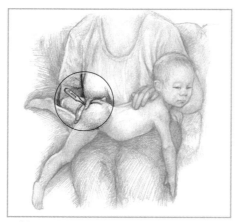

Taking a rectal temperature.
The recommended position for your baby is lying on her tummy over your legs or on a firm surface such as a changing table. This lets you control your baby's movements and prevents her from rolling onto the thermometer, which could cause an injury.

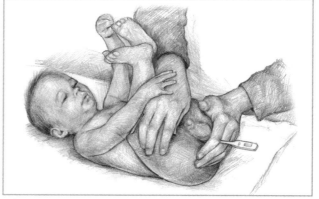

After your baby is home and if you suspect that your baby has a fever, your baby's care provider will probably ask you to take a rectal temperature.

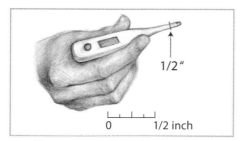

The thermometer should be inserted 1/2 inch into the rectum. Never force a rectal thermometer.

Outings

Use common sense when deciding about outings. There's probably no reason why your baby can't sit outside in the shade with you on a nice spring day or go with you to a friend's house for lunch. If you're debating over whether it's wise to take your baby someplace with you, ask yourself about chances for exposure to illness.

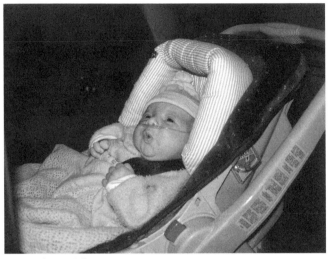

Going for a ride.
Learn safe and proper use of your baby's car safety seat. (See Appendix C for information on car safety seat use.)

Although recommendations vary, most health care providers suggest limiting your baby's public outings for the first 1 to 2 months at home. Fall and winter months are particularly bad for respiratory and flu viruses that could put your preterm or special needs infant back into the hospital. If you do take your baby out, avoid crowded places like shopping malls, grocery stores, and religious services. Many parents find these places frustrating anyway because well-meaning people continually stop them to inquire about the baby. One mother of triplets stated, "You get tired of people stopping you at every corner to look at the babies. Once someone said to me, 'I'm glad they're yours and not mine,' and I said, 'I'm glad they're mine and not yours too!' "

Babysitters and Child Care

Because the recommendation is to limit your baby's outings and visitors for the first few months at home, you may be wondering what to do when you need to go out. Anyone who watches your baby while you are away, whether that person is a babysitter, grandparent, or other relative or friend, should not only know how to manage your baby's special needs, but also be trained in infant CPR. If your hospital does not offer infant CPR, then it is important to ask your discharge coordinator or social worker where in your area you (and your family or babysitter) can get this important training prior to your baby's discharge.

If you are hiring a babysitter that is not a family member, then you need to make sure you check carefully her or his child care experience—that she or he is CPR certified and comes with a list of recent references that you can call directly. Some babysitters have taken special child care and/or child development classes along with CPR.

Infant CPR and the Back to Sleep recommendations discussed earlier are some of the most important safety measures you and other caregivers can learn in order to help decrease the risk of your baby having a potentially life-threatening event.

If you are returning to work and need to use out-of-home child care sooner than what is recommended, it is important that you look carefully at the child care facilities in your area and consider some important points.

- It is important that the facility you choose is certified as a child care facility by the state and that every child care worker is certified in infant and child CPR and first aid according to the American Heart Association's guidelines.
- Check also with your local better business bureau to make sure there have been no unresolved complaints or health violations made against this agency.
- Question the director on their infant sleep position practices and if they have ever cared for infants who were born premature or have special needs.
- Ask about visitation policies. Can you visit the facility anytime (so that you can really see how the staff interact with the infants and toddlers) or must you call first? Some facilities now have special Webcams set up so you can view your baby at any time during the day while you are at work.
- Pay particular attention to their hand washing practices and whether or not they use gloves when changing diapers. Are there sinks and soap near the cribs?
- Look at the storage area for breast milk and formula. Are bottles clearly labeled so there is less risk of feeding a baby the wrong formula or someone else's breast milk?
- What is the caregiver-to-baby ratio? The lower the ratio, the better it is for your premature baby or NICU graduate. Keep in mind that child care centers that foster developmental care and offer low worker-to-baby ratios tend to be more expensive and have longer waiting lists.

Even in the best facility, babies who require child care are more likely to get sick than those babies who stay at home. This can be particularly detrimental if your baby still has unresolved medical issues from prematurity or her NICU stay. That is why out-of-home child care is typically recommended as a last option. Working parents should begin their child care search during the pregnancy, along with interviewing health care providers, in the event that there is a waiting list. Remember not to wait until too close to the end of your pregnancy because one cannot always predict a premature or complicated delivery. For more information on choosing quality child care, visit the AAP's Web site.

Managing Advice

The phrase "If I were you…" may already make your cheeks burn. As they did when you were pregnant, well-meaning individuals will continue to give you advice, only this time about your baby. Only you can decide what will work for you.

Your health care team has also given you recommendations for the care of your baby at home. A bulletin board and calendar (see Chapter 15) may help you organize the instructional information you received from the hospital. Trust your instincts. You will soon know what needs to be done now and what can wait. Above all, let yourself enjoy the time you spend with your baby now that she is finally home and you're becoming a family.

Parent or Paramedic?

Most parents feel like paramedics in training throughout their children's lives. The first fever, the first rash, the first fall off the tricycle—all present new experiences in assessment and treatment. Most parents learn, through experience, the difference between serious and minor problems. The table on page 497 lists injury prevention strategies. The following section discusses some of the special circumstances of illness in NICU graduates.

Protecting Your Baby From Illnesses

"I was trying to be a good mom, but how would I know if I was doing everything right? Then the pediatrician told me that Adam was doing well because of my 'strong mothering skills.' Wow! That one comment was a turning point for me—I could do this!"

It's too bad that we can't wave a magic wand and protect our babies from illness and injury once they're home. The possibility of illness is especially frightening for parents of preterm infants or infants with special needs, who have already had to overcome many obstacles just to get home.

You know to limit visitors soon after your baby's arrival home, especially children who attend child care or school, and to ask that friends or family with illnesses not visit. But what if you or someone in your household gets sick? How do you keep your baby from getting the illness?

Good hand washing is the best way to prevent the spread of infection. This includes washing your hands after you blow your nose, after you sneeze or cough into your hands, and before you pick up your baby. Good hand washing is a must if you or someone in your family has a cold, the flu, a fever, or a stomach/diarrhea illness. Avoid kissing or getting too close to your baby's face, especially if you have a respiratory illness or cold sore (herpes simplex virus).

It may help protect your baby during the more acute phase of your illness if another caregiver is available to provide most (but not necessarily all) of your baby's care. Some

Injury Prevention Basics[a]

Injuries are the number one killer of our infants and children in the United States. Here are some ways to keep your precious little ones safe.	
Type of Injury	**Prevention Measures**
Airway obstruction *Choking*	**Never** prop your baby's bottle. Use only 1-piece pacifiers; **do not** "make" a pacifier from a baby bottle nipple. Keep small objects and balloons out of your baby's reach (this includes such items as button eyes glued or sewn onto stuffed animals that may be pulled off). Do not feed your infant hard pieces of food such as hot dogs, raw carrots, grapes, peanuts, or popcorn. As your infant gets older, and ready for finger foods, cut food into thin slices. **Learn first aid for a choking baby.**
Strangulation	**Do not** place the crib close to window drapery cords; gather cords up and out of reach on hooks. **Never** tie pacifiers or other items (for example, jewelry) around your baby's neck. Remove drawstrings from your baby's clothing. **Do not** place electrical cords or extension cords where infants or children can become entangled in them.
Suffocation	Place your baby on her back to sleep if not contraindicated. **Do not** place pillows, quilts, comforters, sheepskin, or other soft objects in your baby's crib (especially large stuffed animals). **Do not** place your baby on a water bed, beanbag or other soft chair, or sofa. Store and dispose of plastic bags safely. Learn infant CPR (or pediatric basic life support).
Car related	Follow instructions on proper use of car safety seats (see Appendix C). Your infant must always ride in a rear-facing car safety seat until she is at least 1 year of age, is at least 20 pounds, and has good head control. All infants and children younger than 12 years should be placed in the backseat whenever possible as long as the backseat permits them to be secured with a restraint that is appropriate for their age and size. Never leave your infant or child alone in a car. Death from excessive heat/cold may occur in a short time. Use child safety locks and keep your vehicle and its trunk locked at all times.
Crib related	**Never** leave your baby in a crib with the side rail lowered. Cornerposts should **not** extend above the crib end panels because older infants can use them to climb up and over the railing. The headboard and footboard should **not** have cutouts. Spacing between crib slats should not exceed 2 3/8 inches. Crib hardware should be secure. The mattress should be firm and snug fitting (**no** gaps between the frame and mattress to entrap the infant). The bottom sheet should be fitted. If blankets are used, they should be tucked in and around the crib mattress and they should not reach any higher than your baby's chest. Bumper pads should be thin, firm, and well-secured. Remove mobiles, crib gyms, and bumper pads from crib rails as soon as the infant can crawl or kneel. Check for peeling paint and rough edges or splinters.

Injury Prevention Basics[a], continued

Type of Injury	Prevention Measures
Drowning	**Never** leave your baby alone in or near a bathtub, pail of water, wading or swimming pool, or any body of water—not even for a minute. Stay within an arm's reach of your infant around water. Drowning can happen in less than 2 inches of water. Empty buckets or containers of fluid immediately after use; never leave them unattended. Keep the bathroom door closed; use doorknob covers. Use lid-locks for toilets. Install a barrier (fence) between the swimming pool and house. The pool should be fenced in on all 4 sides.
Falls	**As your baby's motor skills improve, she will fall often so protect her from injury.** **Do not** use a baby walker. Your baby may tip it over, fall out of it, fall down the stairs, or get to places where she may be injured. When your baby is on a high surface (eg, changing table, couch, bed), always place one hand on your baby, and **never** leave her unattended. Use gates at the top and bottom of stairways and doors. Use window guards. **Never** put a crib or playpen near a window. Use nonslip area rugs. Use a rubber mat or another nonslip device in the bathtub. Remove coffee tables with sharp edges or other hard furniture from the room where your baby plays, especially once she is able to pull herself up to stand. Stabilize or remove from tables or shelves heavy items that a child could pull down on herself—such as lamps, TV sets, VCRs. **If your child has a serious fall and is not acting normally afterward, call your health care provider or 911 (local emergency number).**
Fire, scald burns, and electrical injuries	**Do not** carry your baby and hot items at the same time. Keep hot beverages out of the baby's reach. **Do not** use placemats or tablecloths—infants and children can tug on them. Keep your baby in a safe place (such as a playpen, crib, stationary activity center, or buckled into a high chair) while you are cooking, eating, or unable to provide her with your full attention. Turn pot handles to the stove's back or side so the child can't pull down pots. Keep small appliances out of reach and unplugged. Have a fire extinguisher handy. Have working smoke detectors in your home. Maintain your hot water heater temperature at no more than 120°F. When preparing a bath, turn cold water on first, and then add hot water. Block fireplaces, space heaters, and kerosene lamps with gates or another barrier. Keep lighters and matches out of children's reach. Use safety plugs on all outlets. Install ground fault circuit interrupters in electrical outlets in bathrooms, kitchens, and laundry rooms.

Injury Prevention Basics[a], continued

Type of Injury	Prevention Measures
Fire, scald burns, and electrical injuries, cont.	**Do not** place electrical cords or extension cords where infants or children can bite or chew on them. **If your baby does get burned:** Rinse the area with cold (but not ice cold) water or place the area in cold water for a few minutes to cool it off. Do not put ice, lotion, petroleum jelly, or any topical medicine on the burn. Cover it with a clean, dry bandage or cloth and call your health care provider (or 911 if the burn is severe). Do not break any blisters that may form after the burn.
Poisoning	Store household cleaners, medicines (especially iron pills and food supplements containing iron), cosmetics, toiletries, kerosene, lighter fluid, furniture polish, turpentine, products containing lye and acids, and other chemicals in high, locked cabinets. **Do not** store these items near food. Keep all of these items in their original containers (**do not** transfer to soda or other food bottles). Use child-protective caps whenever possible. **Do not** call medicine candy. **Do not** flush old medicines down the toilet or drain since recent studies have identified trace levels of human medicines in our lakes, rivers, oceans, surface water, ground water, and even drinking water. Dispose of old medicines by returning them to your local pharmacy for proper disposal (ask your pharmacist if they have a return policy for disposal of old medicine). Otherwise, contact your health care provider or local household hazardous waste collection in the government section of your local white pages. Consult your pharmacist for ways to safely dispose of old medicines in your home trash (although this is controversial). Be sure all medicines and household products are labeled properly. Read the label before using. When giving or taking medicine, always turn on the light, check that you have the correct medicine, and read the directions to ensure correct dosing. **Do not** use syrup of ipecac. This drug was used in the past to make children vomit if they swallowed a poison. Do not make your child vomit; this is no longer recommended and can be dangerous. Place household plants out of reach—some are poisonous (check with your local poison control center or American Heart Association, Pediatric Basic Life Support Program). Keep the local (and national) poison control center phone number by your phones. Install carbon monoxide detectors in your home. **The US National Poison Control Center phone number is 800-222-1222.**
Other injuries	Keep all firearms unloaded and locked up and out of reach of children of all ages (preferably out of the house). Install safety latches on cabinets, particularly those containing sharp utensils and poisons. Make basements, utility rooms, and garages off limits.
As your child grows, check with your health care provider for more age-appropriate injury prevention information.	

[a]Courtesy of Kathleen Southerton, RNC, PhD, University Hospital, Stony Brook, New York. Adapted by permission.

parents request a box of face masks from the hospital to take home with them in the event of a family illness. This is really not helpful because once the mask is moistened from breathing, it doesn't provide much protection.

Keeping ill siblings away from their baby sister or brother can be difficult; it may be easier to keep the baby away from them. A careful explanation may help if the ill child is old enough to understand cause-and-effect relationships. Washing the sibling's hands periodically may help, but young children often do not cover their nose and mouth when they cough or sneeze. In addition to good hand washing, common sense helps prevent the spread of most illnesses.

Secondhand and Thirdhand Smoke

Secondhand smoke is exhaled smoke along with the smoke that comes from the tip of a burning cigarette, pipe, or cigar. It contains thousands of dangerous chemicals, with more than 50 of them known to cause cancer. Anytime your baby is near someone smoking she is exposed to these chemicals (as are you).

Infants and children exposed to secondhand smoke have a higher risk of serious health problems than children in nonsmoking households. Infants exposed to secondhand smoke are at increased risk of SIDS. Many preterm and chronically ill infants have residual lung disease that may worsen, or permanent lung changes may occur if exposed to secondhand smoke. Studies have shown that infants and children who breathe secondhand smoke have more ear infections, upper respiratory infections, respiratory problems such as bronchitis and pneumonia, and tooth decay. They are also at greater risk for developing allergies and asthma. Infants and children of smokers also have more colds, they cough and wheeze more, and they frequently have other symptoms, including stuffy nose, headache, sore throat, eye irritation, and hoarseness. Finally, children who grow up with parents who smoke are more likely to smoke themselves, risking later medical problems such as lung cancer, heart disease, and cataracts.

If you are breastfeeding and still smoke, consult your health care provider about smoking cessation programs. If you cannot quit, breastfeed before smoking a cigarette and delay nursing or pump and discard your breast milk after smoking a cigarette. If you've recently quit smoking and are breastfeeding, it is safe to use nicotine gum or nicotine transdermal patches while breastfeeding.

Thirdhand smoke is as hazardous as secondhand smoke. Thirdhand smoke is the contamination that remains after the cigarette has been extinguished. Thirdhand smoke is found, for example, on the clothing and furniture of a smoker and in the car where a smoker uses tobacco. Because children breathe, crawl on, touch, and put their mouths on smoke-contaminated surfaces, they are particularly susceptible to the neurotoxic compounds left behind by tobacco smoke. Smoking should be absolutely banned anyplace your child spends time, and if your baby's caregivers smoke, they should change or cover their clothing after smoking a cigarette and before resuming caregiving.

It is important to create a smoke-free environment for you, your baby, and your family. Ban smoking in your house (put a sign on your front door as a reminder if necessary) and anyplace where your baby spends time. Avoid places that are not smoke-free and be aware that secondhand and thirdhand smoke are both detrimental to your child's health and developmental potential.

Working With Your Baby's Health Care Provider

Babies with special needs usually require more vigilant watching for illness because, for these infants, a simple respiratory infection can be life-threatening. Balance this vigilance with common sense and a dose of reality. Your baby's health care providers probably explained the risks illness may present for your baby before discharge.

If your baby is a healthy NICU graduate with few or no complications, most illnesses will run their course without problems. If your baby has special needs, illness may represent a greater threat. Communicate well with your health care provider to find out when you should call about a suspected illness and to discuss plans for home treatment, examination, or rehospitalization. You need to feel that your health care provider listens to you and takes the time to answer your questions. Seeing your health care provider on a regular basis for the first few months gives you the opportunity to get answers to your questions and concerns about baby care and parenting. The health care provider also closely monitors your baby's weight gain, medical status, and development. Anticipatory guidance in the office often prevents emergency telephone calls, unnecessary trips to the office, or emergency department visits during times of anxiety.

Signs of Illness

Knowing how much care and monitoring your baby required in the NICU, you may be concerned that you won't be able to tell when your baby is getting sick at home. You'll quickly learn, though, what is and what is not normal behavior for your baby. You'll be the best person to determine when something is not right. Trust your instincts. All babies get sick, but not every illness is life-threatening.

Some signs and symptoms of illness include

- Fever (a temperature higher than 99°F [37.2°C] axillary or 100.4°F [38°C] rectally) or a low temperature (less than 97.5°F [36.4°C] axillary) that does not respond to warming efforts or is accompanied by other symptoms of illness. The rectal route is the most accurate way of assessing fever in infants between 0 to 3 months of age. Although the axillary measurement is frequently used for premature and small infants, a careful rectal measurement should be done whenever illness is suspected.

- Lack of interest in eating, or not feeding as well as usual.
- Vomiting most or all feedings (different from the usual amount, if your baby has reflux and especially if the vomitus is green, bloody, or projectile).
- Frequent watery stools (usually more than 5 per day) that soak into the diaper.
- A decrease in wet diapers.
- Behavior that is "just not right" (for example, less activity than usual, more sleeping, or more difficulty awakening).
- Difficulty breathing (breathing may be faster and harder, and your baby may draw in the chest muscles [called *retractions]* with each breath) or noisy breathing.
- More crying and irritability than usual (normal means of calming and comforting don't work) or refusal to sleep.
- Change in color: pale, bluish, or marbled-looking (mottled) appearance.

It's important to be able to recognize when your baby is not acting like herself, but you aren't expected to be the doctor. When you have concerns about illness, call your health care provider. Most offices expect calls from concerned parents and have experienced nurses to help you. Don't be shy, but be ready to supply the following information:

- Baby's name, age, and last appointment date and any concerns noted at that time
- Why you suspect that your baby is ill
- Baby's temperature and your method of measurement (axillary or rectal)
- Current medications, any new medications or recently discontinued medications, and recent immunizations
- Anything else your doctor should know (for example, illnesses in the family or at child care, whether your baby has shown these symptoms before, and what seemed to work last time)

Giving Medications: Missed or Vomited Doses

If your baby must continue on one or more medications at home, you need to know the name, the purpose, the dose (how much), the possible side effects, when to give, and how to administer each medication to your baby. The nurse should have given you this information in writing at discharge. Tack it to your bulletin board for handy reference and keep a copy in your purse.

Give all medications as directed by your baby's health care provider. Most medications work best when a specific level is maintained in the body. Missing one dose of a medication is usually not a problem, however. If you do forget a dose or if your baby vomits shortly after you give a dose, give the normal dose of the medication at the next regularly scheduled time. Some health care providers instruct you to repeat the dose once if your baby vomits within 15 minutes after receiving it. If you did not do so before discharge, check with your baby's doctor or nurse before repeating a dose because *some medications should not be repeated under any circumstances. Never* try to make up for a missed or vomited dose by doubling or increasing the next dose.

Vomiting is a common potential side effect of many of the medications given to babies. It's a sign that there may be too much of the medication in the baby's body or in the blood. Vomiting may also occur if the baby is ill with a stomach virus. Call your health care provider if your baby misses or vomits 2 regularly scheduled doses or if she begins to vomit more feedings than usual. A blood test to check the level of the medication in your baby's body may be needed. Also notify your doctor if your baby experiences any of the potential adverse side effects associated with a medication.

Appendix B contains information about common medications prescribed for infants, including potential side effects.

Don't forget these basic rules about medications.

- Keep all medications out of the reach of children. This is especially important if you have toddlers at home.
- Use a standard pharmaceutical measuring spoon, cup, or dropper to measure medications. Do not use your regular silverware or household measuring spoons to estimate a dosage.
- Do not give your baby nonprescription medicines without consulting your baby's health care provider; especially over-the-counter cough and cold syrups that may have side effects dangerous to your baby.
- Fever is a sign of illness that should not be masked by medicine. Fever reducers such as acetaminophen (Tylenol) or ibuprofen (Advil) should not be given to infants younger than 3 months without consulting a health care provider first. If your health care provider recommends a fever reducer, the AAP recommends that acetaminophen be given to infants younger than 6 months, and ibuprofen for infants older than 6 months. Never give your baby aspirin.
- Do not use old prescription medicines or another child's prescription medicine.
- Find out how to store the medication. For example, some medicines require refrigeration. Other medicines should be stored in a locked, childproof cabinet.
- Always use child-resistant safety caps.
- Do not administer medications in the dark. Be sure you have enough light to read the label, measure the dose, and see that your baby actually receives the medication.

The Biggest Adjustment of Your Life

"I went back to work two weeks after Katie's birth. I finished my maternity leave two months later, when Katie came home from the hospital. That's when we really needed our time together."

Having your baby home at last can seem overwhelming. Trying to establish a home routine while at the same time meeting the unpredictable demands of your baby can be exhausting. There just don't seem to be enough hours in the day.

Amid caring for your baby, making time for your other children, and attending to your partner, it's easy to forget your own basic care needs. Remember that you need to get a haircut once in a while, visit the dentist, and get some exercise. Take advantage of trustworthy volunteers who are willing to watch your baby occasionally so that you can take care of your personal needs.

Even though time alone may be short, partners also need to make time for each other if they are to successfully meet the challenge of caring for a NICU graduate. Unfortunately, the divorce rate among parents of NICU graduates is 30% above the average. One father of a NICU graduate with special needs offers this advice: "Communication is the most important thing between parents. Talk to each other, ask questions and, above all, listen to each other. Share everything and trust your instincts. This will help you get through even the most difficult times."

Special Care for Technology-Dependent Infants

Studies have shown that the discharge of a healthy preterm infant is extremely stressful for most families. The added demands of a chronically ill or technology-dependent infant can intensify this stress and even permanently change the family structure. Parents who wanted to keep their families intact spearheaded the movement to care for infants with special needs at home. But the trade-offs for these families are many.

Infants who are technology dependent most commonly require cardiorespiratory monitoring, respiratory support, or nutritional support in the home. The homecoming of a technology-dependent baby can produce mixed emotions in parents. It's exciting to have your baby home at last and your family reunited. It's also frightening and fatiguing to have to constantly attend to your baby's complex needs.

You may feel overwhelmed, isolated, and exhausted. Not only do you need to manage your baby's care, but you have to understand the equipment, deal with the many people

A Night in the Life of a Special Child

Somewhere in a far-off place, people sleep through the night and wake to a ringing alarm clock. In our house, the alarm can ring or buzz loudly no matter what the clock says. Our little one, and I do mean little, has wriggled free of his monitor's leads again. I sleepily push the wrong button on the monitor, and the intermittent sound changes to a never-ending wail. Oops! My spouse squints open one eye. I smile sorrowfully, shaking my head with guilt, and with open hands pantomime what stupidity it took to set the whole thing off. She squints and covers her ears, burrowing under the covers.

I walk the few steps to David's crib and check wires, leads, baby. The sound continues…. It may never stop…. Then there is silence. But I turn to see my wife holding the monitor's buttons to still the alarm.

My "Sorry, Honey" follows her back to bed, and I am left standing alone.

I touch the lamp to read the daily log sheet, and bright light fills the room, causing me to wince. Even my son turns and covers his eyes with his little hands. Now I have two of them, mother and son, "night-burrowing light eschewers," and I have to ask myself, "Why am I not in bed?" I read the log and it says why. It's time to feed David.

I lean heavily on the rail going downstairs to the kitchen, finding that late-night stiffness, as usual, ends with the last step downward. I think of mixing the formula, but after checking the refrigerator, I am rewarded with a prepared bottle. This means a quick heating, and I am back upstairs. But did I turn off the lights? Back down I go, and up. Did I make sure the refrigerator was closed? This time I check everything and then thump back up the stairs with the bottle…. "Bottle? Where's the bottle?" Up from the kitchen again, I am now a proven competitor in Late-Night Stair Aerobics. Leaning on the crib for support as I gasp for oxygen, I find the angelic David asleep, making cute little facial expressions while his daddy wonders why the room seems so warm.

In any event, little David must be fed. "Come on, Son, try the bottle this time!" But David only opens his mouth to voice his refusal. One look from my wife, now "the frown that lives under the covers," and I realize that David must be fed by his feeding tube. His doctors want him to conserve energy and sleep at night, saving his nippling attempts for the daylight hours.

Actually, tube feeding a child is an easy task, taking only a little dexterity and planning. Once the feeding tube syringe is attached, maneuvering the already-uncapped bottle and pouring is simple. At night and with only a few hours' sleep, I find myself in a slow-motion comedy of errors culminating with the ever-present where-did-I-put-the-feeding-tube-cap routine. Five minutes later, I find the cap just where I left it, only slightly hidden by the written log papers.

I don't spill any this time, and David takes it all. Usually, the last 5 to 10 milliliters just won't go in. But that's when I am allowed to "plunge" the formula slowly into the baby. Another concern is that a cough, burp, or some other stomach motion can "refill" the feeding syringe, and then I must begin the feeding again. We who have mastered the feeding tube find that a little pinch to the tube will hold back the flood, much as the little Dutch boy with the dike.

A Night in the Life of a Special Child, continued

Feeding is over. David is breathing fine, and his skin color is good. His little face nuzzles his blanket. I pause and try to memorize the picture. David is quite a resilient little guy, and that's the key. Without resilience, David would not be home, would not be growing or getting better. Sure, he struggles, but life is a struggle. Together, though, we try to make it better. We try, we fail, we succeed, and the process repeats itself. It's like breathing. You don't think about it a lot. You just do it.

I yawn and smile. David's ok, and I'm tired. I try not to trip over anything, and I crawl beneath the very welcome bedcovers. I roll onto my back, and as my head touches the pillow, I wonder, "Did I turn the monitor back on?" I throw back the covers, march to the crib, and press the button. The buzzer sounds, David starts crying, and I can't shut it off. I pick up the baby to quiet him, and then there is abrupt silence again. My wife breathes heavily, with her hand on the silenced monitor. She pats David gently and signals me to return to bed. The next feeding will be her turn.

Feeding tubes, syringes, nebulizers, monitors and alarms, treatments, therapy, operations, doctors, nurses, social workers, insurance, bills, government programs, etc. Nothing seems to end. But then there are wonderful little milestones every day. David is born, he can breathe, he survives the operation, another operation, he can smile, he can suck, he can lift his head, he can even eat and wet, and these go on. I remember every day that we have been given hope, and every day that our hopes have been crushed. The memories of those earlier days fade as each day with David fills our lives with new hopes and love. I mentioned earlier that resilience was the key to David's survival, and really it's the key for us all. A lot of our resilience comes from the humor that we find even in the struggles of everyday life.

Special thanks and in loving memory of Penn Hendler, who wrote this story for the first edition of this book. A photo of David during his NICU stay appears on page 427. Sadly, Mr Hendler passed away in 2008. David, 17 years old at this writing, is home schooled and is about to get his driver's permit! According to his mother, David loves to ride horses and is involved in a church youth group. He enjoys bowling, girls, and Playstation—not necessarily in that order!

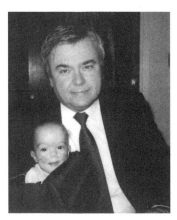 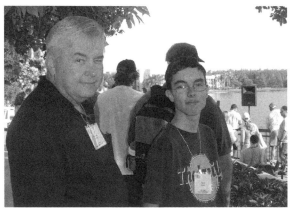

involved in your baby's care, perhaps care for other children, manage career demands, and try to restore some semblance of a normal life.

You cannot do this all alone. Your hospital discharge planning team should have identified community resources available to you and helped you contact them (see also Appendix D). The ability to find resources from the Internet has also helped families with special needs. However, for the safety of your baby and your family, it is important to make sure that agencies found on the Internet are legitimate (licensed and insured, registered with the Better Business Bureau and other agencies your state uses to ensure safety). Use all of the resources available to you. They may provide financial assistance, social services, and personal support.

This section explains some of the devices commonly used in home care. Although the information provided here was current at the time of publication, home care technology is constantly changing. To stay up to date on what is available for your baby, continue to ask questions of your baby's health care providers.

Apnea Monitor

Infants may require cardiorespiratory monitoring in the home for a variety of problems that affect breathing. Apnea monitors do not prevent SIDS and are not prescribed for that purpose (see box below). Because apnea is relatively common in preterm infants, it is the focus of this section.

Apnea is any pause in breathing (respirations) and may cause oxygen desaturation (too little oxygen available to the tissues). Bradycardia is a slowing of the heart rate below what's normal for the baby's age and may be accompanied by cyanosis (a blue color of the

Home Cardiorespiratory Monitoring[a]

- Home cardiorespiratory monitoring should not be prescribed to prevent SIDS.
- Monitoring may be warranted for premature infants who are at high risk of recurrent episodes of apnea, bradycardia, and hypoxemia after hospital discharge.
- Monitoring may be warranted for infants who are technology dependent (tracheostomy, continuous positive airway pressure), have unstable airways, have rare medical conditions affecting the regulation of breathing, or have symptomatic chronic lung disease.
- If a monitor is prescribed, then the monitor should be equipped with an event recorder.
- Parents should be advised that home monitoring does not prevent sudden, unexpected deaths in infants.
- Pediatricians should continue to promote proven practices that decrease the risk of SIDS— supine sleep position, safe sleeping environments, and elimination of exposure to tobacco smoke.

[a]From: American Academy of Pediatrics Committee on Fetus and Newborn. Apnea, sudden infant death syndrome, and home monitoring. *Pediatrics*. 2003;111:914–917.

lips or mucous membranes). Before discharge, the medical team will have ruled out other physiologic causes for your baby's apnea, such as anemia, gastroesophageal reflux disease, bronchospasm related to underlying bronchopulmonary dysplasia, or seizures.

Babies diagnosed with apnea of prematurity are often treated in the NICU with medications such as theophylline or caffeine, which help stimulate the respiratory center in the brain. Babies who have frequent episodes of apnea and bradycardia are not discharged, even with an apnea monitor, until the episodes resolve or become less severe. In most cases, babies outgrow apnea and bradycardia. Clinical observation usually determines whether your baby is breathing well enough on her own to be discharged safely. Newer NICU monitors are able to document breathing and heart rate trends over time, which also validates readiness for discharge.

Some units may perform a sleep study, also called *polysomnography, pneumocardiogram,* or *pneumogram,* before discharge to monitor your baby's breathing and heart rate more over a 12- or 24-hour period. A pneumogram uses a monitor similar to your baby's cardiorespiratory monitor but with additional channels that record your baby's heart rate, respirations, airflow through the nose, and oxygen saturation. If gastroesophageal reflux is suspected as a cause of apnea and/or bradycardia, an additional probe is used to record the acidity of secretions in the esophagus. The baby is attached to this special monitor for a specified period, usually overnight, and specially trained personnel analyze the results. This may help determine the sequence of events that leads to, or triggers, an apneic/bradycardic episode. Institutions vary in their use and interpretation of pneumograms (see also Chapter 15). Many hospitals do not use them at all, but rely heavily on your baby's clinical history (recent episodes) to determine the need for home apnea monitoring.

If the baby is still having significant apneic, bradycardic, or desaturation episodes and is otherwise ready for discharge, a home apnea monitor is ordered from an outside company (sometimes referred to as a *vendor* or a *durable medical equipment [DME] company)* and delivered to the hospital before your baby's discharge. Your discharge planner, case manager, or social worker coordinates this process. The vendor instructs parents in the use of the apnea monitor before the baby's discharge and provides an instruction manual and a phone number for monitor problems once you are home. The vendor should encourage parents to ask questions.

Some hospitals require that parents spend a night rooming-in with their baby before discharge to ensure that the monitor is working properly and that the parents feel comfortable and competent in its operation. Rooming-in is also excellent for practicing the routine care, feedings, and other specialty care (such as medication administration) your baby may need (see Chapter 15). You will learn how to respond to monitor alarms and when to notify your doctor about unusual events. You will also have a chance to get to know your baby's behavior on a 24-hour basis, with nurses and doctors nearby to answer questions.

If your baby has come home with an apnea monitor, you'll want to use it whenever you or your baby is sleeping and when you are busy. It's acceptable to take the monitor off when you're playing with your baby during more alert periods and when you're bathing your baby. This gives her skin a break from the belt that secures the monitor (see figure below). The belt can irritate her skin, especially when the weather is warm. If electrodes are used in place of a belt, they should be changed according to the schedule stated by your health care provider. Because electrodes are adhesive, removing them too frequently, or keeping them in the same place too long, can also irritate your baby's skin.

With advances in monitoring technology in the hospital and improvements in management of apnea of prematurity in general, fewer babies are actually being discharged with home apnea monitors today than a decade ago. When babies are sent home on monitors, parents are often relieved. It makes them feel more secure. After about a week, though, they're ready to throw the monitor out of the window because false alarms are driving them crazy. False alarms are usually set off by abdominal breathing or by a loose belt or incorrectly placed monitor electrodes (leads). The frequency of false alarms tends to increase as a baby grows older and becomes more active. Ignoring the alarms or assuming them to be false can be potentially dangerous.

Health care providers may ask you to keep a log (record) of alarms at home to help them determine when to discontinue monitoring and/or medications. Most babies who come home on both monitor and medications are allowed to outgrow the dose of medication, provided the apnea and bradycardia episodes diminish and then stop. When your baby has been free of apnea and bradycardia for a designated period, your health care provider will stop the medication. The apnea monitor is frequently continued for another month or two. If no episodes of apnea or bradycardia are recorded, the monitor may then be discontinued. Some health care providers will request a "monitor download" (or record of apnea and bradycardia events) from the DME company before stopping the monitor.

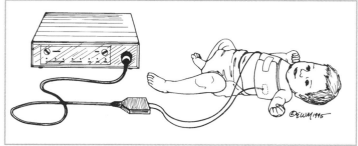

Home apnea monitor.
Use your baby's apnea monitor whenever the baby is sleeping or when you are busy. The soft belt fits over the two leads and around the baby's chest and is connected by a cable to the apnea monitor. The monitor can be removed when you are playing with your baby and at bath time.

Occasionally, a home pneumogram may be done immediately before monitor use is stopped, but this is becoming rare due to lack of payment for this diagnostic test in the home environment from insurance companies and government assistance programs.

An apnea monitor usually has 3 alarms: for apnea, slow heart rate, and fast heart rate. Your health care provider tells the equipment company what alarm settings to use for your baby. Typically, the apnea alarm is set at 15 seconds; slow heart rate, at 80 beats per minute; and fast heart rate, at 210 to 230 beats per minute. The alarm limits are lowered as your baby gets older.

Apnea monitor alarm signals are very loud. It is therefore very important that the apnea monitor not be placed directly next to your baby's head, in order to protect your baby's delicate hearing. Sometimes, the loudness of the apnea monitor alarm itself will startle the baby awake and restart breathing or stop the bradycardia that may have been the cause of the alarm in the first place. Parents sometimes wonder if this was a false alarm, but it is important to check every alarm signal regardless. Therefore, if you are in the shower or vacuuming or performing some other function that might impair your ability to hear your baby's apnea monitor alarm, you may want to use your home baby monitor (kept at the instructed distance from the apnea monitor so the frequencies do not interfere with the monitoring of your baby) as an extra amplifier for the alarm signal.

As with anything electrical, you need to take certain precautions if your infant has a home apnea monitor. Your baby should not be left unsupervised with other children. Infants have been electrocuted by older siblings placing their lead wires into a wall socket. Most monitors today have a protective covering over the lead wires to prevent this from occurring. If your baby's monitor does not have this safety feature, ask for a safer model. Even with a protective design, older children should be specifically warned not to handle the monitor.

Your health care provider will give you letters to send to your telephone company, electric company, and local emergency medical service (EMS) system, alerting them that you have an infant with special needs in your home. This puts your home on a priority list in the event of a power outage or medical emergency.

Oxygen

Babies who are medically stable on supplemental oxygen may go home on oxygen, provided that parents learn the necessary care before discharge. Bronchopulmonary dysplasia (BPD) is the most common condition of babies discharged home on oxygen. With BPD, the lungs are damaged and scarred from long periods on a ventilator and on oxygen. Smaller babies and those born earlier than 32 weeks' gestation are at the greatest risk for developing this complication. The heart and lungs of a baby with BPD must work particularly hard. Fortunately, as the baby grows, so does new lung tissue—and the damaged lung will become less of the total lung tissue.

Other reasons for sending a baby home with supplemental oxygen include

- Evidence of oxygen desaturation when breathing room air while awake, at rest, with activity, or with feedings
- Poor nippling caused by "air hunger" (baby seems to have difficulty catching her breath)
- Apnea or bradycardia that responds to supplemental oxygen
- Poor weight gain
- Airway problems, tracheostomy, or ventilator use

Supplemental oxygen is usually delivered through a nasal cannula—a small tube that fits under your baby's nose and around the head. Three types of oxygen delivery systems are used in the home.

1. **Compressed gas.** Oxygen in the gaseous state is pressurized into cylinders or tanks. A small, portable tank is delivered to the hospital, and a very large, non-portable tank is sent directly to your home. A respiratory care practitioner from the DME company will show you how to read the gauges to determine when you need to refill your tanks. The length of time between tank refillings depends on how much oxygen your baby uses and on the size of the tank. A portable E cylinder set at 1/2 liter of oxygen per minute by nasal cannula, for example, lasts about 20 hours. A smaller D cylinder lasts about 12 hours. The larger H cylinder backup tank at the same setting lasts approximately 175 hours. Larger backup tanks come in a few different sizes as well. Usually the company exchanges your large tank with a full one when the pressure in it reaches 500 pounds per square inch (psi).
2. **Oxygen concentrator.** An oxygen concentrator is a device that separates oxygen out of the air and gives it to your baby. Because a concentrator runs on electricity, a portable backup oxygen tank is necessary when your baby is not near an electrical outlet and in the event of a power outage.
3. **Liquid oxygen.** Oxygen that has been cooled to a liquid state is called *liquid oxygen.* It changes to a gas as your baby breathes it. A liquid oxygen tank takes up considerably less space than a large compressed oxygen tank, which contains oxygen in the gaseous form and is used as a backup oxygen tank. As with a compressed oxygen system, a small, portable tank is delivered to the hospital, and a larger, non-portable tank is sent directly to your home. One drawback of liquid oxygen is that it evaporates when not in use. It's also expensive and may not be covered under insurance provisions. A portable liquid oxygen tank set at 1/2 liter of oxygen per minute via nasal cannula lasts approximately 8 hours. The larger backup tank at the same setting lasts approximately 500 hours.

Regardless of the type of oxygen system in your home, certain safety precautions must be followed. Because oxygen is a highly flammable substance, there should be no smoking in a room where oxygen equipment is located. When your baby is receiving oxygen, keep her at least 6 feet away from open flames, such as heaters, fireplaces, or gas appliances with pilot lights. Oxygen tanks themselves should also be kept at least 6 feet away from an open flame, radiator, or heater. Do not use rubbing alcohol, petroleum jelly, or spray cans near a baby on oxygen. Keep the door to your baby's room open so the room is well ventilated and not stuffy. Finally, make sure the smoke detectors in your home work well, and periodically review your home fire escape plan with your family.

Your instruction in home oxygen use should have begun well before discharge to give you ample opportunity to ask questions and practice operating the equipment. Rooming-in with your baby and the oxygen equipment is an excellent way to achieve these goals. Infants who are oxygen dependent are often discharged home with an apnea monitor to alert parents of potential signs and symptoms of respiratory distress and/or arrest. Rarely, an oxygen-dependent infant will be discharged home on a pulse oximeter (a machine that measures arterial blood oxygenation). Pulse oximeters are known for frequent false alarms, especially when a baby is active, which limits their usefulness and reliability in the home setting. Therefore, most oxygen-dependent babies will have their oxygenation measured periodically by a respiratory care practitioner (using a pulse oximeter) in the home or in a follow-up clinic with their health care provider or pulmonary specialist. They may also need periodic aerosol breathing treatments (medication inhaled directly into the lungs to open breathing passages) and systemic oral medications at home. Rooming-in also provides you with the opportunity to learn these aspects of your baby's care.

Lastly, rooming-in is also a good time to take a planned "road-trip," or walk through the hospital, with your baby in a stroller and the oxygen equipment attached. You will have to travel with your baby by yourself eventually, even if it is only to go to the doctor, and this will give you an opportunity to practice managing all of the equipment attached to the stroller or carried along with your baby. At first it may seem overwhelming, but you will soon become a pro!

Letters from your health care provider will be given to you to send to your telephone company, electric company, and local EMS system alerting them that you have an infant with special needs in your home. Problems with oxygen-dependent infants can be life-threatening. You need to be able to identify potential problems right away and then immediately contact your physician, EMS system, or ambulance service.

After discharge, babies on oxygen may receive home health nursing visits or private-duty nursing if medically necessary. The amount and type of home nursing follow-up is determined by your baby's physician, your individual needs, and your health care coverage.

The decision to begin weaning a baby from oxygen depends on many factors. Some physicians begin weaning when the baby's respiratory effort decreases and oxygen saturation stabilizes. Other physicians keep the baby on oxygen to ensure continued weight gain and attainment of developmental milestones. Studies report fewer respiratory infections in infants on oxygen than in those whose oxygen saturation levels are borderline. Your doctor will take into account these and other factors unique to your baby. Weaning is usually gradual and is accompanied by physical examinations, chest x-rays, and periodic oxygenation measurements (which can be done in your home by a respiratory care practitioner). If at any time your baby fails to progress in the weaning schedule, she will be evaluated to determine the cause. Your baby will be assessed throughout the weaning process to determine her tolerance for increasingly lower levels of oxygen, until the oxygen is finally discontinued.

Feeding Tubes

Although most infants are able to take in adequate nutrition by mouth before discharge, a few cannot. Babies who have problems with their heart, lungs, brain, muscle coordination, esophagus (food pipe), or mouth (such as cleft lip and/or palate) may not be able to suck and/or swallow well. A variety of feeding tubes are available to make sure your infant receives the proper nourishment for growth and development.

Nasogastric and Orogastric Tubes

Use of a nasogastric (NG) tube is generally a temporary measure to supplement your baby's oral intake. An NG tube is often used for infants who are able to nipple some of their feeding but not enough to get adequate calories for growth and development. It is inserted into one nostril of your baby's nose and passed through the esophagus into the stomach, then taped in place for a time. When it's changed, the tube is inserted through the other nostril.

The most common problem with NG tubes is that they can cause nasal irritation and/or bleeding. If this occurs, change the NG tube to the other side until the irritated nostril heals. Rarely, if used for extended periods (usually several months), NG tubes can also cause esophageal irritation and/or erosions, and indentations in the nares. If you note blood when checking residuals or in your baby's vomit, notify the doctor immediately.

If your baby has an NG tube, you may let her nipple as much as possible by mouth first. Then you'll attach a syringe filled with the remainder of the milk to the NG tube and feed the milk to your baby slowly by gravity flow. If your baby has not fallen asleep and is not too stressed, you may want to offer a pacifier during the gavage portion of the feeding. This helps your baby to associate sucking with the feeling of getting a full stomach.

Some babies can't tolerate an NG tube because it blocks part of one nostril and may interfere with breathing. An orogastric (OG) tube, which is inserted into the baby's mouth, may be used instead. Parents who do not wish to have anything taped to their baby's face may prefer the OG tube, which is usually inserted before each feeding and removed afterward. Frequent insertion of an OG tube can stress some babies, however, and an NG tube that remains taped in place is more convenient for a baby who requires frequent gavage feedings. Both NG and OG tubes can cause gagging and vomiting on insertion and removal.

If your baby has an OG tube, you may insert the OG tube and gavage feed your baby first, then remove the tube and let her finish the feeding by sucking. If the OG tube is inserted after feeding, the baby may gag and vomit everything she worked so hard to eat. As your baby's feeding abilities improve, you will gavage feed less and allow your baby to suck more. It's preferable to end your baby's feeding with the pleasant association of sucking.

Before discharge, your baby's health care providers should have given you written instructions for gavage feedings. The instructions should cover gathering equipment, measuring and inserting the tube, checking for correct placement of the tube, checking any residual from the previous feeding, feeding your baby, removing the tube, and cleaning the equipment. Again, there should also be ample time for you to practice this procedure many times under the watchful eyes of an experienced nurse during your rooming-in experience. Some hospitals do not allow babies to go home on gavage feedings and require that the baby gets some type of gastrostomy tube—whether it be a surgical procedure performed or a percutaneous endoscopic gastrostomy tube inserted by a gastroenterologist. Each type of gastrostomy tube and procedure is described below.

Gastrostomy Tubes

An ostomy is formed by surgically creating an artificial opening in the gastrointestinal tract. This opening in the stomach (gastrostomy) or the intestine (jejunostomy, ileostomy, or colostomy) is attached to the skin covering the abdominal wall.

When health care providers anticipate that your infant will have long-term feeding difficulties, your baby will go to surgery for placement of a gastrostomy tube (GT). A rubber tube is inserted into your baby's stomach through a hole made in the stomach by a surgeon. You can then feed the prescribed amount of formula through the tube directly into your baby's stomach. If your baby has problems with gastroesophageal reflux (see Chapter 14), a surgical procedure called a *fundoplication* is sometimes done at the same time the GT is placed. A fundoplication tightens the surrounding muscle in the opening between the esophagus (food pipe) and the stomach. This prevents food from moving back up into the baby's esophagus. Feedings are usually started slowly, using the gastrostomy tube, 2 to 3 days after surgery.

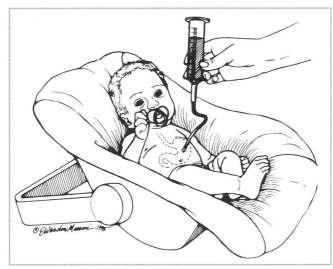

Gastrostomy tube feeding.
Your baby's gastrostomy tube ensures that she receives adequate nutrition. A feeding syringe attaches to the gastrostomy tube, and the formula flows into the baby's stomach by gravity. Most health care professionals recommend offering the baby a pacifier to suck during the feeding so that she learns to associate sucking with the feeling of a full stomach.

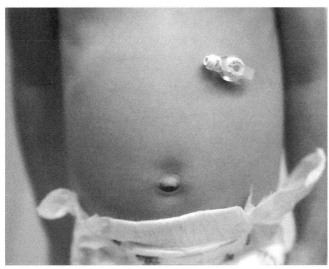

Button gastrostomy.
A button gastrostomy allows removal of the feeding tube attachment after feeding. A button is not obvious under clothing and can even be submerged at bath time.

From: Pediatrics. *2000;105:e80.*

Your baby may also eat by mouth if she can and if there are no other medical reasons not to. A GT, like an NG tube, may be used to supply what your baby cannot take by mouth. You attach a syringe filled with the remaining formula or breast milk to the GT and feed the milk to your baby slowly by gravity flow. It's beneficial to give your baby a pacifier during the GT feeding so that she learns to associate sucking with the feeling of getting a full stomach. This technique, called *nonnutritive sucking,* is particularly important for babies who cannot nipple feed at all but will accept a pacifier. When your baby's nippling ability improves to the point that she is getting adequate nutrition orally, the GT may be removed. The opening in the skin of the stomach eventually scars over without the need for further surgery or stitches.

Button Gastrostomy

If you and your doctor feel your baby may have difficulty feeding over a longer period, the GT may be converted to a button gastrostomy after your baby reaches a certain weight (usually about 4,500 grams, or 10 pounds). This procedure can usually be done in your doctor's office. Some health care providers will directly place a button gastrostomy, regardless of weight; thus bypassing the GT altogether.

A button gastrostomy allows you to remove the feeding tube attachment after the feeding. A flap, which looks similar to a valve on a beach ball when it's pushed in, then closes the button and prevents feeding loss. Button gastrostomies are less obvious under shirts and are easy to care for.

Percutaneous Endoscopic Gastrostomy Tube

If your baby has no problems with reflux and does not require surgery for a fundoplication but is a weak feeder, she may have surgery to place a percutaneous endoscopic gastrostomy (PEG) tube. Percutaneous means "through the skin." An endoscope is a floppy tube with a light on the end that is used to place the PEG tube properly through the baby's mouth and into the stomach. The tube is then advanced up out of the stomach through a small hole made through the skin of the abdomen. A PEG tube requires only a small opening (stoma) in the stomach. If long-term feeding problems are anticipated, a PEG tube may be replaced with a button gastrostomy after 2 to 3 months or when your baby weighs about 4,500 grams, or 10 pounds. As with a GT tube, some health care providers prefer to directly place a button gastrostomy, regardless of weight, bypassing use of a PEG tube.

The procedures for feeding with and care of a PEG tube are similar to those for a GT. They include gathering equipment, checking for any residual from the previous feeding, feeding your baby, removing the syringe, and cleaning the equipment. Gastrostomy, button, and PEG tube care also includes routine cleaning around the stoma (insertion site). Your doctor may order cleaning once or twice a day and as needed. You may be instructed to clean the site with a mild soap and water and/or half-strength hydrogen peroxide (full strength hydrogen peroxide can dry and irritate the skin). You should receive written instructions before discharge. Local skin irritation and drainage from the stoma site are the most common complications of GTs. If either occurs, your doctor may recommend a topical antibiotic ointment or a drying powder. Accidental removal of the tube and tube movement within the stomach are occasional complications. Accidental removal of your baby's GT is not a medical emergency. You will be taught how to replace it or instructed to call your baby's doctor if this occurs.

Continuous Feedings

Infants unable to nipple feed or handle bolus feedings (the entire feeding given at once instead of over a long period) may require continuous feedings using a feeding pump. Continuous feedings may be given through any of the feeding tubes just discussed. Continuous feedings are also sometimes used at night to supplement daytime bolus or bottle feedings. This technique may be used for infants unable to get adequate nutrition by either of these forms alone. Fundoplication (see Gastrostomy Tubes on page 516) may be needed to lessen the potential risk of aspiration. You should have received instruction in the use of the equipment before your baby's discharge. Equipment and supplies for home tube feedings, as well as home nursing follow-up, are also arranged before discharge based on your baby's medical condition, your individual needs, and your health care coverage.

Ileostomy and Colostomy

An ileostomy or a colostomy is most commonly performed after surgical removal of a portion of the small or large intestine, respectively. One of these procedures may have been necessary if your baby had necrotizing enterocolitis (NEC) (see Chapter 9), an imperforate anus (or anal atresia), Hirschsprung disease, an intestinal obstruction, or some other problem with the gastrointestinal tract. In both of these procedures, an opening (stoma) is made in the abdominal wall, and a portion of the intestine is brought to the surface and attached to the skin. Your baby's bowel movements will come through this hole instead of from her rectum. The stoma is covered with a bag or pouch to collect the stool, which is more liquid than what you would find in a diaper. Ostomies are often temporary. When your baby is big enough and the intestines are healed enough, the cut sections may be surgically put back together again.

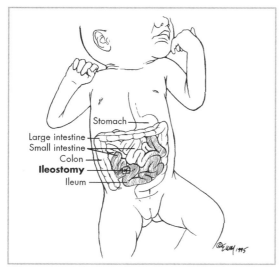

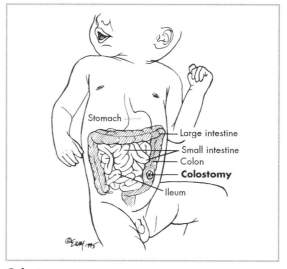

Ileostomy.
A portion of the small intestine is brought to the surface and attached to the skin. The baby's bowel movements will come through this hole instead of through her rectum. A plastic bag fits over the stoma and collects the stool.

Colostomy.
A portion of the large intestine is brought to the surface and attached to the skin. As with an ileostomy, the stoma of the colostomy is covered by a disposable plastic bag that collects the baby's bowel movements.

Before discharge, you were taught how to empty and change your baby's ostomy bag and do skin care. Post the written instructions you were given on your bulletin board for reference. Basic care is reviewed here. Hold the opened bottom of the ostomy bag over a container to empty the stool, or use a large syringe to empty stool that is more liquid. Use a squeeze bottle or large syringe filled with cool water to rinse the stool out of the bag. Then dry the bottom of the bag and close it with the twist tie provided or with a rubber band. Ostomy bags need to be changed routinely every few days or if leaking occurs. Once the old bag is removed, wash the skin with a mild soap and water, rinse and pat dry, and inspect the skin for redness or sores. Antibiotic ointments or adhesive powders and pastes are sometimes needed to remedy problems of skin irritation, bleeding, or leakage of stool. Call your health care provider if these problems persist. Ostomy bags are attached to adhesive backings cut to fit around your baby's stoma. The new bag fits over the stoma and sticks with adhesive backing onto the skin.

Equipment and supplies for home ostomy care and home nursing follow-up are arranged before discharge based on your baby's medical condition, your individual needs, and your health care coverage.

Tracheostomy

A tracheostomy is a surgical opening made through your baby's neck and into the windpipe (trachea). Your baby then breathes through a tube inserted in this artificial

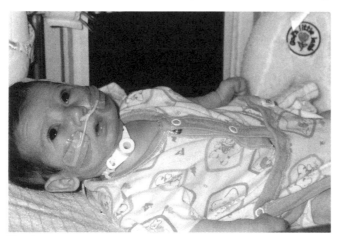

Tracheostomy.
A tracheostomy is a surgical opening made through the baby's neck and into the windpipe (trachea). The baby breathes through a tube inserted into this opening instead of through her nose or mouth.

opening instead of through the nose or mouth. The most common reasons babies require a tracheostomy include

- Birth defects that affect the airway
- Upper airway obstructions, such as tracheomalacia (a soft airway that collapses with respirations) or subglottic stenosis (a narrowing of the trachea caused by a congenital defect, prolonged ventilation, or repeated intubations)

- The need for continued ventilation (ventilator dependence)
- Neuromuscular disorders that affect the ability to swallow and handle saliva, thus interfering with breathing

A tracheostomy is not always permanent. The tube may be removed once the underlying problem is corrected or your baby grows big enough and no longer needs help breathing.

Home care for a baby with a tracheostomy (or trach, pronounced "trake") is quite involved and requires a significant commitment to learning on the family's part. Having more than one family member learn tracheostomy care helps to ensure that the primary caregiver will get much-needed relief and support. This is not always possible, however, and the issue is generally addressed with your doctors, nurses, and social workers during discharge planning.

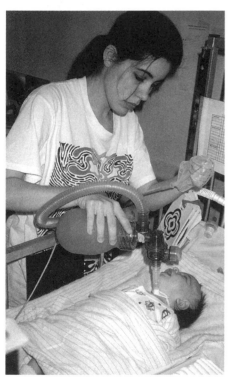

Suctioning the tracheostomy at home. This baby's mother hand-bags through the baby's tracheostomy during suctioning. When she is finished, she reattaches the tracheostomy to a home ventilator. Care of a ventilator-dependent baby requires help from many community services and a tremendous commitment on the part of the baby's family.

Home tracheostomy care includes

- Routine suctioning of the tracheostomy tube to clear the artificial airway of secretions (mucus).
- Use of a self-inflating oxygen bag (a device that, when squeezed, delivers a breath of air and/or oxygen through the tracheostomy tube) and saline (a sterile saltwater solution) to assist with breathing and secretion removal. If the tracheostomy tube is not functioning in an emergency, the baby would be ventilated with a face mask and self-inflating bag.
- Daily cleaning of the skin around the tracheostomy opening (stoma) with either mild soap and water or half-strength hydrogen peroxide (as recommended by your doctor) and assessment of the skin for irritation.
- Daily changing of the tracheostomy ties or tracheostomy tube holder.
- Routine changing of the tracheostomy tube itself (usually recommended every 1–4 weeks) or daily changing and cleaning of the inner cannula (inner cannulas are used with larger tracheostomies in older children).
- Operation and cleaning of equipment and supplies.
- Special attention to general baby care and safety because a baby with a tracheostomy cannot make any crying or cooing sounds.

Babies discharged home with a tracheostomy tube also often require some type of humidification; a home cardiorespiratory monitor to alert parents to potential problems, such as plugging or dislodgement of the tube; aerosol or breathing treatments; and medications.

At discharge, parents of babies with a tracheostomy tube learn what is normal breathing for their baby by observing and participating in the baby's care. This knowledge helps you watch for signs of breathing problems, which may include

- Irritability, restlessness, and/or sweating
- Increased respiratory rate
- Noisy respirations (grunting, gurgling, or whistling from the tracheostomy)
- Nasal flaring
- Retractions (sinking in of the chest and skin, making the breastbone and ribs visible)
- Color change (to pale, dusky, or blue)

Problems with a tracheostomy tube can be life-threatening. You need to be able to identify potential problems right away and then immediately contact your physician, EMS system, or ambulance service. Plugging of the tracheostomy with mucus, vomit, or blood requires quick thinking and fast action by the parent to prevent a life-threatening event. A clean tracheostomy tube and scissors (to cut the ties) should be taped at the head of the bed for such emergencies. Before discharge, care providers should have discussed actions to take in emergencies, and you may even have been asked to play-act your responses. It's also important that you know how to ventilate your baby using a self-inflating resuscitation bag or by mouth-to-tracheostomy tube ventilations. For acute emergencies, parents should also know how to perform infant CPR modified for a baby with a tracheostomy. Post your emergency instructions on a kitchen cupboard or closet door or at the head of your baby's bed.

The more you learned about your baby's tracheostomy care and other needs through rooming-in and independent caretaking during your infant's hospital stay, the smoother the transition to home will be. Again, prior to discharge, a planned "road-trip" throughout the hospital should be recommended during the rooming-in period so you get experience transporting your baby and all of her necessary equipment independently before you actually have to do it on your own.

Your health care provider will work closely with the specialist who placed your baby's tracheostomy tube to determine the timing of weaning and decannulation (removal of the tube). Once your baby is big enough or the problem that necessitated the tracheostomy is corrected, the weaning process may begin. Frequently, your baby will be weaned to a tube that is a size smaller than the one in place or be allowed to outgrow the tube in place without changing to a larger size. If she is able to tolerate the smaller tube for the designated trial period (weeks or months), then she may be weaned to the next smaller size, if necessary. As your baby gradually begins to breathe around the smaller tube, you may be able to hear her make sounds. Before decannulation occurs, your baby's tracheostomy may be capped to see if she can tolerate the full work of breathing on her own. Capping is often done in the hospital overnight so that your baby's respiratory rate, heart rate, and oxygen saturation can be monitored. A blood gas analysis of your baby's oxygenation and carbon dioxide levels may also be performed. If all parameters remain within normal limits for your baby, the tracheostomy tube will be removed. The hole in the neck is usually left to heal gradually on its own without surgical repair. It will leave a small scar.

Home Ventilator

"No matter what happens to your baby at home, you have enough time to make a plan. Stop and think things through in an emergency. Don't run; walk. Don't panic; direct someone to help. When you use the first moments of an emergency to get organized, you save precious seconds when they matter the most."

Some infants who need long-term ventilatory support can be cared for at home. There are several important factors to consider regarding the practicality of home ventilation, however.

First, other than being unable to wean from the ventilator, is your baby basically stable? Her ventilator settings should be stable for at least 1 week using an inspired oxygen concentration of 40% or less. Is the disease or condition causing the need for ventilation under control? Your baby's doctor will determine the answer to this question.

Second, what are your own feelings? A 24-hour-per-day, 7-day-per-week commitment can place a tremendous strain on even the best-functioning families. A parent and at least one other person (parent or other family member or home health nurse) should be trained in home ventilator care prior to discharge. Sometimes the decision must be made in the best interest of the family as a whole, not necessarily in the best interest of one member. You should not feel pressured into taking your ventilator-dependent infant home. Skilled nursing facilities that accept ventilator-dependent children may be available in your area.

Third, is your home suited for ventilator care? Do you have enough space to handle the equipment and supplies? Are there enough electrical outlets? The company supplying the ventilator and supplies can assess your home's electrical capability.

Finally, what community support systems are available in your area? These may include appropriately trained home nurses, 24-hour servicing of equipment and supplies, emergency medical services, other support persons to provide backup or respite care, early intervention programs, and financial resources. Home health nursing or private duty nursing services are recommended for at least 16 hours per day on discharge in order to assist the family with safe transition and ongoing education of the infant at home. Ideally, members of the home nursing agency will be able to come to the hospital prior to your baby's discharge for training specific to your baby's needs (some agencies will do this at no charge since most insurance companies won't cover this service). Home health nursing coverage is becoming difficult to get approved through private insurance and government assistance programs. Letters of medical necessity must be written well in advance of discharge along with home health/private duty nursing orders documenting the extensive amount of care your baby will need at home; thus justifying the need for nursing services. Your social worker or discharge planner will be responsible for getting these services approved with the help of your health care provider.

If your infant is ventilator dependent, you'll have been trained in use of a home ventilator (which is different from the NICU ventilator), but you'll also learn about tracheostomy care, use of a cardiorespiratory monitor, home oxygen therapy (possibly) and, if your baby has a feeding problem, gastrostomy care. This specialized training is usually provided through your NICU or at a transitional care facility. Training usually takes several weeks, during which you room-in with your baby to learn the necessary care. In many urban areas, only one hospital (often a children's hospital) has a home ventilator program. Your baby may have to be transferred to this hospital to spend several weeks with new health care providers who will assist with discharge teaching for you and the necessary preparations for your baby going home on a ventilator. This change of care is often difficult for parents, who must adjust to new care providers, and the NICU staff, who must say good-bye to you and your baby. It is important that the lines of communication remain open among parents and both institutions' staff members to ensure a seamless transition of care.

After discharge, you and your baby will be closely followed by a variety of services. Your baby may initially require home health or private duty nursing services for 16 to 24 hours per day. Once you are comfortable with your baby's care at home, and a backup caregiver has learned your baby's care, the home health nursing services may be decreased to daily visits. A respiratory care practitioner from the equipment supply company will do periodic ventilator checks and assist you with other equipment and supply needs. An education specialist from the early intervention program (explained in Chapter 17) may visit to do an individual family service plan.

Several doctors may follow your baby closely. Often a pediatric pulmonologist manages the ventilator care. If weaning from the ventilator becomes possible as your baby grows, it will be done in small increments as your baby can tolerate it. You, the respiratory care practitioner, and your baby's nurses will need to monitor your baby closely as she is weaned from the ventilator. Frequent visits to doctors' offices and an occasional readmission to the hospital for pulmonary function tests may also be required.

The Key: Coordination

For a technology-dependent infant, it's crucial that coordination of care continues after discharge. As a parent, you need to identify one person who will coordinate your infant's medical care now that you are home. That person most often is your primary health care provider. Teamwork is essential in caring for your special baby. Work closely with your health care professionals, and stay in close touch with your insurance case manager or social worker.

Pulling It All Together

Now that you're home at last, your feelings and family structure may be changing. The anxiety and fear about making it through each day of hospitalization are replaced by exhaustion and perhaps sleepless nights. You may be about ready to send back the baby you couldn't wait to bring home.

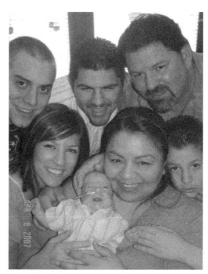

Have confidence in what you've learned about your baby's care. Identify helpful resources and use them. The challenge of establishing a home routine remains yours, however. As one mother put it, "My life has never been in such chaos, and yet it's never been more rewarding!"

Family support.
The entire family is affected by your baby's homecoming. This NICU graduate and his parents will benefit from family members eager to help with the baby's transition from hospital to home.

Chapter 17
Looking Ahead

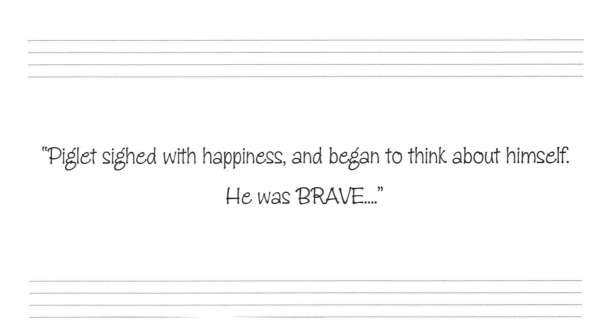

"Piglet sighed with happiness, and began to think about himself. He was BRAVE...."

TrezMarie T. Zotkiewicz, RNC-NIC, MN, APRN

The neonatal intensive care unit (NICU) experience doesn't end at discharge. Many parents describe their baby's first year of life as the longest roller-coaster ride of their lives.

The first weeks at home are filled with mixed emotions, new challenges, and changes within your family. Now that you're home and settling into a routine, you'll begin looking to the future.

Developing Normally

Having a baby in the NICU is frightening. Your initial concern is survival. Once your baby is medically stable, though, it's only natural to wonder, "Will my baby be normal?" This section addresses medical and environmental risk factors that can affect your child's development and also looks at the potential for behavioral and learning problems.

Perinatal Risk Factors

Although it's difficult to talk in absolutes about developmental outcome among NICU graduates, it's safe to say that most NICU infants do not have significant disabilities. Even so, many parents worry about their baby's risk of having physical and/or developmental delays, cerebral palsy, or visual or hearing losses. Studies that look at health-related outcomes during infancy and childhood show that more health problems and quality of life concerns occur in children who required NICU care versus those who did not. Usually, the lower an infant's birth weight and the more complicated the hospital course, the greater the risk of future problems. Factors related to your baby's experience in the uterus, during labor and birth, and in the early days of life that predispose infants to developmental, physical, visual, or auditory challenges include

- Prematurity (born before 37 completed weeks of gestation) and low birth weight, categorized as follows
    - Low birth weight (LBW): 5 pounds, 8 ounces (2,500 grams)
    - Very low birth weight (VLBW): less than 3 pounds, 5 ounces (1,500 grams)
    - Extremely low birth weight (ELBW): less than 2 pounds, 4 ounces (1,000 grams).
- Intraventricular hemorrhage (IVH) (bleeding in the brain) and periventricular leukomalacia (brain cysts that can result from brain injury)
- Perinatal asphyxia, with or without seizures and brain damage; hypoxic-ischemic encephalopathy (see Chapter 10)

- Bronchopulmonary dysplasia (BPD) (also called *chronic lung disease)* and long-term mechanical ventilation with prolonged need for supplemental oxygen
- Other chronic illnesses, such as short bowel or short gut syndrome resulting from necrotizing enterocolitis or congenital abnormalities of the intestine
- Significant intrauterine growth restriction fetus/small for gestational age newborn
- Microcephaly (head too small) or macrocephaly (head too large) for gestational age
- Multiple birth defects and known genetic syndromes, especially defects of the head and neck
- Neonatal infections: TORCH (toxoplasmosis, other agents, rubella, cytomegalovirus, herpes simplex) or other infections such as group B streptococcus, human immuno-deficiency virus, central nervous system infections, and others
- Abnormal neonatal neurologic examination: hypotonia (low muscle tone or limp) or hypertonia (high muscle tone or stiffness) for gestational age
- Failure to thrive/grow
- Hyperbilirubinemia (jaundice) requiring exchange transfusion
- Receiving an ototoxic medication (one with side effects that can negatively affect hearing, such as certain antibiotics) for more than 5 days
- Substance abuse during pregnancy
- An extended NICU stay

You'll find more information on most of these factors in Chapters 8 through 10.

Environmental Risk Factors

A baby's medical problems are not the only factors that play a role in determining his developmental outcome. The family's socioeconomic status also influences childhood development. The risk of developmental delays and other health problems is greater for both term and preterm infants on the lower rungs of the socioeconomic ladder than for those from more affluent families. The significant financial pressures and other stressors that less-advantaged families must face can affect the development of their children.

The caregiver's educational level and the quality of the care given also influence a baby's development. If the mother is younger than 16 years, or if there is a parent history of mental retardation, psychiatric disorder, or substance abuse, then the baby is not only at risk for developmental delay, but also inadequate parenting and child abuse. The amount of attention and stimulation a baby receives at home and the types of opportunities a baby has to learn new skills all play a part in developmental outcome.

The impact of your baby's environment on his development can't be emphasized enough. Infants with known developmental risk factors, such as IVH, may develop normally with early intervention and appropriate stimulation at home. Conversely, babies discharged as "well preemies" may return to follow-up clinics with significant delays, in part because of lack of learning opportunities at home. An environment rich in learning opportunities is of utmost importance to your baby's developmental progress.

Developmental tests are often used to measure a child's mental, social, speech and language, and physical skills. Activities such as playing pat-a-cake, using a spoon to stir pretend coffee, pointing to body parts on a doll, drawing, and playing with simple puzzles are used to elicit responses that help testers determine a child's developmental progress. But children who have never played pat-a-cake or put together a puzzle may fail these parts of developmental tests because they have never had the opportunity to learn these skills. This type of developmental delay is related to lack of learning opportunities provided by parents and other caregivers—and is preventable.

Potential for Behavior Problems

Behavioral challenges may be evident in early infancy. Infants who are preterm or chronically ill are often irritable and show unpredictable feeding, crying, and sleeping patterns. They are less responsive than their well, term counterparts and therefore require understanding of their behavioral cues to prevent overstimulation.

Not all premature or chronically ill babies have behavior problems in childhood, but some do. Behavior problems seen in early childhood include frequent temper tantrums, over-aggressiveness in play, hyperactivity, and exaggerated separation anxiety. These behavioral problems may be attributable to sensory over-sensitivity (for example, being extra sensitive to loud sounds or certain textures that are touched or eaten), or may be a result of problems with movement or muscle tone. As these children reach school age, their behaviors may worsen or improve with maturity. Some may have discipline problems because of a short attention span, hyperactivity, and aggressive or disorganized behavior. Others may show more introverted behavior marked by extreme shyness and passivity, anxiety, or depression. Close follow-up and teamwork with your child's teachers, counselors, and health care provider is important if your child is to reach his full potential.

"Why must parents use their children's growth and development for comparison and competition? My child is her own person, and her achievements belong to her, not to me, and not to anyone else."

Potential for Learning Problems

Some NICU graduates experience learning problems. Risk factors include VLBW (less than 3 pounds, 5 ounces), ELBW (less than 2 pounds, 4 ounces), neonatal complications, and a poor environment for growing and learning. Some children may have problems with drawing and writing, difficulty with language and following directions, or reading comprehension, and may have attention-deficit/hyperactivity disorders. Children who experience problems such as these in school may require special education classes to facilitate learning. Approximately 50% of VLBW infants receive some form of special education in school. In the ELBW population, 50% to 70% have learning disabilities requiring special education even if they have a normal IQ (greater than 85).

You play an important role in determining your child's potential. Knowing what resources are available and using them is just as important for enhancing your child's development as for preventing medical complications. Your child also needs to be loved, nurtured, and made to feel important. You don't have to purchase every developmental toy on the market. Children can learn a lot from the people around them and from an environment that's naturally rich with learning opportunities for a curious mind.

Potential for Vision Problems

Once again, the tiniest and most premature babies are most at risk for future vision problems. Infants at risk are typically those that have a history of retinopathy of prematurity (ROP). Fifty percent of infants diagnosed with ROP in the NICU show decreased visual acuity, myopia (nearsightedness), glaucoma (an increase in eye pressure), strabismus (crossed eyes), and amblyopia (a lazy eye) in early childhood.

More than likely, if your baby was significantly premature, he will need glasses at some point in his life, since more than 85% of preterm infants and children become myopic (nearsighted)—20% by 1 year of age. For babies with severe (threshold) ROP, most will have serious visual impairments, even with glasses, resulting in developmental challenges as well. The potential for late retinal detachment is even greater in this population. And finally, blindness has been reported in approximately 6% of ELBW infants.

Fortunately, recent advances in the treatment of ROP have greatly minimized the number of infants with severe ROP and/or blindness. Infants born after 28 weeks weighing more than 3 pounds, 5 ounces (1,500 grams) have a very low risk of ROP compared with infants born weighing less than 2 pounds, 4 ounces (1,000 grams). Occasionally, LBW infants (weighing less than 2,500 grams) will develop ROP as a result of an unstable NICU course. Visual problems may also occur as a result of IVH, periventricular leukomalacia (PVL), neonatal infections, or other neonatal medical conditions. Cortical visual impairment or blindness may result from a serious IVH or other injury to the brain. In other words, the eyes may be able to "see," but the brain cannot interpret or understand the picture being sent.

The American Academy of Pediatrics has a protocol for routine ophthalmology screening of premature infants based on gestational age that is done at regular intervals while in the NICU. Follow-up visual examinations must be continued on schedule once your baby goes home in order to optimize functional vision and minimize problems. These follow-up eye appointments will ideally be scheduled for you prior to your baby's discharge. It is important that you know when your baby's follow-up eye appointments are due so you do not miss any appointments. Timing is everything! It is not acceptable to wait a week or two past the scheduled due date for your baby's eye appointments. For babies with suspected cortical vision problems, developmental follow-up and early intervention referrals will also be necessary.

Potential for Hearing Problems

Low birth weight infants are at increased risk for both sensorineural hearing loss (from damage to the sensory nerves that supply the inner ear) and conductive hearing loss (a problem conducting sound waves through the outer ear, tympanic membrane [eardrum], or middle ear [ossicles]). Studies show that 2% to 3% of LBW infants and between 1% to 9% of ELBW infants will have a hearing loss significant enough to require hearing aids and assisted communication. This increases to 11% of ELBW infants if conductive hearing losses are included.

The potential for hearing impairments is not restricted to premature or LBW infants. In fact, infants diagnosed with persistent pulmonary hypertension of the newborn, perinatal asphyxia, significant hyperbilirubinemia, or infections, or who received ototoxic drugs, have an even higher risk for hearing loss. All VLBW and ELBW infants, along with those neonates with medical conditions or risk factors (listed previously) should have a brain stem auditory evoked response newborn hearing screening before 1 month corrected age or prior to discharge from the NICU.

If your baby has a mild hearing loss, he will have difficulty hearing soft or distant speech. Because most infants are held close, this is usually not a problem, or may not even be apparent, until he becomes a toddler. A hearing aid may be needed at that time. If your baby has a moderate hearing loss, he may understand face-to-face conversation, but have trouble with group discussions. Children with severe hearing losses can only hear very loud sounds and close voices. Hearing aids and speech therapy work best for children with moderate to severe hearing loss.

Lastly, children with profound hearing loss will only perceive very loud sounds or vibrations. Hearing aids do not work as well for these children, so ask your health care provider if your child would be a candidate for a cochlear implant (a device surgically implanted in the inner ear that picks up sounds from the environment and directly stimulates the auditory nerve). Your child would actually wear a "receiver" device on his body that electronically codes incoming sounds and transmits them to the cochlear implant. The National Institutes of Health, the American Medical Association, and most hearing specialists recognize cochlear implantation as standard treatment for profound deafness.

Children with hearing impairments often have associated speech and language problems. The more severe the hearing loss, the greater the risk for speech and language delays. They are also at risk for education failure as they enter preschool and school. Graduates of the NICU who are not performing well in school should have their hearing rechecked in the event anything has changed since their last evaluation. Since there are a variety of hearing aids, an audiologist will assist you to find the best one for your child. Likewise, there are several approaches to language education for children with hearing loss. A speech and language therapist (often called a *speech pathologist)* will assist you and your child with the communication skills necessary to support your child's optimal development.

Potential for Cerebral Palsy

Cerebral palsy (CP) is the most common cause of abnormal posture and movement in children (both term and preterm births). It is a diagnosis that many parents of premature infants fear. Cerebral palsy does not mean there is a problem with intelligence, although some children with CP will also have intellectual disability and/or learning disabilities.

The actual incidence of CP in the general population is a little more than 3 cases per 1,000 live births. Prematurity and multiple births are 2 of the leading risk factors for CP, followed by perinatal asphyxia and intrauterine infection. However, in most of the cases of CP no direct cause can be found. The incidence of CP in prematurity is once again higher in the smallest and most premature babies, with a prevalence as high as 20% in the smallest ELBW infant to 6% to 8% of LBW infants. See Chapter 9 for a discussion of CP related to prematurity. Chapter 10 discusses CP related to brain injury due to other causes.

Cerebral palsy is defined as an abnormality of posture or movement generated from non-progressive damage to the brain. The child's difficulties, however, often change over time during early infancy and childhood. Spastic diplegia, or stiff muscle tone of all 4 extremities with more involvement of both legs and feet, is the most common form of CP among premature infants. Many premature infants with spastic diplegia have normal to near-normal intelligence.

Occasionally, one arm and hand may be uncoordinated as well, which some clinicians call *spastic triplegia* (stiffness of 3 extremities). Spastic quadriplegia is when all 4 extremities, along with the head and trunk, are fairly equally affected. This is the most severe form of CP and can often be diagnosed before the first year of life. Spastic quadriplegia is frequently associated with intellectual disability.

When muscle tone changes (from moment to moment) from too low (like a noodle) to too high (stiff), this is called *athetoid CP*. Children with athetoid CP often have difficulty with mobility and posture and have frequent involuntary, often jerky, movements. They often need a wheelchair, but have normal to above-average intelligence.

Children diagnosed with ataxic CP may look normal to the untrained eye. If you did not know the child's birth history, you might think he was just clumsy, uncoordinated, or had poor balance. Children with ataxic CP often look normal until they have to walk on an uneven surface (very deliberately) or run (which may be on their toes).

The diagnosis of CP is generally not made until the premature infant is 12 to 18 months corrected age unless the child's problems are severe. The same is true for term infants. As you can see, the characteristics of CP can range from mild muscle tone abnormalities with normal or above-average intelligence to severe physical disability and intellectual disability. Severe lung disease, Grade III through IV IVH or PVL, and severe ROP are independent risk factors that increase the likelihood and severity of CP in VLBW children. Cerebral palsy is also more prevalent and more severe in male infants.

All children diagnosed with neonatal hypertonia or who are at risk for CP need close developmental follow-up and referrals into early intervention programs. Occupational therapy and/or physical therapy may be prescribed at hospital discharge since it takes some time before early intervention programs get started. As a parent of a child with special needs, you may have to advocate to get these needed services for your child.

In addition to a developmental pediatrician or specialist, your child may be referred to neurology and/or orthopedics once a diagnosis of CP is made. Various treatment options are available for children with CP to help decrease the spasticity. These include proven treatments such as physical therapy, which may or may not be combined with Botox injections, braces, and heel tendon releases (surgery), and adjunct therapy such as horseback riding. School-aged children diagnosed with CP will often receive "adaptive physical education" aimed at "adapting" the sport or physical activity to include the child to the best of his ability. Consult your health care provider before trying any new therapies claiming to "cure" CP, such as hyperbaric oxygen therapy, which may be dangerous, is extremely expensive and has been shown not to be effective in improving outcomes of children with CP. It is important that you work with your health care provider to find the best treatment option that will minimize the effects of CP and other developmental delays.

Potential for Intellectual Disability

Intellectual disability (sometimes referred to as *mental retardation)* is defined as "impairment of adaptive function and a standard intelligence quotient (IQ) of more than 2 standard deviations (SD) below the mean." In other words, a child who scores less than 70 on a standard IQ test is diagnosed with mental retardation. Because the normal range for IQ scores is 85 to 115, there are varying degrees of intellectual disability. Borderline intelligence (previously called *slow learners)* is an IQ score of 70 to 85. This is not intellectual disability, and it often goes unrecognized. Moderate intellectual disability is an IQ score of 50 to 70; severe intellectual disability is an IQ score of 0 to 50. When parents hear the diagnosis of CP, they often automatically assume intellectual disability as well. Intellectual disability is a separate diagnosis that may occur with or without CP.

The percentage of infants diagnosed with intellectual disability increases as gestational age and birth weight decreases. At school age, intellectual disability is seen in 4% to 6% of LBW NICU graduates. That percentage jumps dramatically to 15% in infants born weighing between 750 to 1,499 grams and 37% in infants born weighing less than 750 grams. The incidence of term infants with an IQ score of less than 70 at school age is similar to LBW infants (6%). It should be noted that formal IQ testing cannot be done until the child is at least 3 years old. A variety of developmental testing tools are available to evaluate young infants and toddlers. Close developmental follow-up and referrals to early intervention programs are again essential in identifying and/or minimizing the effects of prematurity and the potential for developmental delay.

Optimizing Your Baby's Development

Knowing what to expect in the way of follow-up for your NICU graduate and how you can contribute to your baby's progress are important and rewarding aspects of parenting a NICU graduate. You play a vital role in your baby's growth and development.

Developmental Follow-Up

Infants with any of the neonatal factors listed earlier in this chapter may be at risk for developmental delay. At discharge from the NICU, you and your baby may be referred to a developmental follow-up clinic, often along with a referral to your community early intervention program. If your hospital does not have an infant high-risk clinic, your health care provider will be responsible for monitoring your child's development and making any necessary referrals.

Your baby's follow-up should include basic monitoring of hearing, vision, and growth, including height, weight, and head circumference. If your baby weighed less than 3 pounds, 5 ounces (1,500 grams) or had a difficult hospital course, you should expect

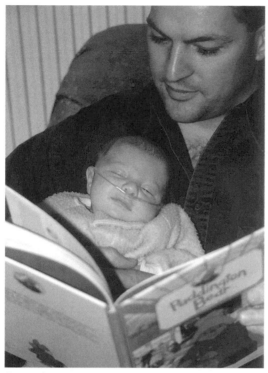

Story time.
It is never too soon to begin reading aloud to your baby.

additional developmental screening tests. If your baby weighed less than 2 pounds, 4 ounces (1,000 grams) at birth, know that he is at risk for the same health and neurodevelopmental problems as children born with LBW, but at a greater percentage and greater severity. Therefore, all LBW infants need close monitoring after discharge—paying close attention to developmental milestones for corrected age. (Corrected age is explained in Chapter 15.) They should also receive automatic referrals to early intervention programs in their area.

It is a good idea to keep your own record of your child's developmental progress. Most of the baby books available commercially have places to keep track of developmental milestones. This book should be brought to all follow-up appointments so that information can be shared with your health care provider.

Many screening tests are available, and health care professionals have individual preferences as to which they use. You may hear any of these names: the neonatal neurodevelopmental examination, the Denver Developmental Screening Test II, the Early Screening Inventory, the Battelle Developmental Inventory Screening Test, the Bayley Infant Neurodevelopmental Screener, the Bayley Scales of Infant and Toddler Development, or the McCarthy Scales of Children's Abilities (an early IQ test). Screening test results that suggest problems indicate a need for further evaluation.

Some of the specialists your baby may need to see include a developmental and/or educational specialist, physical and/or occupational therapist, neurologist, psychologist, ophthalmologist, audiologist, nutritionist, orthopedist, otolaryngologist (ear, nose, and throat doctor), and surgeon, to name a few. Your knowledge of what is normal for your baby, both medically and developmentally, will assist these professionals in enhancing your baby's health, growth, and development.

Early Intervention Programs and the Individuals with Disabilities Education Act

The foundation for learning begins in early infancy. Therefore, every infant identified as at risk for developmental delay should receive intervention as early as possible. Early intervention programs seem to influence developmental outcome by helping not only the baby, but the baby's family as well.

The Individuals with Disabilities Education Act (IDEA) was formerly Public Law (PL) 94-142, the Education for all Handicapped Children Act (1975) and its 1986 Amendments, PL 99-457, Part H. The general purpose of IDEA states that all children with disabilities who qualify may receive special education and related services.

Infants and children up to age 3 years are covered by Part C of IDEA. Early intervention services are ideally provided to children in this age group in the child's home or child care setting. Occasionally, these services may occur in a hospital or rehabilitation center. Individuals with Disabilities Act Part C is not only focused on helping the family meet the developmental needs of their child, but also to provide support and assistance to the family.

Your baby may be eligible for services if he is experiencing any difficulties with physical, mental, language, social, hearing, visual, behavioral, or emotional skills. You may have received a referral to your local early intervention program before your baby was discharged from the hospital. Your social worker may have filled out a multidisciplinary evaluation form, which would have also been signed by you and by your baby's physician or nurse. Your health care provider may make a referral if any developmental concerns arise during office visits. Finally, you may request a referral if you feel your infant or child needs help. To do so, contact your local school system, your state department of education, or your state office for children with disabilities (sometimes called *children with special health care needs*). You may need to ask specifically for the person in charge of the special education programs. Some states have toll-free telephone numbers to call for information about services in your area. Services vary from state to state.

Once a referral is made, a team of professionals will gather information about your baby and family to determine your needs. If the team determines that your infant needs services, an individualized family service plan (IFSP) will be developed. The IFSP is based on the information from the assessment and on your perception of intervention needs.

Services, such as occupational therapy, physical therapy, speech therapy, or nursing care, may be provided to your baby and family in your home or at a center. Location of services and the type of instruction (individual or group) provided varies from area to area and from state to state. The quality of available services also varies, which can be a source of frustration for parents. Your IFSP should be reviewed by you and your service coordinator at least every 6 months and modified as your baby's needs change. You may request a review earlier if you feel your baby needs more services or has outgrown his need for therapy.

You are the most valuable member of your baby's team. You are your baby's advocate and know him better than anyone else. It's important that you become actively involved in his growth and development. A good quality program helps both parents and baby. Some parents think that early intervention is the sole responsibility of trained professionals; but in reality, parents can make the biggest difference in a child's life. Many times the state (social security benefits) or insurance companies deny services to a child because he does not meet certain predetermined criteria for coverage. Sometimes there are financial reasons for this denial, but often the reasons are unclear. You must appeal any denial of services in writing and advocate for your child to get these needed services.

Professionals can instruct you in developmentally appropriate activities to play with your baby. They may teach you special exercises to strengthen your baby's muscles or positioning techniques if your child has any physical disabilities. Enjoy working with your child, and take pride in knowing that you are making a difference in his development.

Once your child turns 3 years, he will transition from early intervention and an IFSP to an individualized education program (IEP) and preschool services, which are covered in the Part B section of IDEA. Your family service coordinator will help you with this transition. Although providing free special educational services to children with disabilities is required by law, it becomes exceedingly challenging for local school systems to continue the "related services" still required, such as transportation and mobility services, developmental and psychological services, various therapies, school health nursing, and social work counseling, to name a few. As parents, it is important that you understand the laws regarding early intervention and special education, as well as your rights and the rights of your child. The Internet and local library are good resources for IDEA legislation. Contact your local school system or state department of education (they are required to give you material on your rights under IDEA) to discuss where your child should receive early childhood special education services, such as your local preschool, Head Start, or pre-kindergarten program.

Developmental Milestones and Your Baby

"Because of our baby's disabilities, we measure her progress in small steps. We won't worry about when she'll walk until we celebrate the fact that she can crawl."

As you monitor your baby's development, bear in mind that all children do not learn the same things at the same times. Even healthy term babies achieve developmental milestones over a range of ages. See pages 538 through 540 for a list of developmental milestones and potential problems that you should call to the attention of your health

Typical Speech Development*

Early Detection is the Best Prevention!

Important Parent Ideas:

☐ Keep a **notebook** for your concerns and observations.

☐ Review **this chart** and check the signs you see in your baby.**

☐ **Share your concerns,** this chart and your notebook with your child's doctor or health care professional.

***It is okay to check boxes in both the areas of "Typical Development" and "Signs to Watch for."*

BY 3 MONTHS

☐ Sucks and swallows well during feeding
☐ Quiets or smiles in response to sound or voice
☐ Coos or vocalizes other than crying
☐ Turns head toward direction of sound

BY 6 MONTHS

☐ Begins to use consonant sounds in babbling, e.g. "dada"
☐ Uses babbling to get attention
☐ Begins to eat cereals and pureed foods

BY 9 MONTHS

☐ Increases variety of sounds and syllable combinations in babbling
☐ Looks at familiar objects and people when named
☐ Begins to eat junior and mashed table foods

BY 12 MONTHS

☐ Meaningfully uses "mama" or "dada"
☐ Responds to simple commands, e.g. "come here"
☐ Produces long strings of gibberish (jargoning) in social communication
☐ Begins to use an open cup

BY 15 MONTHS

☐ Vocabulary consists of 5-10 words
☐ Imitates new less familiar words
☐ Understands 50 words
☐ Increases variety of coarsely chopped table foods

* Remember to correct your child's age for prematurity.

Typical Play Development*	**Typical Physical Development***

While lying on their back...
- ❑ Visually tracks a moving toy from side to side
- ❑ Attempts to reach for a rattle held above their chest
- ❑ Keeps head in the middle to watch faces or toys

While lying on their tummy...
- ❑ Pushes up on arms
- ❑ Lifts and holds head up

- ❑ Reaches for a nearby toy while on their tummy

While lying on their back...
- ❑ Transfers a toy from one hand to the other
- ❑ Reaches both hands to play with feet

- ❑ Uses hands to support self in sitting
- ❑ Rolls from back to tummy
- ❑ While standing with support, accepts entire weight with legs

- ❑ In a high chair, holds and drinks from a bottle
- ❑ Explores and examines an object using both hands
- ❑ Turns several pages of a chunky (board) book at once
- ❑ In simple play imitates others

- ❑ Sits and reaches for toys without falling
- ❑ Moves from tummy or back into sitting
- ❑ Creeps on hands and knees with alternate arm and leg movement

- ❑ Finger feeds self
- ❑ Releases objects into a container with a large opening
- ❑ Uses thumb and pointer finger to pick up tiny objects

- ❑ Pulls to stand and cruises along furniture
- ❑ Stands alone and takes several independent steps

- ❑ Stacks two objects or blocks
- ❑ Helps with getting undressed
- ❑ Holds and drinks from a cup

- ❑ Walks independently and seldom falls
- ❑ Squats to pick up toy

Signs to Watch for in Physical Development*

- ❏ Difficulty lifting head
- ❏ Stiff legs with little or no movement

- ❏ Pushes back with head
- ❏ Keeps hands fisted and lacks arm movement

- ❏ Rounded back
- ❏ Unable to lift head up
- ❏ Poor head control

- ❏ Difficult to bring arms forward to reach out
- ❏ Arches back and stiffens legs

- ❏ Arms held back
- ❏ Stiff legs

- ❏ Uses one hand predominately
- ❏ Rounded back
- ❏ Poor use of arms in sitting

- ❏ Difficulty crawling
- ❏ Uses only one side of body to move

- ❏ Inability to straighten back
- ❏ Cannot take weight on legs

- ❏ Difficulty getting to stand because of stiff legs and pointed toes
- ❏ Only uses arms to pull up to standing

- ❏ Sits with weight to one side
- ❏ Strongly flexed or stiffly extended arms
- ❏ Needs to use hand to maintain sitting

- ❏ Unable to take steps independently
- ❏ Poor standing balance, falls frequently
- ❏ Walks on toes

Reprinted with permission from Pathways Awareness (800/955-2455; www.pathwaysawareness.org).

care provider. Continue to use corrected age for the first 2 years of your baby's life when looking at developmental milestones. Remember that every baby is different—some babies are walking by 9 months; others not until 15 months. Some babies are more assertive, more active, and quicker to learn—and therefore may develop at a faster pace than babies who are content to observe and socialize. These temperament differences may also be evident later in life in children's behavior.

Another important factor in developmental progress is the presence of chronic illness. Even if brain development is normal, children with severe lung disease, heart disease, or intestinal problems may have delays because they cannot physically handle some activities. This is especially apparent in the baby's gross motor (large muscle movement) development.

Infants who receive more frequent attention and more sensitive social responses achieve developmental milestones more rapidly. Studies have shown this to be true in both the term and preterm populations. Quality care from loving, attentive parents can help infants born preterm, at risk, or with certain neonatal problems achieve optimum development.

Dr Kathryn Barnard, professor emeritus at the University of Washington School of Nursing, directed the development of important assessment tools to measure "the health and caregiving environments of infants and young children." Specially trained health care professionals use this system to help parents and other health care professionals identify strengths and problem areas in parent-child interaction that research has found to be predictive of a child's later development. By observing the child's environment and noting behavioral components of the interaction between parent and child during a home visit, a feeding session, and a "teaching" session, the health care professional is able to identify areas of parent strength, problem areas to work on, and areas of concern that may require further assessment. Originally designed for use with term infants and their families, these scales have also shown positive correlations with the intellectual and behavioral development of preterm infants and their families.

Not everyone has the advantage of a visiting nurse who has the special training required to use these tools for home care and follow-up. Therefore, selected components of the scales are shown on pages 545 through 546 to guide you in ways to foster your baby's development. If many of the suggestions in these boxes seem to you like simple common sense, know that you are already on the right track to optimizing your baby's development.

As your baby grows, you'll have many opportunities to teach different skills. You are your child's most important teacher. You'll learn to couple realistic expectations of your child's abilities with support and inspiration for your child to stretch those abilities to their greatest potential.

Child Development

Average Age[a]	Developmental Milestones	Ways to Optimize Your Baby's Development
0–1 month	Lifts head Briefly watches and follows face or object with eyes Responds to sounds Smiles spontaneously Vocalizes ("talks")	Talk to your baby. Place your face or a bright/shiny object 8–12 inches in front of your baby's face. Provide bells or rattles. Hang mobiles. Position baby on stomach for play.
2 months	Holds head erect, bobbing when supported in sitting position Follows face or object with eyes as it moves to left or right over midline Smiles responsively Coos, laughs, squeals	Talk to your baby. Get your baby to follow your face or an object (a colorful puppet is nice) by moving left, right, up, and down. Smile and make happy sounds. Sing songs. Give your baby different textures (stuffed animals, plastic toys, terry cloth) to feel.
3 months	Lifts head and chest when lying on stomach, supports self on arms Has improved control of head Shows vigorous body movements Recognizes bottle or breast Plays with rattle Reaches for objects Glances from one object to another Coos, laughs, squeals	Talk, smile, socialize with your baby. Position baby on stomach for play; support in sitting position. Offer toys/objects that your baby has to reach for or work to get at. Offer rattle or small toy that your baby can grasp. Shake a rattle in your baby's hand if he doesn't do it by himself (babies learn by doing).
4 months	Has good head control Rolls from stomach to back Reaches for and may grasp rattle or plastic rod if held near hand Pulls to sitting position without head lagging behind When held in sitting position, follows moving object Turns to sounds Laughs aloud Enjoys play	Talk, smile, socialize with your baby. Change positions during play— sitting, lying on back or stomach. Encourage rolling over by offering toys on the side opposite your baby's position. Bring your baby's hands together to the center of his body; let your baby bring his hands to his mouth. Shake a rattle or bell to elicit a response.

Child Development

Average Age[a]	Developmental Milestones	Ways to Optimize Your Baby's Development
6 months	Sits briefly with no support Rolls over from back to stomach Transfers objects from hand to hand and from hand to mouth Bangs toys Babbles	Continue talking, singing, smiling, and laughing with your baby. Position your baby on his back and place toys out of reach to one side to encourage rolling over onto his stomach. Let your baby explore the environment by placing toys and objects into his mouth (as long as they are clean and safe). Encourage banging and sound production.
9 months	Waves bye-bye Plays pat-a-cake Says "Ma Ma" and "Da Da" Indicates wants Sits alone, pulls to stand, changes positions without falling Plays with 2 toys at the same time	Play social games with your baby. Name objects to encourage vocabulary development. Place your infant on the floor with several toys to play with.
12 months (1 year)	Jabbers expressively; may say 2 or 3 words Drinks from cup Can pick up toys using thumb and forefinger Likes to imitate Turns pages in book Stands and walks alone, although may be somewhat unsteady Gives affection Follows simple directions accompanied by gestures	Continue to name objects. Offer a cup with a lid or a partly filled standard cup. Praise his efforts to imitate. Read to your child and let him turn the pages (children's books with thick pages work best). Give simple directions ("Give Mommy the book.") and praise if your request is followed.

Child Development, continued

Average Age[a]	Developmental Milestones	Ways to Optimize Your Baby's Development
15 months	Vocalizes with pitch, as in conversation May say 4 or 5 words Walks steadily without support Runs Throws ball Helps feed and dress self (can probably only remove garments); "helps" with housework Scribbles	Have conversations with your child. Offer finger foods; let your child try to feed and dress himself with your help. Praise his efforts to help with housework. Let your child color with crayons or use soap-based finger paints with supervision.
18 months	May say 5 to 10 words Walks, runs, climbs up and down stairs with help Likes pull toys Likes being read to Continues to try to feed, dress, and wash himself Points to body parts when asked Stacks blocks	Encourage conversation. Play ball: throw and kick. Offer blocks. Read books together. Encourage and praise his attempts to feed, dress, and wash (including to brush teeth).
24 months (2 years)	Uses 2 or 3 words together to communicate needs ("more milk") Recognizes familiar pictures; can point to and name pictures or objects in a book May ask for items by name: ball, doll, cup Can tell the difference between objects Improving at feeding, dressing, washing, and imitating housework skills Beginning to play with 2- or 3-piece puzzles	Encourage your child to vocalize his needs instead of pointing. Read together—have your child point to and name pictures in a book (doggie, kitty cat, ball, house, and so on). Continue to praise his attempts at dressing, washing, feeding, and housework. Encourage the use of a spoon and fork. Offer simple puzzles to encourage size and shape differentiation. Play games that encourage large-muscle development and interactive skills (tag, hide-and-seek, ball). Encourage cooperation with other children. Plan outings (to the store or zoo, for example) for more learning experiences.

[a]Note: If your baby was born preterm, calculate corrected age (see pages 437–438). Use that number to monitor development.

Feeding Your Baby[a]

You provide your baby with an opportunity for socializing and learning during feeding when you make sure that
• Your baby feels safe and comfortable.
• Your baby's head is higher than his hips.
• Your baby's trunk is touching yours for at least half the feeding.
• The 2 of you can make eye contact.
• Your face is at least 7–8 inches away from your baby's face except during kissing, caressing, or burping.
• Your baby can move his arms.
• You pay more attention to your baby during the feeding than to other people or things around you.
• You smile and gently touch your baby during the feeding.
• You let your baby touch and explore your breast or the bottle.
• You talk to your baby about the feeding. ("Are you ready to eat?" "Do you need a break?" "This is nice warm milk!" "Are you feeling full?")
• You also talk to your baby about things other than the feeding ("It's so warm and sunny today!" "Do you hear that dog barking?") and do not use baby talk.
• You respond to your baby's smile or "talking" with your own smile, touch, or voice.

Your baby learns that feeding is safe and enjoyable when you
• Briefly stop the feeding when your baby shows distress.
• Do not interrupt your baby's sucking by removing or jiggling the nipple.
• Comfort your baby in response to distress with a gentle voice and touch, a position change, and general soothing.
• Stop the feeding when your baby falls asleep, pushes the food away, or turns his head away and your attempts to continue the feeding (repositioning, burping, waiting) prove unsuccessful.

[a]Adapted from Barnard KE. Feeding scale (birth to one year). In: *Nursing Child Assessment Feeding Scale.* Seattle, WA: University of Washington, NCAST-AVENUW Programs; 1994. Reprinted by permission.

Teaching Your Child[a]

Your child understands that you are a loving and supportive teacher and feels good about testing his abilities when you
• Position and support your child so that he can reach toys and make eye contact with you.
• Provide a learning area that is free from distractions.
• Let your child touch and play with toys before you start to give instructions.
• Describe toys to your child before beginning. ("Look at this smooth red block.")
• Have your child's attention before you begin a lesson. ("Matthew, are you ready to start?")
• Are relaxed and laugh and smile with your child while teaching.
• Make encouraging statements and gently pat, stroke, hug, or kiss your child during the lesson.
• Give clear instructions as you demonstrate a task. For example, "See how the green block stacks on top of the red block?" is more helpful than, "Put this one up here."
• Give your child at least 5 seconds to try a skill before you help.
• Praise your child for effort and improved performance by commenting, smiling, and/or nodding.
• Respond to your child's smiles and "talking," but do not interrupt his vocalizing.
• Change your child's position or the position of the toys after an unsuccessful try.
• Do not force your child to complete a task or make your child perform a task repeatedly after successfully completing it once.
• Respond to your child's distress by stopping, soothing, or diverting attention to a different task.
• Let your child know when the "teaching session" is over.
• Spend no more than 5 minutes and no less than 1 minute teaching your child.

[a]Adapted from Barnard KE. Teaching scale (birth to three years). In: *Nursing Child Assessment Teaching Scale.* Seattle, WA: University of Washington, NCAST-AVENUW Programs; 1994. Reprinted by permission.

Chances of Hospital Readmission

Technological advances in perinatal and neonatal medicine are creating a growing population of infants with special medical needs, both in the hospital and at home. Babies are going home sicker and quicker than ever before. Despite parental training in special care and close medical follow-up, these infants are at significant risk for rehospitalization. A baby born weighing less than 3 pounds, 5 ounces (1,500 grams) has almost a 40% chance of being rehospitalized during the first year of life. Depending on the underlying disease, statistics are similar for chronically ill or technology-dependent infants. This rate drops to about 10% after the first year.

These statistics are not meant to frighten you. Rather, they are to remind you that your baby may still have special health needs at discharge and that going home, in reality, is just the beginning of a whole new set of challenges for you and your family.

Common Reasons for Rehospitalization

"Tommy was rehospitalized three times during his first year at home. Each time was discouraging and exhausting for the whole family. But now that he's two years old, and he gets sick less often. I think we've turned the corner."

Common childhood diseases can be potentially life-threatening for VLBW infants, those with BPD or other chronic illnesses, and technology-dependent infants. Immunizing your NICU graduate (discussed later in this chapter and in Chapter 15) is an important step in preventing many potentially serious diseases.

Respiratory infections are the most frequent cause of hospital readmission among NICU graduates. They may result in continued need for supplemental oxygen, ventilator support, respiratory treatments, and/or medications for reactive airway disease (similar to asthma). The common cold, which is an upper respiratory infection, may cause your baby significant respiratory distress. Infections of the lower respiratory tract, such as pneumonia, can have the greatest impact on your baby, possibly requiring an extended hospital readmission. Respiratory infections occur more frequently in babies who are exposed to smoking in the home than those who are not.

Feeding difficulties and unmet nutrition needs may also lead to repeated hospital admissions. Your baby may not be meeting his nutritional requirements if he is nippling poorly, burning up too many calories working to breathe, or experiencing gastroesophageal reflux disease (see Chapter 14). When conventional treatment methods for increasing nutritional intake fail, your baby may be referred to an occupational or speech therapist who is specially trained in oral-motor issues if oral feeding is the problem. If reflux is the problem and is severe, your baby may be readmitted for further evaluation and/or for a surgical procedure called a *fundoplication* (see page 514). Optimal nutrition and weight gain are necessary to help your baby fight infections, decrease the work of breathing, lower oxygen requirements, and attain developmental milestones.

If your NICU graduate is on an apnea monitor at home, you may at some point notice more frequent or intense episodes of apnea and bradycardia. Report this trend to your pediatrician immediately. In some cases, a test to check the theophylline or caffeine level in your baby's blood may be done in your doctor's office. If the episodes of apnea and bradycardia are severe or are accompanied by other signs of illness, your baby may need to be readmitted to the hospital for closer monitoring, further evaluation, and/or medication adjustments.

Neurodevelopmental problems, vision and hearing impairments, and cosmetic surgeries may also require hospital readmission, especially when your child is older. A child with CP may require orthopedic surgeries to release tight tendons. A child with a blocked tear duct may need a minor surgical procedure to open it up. If your baby has scars from NICU procedures (chest tubes or major line placement), you may want to consider cosmetic surgery when he is older and his medical risks have lessened or resolved.

Your Part in Preventing Rehospitalization

You can't necessarily control the progress of your baby's medical recovery, but you can take steps to reduce the risks for rehospitalization. Here are some suggestions.

Providing Adequate Care

Prevention of rehospitalization actually begins before discharge as you learn about your baby's special care needs. Ask questions and practice until you feel comfortable with and competent at providing your baby's care. Speak up if you have questions or feel that you are being hurried out the door. It's normal to feel somewhat apprehensive when your baby first comes home, but it helps to know that you are familiar with your baby's care and understand how to monitor for potential problems.

Working With Your Health Care Provider

Selecting a health care provider who understands the complex needs of a NICU graduate also helps prevent rehospitalization. Weekly visits to the office may be necessary for the first month to monitor your baby's weight gain and general progress and to address your questions and concerns. Early identification of illness and good communication with your health care provider can prevent a minor illness from turning into a major hospitalization.

Hand Washing

Good hand washing is the easiest and most effective way to prevent the spread of infection. Wash your hands after changing diapers, after blowing or wiping your nose, and before preparing food. Make it a habit to wash when you return from work or running errands, and encourage siblings to wash immediately when they come home from school, child care, or a friend's house. Hand washing is not only important for family and visitors, though. As your baby grows and begins to touch and hold objects, wash your baby's hands after an outing, before he eats finger foods, and when common sense tells you it is a good idea. Use mild soap and warm water and make hand washing fun for your baby. Do not use waterless hand sanitizer because the chemicals are quickly absorbed into your baby's skin.

Immunizations

Another important measure in preventing infection and rehospitalization is making sure that your baby is immunized on schedule and that he receives boosters as appropriate. Your health care provider will give you written information about each immunization your baby should receive so that you can ask questions and discuss any concerns. See Chapter 15 for information about recommended immunizations that will keep your baby healthy and decrease the risk of rehospitalization.

Coping With Rehospitalization

If your baby's rehospitalization is planned and anticipated (a hernia repair, for example), you may consider it a milestone and look forward to continued progress at home. If your baby is rehospitalized with an illness or emergency, though, you may feel angry, guilty, frustrated, and inadequate as a parent. Even when forewarned, parents often blame themselves when their baby has to be rehospitalized. They feel as if they have failed to provide adequate care for their baby at home. "If only I had…" is a familiar phrase. It may help to realize that rehospitalization often occurs despite all of your good care and precautions. It is not an indication that you did something wrong. Recognize that your NICU graduate has the potential for many medical problems beyond your scope of caregiving and that hospitalization is sometimes necessary to get him back on the road to progress.

If your baby's rehospitalization is unanticipated, take this opportunity to examine your management of the events leading up to the readmission. Instead of asking yourself, "What did I do wrong?" ask yourself, "How did I manage this crisis?" Here are some questions to consider.

- Did I have enough information to know what signs and symptoms to report?
- Did I know who to talk to about my concerns? Did that person really listen to me?
- Did I report my concerns to my health care provider in a timely manner?

- Did everyone involved in this hospitalization (myself and the health care professionals) communicate well to define the problem and decide on treatment?
- Did I learn something from this experience?
- What aspects of this experience did I manage well?
- What, if anything, would I do differently next time?

Your answers to these questions may reveal that you need more support and information to monitor your baby's special care needs. You may want to discuss your need for better communication with your baby's health care professionals. Or you may discover, as is true for most parents, that you did everything you knew to do.

Before discharge, you may not have known what you didn't know—and that made it difficult to ask questions. It's often after you get home or after an unanticipated rehospitalization that your learning needs become clear.

Every parenting crisis presents an opportunity to learn. Even though rehospitalization is not an experience you'd deliberately seek, try to look at it as a chance to manage a difficult situation, advocate for your baby's needs, and grow as a responsible and caring parent.

Working With Your Baby's Health Care Providers

Learning to communicate and negotiate effectively was important to your survival and involvement in the NICU (see Chapter 3). Communication skills will continue to serve you well as you meet and work with numerous health care providers in your community. Because you and members of your baby's caregiving team may have different expectations, it's important to create the best possible working relationship.

Developing a Partnership and a Medical Home

The concept of a medical home means that you and your baby's primary health care provider have a trusting relationship and work together as partners to coordinate all of your baby's health care needs. (See Chapter 15 for more discussion about medical home.) Begin by being honest and expressing your needs and expectations. Your health care providers will appreciate the fact that you value and depend on their experience and advice, but they should also realize that you have experience and information that will influence your child's health care. Over time, you will work out a relationship that allows for negotiation and polite disagreement. You should be able to trust one another enough so that it is acceptable for either of you to say "I don't know" or "You were right." Your relationship will grow strong enough to survive small disagreements if you also remember to express your appreciation when your health care provider's expertise has been especially helpful. Everyone likes to feel successful. Your acknowledgment of a job well done helps inspire future problem-solving and keeps your partnership strong.

Changing Health Care Providers

At some point in your child's care, you may find yourself thinking about switching health care providers. To stay in control, plan ahead and try to avoid an abrupt termination of this important relationship.

Laying the Groundwork

Before switching health care providers, try to discuss your concerns. Unmet expectations are the source of many problems, and honest communication may help resolve the situation. Be specific about your concerns, write them down, and look for a respectful and courteous response. Be prepared to participate in mutual problem-solving. Most problems have 2 sides. Just as you expect the health care provider to consider your side of the story, you need to give the professional's perspective equal consideration. Most health care providers prefer to discuss concerns in person; however, if this seems impossible for you, write your health care provider a letter stating why you are dissatisfied.

There is rarely a reason for hostility when terminating a relationship with a health care professional. Also, despite the fact that the health care provider has been an authority figure in your situation, there is no reason to feel intimidated in this process.

Before you end your relationship with your current caregiver, find another. You don't want to be caught in the awkward situation of needing care and not having someone familiar with your baby.

Making a Wise Choice

Choose your new health care professional with care. In your efforts to find answers to your baby's complex needs, it's possible to be taken in by the promise of a fast cure. Review the basic rules of interviewing and selection (see Chapter 15), and this time focus some of your questions on the areas in which you are having problems with your current health care professional.

The Overprotective Parent

Graduates of a NICU may come home with nursing support, equipment, supplies, medications, and a long list of caregiving requirements. You've been given a list of dos and don'ts for your baby's care and warned of the potential for rehospitalization. It's no wonder that at first you tend to overprotect your baby. In some cases, though, this sheltering continues well past the point of necessity and beyond what is healthy for you and your child. The psychological damage of overprotecting a child can be more limiting than any diagnosed disability.

Vulnerable Child Syndrome

When parents continue to view their child as sickly despite healthy findings on physical examinations, professionals describe this attitude as *vulnerable child syndrome*. When the child reaches school age, he is not allowed to participate in sports or special events. The parents don't encourage high academic standards, and so their healthy, mentally normal child performs below his potential.

The psychological impact of overprotection can be devastating to children. Overprotection stunts children's efforts to develop skills appropriate for their age. They may continue to experience separation anxiety. They may have temper tantrums whenever they do not get their way. They may have difficulty playing with or participating in social games with other children. They may bite or hit other children during outbursts of anger. School grades tend to be below average, possibly because of frequent absences from school with real or imagined illness to blame. Children may actually feed into parental overprotection by complaining of nonspecific symptoms or of a problem with one organ to focus the parents' anxiety on a specific area.

Children who are severely overprotected by their parents are more likely than not to have had special medical needs as infants—for example, a medical history of prematurity, apnea and bradycardia, failure to thrive, or another chronic illness. Professional intervention is often necessary to help parents recognize and accept that the illness event, which took place years earlier, is now over. Only then can these parents begin to view their child as a healthy individual and encourage his social development.

A Difficult Balance

Because your baby spent time in the NICU, he is at risk for overprotection. Close watchfulness may be necessary and appropriate early in life because of continued medical problems. Listen to your health care provider and to other child care specialists when they tell you that your baby is medically stable and developmentally ready for new challenges, however. They can educate you about normal infant behavior and basic parenting. Ask your health care professional the following questions to avoid becoming overprotective parents:

1. Does the fact that my baby has had this problem mean that he is in any way worse off than a baby born without any problems?
2. If my baby is more at risk, what can I do to reduce the risk? What signs and symptoms should I watch for? For how long will my baby continue to be at risk?
3. Is my baby fully recovered?

Share your anxiety with your health care provider. She may be in the best position to alleviate your fears and help prevent you from sheltering your child for longer than is necessary. Don't hesitate to call or visit your health care provider more frequently than usual if you're experiencing undue stress over your child's health. You may also benefit from

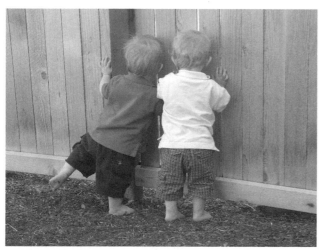

A difficult balance.
Caring for and protecting your baby without providing too much care and protection is indeed a tricky balancing act.

speaking with other parents of NICU graduates. Getting involved with people and/or support groups who have experienced or are feeling similar fears can help you learn to cope with these feelings in a positive way. Be wary of online NICU chat rooms where other parents are only sharing complaints or "bad advice." Remember that no 2 babies are alike—even if they are the same gestational age—so always ask your health care provider before adopting advice from strangers.

Caring for and protecting your baby without providing too much care and protection is indeed a tricky balancing act. You've worked hard to get to this point, and it's only natural to want to safeguard your special baby. But part of being a parent is growing with your child and realizing when it's time to loosen your grip in some areas and to expect your child's cooperation in others.

As your child explores the world, fights his own battles, and begins to feel accomplished as an individual, he will grow healthier. You'll find your own way as you give your child's potential abilities a chance to unfold. Through trial and error, you'll learn how much to expect from your child and when the time is right to stretch your expectations a bit further. Every child's needs are different, but most benefit from parents who expect socially acceptable behavior and accomplishments that reflect their child's fullest abilities.

Planning Another Baby

The decision to have another baby is very personal and usually involves emotion more than logic. As you think about the future, look closely at your reasons for wanting another baby. Because 50% of pregnancies in the United States are unplanned, use of a reliable family planning method is key for ensuring that your next pregnancy is intentional. Once you've had one premature infant, there is a 30% chance that your next baby will also be premature. Therefore, if you are considering another baby, it is important to seek the services of a perinatologist, a doctor who specializes in high-risk pregnancies. It is equally important that you make arrangements to potentially deliver your baby in a health care facility that has a Level III NICU capable of caring for preterm infants if that is in fact needed.

The birth of a preterm or sick baby may change the way you look at future pregnancies. A complicated pregnancy or a baby's prolonged NICU stay is enough to make some women decide against additional pregnancies. This is especially true for women who have had more than one complicated or premature birth. On the other hand, some women feel as if they've "failed" in this pregnancy and want another pregnancy as a chance to "do it right." Families of a NICU graduate with special needs sometimes find that having other children makes their life more normal and that a healthy child makes them more aware of healthy aspects of their ill child.

Questions to Ask Yourself

Do you truly want another child, or are you trying to make up for a pregnancy and birth that did not proceed quite as you planned? Does your partner want another child? What about your family, including your other children? Will you be able to keep up with the stressful caregiving demands of your NICU graduate while you're pregnant?

Also consider your personal finances, home environment, and employment situation before deciding to become pregnant again. If you are restricted to home or put on bed rest during your next pregnancy, will employment disability insurance be necessary or available to you? What child care arrangements will you make if you must be hospitalized or are restricted to bed during your pregnancy? Is your partner willing to make some sacrifices for another pregnancy? Perhaps the most important question to ask is this one: Are you ready for another pregnancy knowing that you may face complications and another NICU experience?

Every pregnancy is different. All of the anticipatory planning in the world will not prevent unexpected events from occurring. A woman with no obvious risk factors may experience a complicated pregnancy and birth, and a woman with previous pregnancy and birth complications may later deliver a healthy term baby. In any case, if you decide to have another baby, plan your pregnancy and seek preconception counseling and genetic counseling if appropriate. Once you're pregnant, get early prenatal care and follow the basic guidelines of a healthy diet, moderate exercise, rest, and relaxation to give your baby the best chance for a healthy beginning.

Believing in Yourself

Many parents of NICU graduates are a bit frightened to look far ahead. In fact, fear of the unknown contributes to chronic stress in many families. The potential for rehospitalization, future health problems, and overprotection of your baby is very real.

The NICU experience does not make for an easy transition to parenthood. As your baby grows, you'll continue to discover important parenting resources within yourself—for managing stress, for advocating your baby's needs, and for seeking support and lending it to those around you. For you, parenthood has brought with it unique changes—different from those felt by parents whose baby was born healthy. It's given you opportunities for strengthening relationships, uncovering hidden strengths, and reordering priorities.

On those occasions when you are coping well, take a moment to congratulate yourself for a job well done. You may face many challenges ahead. But you can feel good about your abilities as a parent as long as you continue to ask questions and actively participate on the health care team as your baby's advocate.

Your baby's growth and development will reflect not only his medical legacy, but the way you bring him up as well. A parent's most difficult task is knowing when to offer a helping hand—and when to provide a gentle push forward. Your job is to inspire achievement and independence, while realizing that some of life's most valuable lessons come from disappointment. Your success as a parent depends on your ability to trust yourself to make a positive impact on your child's life.

Your child's success will depend largely on your outlook on life—and what you teach your child about achieving his personal best.

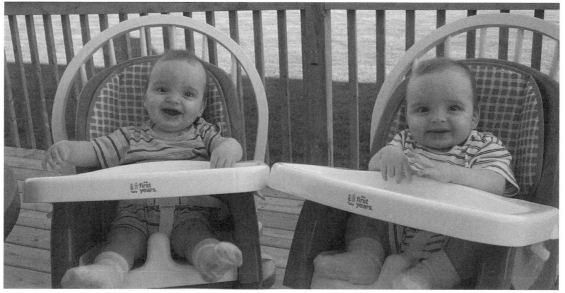

Enjoying life.
The NICU experience creates unique challenges for parents and babies. Take a moment to congratulate yourself for a job well done.

Appendix A
Weights and Measures: Conversion Charts

"There you are," said Piglet.

"Inside as well as outside," said Pooh proudly.

Conversion of Pounds and Ounces to Grams

Pounds \ Ounces	0	1	2	3	4	5	6	7	8	9	10	11	12	13	14	15
0	—	28	57	85	113	142	170	198	227	255	283	312	340	369	397	425
1	454	482	510	539	567	595	624	652	680	709	737	765	794	822	850	879
2	907	936	964	992	1,021	1,049	1,077	1,106	1,134	1,162	1,191	1,219	1,247	1,276	1,304	1,332
3	1,361	1,389	1,417	1,446	1,474	1,502	1,531	1,559	1,588	1,616	1,644	1,673	1,701	1,729	1,758	1,786
4	1,814	1,843	1,871	1,899	1,928	1,956	1,984	2,013	2,041	2,070	2,098	2,126	2,155	2,183	2,211	2,240
5	2,268	2,296	2,325	2,353	2,381	2,410	2,438	2,466	2,495	2,523	2,551	2,580	2,608	2,637	2,665	2,693
6	2,722	2,750	2,778	2,807	2,835	2,863	2,892	2,920	2,948	2,977	3,005	3,033	3,062	3,090	3,118	3,147
7	3,175	3,203	3,232	3,260	3,289	3,317	3,345	3,374	3,402	3,430	3,459	3,487	3,515	3,544	3,572	3,600
8	3,629	3,657	3,685	3,714	3,742	3,770	3,799	3,827	3,856	3,884	3,912	3,941	3,969	3,997	4,026	4,054
9	4,082	4,111	4,139	4,167	4,196	4,224	4,252	4,281	4,309	4,337	4,366	4,394	4,423	4,451	4,479	4,508
10	4,536	4,564	4,593	4,621	4,649	4,678	4,705	4,734	4,763	4,791	4,819	4,848	4,876	4,904	4,933	4,961
11	4,990	5,018	5,046	5,075	5103	5,131	5,160	5,188	5,216	5,245	5,273	5,301	5,330	5,358	5,386	5,415
12	5,443	5,471	5,500	5,528	5,557	5,585	5,613	5,642	5,670	5,698	5,727	5,755	5,783	5,812	5,840	5,868

To Convert Pounds and Ounces to Grams

Find the baby's weight in pounds down the left side of the table. Find the ounces across the top of the table. The intersection of the 2 measurements equals the equivalent weight in grams. For example, 3 pounds, 8 ounces equals 1,588 grams.

To Convert Grams to Pounds and Ounces

Find the baby's weight in grams on the chart. Look to the far left line for the pound measurement and to the top of the gram column for the ounces.

Conversion of Centimeters to Inches

Centimeters	Inches	Centimeters	Inches	Centimeters	Inches
25.4	10	43.2	17	61.0	24
26.7	10-1/2	44.4	17-1/2	62.2	24-1/2
27.9	11	45.7	18	63.5	25
29.2	11-1/2	47.0	18-1/2	64.8	25-1/2
30.5	12	48.3	19	66.1	26
31.8	12-1/2	49.5	19-1/2	67.4	26-1/2
33.0	13	50.8	20	68.7	27
34.3	13-1/2	52.1	20-1/2	69.9	27-1/2
35.6	14	53.3	21	71.2	28
36.8	14-1/2	54.6	21-1/2	72.5	28-1/2
38.1	15	55.9	22	73.8	29
39.4	15-1/2	57.2	22-1/2	75.1	29-1/2
40.6	16	58.4	23	76.4	30
41.9	16-1/2	59.7	23-1/2	77.6	30-1/2

Conversion of Temperature (Fahrenheit and Centigrade)

To convert degrees Fahrenheit to degrees centigrade, subtract 32, multiply by 5, and divide by 9.
To convert degrees centigrade to degrees Fahrenheit, multiply by 9, divide by 5, and add 32.

Fahrenheit	Centigrade
96.1	35.6
96.4	35.8
96.8	36.0
97.7	36.5
98.6	37.0
99.5	37.5
100.4	38.0
101.3	38.5
102.2	39.0
103.1	39.5
104.0	40.0
104.9	40.5
105.8	41.0
106.7	41.5
107.6	42.0

Medications and Your Baby

"To make you grow big and strong, dear.

You don't want to grow up small

and weak like Piglet, do you?"

—Kanga

Debbie Fraser Askin, MN, RNC-NIC

Many drugs are used in the treatment of sick or premature infants. Some have been used for many years.

All have undergone careful testing in children and have been given to thousands of newborns since their introduction. Other drugs have been developed more recently but have again been tested first in animals and then in adults and children before they are approved for use in the United States or Canada. This appendix will briefly describe some of the more common drugs used to treat infants.

Reasons for Giving Medications

Your baby may receive medications in the neonatal intensive care unit (NICU) for many reasons. Some drugs, such as phenobarbital or vitamin K, may be given to keep your baby from developing certain conditions or complications. Others, such as caffeine or antibiotics, are given to treat a problem that your baby has developed. Drugs such as vitamins and iron are given as supplements to breast milk or formula. Certain drugs—antibiotics, for example—may be given for a short time, whereas others, such as caffeine and phenobarbital, may be needed for many weeks or months.

The decision to give medication to an infant comes after careful thought. Your baby's medical provider will weigh the benefits of giving a drug against any risks or possible side effects the drug may produce.

All drugs have a desired effect—that is, a reason for which they are given. Desired effects may include fighting infection, increasing blood pressure, or relieving pain.

Many drugs also have possible side effects. That means that, in addition to the action they are intended to produce, they can cause changes—ranging from minor to major—in other body functions. Minor side effects of some drugs may include loose stools or skin irritation. Major side effects—such as depression of breathing or lowering of the blood pressure—can be serious enough in some infants that the drug must be discontinued. Potential major side effects are especially of concern in ill or very premature babies. Note though, that each baby reacts differently to a given medication. Some experience no side effects from a specific drug; others show some of the side effects described for the drug in the listing later in this appendix.

Many of the side effects seen in children and adults are difficult to diagnose in a newborn (headache or nausea, for example) or, in the case of rashes or allergic reactions, may not occur in babies because of the immaturity of their bodies.

Finally, some drugs can have toxic effects. They can cause damage to the body's organs if given in too large a dose (an overdose) or if the concentration of the drug in the blood becomes unexpectedly high. When drugs with potentially toxic effects are given, levels in the blood are monitored closely to guard against toxicity.

Methods of Giving Medications

Various methods (routes of administration) are used to give drugs to infants in the NICU. The route used may depend both on the drug being given and on the infant's condition.

Intravenous

In sick infants, many drugs are given directly into a vein through an intravenous (IV) infusion. This route allows the baby's body to quickly begin to use the medication.

Oral

Some drugs are easily absorbed by the baby's digestive system and are well tolerated by the stomach; these drugs may be given orally (by mouth). Others cannot be given orally because the baby's digestive system cannot absorb them or because they will upset the stomach or the bowel. In some cases, very ill infants may not receive any fluid or medication orally because of concerns about their digestive system.

Intranasal

A few drugs for babies are given by spraying the drug into the nose. The nose is well supplied with blood vessels, allowing drugs to be absorbed and transferred to the bloodstream.

Inhalation

Drugs given by inhalation—those that are breathed in—are usually intended to treat lung problems. Medication given directly into the lungs may produce fewer side effects than if it were given intravenously. The lungs have a rich blood supply and therefore can absorb some medications quite well. Inhalation drugs may be given by face mask, by nebulizer (puffer), or through the endotracheal tube.

Rectal

In some cases, drugs may be given through a thin tube or a suppository (specially prepared capsule) placed in the baby's rectum. This may be done if an oral drug is desirable but cannot be given because of surgery or feeding problems.

Intramuscular

Intramuscular (IM) drugs—those given by needle—are often poorly absorbed by babies because of their immature muscle mass and poor circulation. Drugs that may be given intramuscularly include vitamin K (given routinely to newborn infants) and some drugs needed in emergency situations when an IV route may not be available.

Transdermal

The transdermal route—literally "across or through the skin"—involves the use of skin patches. This route is becoming more popular in adults. Because infants have thin skin, drugs cross into the bloodstream quite readily. At this time, few drugs are available in patches for use in the NICU; therefore, this route is not frequently used.

Safety of Medications

Most drugs given to newborn babies have been used for a number of years. New drugs are also being developed and tested. Most of these drugs are used in adults and older children for some time before they are given to babies.

All new medications used in the United States and Canada must be approved by these federal governments before they become available. Manufacturers of drugs must complete a series of steps before this approval is given. In the United States, manufacturers submit information and animal study results for each new drug to the Food and Drug Administration (FDA), which then grants the drug investigational status. At that time, the drug is tested on healthy adults and then on small numbers of patients for whom it is intended. Finally, clinical trials occur, in which the new drug is tested on larger groups of patients. In Canada, this process is handled by the Health Protection Branch of Health Canada. If your baby's doctor would like your infant to receive an investigational drug, the doctor will explain the situation to you and obtain your permission.

The members of your health care team have all received special training in the safe administration of medications. As a partner in your baby's health care team, you can also play a role in ensuring that medications are given correctly. When medications are being given to your baby you should feel welcome to ask for information about the purpose of the medication and any side effects that might be expected. The health professional giving your baby a medication will have checked to ensure that the medication has been ordered correctly and is being given at the correct time and through the correct route. If you wish, you can double-check these points with the person giving the medication.

Monitoring Drug Levels

When certain drugs are given, it's necessary to monitor the amount of the drug that is present in your baby's blood (called the *serum drug level)*. Drugs requiring monitoring of levels are those with a narrow range between desired effects and toxic side effects. Levels are monitored to ensure that an adequate amount of the drug is present to achieve the desired effect but that the level is not so high as to cause side effects.

Discontinuation of a Baby's Medication

The decision to stop a medication depends on a number of things. For some drugs, such as an antibiotic, the medication is stopped when your baby is free of infection. Other drugs may be given for a certain number of doses. Still others may be given over a period of weeks or months, depending on the problem being treated. Some drugs can be stopped at any time; others cannot be stopped all at once. Instead, the baby must be slowly weaned from the medication. The amount given or the frequency with which the drug is given is reduced over time so that the baby's body becomes used to being without the drug. With some medications the baby is weaned by being allowed to outgrow the dose. Be sure your baby's caregiver explains your baby's medication plan to you.

Common Drugs in the NICU

This section lists some of the drugs that may be given to babies who are sick or premature. The drugs are arranged alphabetically by common (generic) name. Trade or brand names follow the common name in parentheses. The entry for each drug describes what the drug is used for; what side effects it might produce; contraindications, if any, for its administration (medical conditions a health care provider considers when weighing the risks and benefits of a particular drug); information about monitoring, if available; and special notes. The information provided here is general, and every baby's medication needs are unique. Be sure to discuss your baby's medications with his medical and nursing providers.

General Categories of Drugs

Antibiotics: Agents that inhibit or stop the growth of microorganisms—usually bacteria. The best-known antibiotics are members of the penicillin family. Broad-spectrum antibiotics are those that are effective against a wide range of bacteria. Gentamicin is one of these.

Anticonvulsants: Agents that prevent, control, or relieve convulsions (seizures). Seizures are explained in detail in Chapter 10. Anticonvulsants include fosphenytoin, lorazepam, phenobarbital, and phenytoin.

Diuretics: Agents that help the kidneys get rid of excess water in the body by increasing urine excretion. Two examples are hydrochlorothiazide/spironolactone and furosemide.

Narcotics: Agents that relieve pain. Narcotics also dull the senses, bring on a stuporous state, and affect the central nervous system. Medical personnel may refer to them as opioid analgesics. They include fentanyl and morphine sulfate.

Sedatives: Agents that calm by reducing nervousness, excitement, and activity. They work by depressing the activity of tissue in the central nervous system. Called sedative-hypnotics by medical personnel, these agents do not directly reduce pain. They include chloral hydrate, midazolam, and phenobarbital, as well as the anticonvulsant agents diazepam and lorazepam.

Steroids: Agents that decrease inflammation and raise blood pressure. Dexamethasone is one of these.

Stimulants: Agents that increase the functional activity or efficiency of an organ or system. They act on the tissue of the nervous system to increase tension in the muscles, thus increasing stimulation to the tissue. Caffeine is included in this category. Many stimulants target their effect to a specific organ or body system.

Common Specific Drugs

Acetaminophen (Tempra, Tylenol)
Use: A mild pain reliever that also reduces fever; available as an oral medication or as a rectal suppository.
Side effects: Rash (very uncommon in neonates).

Acyclovir (Zovirax)
Use: A medication that helps babies fight infections caused by some viruses; in particular, may be used to treat herpes or chickenpox.
Side effects: Irritation at the IV site; temporary decrease in kidney function.

Albuterol (Salbutamol, Ventolin)
Use: A drug used to treat airway constriction, as can occur in some babies with bronchopulmonary dysplasia; works by relaxing, or "opening up," the breathing tubes in the lungs.
Indications: Wheezing or airway spasms.
Side effects: Increased heart rate, increased blood pressure, headache, tremors, hyperglycemia (high blood sugar).

Aldactazide. See Hydrochlorothiazide/Spironolactone

Aldactone. See Spironolactone

Alteplase (Activase)
Use: A drug given to clear a blocked central line or to treat a blood clot in a vein.
Side effects: Bleeding

Aminophylline (IV) and Theophylline (Oral) (Note: These drugs are now rarely used in neonates. Caffeine is the drug of choice for apnea, and bronchoconstriction is treated with drugs such as albuterol.)
Use: Medications usually used in 2 groups of infants: those with apnea and those with bronchopulmonary dysplasia (BPD). Older infants or children with asthma may also receive theophylline. Used in the treatment of apnea of prematurity, theophylline stimulates the baby's breathing center to make breathing more regular. In BPD and asthma, theophylline helps to dilate the breathing tubes (bronchi) in the lungs and relieve muscle spasms in the bronchi. In some critically ill infants, aminophylline may be used to help the kidneys produce urine.
Side effects: Diuresis (increased urine production), increased heart rate, vomiting, increased activity, irritability.
Monitoring: Blood levels of these drugs are monitored.

Amoxicillin
Use: A member of the penicillin family; an oral antibiotic used against infection caused by an organism sensitive to it.
Side effects: Allergic reaction (very uncommon in young babies because their immune system is not fully developed), vomiting, diarrhea.

Amphotericin B (Fungizone)
Use: A strong drug used to treat blood infections caused by yeast or other fungi.
Side effects: Fever (very rare in neonates), vomiting, and chemical imbalances in the blood; may also interfere with kidney function and blood clotting.
Cautions/Contraindications: Usually not given to babies with kidney failure.

Ampicillin
Use: An antibiotic from the penicillin family; effective against a number of bacteria that cause infection in infants.
Side effects: Allergic reaction (uncommon in young babies), diarrhea.

Ancobon. See Flucytosine

Ativan. See Lorazepam

Azithromycin
Use: An antibiotic used to treat infection caused by *Chlamydia*.
Side effects: Diarrhea, rash, blood in the stool

Bactrim. See Co-Trimoxazole

Beractant (Survanta)
Use: A surfactant made from cow lungs used to reduce the severity of respiratory disease in premature infants. Also used in infants with meconium aspiration and pneumonia.
Side effects: Blockage of the endotracheal tube and, rarely, bleeding from the lungs (pulmonary hemorrhage).
Cautions: Some babies have brief periods of oxygen desaturation during administration.

Caffeine
Use: A stimulant that acts on the baby's breathing center; used to treat apnea of prematurity.
Side effects: Restlessness, vomiting (rare in neonates), high heart rate.
Monitoring: Blood levels of this drug are monitored.

Capoten. See Captopril

Captopril (Capoten)
Use: A medication used to treat high blood pressure and manage congestive heart failure.
Side effects: Low blood pressure, increased heart rate, chemical imbalances in the blood.
Cautions/Contraindications: Usually not given to babies with kidney failure.

Carnitine (Carnitor)
Use: A nutrient given to treat carnitine deficiency common in very small babies.
Side effects: (uncommon) nausea, diarrhea.

Cefotaxime Sodium (Claforan)
Use: A cephalosporin antibiotic used to treat suspected sepsis (infection in the blood).
Side effects: Rash, diarrhea.

Ceftazidime (Fortaz, Tazicef)
Use: A cephalosporin antibiotic used to treat infections by certain gram-negative bacteria.
Side effects: Rash, low white blood cell count, low platelets.
Cautions/Contraindications: Some bacteria are resistant to this antibiotic.

Cerebyx. See Fosphenytoin

Chloral Hydrate (Noctec)

Use: A sedative that can be given for restlessness or agitation; not used to relieve pain. Only given orally or rectally.

Side effects: Nausea, diarrhea, drowsiness, respiratory depression.

Cautions/Contraindications: Only given orally or rectally; can't be used if these routes aren't available. Usually not given to infants with severe liver or kidney disease. Other more serious toxic effects occur with repeated doses.

Cimetidine (Tagamet) (Note: Rarely used now. Drug of choice is ranitidine [Zantac].)

Use: An antacid used to treat bleeding in the stomach.

Side effects: Diarrhea, rash.

Claforan. See Cefotaxime Sodium

Cleocin. See Clindamycin

Clindamycin (Cleocin)

Use: An antibiotic used to treat certain types of bacterial sepsis (blood infections) or used in combination with other antibiotics in the treatment of necrotizing enterocolitis.

Side effects: Rash, diarrhea.

Cautions/Contraindications: Infections of the fluid around the baby's brain.

Cloxacillin (Note: Rarely used in the NICU.)

Use: An oral antibiotic from the penicillin family used to fight infection caused by an organism sensitive to it.

Side effects: Allergic reaction (uncommon in young babies), vomiting, diarrhea, occasional rash.

Co-Trimoxazole (Septra, Bactrim)

Use: An oral antibiotic used to treat susceptible bacteria—in particular, those that cause many ear and urinary tract infections.

Side effects: Rash, nausea, diarrhea.

Cautions/Contraindications: Usually not given to infants younger than 1 month.

Decadron. See Dexamethasone

Dexamethasone (Decadron)

Use: A form of steroid with anti-inflammatory properties; has been shown to improve lung function of some infants with BPD. Also used to treat tracheal edema. Following placement of an endotracheal tube, some infants develop swelling of the vocal cords, which makes breathing after extubation more difficult. Dexamethasone is used in these infants to reduce swelling around the cords. This course of dexamethasone is short, lasting 24 to 48 hours.

Side effects: High blood pressure, high blood sugar, suppression of growth, fluid and blood chemistry imbalances, increased risk of infection.

Note: The benefits and risks of this drug must be considered in infants with infection or high blood pressure.

Diazepam (Valium)

Use: A medication given either as a sedative or as treatment for neonatal seizures.

Side effects: Low blood pressure, drowsiness, slowed breathing efforts.

Digoxin

Use: A medication used to help strengthen the muscle of the heart; used in the treatment of congestive heart failure or in certain types of tachycardia.

Side effects: Low heart rate, changes in the rhythm of the heart, nausea and vomiting.

Cautions/Contraindications: Cannot be used in infants with low potassium levels in the blood or with severe kidney or liver disease; should not be given to babies with a low heart rate.

Monitoring: Blood levels of this drug are monitored. The amount of drug the baby is receiving may need to be adjusted often in the first week to 2 weeks of treatment until drug blood levels stabilize.

Note: If your baby is going home on this drug, you will be taught how to watch for signs that he is receiving too much medication.

Dilantin. See Phenytoin

Dobutamine/Dopamine

Use: Two drugs used to improve low blood pressure and low urine output; given intravenously in a continuous infusion.

Side effects: Increased heart rate, changes in heart rhythm. When given through IV placement in the limbs, the drug can cause skin damage.

Monitoring: Heart rate, blood pressure, and urine output are monitored carefully.

EMLA cream

Use: A cream used to numb the skin prior to a painful procedure such as the insertion of a catheter into a vein.

Side effects: Rarely occur. Local skin redness occasionally seen.

Contraindications: Should not be used on open wounds.

Note: Should be applied 20 to 30 minutes prior to the procedure.

Epinephrine

Use: A powerful heart stimulant used to help strengthen the heart muscle and/or to treat cardiac failure and low blood pressure.

Side effects: Heart rhythm changes, high blood pressure, local irritation at the IV site.

Monitoring: Heart rate and blood pressure are monitored closely.

Epogen. See Erythropoietin

Erythromycin
Use: An ointment that may be used in the newborn's eyes just after delivery to prevent infection caused by gonorrhea; an antibiotic used to treat infections caused by organisms sensitive to it.
Side effects: Vomiting, diarrhea, discomfort at site if given by injection. (Note: These side effects are not associated with erythromycin eye medication.)

Erythropoietin (Epogen, recombinant human erythropoietin, HuEpo)
Use: A drug that helps the body to produce red blood cells. In premature babies, it may reduce the need for blood transfusions. Erythropoietin may be given every day or every other day for a time. It is injected just under the skin (or rarely into the baby's IV line).
Side effects: Swelling, fever, diarrhea, increased blood pressure.
Cautions/Contraindications: May not be used if your baby has high blood pressure.

Famotidine
Use: An antacid used to treat bleeding in the stomach or irritation of the esophagus (tube leading from the mouth to the stomach).
Side effects: Constipation or diarrhea, insomnia or sleepiness

Fentanyl (Sublimaze)
Use: A synthetic opioid used for pain relief, sedation, or anesthesia; may be used in the nursery or in the operating room during surgery.
Side effects: Decreased breathing efforts, muscle rigidity (when high doses are administered as a bolus), some risk of lowered blood pressure. Withdrawal symptoms can occur if the drug is discontinued abruptly after several days of use. Gradual weaning of the drug is recommended.
Note: Fentanyl is usually used only in infants receiving mechanical ventilation because it can produce respiratory depression (decreased breathing efforts).

Fer-In-Sol. See Ferrous Sulfate

Ferrous Sulfate (Fer-In-Sol, Iron)
Use: A mineral that helps to overcome anemia. As premature infants approach 6 to 8 weeks of age, their iron stores become depleted as their bodies begin to produce hemoglobin, and they need extra iron.
Side effects: Constipation, nausea.

Flagyl. See Metronidazole

Fluconazole (Diflucan)

Use: Given to treat infections caused by fungus or yeast.

Side effects: Vomiting, diarrhea, rash.

Flucytosine (Ancobon)

Use: A drug used to treat blood infections caused by a fungus.

Side effects: Nausea, vomiting, diarrhea, anemia, chemical imbalances in the blood.

Folic Acid/Folate

Use: One of the B vitamins; given to correct a deficiency, common in premature infants, that results in a type of anemia.

Side effects: Skin redness or rash (rare).

Fortaz. See Ceftazidime

Fosphenytoin (Cerebyx) (Note: This drug is replacing phenytoin [Dilantin] in the NICU.)

Use: An anticonvulsant used to treat seizures; usually added if the phenobarbital does not control the seizures.

Side effects: Drowsiness, irritation at the IV site, changes in blood pressure.

Note: This drug is similar to phenytoin (Dilantin). It is sometimes used in place of Dilantin because it is easier to administer than Dilantin.

Fungizone. See Amphotericin B

Furosemide (Lasix)

Use: A diuretic that helps the kidneys get rid of excess water; used to treat conditions such as congestive heart failure, patent ductus arteriosus, fluid in the lungs, bronchopulmonary dysplasia, and some kidney diseases.

Side effects: Chemical imbalances in the blood, kidney stones (with prolonged use). If given with other potentially ear-damaging drugs, hearing damage may occur.

Gentamicin

Use: An antibiotic that is effective against most kinds of bacteria that occur in babies; used when infection is suspected or when infection with a bacterium sensitive to it is identified.

Side effects: At high blood levels, damage to the kidneys and hearing.

Monitoring: Blood levels of this drug are monitored.

Heparin

Use: An anticoagulant used to prevent clotting of the blood; may also be used to prevent catheters from blocking.

Side effects: Hemorrhage.

Cautions/Contraindications: Not usually given to infants with bleeding in the stomach.

HuEpo. See Erythropoietin

Hydrochlorothiazide/Spironolactone (Aldactazide)

Use: An oral diuretic that helps the kidneys to remove excess water from the body; used in longer-term treatment of conditions such as BPD, edema, and congestive heart failure.

Side effects: Diarrhea, lethargy, chemical imbalances.

Cautions/Contraindications: Cannot be given to some babies with kidney problems.

Hydrocortisone (Solucortef)

Use: A steroid used to treat low blood sugar or low blood pressure.

Side effects: High blood pressure, high blood sugar.

Ibuprofen (Neoprofen)

Use: Used to close a patent ductus arteriosus.

Side effects: Small increased risk of bleeding, may decrease urine production.

Caution: Cannot be given to babies with an active infection, active bleeding, low platelets, kidney problems, or necrotizing enterocolitis.

Imipenem-Cilastatin (Primaxin)

Use: A strong antibiotic used to treat blood infections caused by a number of bacteria.

Side effects: Diarrhea, irritation at the IV site.

Indocin. See Indomethacin

Indomethacin (Indocin) (Note: Use in the neonate is more common in Canada than the United States.)

Use: A medication used to close a patent ductus arteriosus. Some centers are studying the use of this drug to prevent intraventricular hemorrhage.

Side effects: Temporary decrease in urine production, resulting in swelling (edema) and fluid imbalances.

Cautions/Contraindications: Cannot be given to babies with active kidney problems, bleeding problems, high bilirubin, or necrotizing enterocolitis.

Insulin

Use: A drug used to treat high blood sugar. Premature infants frequently develop imbalances in their blood sugar. This is a temporary problem related to immaturity and is not a sign of diabetes.

Side effects: Possible high or low blood sugar levels as the medication level is adjusted or when the medication is stopped.
Monitoring: Frequent blood sampling needed when insulin is started or adjusted to monitor blood sugar levels.

Iron. See Ferrous Sulfate

Keppra. See Levetiracetam

Lasix. See Furosemide

Levetiracetam (Keppra)
Use: An anticonvulsant used to treat seizures; usually added if phenobarbital does not control the seizures.
Side effects: Drowsiness.

Lorazepam (Ativan)
Use: A medication given either as a sedative or as a treatment for neonatal seizures.
Side effects: Low blood pressure, nausea and vomiting, drowsiness, slowed breathing efforts.
Cautions/Contraindications: Cannot be given to some babies with kidney or liver disease.

Meropenem (Merrem)
Use: A strong antibiotic used to treat serious infections in babies.
Side effects: Diarrhea, redness at IV site.

Metoclopramide (Reglan)
Use: A drug used to help the stomach empty more rapidly; may be given to some infants with reflux (regurgitation or vomiting after feedings).
Side effects: Unusual muscle activity.
Cautions/Contraindications: Can be used only for short periods.

Metronidazole (Flagyl)
Use: An antibiotic used to treat suspected infections or cases of necrotizing enterocolitis.
Side effects: Nausea, vomiting.

Midazolam (Versed)
Use: A short-acting sedative used especially before major procedures for its calming effects.
Side effects: Apnea, increased heart rate, drowsiness, cough, low blood pressure.

Morphine Sulfate

Use: A narcotic used for pain relief and sedation; may be given as a continuous or intermittent IV infusion.

Side effects: Low blood pressure, respiratory depression (slowed breathing), urine retention, physical tolerance and dependence possible after prolonged use.

Mycostatin. See Nystatin

Naloxone (Narcan)

Use: A drug that reverses the effects of narcotic agents such as morphine or meperidine (Demerol); may be given after delivery to newborns with decreased breathing efforts whose mothers received meperidine shortly before delivery or to reverse the effects of narcotics given to infants for sedation or pain relief.

Side effects: Tremors, rapid breathing.

Narcan. See Naloxone

Neoprofen. See Ibuprofen

Noctec. See Chloral Hydrate

Nystatin (Mycostatin)

Use: A medication used in a cream or oral form to treat yeast *(Candida)* infections. These infections appear as a pebbly rash, usually in the diaper area, or as white patches in the mouth (thrush).

Side effects: Nausea, diarrhea, local irritation.

Palivizumab (Synagis)

Use: An antibody that helps to protect infants from developing respiratory syncytial virus (RSV) (an upper respiratory virus). Infants considered at risk for RSV include those born before 32 weeks' gestational age and those with chronic lung problems. This drug is injected monthly during the RSV season (usually November through April).

Side effects: Mild pain and redness at the injection site.

Pancuronium Bromide (Pavulon)

Use: A medication that causes temporary paralysis of muscles; used to keep critically ill babies from breathing against, or "fighting," the ventilator; may be used to attempt to improve oxygen levels in the blood. (Note: This drug does not independently improve oxygen levels, and sometimes its use results in worsening oxygen levels that then require increased ventilator support.)

Side effects: Increased heart rate, swelling (edema) of the limbs, increased saliva production, low blood pressure.

Note: Because pancuronium keeps infants from making any breathing efforts, it is given only to infants on mechanical ventilation. Babies receiving pancuronium cannot move, but they can hear your voice and feel your touch.

Pavulon. See Pancuronium Bromide

Penicillin

Use: An antibiotic used to treat susceptible bacteria, especially group B beta-hemolytic *Streptococcus* (group B strep or GBS).

Side effects: Diarrhea.

Phenobarbital or Phenobarb

Use: An anticonvulsant used to treat neonatal seizures; also used as a sedative in some instances.

Side effects: Drowsiness, lethargy, low blood pressure, depressed respirations, nausea.

Monitoring: Blood levels of this drug may be monitored.

Phenytoin (Dilantin) (Note: Fosphenytoin [Cerebyx] is replacing this drug in the NICU.)

Use: An anticonvulsant used to treat seizures; usually added if phenobarbital does not control the seizures.

Side effects: Low blood pressure, nausea, constipation, jaundice, rash, drowsiness.

Cautions/Contraindications: Cannot be given to babies with severe liver or kidney disease.

Monitoring: Blood levels of this drug are monitored.

Prostaglandin E1 (PGE1)

Use: A medication used to improve oxygenation and circulation in newborns with cyanotic congenital heart disease. Maintains blood flow through the ductus arteriosus until surgery can be performed.

Side effects: Elevated temperature, apnea, low blood pressure, skin flushing, bradycardia, tachycardia.

Ranitidine (Zantac)

Use: An antacid used to prevent or treat bleeding in the stomach.

Side effects: Nausea, diarrhea, constipation, vomiting.

Recombinant Human Erythropoietin. See Erythropoietin

Reglan. See Metoclopramide

Salbutamol. See Albuterol

Septra. See Co-Trimoxazole

Sildenafil

Use: A drug used to help dilate the blood vessels in the lungs in babies with persistent pulmonary hypertension.

Side effects: Low blood pressure, bleeding (rare).

Spironolactone (Aldactone)
Use: An oral diuretic that helps the kidneys get rid of excess water; used to treat congestive heart failure and BPD. Also may be used in the combination medication Aldactazide (see Hydrochlorothiazide/Spironolactone).
Side effects: Rash, vomiting, diarrhea, chemical imbalances in the blood.
Cautions/Contraindications: Used cautiously in infants with kidney problems.

Sublimaze. See Fentanyl

Synagis. See Palivizumab

Tagamet. See Cimetidine

Tazicef. See Ceftazidime

Tempra. See Acetaminophen

Theophylline. See Aminophylline

Tri-Vi-Sol
Use: A combination of vitamins A, C, and D that comes in liquid drops and is used to supplement the formula or breast milk that your baby is receiving.

Tylenol. See Acetaminophen

Ursodiol (Actigal)
Use: A drug used to treat high bilirubin levels caused by the use of total parenteral nutrition.
Side effects: Vomiting, constipation.

Valium. See Diazepam

Vancomycin
Use: An antibiotic used to treat suspected or confirmed neonatal infections, most commonly used to treat staphylococcal infections that are resistant to oxacillin or methicillin.
Side effects: Diarrhea, vomiting; at high blood levels, possible kidney or hearing damage.
Monitoring: Blood levels of this drug are monitored.

Vecuronium Bromide

Use: A drug used to cause temporary paralysis of muscles and to keep critically ill babies from breathing against, or "fighting," the ventilator; may be given to attempt to improve oxygen levels in the blood. (Note: See note under Pancuronium Bromide.)

Side effects: Increased heart rate, swelling (edema) of the limbs, increased saliva production, low blood pressure.

Note: Because vecuronium keeps infants from making any breathing efforts, it is given only to infants on mechanical ventilation. Babies receiving vecuronium cannot move, but they can hear your voice and feel your touch.

Ventolin. See Albuterol

Versed. See Midazolam

Vitamins. See also Folic Acid/Folate, Tri-Vi-Sol

Use: Various combinations of vitamins may be prescribed for your infant. Vitamin solutions may or may not be prescribed for your baby after discharge. Discuss this with your health care provider.

Vitamin D

Use: Liquid drops given to premature infants to supplement the vitamin D in breast milk or formula, or to infants with calcium deficiency; shortage may lead to weakening of the bones.

Vitamin K

Use: An injection routinely given to all newborns soon after birth to help the body form clotting substances that help prevent bleeding.

Side effects: Pain or swelling at the injection site.

Zantac. See Ranitidine

Zovirax. See Acyclovir

Appendix C
Car Safety Seats

"I must move about more. I must come and go."

—Eeyore

Jeanette Zaichkin, RN, MN, NNP-BC

When your baby is in the hospital, her safety depends largely on the vigilance and expertise of the nurses, physicians, and other professionals who care for her.

When she leaves the hospital and comes home, her safety depends on the steps you take to protect her from harm. This safekeeping begins on discharge day when you buckle your baby into her car safety seat for a safe trip home.

A car safety seat is also called a *child safety seat* or *child restraint*. It doesn't matter what term you use—the fact remains that using a car safety seat every time your baby is in the car is one of the most important things you can do to protect her. Many parents convince their children when they are very young that the car engine will not start until every person is buckled up. This routine may also offer an opportunity to convince other family members of the importance of using seat belts.

This appendix provides car safety seat information that will be helpful as you prepare for your baby's hospital discharge. The list on the next page provides questions to ask the neonatal intensive care unit (NICU) team about car safety seats and suggestions for how to learn to use your baby's car safety seat before the baby's discharge. The remainder of this appendix provides important information about car safety seat use and safety.

Car Safety Seat Trial

Ask NICU team members if your baby will have a car safety seat trial prior to discharge. The American Academy of Pediatrics (AAP) recommends this evaluation if your baby is born premature (less than about 37 weeks' gestation) or is discharged from the hospital with cardiac, respiratory, neurologic, or musculoskeletal problems. During a car safety seat trial, which takes place in the NICU, your baby is positioned properly in her car safety seat while a member of the NICU team monitors her color, heart rate, breathing, and oxygen saturation. The car safety seat trial will determine if the baby can tolerate the upright position of the car safety seat and also if the baby could tolerate the same position in an infant carrier, baby seat, or swing. If the trial indicates that she cannot tolerate an upright position in a car safety seat, the team will advise against use of similar positioning in an infant carrier, baby seat, or swing and may suggest a different type of car safety seat that allows the baby to lie flat while traveling.

Preparing for Car Safety Seat Purchase and Use

As hospital discharge nears, you may become very busy in a flurry of activities to prepare for your baby's homecoming. By planning ahead, you can avoid stress or even delayed discharge due to a car safety seat that does not fit your baby or your vehicle. Talk with you baby's primary nurse or discharge coordinator to ensure that your responsibilities related to car safety seat usage are clear and that you are prepared and educated about car safety seat use before discharge day.

1. Ask your baby's nurse if your baby will have a car safety seat trial prior to discharge. If yes, ask when you should be prepared to bring your baby's car safety seat in for use during this car safety seat evaluation. It may not be possible to give you an exact date, but it will help to know approximately when you should be ready. If your baby does not require a car safety seat evaluation, your approximate date of discharge will be your "ready" date.

2. If you cannot afford to purchase a car safety seat, ask your baby's nurse or your social worker about resources for car safety seat loan or rental.

3. Ask the NICU team if your baby has any special needs that will influence your selection of a car safety seat. Some babies need a car safety seat that allows the baby to lie flat. (See page 594.) Smaller babies need car safety seats with certain dimensions for correct harness fit. (See page 587.)

4. Ask NICU staff for recommendations for different models of car safety seats. Models change from year to year, and some car safety seats are easier to use than others. The AAP offers a helpful pamphlet for parents every year titled "Car Safety Seats: A Guide for Families." (Visit the AAP Web site at www.aap.org.)

5. Follow the recommendations presented in this chapter and shop for a car safety seat that might fit your vehicle and your baby. Check the store's return policy and keep your receipt! It's possible that you may need to try a few models before finding one that works best. (See page 591.)

6. Read the car safety seat installation instructions and your vehicle owner's manual and install the car safety seat in your car. If possible, get a certified child passenger safety technician to check that your car safety seat is installed properly and make corrections as needed (see Resources on page 596.)

7. Make arrangements with your baby's nurse or discharge coordinator to bring the car safety seat to the hospital on a day the nurse or designated NICU team member will teach you how to position your baby safely in the car safety seat. This may happen at the time of the car safety seat evaluation. Some nurseries will refer you to a child passenger safety technician for this type of assistance.

8. If possible, have a certified child passenger safety technician check the car safety seat installation and the baby's positioning in the car safety seat every few months. (See Resources on page 596.) Adjustments will be necessary as your baby grows to keep her safe in the car.

Basic Information About Car Safety Seats

Car safety seats come with many features and often involve complex installation. Learn about car safety seats before your baby's discharge is imminent, especially if this is your first experience.

- The safety seat must be the right size for the baby. Many car safety seats are too large to fit premature or small babies. Read about recommendations for safety seat dimensions in the Special Considerations section.

- Experts recommend that you select an infant-only seat if your baby was premature or of low birth weight. You may also choose a convertible car safety seat with a rear-facing weight limit of at least 30 pounds. Otherwise, buy a convertible seat when your baby is approaching the weight or height limit of her infant-only seat. Move her to a convertible seat before her head reaches the top of the infant-only car safety shell and keep her rear-facing.

- Household carriers or feeding seats are not strong enough to protect a baby in a crash. The car safety seat must meet current federal motor vehicle safety standards.

- Do not use a car safety seat that is too old. The manufacturer determines the life span of the car safety seat, which is typically 6 years. Check the label.

- The AAP recommends that preterm and low birth weight "infants ride rear-facing as long as possible and to the highest weight and length allowed by the manufacturer of the seat." At a minimum, infants must ride rear-facing until they are at least 1 year of age and weigh at least 20 pounds. This position best protects a baby's weak neck and large head.

- Read your automobile owner's manual for special instructions regarding car safety seat use. Every make and model has specifications for proper car safety seat installation. Most vehicles built after September 1, 2002, are equipped with lower anchors that can be used for installation. If you use the seat belt for installation, check both the car safety seat manual and vehicle owner's manual to be sure the seat belt is compatible.

- Read the car safety seat instructions before it is time to buckle your baby into the car. Practice securing your car safety seat in the car and taking it out again. (See Installation Tips for Rear-facing Seats on page 586.)

- Install the car safety seat in the back seat of your vehicle. Babies and young children riding rear-facing must never ride in the front seat. If there is a passenger-side air bag, riding in the front seat could be deadly for a baby in a crash.

- Be sure that safety belts securing safety seats lock tightly and hold the seat firmly in place. Make sure the baby's seat cannot be moved side to side or forward more than 1 inch.

- Use baby clothes with legs (not outfits that enclose the baby's legs like a sleeping bag) so the crotch strap can go between her legs. To keep the baby warm, tuck a blanket over her after buckling the harness.

- If you use a car safety seat with a carrying handle, check your instruction manual for information about what handle positions are allowed during travel.
- If necessary, learn how to secure special care items, such as your baby's oxygen cylinder or apnea monitor. (See Travel Guidelines for Infants With Special Health Care Needs on page 590.) Decide where to position the baby and other passengers so that the baby is supervised and in a safe place in the car.
- If your baby needs attention while you are driving, pull over and stop the car. In addition, know that some air bags may inflate on impact even if the vehicle engine is turned off. When you care for your baby in a parked car, do so in the back seat.
- Attend a car safety seat safety clinic or class if one is offered in your area. Proper car safety seat use can be difficult without help. (See Resources on page 596.)

Installation Tips for Rear-facing Seats[a]

When using a rear-facing seat, keep the following in mind:
• Make sure the car safety seat is installed tightly in the vehicle and that the harness fits the child snugly.
• Never place a rear-facing car safety seat in the front seat of a vehicle that has an active front passenger air bag. If the air bag inflates, it will hit the back of the car safety seat, right where your baby's head is, and could cause serious injury or death.
• If your rear-facing seat has more than one set of harness slots, make sure the harnesses are in the slots at or below your baby's shoulders.
• Be sure you know what kind of seat belts your vehicle has. Some seat belts need locking clips. Locking clips come with all new car safety seats. If you're not sure, check the owner's manual that came with your vehicle. Locking clips are not needed in most newer vehicles.
• If you are using a convertible seat in the rear-facing position, make sure the seat belt is routed through the correct belt path. Check the instructions that came with the car safety seat to be sure.
• If your vehicle was made after 2002, it may come with the LATCH system, which is used to secure car safety seats. See page 593 for information on using LATCH.
• Make sure the seat is at the correct angle so your infant's head does not flop forward. Many seats have angle indicators or adjusters that can help prevent this. If your seat does not have an angle adjuster, tilt the car safety seat back by putting a rolled towel or other firm padding (such as a pool noodle) under the base near the point where the back and bottom of the vehicle seat meet. (See page 589.)
• Be sure the car safety seat is installed tightly. If you can move the seat more than an inch side to side or front to back, it's not tight enough.
• Still having trouble? There may be a certified child passenger safety (CPS) technician in your area who can help. If you need installation help, see page 596 for information on how to locate a CPS technician.

[a]From American Academy of Pediatrics. Car safety seats: a guide for families 2009 [brochure]. Elk Grove Village, IL: American Academy of Pediatrics; 2009.

Special Considerations for NICU Graduates

Correct selection of a restraint device is particularly important for newborn infants who are preterm or weigh less than 5 1/2 pounds (2,500 grams) or have certain conditions, such as spina bifida, hydrocephalus, Pierre Robin sequence, or neuromuscular disorders. In some cases, the use of some or all conventional infant/child safety seats may be unsuitable. However, devices are available to accommodate virtually all special needs.

Selecting the Car Safety Seat for Infants With Special Needs

- Some babies may have trouble breathing when they sit in a semireclined seat, such as a car safety seat, swing, and other upright equipment such as backpacks, slings, and infant carriers. These babies should ride lying flat in a special bed made for use in the car until the child's respiratory status is stable. (See page 594.)
- Babies with tracheostomies should not be placed in child restraint systems with a harness-tray/shield combination or an armrest. On sudden impact, the child could fall forward, causing the tracheostomy to contact the shield or armrest, possibly resulting in injury and a blocked airway. A child safety seat with a 5-point harness should be selected for children with tracheostomies. (See page 592.)
- Child safety seats with a 5-point harness (at both shoulders, both hips, and between the legs) can be adjusted to provide good upper torso support for many children with special needs.

Safety Seat Dimensions

Many car safety seats are simply too large to safely restrain a very small baby.

- Take a measuring tape with you to the store. Be sure that the car safety seat meets the AAP recommended measurements for crotch to seat back. Car safety seats with a space of 5 1/2 inches or less between the crotch strap and the seat back will keep your baby from slouching too much.
- If you already own a car safety seat, you may be able to use it, depending on how it fits your baby. Many models can be adapted with removable inserts for small babies that help the seat fit them better. Rolled receiving blankets can be used outside of the harness system to give lateral support, as described on page 588.

Positioning the Baby in the Car Safety Seat

All infants need special attention to be comfortable and safe in the car. To function properly, the safety restraint must fit the infant's body. The restraint must be installed securely, and the infant must be buckled in with adequate support.

- Your baby should ride facing the back of the vehicle for as long as possible and to the highest weight and length allowed by the manufacturer of the seat. When your baby weighs 20 pounds or reaches the top length allowed by the seat manufacturer, she should continue to ride facing the rear in an infant seat or convertible car safety seat approved for rear-facing use at higher weights and lengths. Most convertible car safety seats are approved for rear-facing use up to 30 to 35 pounds and 36 inches tall.
- The safety seat should recline halfway back, at no more than a 45-degree tilt, so the baby's head does not flop forward. If the vehicle seat slopes so that the infant's head falls forward, the safety seat should be tipped back so the baby's head is upright. (Some infant safety seats also have tilt indicators to indicate how the seat is angled.) Many infant seats have built-in recline adjusters. If yours does not or if more recline is needed, wedge a firm roll of cloth or newspaper, or place a pool noodle of closed-cell foam, under the base below the infant's feet. (See Figure 1.) Don't recline the seat back farther than 45 degrees.
- The infant's buttocks and back should be flat against the back of the safety seat. Rolled-up diapers or small blankets along the sides can help center the baby in the car safety seat. (See Figure 2.) If she slips down, add a rolled washcloth between her crotch and the harness. Do not use padding under the baby's buttocks or behind the back and head.
- Shoulder straps must be in the lowest slots, the harness snug, and the harness retainer clip at the midpoint of the infant's chest, not on the abdomen or in front of the neck.
- Any blankets used must be put over the infant after the harness has been adjusted snugly.
- Do not use an add-on infant head support. A head support that came in the box with the seat may be used as long as it has slots through which harness straps can be pulled. It must not have thick padding behind the infant's back because this could make the harness too loose in a crash, allowing the baby to be thrown out of the car safety seat.
- Infants who must ride lying flat in a special car bed because of potential breathing problems should be positioned with their head as far as possible from the side of the vehicle. The baby's health care provider will indicate whether the baby should lie on her back or tummy.
- If your baby is riding flat in a car bed, the harness should be snug. Unfortunately, a flat car bed does not rest securely on the contoured seats of many vehicles.

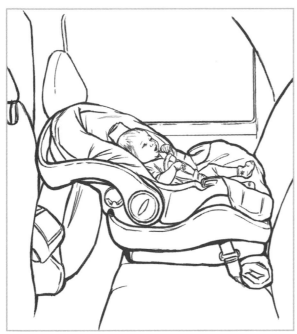

Figure 1. Wedge to tilt safety seat.
A firm roll is wedged under the safety seat below the infant's feet to make the base of the seat horizontal.

From: American Academy of Pediatrics Committee on Injury, Violence and Poison Prevention and Committee on Fetus and Newborn. Safe transportation of preterm and low birth weight infants at hospital discharge. Pediatrics. 2009;123;1424–1429.

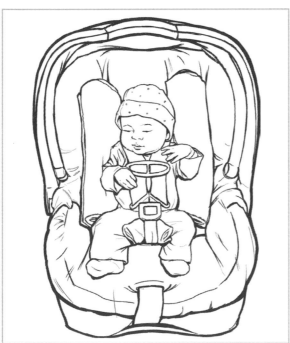

Figure 2. Padding placement for a small baby.
Padding beside head and torso and in crotch of newborn infant in infant-only safet y seat. No padding should be placed under the infant's buttocks.

From: American Academy of Pediatrics Committee on Injury, Violence and Poison Prevention and Committee on Fetus and Newborn. Safe transportation of preterm and low birth weight infants at hospital discharge. Pediatrics. 2009;123;1424–1429.

Travel Guidelines for Infants With Special Health Care Needs

(Adapted from http://www.aap.org/publiced/BR_SpNeedsCarSeats.htm.)

- Depending on your child's condition, it may be wise to limit the amount of car travel.
- Stop often if your trip is long.
- When possible, an adult should ride in the back seat next to your child to watch her closely.
- Develop a medical care plan in case your child has a medical emergency during travel. Some parents attach a copy of the plan to the child's car safety seat/restraint.
- Carry with you an emergency kit that includes any special medications or supplies that your child may need. A checklist will help you ensure that the right medications and supplies are always with you. Do not leave this kit in the vehicle.
- Keep a cellular phone with you to contact help, if needed. Cellular phones can dial 911 even if you do not purchase a service contract.
- Never use a reclined vehicle seat to transport a child. In a crash, the child can slip out of position and not be protected by the seat belt.
- Apply for a handicap parking permit on behalf of your child if it is hard to get her in and out of the car safety restraint. Handicap parking often allows more space to maneuver.
- Never leave your child alone in a vehicle, even to do an errand that should only take a minute. Your child's safety is worth the effort to remove her from the car safety seat/restraint, take her with you, and then secure her again when you return.
- Some children must travel with devices such as apnea monitors, oxygen tanks, ventilators, walkers, and crutches. Secure these in the vehicle so that they do not become flying objects in the event of a crash or sudden stop. At this time, there is no single product available to secure medical devices. Try wedging the equipment on the vehicle floor with pillows or securing it with seat belts not being used by a passenger. Make sure that any devices that use batteries have enough power for at least double the length of your trip.

Shopping for Car Safety Seats[a]

When shopping for a car safety seat, keep the following tips in mind:

- **No one seat is the "best" or "safest."** The best seat is the one that fits your child's age and size, is correctly installed, fits well in your vehicle, and can be used properly every time you drive.

- **Don't decide by price alone.** A higher price does not mean the seat is safer or easier to use.

- **Avoid used seats if you don't know the seat's history.** Never use a car safety seat that
  - **Is too old.** Look on the label for the date it was made. Check with the manufacturer to find out how long it recommends using the seat.
  - **Has any visible cracks on it.**
  - **Does not have a label with the date of manufacture and model number.** Without these, you cannot check to see if the seat has been recalled.
  - **Does not come with instructions.** You need them to know how to use the seat.
  - **Is missing parts.** Used car safety seats often come without important parts. Check with the manufacturer to make sure you can get the right parts.
  - **Was recalled.** You can find out by calling the manufacturer or by contacting the National Highway Traffic Safety Administration (NHTSA) Vehicle Safety Hotline at 888/327-4236. You can also visit the NHTSA Web site at www-odi.nhtsa.dot.gov/cars/problems/recalls/childseat.cfm.

- **Do not use seats that have been in a moderate or severe crash.** Seats that were in a minor crash may still be safe to use. NHTSA considers a crash minor if all of the following are true:
  - The vehicle could be driven away from the crash.
  - The vehicle door closest to the car safety seat was not damaged.
  - No one in the vehicle was injured.
  - The air bags did not go off.
  - You can't see any damage to the car safety seat.

[a]From American Academy of Pediatrics. Car safety seats: a guide for families 2009 [brochure]. Elk Grove Village, IL: American Academy of Pediatrics; 2009:14.

The Right Car Safety Seat[a]

Infants—rear-facing

The American Academy of Pediatrics (AAP) recommends that all infants should ride rear-facing starting with their first ride home from the hospital. They should remain rear-facing until they reach the highest weight or height allowed by their car safety seat's manufacturer. At a minimum, children should ride rear-facing until they have reached at least 1 year of age *and* weigh at least 20 pounds.

There are 2 types of rear-facing car safety seats: infant-only seats and convertible seats.

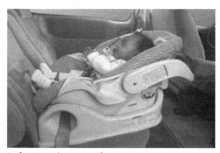
Infant-only car safety seat

Infant-only seats

- Are small and have carrying handles (and sometimes come as part of a stroller system).
- Are used only for travel (not for positioning outside the vehicle).
- Are used for infants up to 22 to 32 pounds, depending on the model.
- Many come with a base that can be left in the car. The seat clicks into and out of the base so you don't have to install the base each time you use it. Parents can buy more than one base for additional vehicles.

Convertible seats (used rear-facing)

- Can be used rear-facing, then "converted" to forward-facing for older children. This means the seat can be used longer by your child. They are bulkier than infant seats, however, and do not come with carrying handles or a separate base.
- Have higher rear-facing weight and height limits than infant-only seats, which makes them ideal for bigger babies.
- Have 2 types of harnesses.

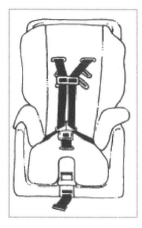
5-point harness— attach at the shoulders, at the hips, and between the legs

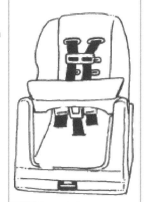
Overhead shield— a padded tray-like shield that swings down over the child (not recommended for very small babies or babies with tracheostomies)

[a]From American Academy of Pediatrics. Car safety seats: a guide for families 2009 [brochure]. Elk Grove Village, IL: American Academy of Pediatrics; 2009:2, 4, 5.

Installing Car Safety Seats Correctly

What You Should Know About Air Bags

All new cars come with front air bags. When used with seat belts, air bags work very well to protect teenagers and adults. However, air bags can be very dangerous to children, particularly those riding in rear-facing car safety seats and to child passengers who are not properly positioned. If your vehicle has a front passenger air bag, infants in rear-facing seats *must ride in the back seat.* Even in a relatively low-speed crash, the air bag can inflate, strike the car safety seat, and cause serious brain and neck injury and death.

Vehicles with no back seat or a back seat that is not made for passengers are not the best choice for traveling with small children. However, the air bag can be turned off in some of these vehicles if the front seat is needed for a child passenger. See your vehicle owner's manual for more information.

Side Air Bags

Side air bags improve safety for adults in side-impact crashes. Read your vehicle owner's manual for more information about the air bags in your vehicle. Read your car safety seat manual for guidance on placing the seat next to a side air bag.

LATCH (lower anchors and tethers for children) is an attachment system that improves safety by eliminating the need to use seat belts to secure the car safety seat. Vehicles with the LATCH system have anchors located in the back seat. Car safety seats that come with LATCH have attachments that fasten to these anchors. Nearly all passenger vehicles and all car safety seats made on or after September 1, 2002, come with LATCH. However, unless both your vehicle *and* the car safety seat have this anchor system, you will still need to use seat belts to install the car safety seat.

If You Need Installation Help

If you have questions or need help installing your car safety seat, find a certified CPS technician. Lists of certified CPS technicians and child seat fitting stations are available on the National Highway Traffic Safety Administration (NHTSA) Web site at www.nhtsa.gov or at www.seatcheck.org. You can also get this information by calling 866/SEATCHECK (866/732-8243) or the NHTSA Vehicle Safety Hotline at 888/327-4236.

Car Beds[a]

Car beds are restraints that allow infants to travel lying down. There are three different kinds of car beds, the Dream Ride SE by Dorel Juvenile Group, the Angel Ride car bed by Angel Guard, and the Snug Seat car bed by Snug Seat (no longer being manufactured but available through some hospital car safety seat programs). Although there are variations in design, all of the beds must be used with the infant's head facing toward the center of the vehicle, away from any side or door. When positioning an infant in a car bed, it is important to ask the medical staff if the baby should lie on his or her stomach, back, or side. Due to concerns about placing babies on their belly increasing the risk of sudden infant death syndrome (SIDS), babies should **not** be positioned on their stomach unless prescribed by their physician to be medically necessary.

For specific product information, contact:

Dorel Juvenile Group, Inc.
2525 State Street
Columbus, IN 47201-7494
800-544-1108
www.djgusa.com

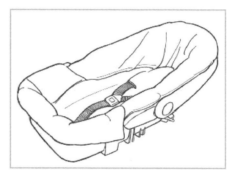

Dream Ride SE
Weight: 5-20 pounds
Height: 19-26 inches

Mercury Distributing
7001 Wooster Pike
Medina, OH 44256
800-815-6330
www.mercurydistributing.com

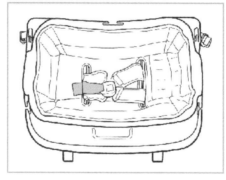

Angel Ride Car Bed
Weight: less than
9 pounds
Height: less than
20 inches

Snug Seat, Inc.
12801 East Independence Blvd.
P.O. Box 1739
Matthews, NC 28106
800-336-SNUG (7684)
www.snugseat.com

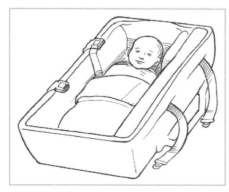

*Snug Seat Car Bed
Weight: up to
21 pounds
Height: up to
29 1/2 inches
*Discontinued

Car Beds[a], continued

Specialized restraints for children in hip casts.

The Snug Seat Hippo is a convertible safety seat specifically for children in hip casts. The modified E-Z-ON Vest may be an option for those children who do not fit in the Hippo.

The Hippo convertible car safety seat by Snug Seat is designed for infants and toddlers in hip casts. Unlike conventional convertible seats, the Hippo has a shallow seating surface and low sides in order to accommodate hip casts. The Hippo convertible seat also has a wedge positioning system for children in casts to assist in achieving a snug fit in the seat.

The Hippo is used rear-facing in the reclined position and with the harness straps at or below the shoulders for infants from 5-33 pounds. The seat is used forward-facing, upright or semi-reclined for toddlers from 20-65 pounds and up to 49 inches. In the forward facing position the seat can be used reclined or upright to 40 pounds and must be upright 40-65 pounds. The weight of the cast is included in the child's weight. Always use the tether for children who weigh more than 40 pounds.

For specific information about this product, contact:

Snug Seat, Inc.
12801 East Independence Blvd.
P.O. Box 1739
Matthews, NC 28106
800-336-SNUG (7684)
www.snugseat.com

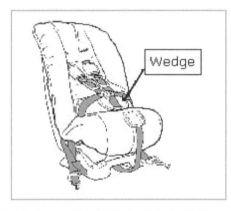

Snug Seat Hippo
Weight: 5-33 pounds rear facing/1 year old and 20-65 pounds forward facing
Height: up to 49 inches
For infants and toddlers in hip casts.

[a]Reprinted with permission from Automotive Safety Program. Special needs transportation: restraints. http://www.preventinjury.org/SNTrestraints.asp.

Important Reminders

1. **Be a good role model.** Make sure you always wear your seat belt. This will help your child form a lifelong habit of buckling up.

2. **Never leave your child alone in or around cars.** Any of the following can happen when a child is left alone in or around a vehicle:
    -   Temperatures can reach deadly levels in minutes, and the child can die of heat stroke.
    -   He can be strangled by power windows, sunroofs, or accessories.
    -   He can knock the vehicle into gear, setting it in motion.
    -   He can be backed over when the vehicle backs up.
    -   He can become trapped in the trunk of the vehicle.

3. **Always read and follow manufacturer's instructions.** If you do not have the manufacturer's instructions for your car safety seat, write or call the company's customer service department. They will ask you for the model number, name of seat, and date of manufacture. The manufacturer's address and phone number are on the label on the seat. Also be sure to follow the instructions in your vehicle owner's manual about using car safety seats.

Resources

1. **National Highway Traffic Safety Administration (NHTSA)**
    Toll-free: 888/327-4236   www.nhtsa.dot.gov

2. **Ease of Use Ratings**
    The NHTSA has put together a system to educate parents and caregivers about car safety seat features and to assist them in finding the appropriate seat for their needs. You can view this list at www.nhtsa.dot.gov/CPS/CSSRating/Index.cfm.

3. **Certified Child Passenger Safety (CPS) Technicians**
    A list of certified CPS technicians is available by state or ZIP code on the NHTSA Web site at www.nhtsa.dot.gov/people/injury/childps/contacts. A list of inspection stations—where you can go to learn how to correctly install a car safety seat—is available in English and Spanish at www.seatcheck.org or toll-free at 866/SEAT-CHECK (866/732-8243). You can also get this information by calling the toll-free NHTSA Auto Safety Hot Line at 888/DASH-2-DOT (888/327-4236), from 8:00 am to 10:00 pm ET, Monday through Friday.

4. **Automotive Safety for Children Program**
    Riley Hospital for Children
    317/274-2977
    www.preventinjury.org

5. **American Academy of Pediatrics**

   The AAP offers more information in the brochure "Car Safety Seats: A Guide for Families." Ask your pediatrician about this brochure or visit the AAP Web site at www.aap.org.

6. **The Children's Hospital of Philadelphia**

   Keeping Kids Safe During Crashes: http://stokes.chop.edu/programs/carseat/

   This site was developed by the Center for Injury Research and Prevention at The Children's Hospital of Philadelphia to help parents and caregivers learn more about child safety seats, booster seats, and seat belts. Read or watch videos about safe use of infant car safety seats.

7. **Safe Ride News**

   www.saferidenews.com/srndnn/

   425/640-5710 or 800/403-1424

   The goal of Safe Ride News publications is to help save lives and prevent injury to children in traffic.

Appendix D
Parent Resources

"Hallo!" said Tigger.

"I've found somebody just like me.

I thought I was the only one of them."

Medicine and the Media:
How to Make Sense of the Messages

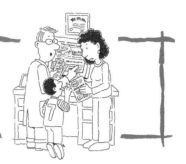

Your child is sick or hurt and the first thought on your mind is, "How can I make my child better?" That's natural. No parent wants his or her child to suffer. So how do you decide what medicines to give or treatments to try?

Aside from your pediatrician, what sources can you trust? Commercials and magazine ads claim products help and heal. Web sites claim to have "cutting-edge" health information. TV programs and newspapers report on the "latest" studies showing which treatments work and don't work.

One challenge of parenting is sorting through all available information about children's health. Some sources can be trusted, while others should be questioned. Read more to learn about the language of advertisers, good science, questioning your sources, using the Internet, Web site addresses, and evaluating new treatments or medicines.

The language of advertisers

Advertisers try many ways to get you to buy the products they are selling. They may use certain words or phrases to interest you, such as

- **"#1 Pediatrician Recommended" or "Doctor Recommended"**
  These are marketing terms that try to get you to buy a product. Although the product may be recommended by a group of doctors, what the advertisers don't tell you is how many doctors or how long ago the recommendation was made. It could be 5 or 100 doctors surveyed 10 years ago.
- **"Patented Design"**
  A patent means that the maker or inventor of a product has proven to the government that he or she was the first to create the product. In return, the government gives a patent and says that only the patent holder can make or sell the product for a certain period. A patent doesn't necessarily mean that the product is the best, is safe, or will work.
- **"Clinically Shown"**
  This phrase means that the product was tested on patients as part of a study to see if the product worked. There are many ways to conduct studies. However, if the people doing the study don't follow strict scientific rules for doing research, the study results may have little meaning.

Good science

Scientific studies require careful planning. Researchers need to follow specific procedures and processes. Studies must follow certain rules to be considered scientifically credible, including the following:
- The testing must take place in carefully **controlled conditions.** Researchers have to make sure to control factors that could affect the results. For example, if researchers want to know how a medicine affects a child, they have to make sure the child isn't taking any other medicines at the same time.

- Researchers need to determine how many people should be included in the study. **Study size** varies according to the kind of study and number of people needed to demonstrate an effect.
- The group of people receiving treatment should be compared to a **control group** to truly test if the treatment has any effect. A control group doesn't receive the new treatment, but instead may be given a placebo (sugar pill) or an alternative treatment.
- Good clinical studies should be **replicated.** That means other researchers should be able to do the same study again using different subjects and get similar results. We know we can trust the findings when different studies come to the same conclusions.
- Well-done, scientifically sound studies should go through **peer review.** This means other experts on the topic being studied should review each study and make sure that all proper scientific standards were met.

Questioning your sources

It's important to ask the following questions when evaluating a source:
1. **What is the source?**
   In general, sources you can trust include accredited medical schools, government agencies, professional medical associations, and recognized national disorder/disease-specific organizations. However, don't rely mainly on the name of the organization—do your own research.
2. **Who is the expert?**
   The doctors or researchers being interviewed may sound like experts, but what are their credentials? What expertise and experience do they have? They may be doctors, but are they experts on the particular issue being talked about? Are there conflicts of interest? Are they working for a company that may benefit from their "expert" support? Are they being paid for their support of a product? If so, this could influence what information these experts choose to share.
3. **What are the facts?**
   Know the difference between preliminary and confirmed findings—a "breakthrough" finding may seem promising but still has to be replicated and reviewed over time. Don't let a headline make you think that "new study" is the same as "proven." Another word of caution: "new" doesn't mean improved. Sometimes newer medicines are not an improvement over older medicines and cost much more.

Using the Internet

The Internet can be a valuable source of medical information and advice, but you can't trust everything you read. The Internet also is the source of a lot of health-related theories and opinions that haven't been proven.

Begin your search for information with the most reliable, general-information Web sites and expand from there. The Web site for the American Academy of Pediatrics (AAP), www.aap.org, is a good starting point.

Web site addresses

The last 3 letters in a Web site address can tell you what type of organization or company set up the site.

- **.gov**—Government Web sites often provide large amounts of information for the general public.
- **.org**—Nonprofit organization Web sites may contain useful information. However, not all organizations put out reliable materials. Search for information on nonprofit Web sites that you have heard of and have good reputations.
- **.edu**—Academic or education-based Web sites may have educational materials for parents.
- **.com**—Commercial Web sites often are designed to sell you something. They are not necessarily a source of reliable information.

Evaluating new treatments or medicines

When you come across a new treatment or medicine, ask yourself the following questions:

1. Will it work for my child?

Be suspicious if the information describing the treatment or medicine

- Claims it will work for everyone.
- Uses a story about one person's experience or testimonials as proof that it works.
- Cites only one study as proof.
- Cites a study without a control (comparison) group.

2. How safe is it?

Be suspicious if the treatment or medicine

- Comes without directions for proper use.
- Doesn't list contents or ingredients.
- Has no information or warnings about side effects.
- Is described as "harmless" or "natural." Remember, most medication is made from natural sources. A "natural" treatment doesn't necessarily work and, worse yet, actually may be harmful to your child. Being "natural" does not necessarily mean it is good or safe.
- Isn't approved by the Food and Drug Administration (FDA).
- Appears on an infomercial.

3. How is it promoted?

Be suspicious if the ad for the treatment or medicine

- Claims it's based on a secret formula.
- Claims it works immediately and permanently.
- Claims it's a "miraculous" or an "amazing" breakthrough.
- Claims it is a "cure."
- Indicates it's available from only one source.

Remember

You shouldn't trust everything that you read or hear. Make sure that your pediatrician knows about your questions and concerns; share the information you've found. You and your pediatrician are partners in your child's health.

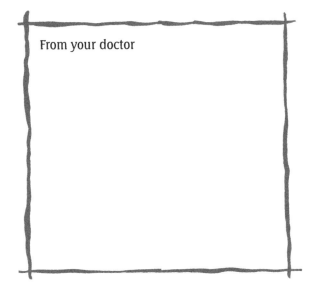

From your doctor

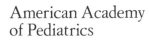

American Academy of Pediatrics

DEDICATED TO THE HEALTH OF ALL CHILDREN™

The American Academy of Pediatrics is an organization of 60,000 primary care pediatricians, pediatric medical subspecialists, and pediatric surgical specialists dedicated to the health, safety, and well-being of infants, children, adolescents, and young adults.

American Academy of Pediatrics
Web site—www.aap.org

Copyright © 2004
American Academy of Pediatrics

Most neonatal intensive care unit (NICU) parents seek additional information and resources on the Internet. Listing Web sites for each aspect of NICU care and parenting would be impossible; however, the following suggestions will get you started. Begin with the section titled "Places to Begin" and go from there to find additional links to your area of interest, including books and other media formats.

Listing a Web site here does not imply an endorsement and this is by no means an all-inclusive list. Use the American Academy of Pediatrics recommendations ("Medicine and the Media") for finding safe and credible Web site information every time you seek resources online.

Places to Begin: Information About NICU Babies and NICU Graduates

American Academy of Pediatrics (AAP)
www.aap.org/

AAP Section on Perinatal Pediatrics
www.aap.org/sections/perinatal/families.html

American Self-Help Group Clearinghouse
(find any type of online support group)
www.mentalhelp.net/selfhelp/

Centers for Disease Control and Prevention
www.cdc.gov/

**Family Village: For Families of Children with Special Needs
An Internet Guide**
www.familyvillage.wisc.edu/websites.html

March of Dimes
www.marchofdimes.com/

Books

Amazon.com or any major bookstore lists books for NICU parents. Keywords for book title search include NICU, premature, premie, preemie, neonatal intensive care, special needs child, sibling, breastfeeding, breast milk, or list the specific condition or disease.

Birth Defects

March of Dimes: Birth Defects and Genetic Conditions
www.marchofdimes.com/4439.asp

TERIS (online database designed to assist physicians or other health care professionals in assessing the risks of possible teratogenic exposures in pregnant women)
http://depts.washington.edu/terisweb/teris/

Breastfeeding

AAP: Breastfeeding and the Use of Human Milk Policy Statement
http://aappolicy.aappublications.org/cgi/content/full/pediatrics;115/2/496

African-American Breastfeeding Alliance
www.aabaonline.com/tp40/default.asp?ID=24582

Ameda-Evenflow
www.ameda.com or www.evenflo.com
866/99-AMEDA

Baby Friendly Hospital Initiative in the US
www.babyfriendlyusa.org/eng/index.html

Book: Best Medicine: Human Milk in the NICU (2008)
Authors: Nancy E. Wright, Jane A. Morton, and Jae H. Kim

Breastfeeding After Breast and Nipple Surgeries (BFAR)
(information and support for low milk supply)
www.bfar.org/

Breastfeeding Canada
www.breastfeedingcanada.ca

Breastfeeding.com
www.breastfeeding.com/

CDC Breastfeeding Resources
www.cdc.gov/breastfeeding/

Human Milk Banking Association of North America
www.hmbana.org/
919/861-4530

INFACT Canada (Infant Feeding Action Coalition)
www.infactcanada.ca/
416/595-9819

International Lactation Consultant Association
www.ilca.org
Find a lactation consultant: http://www.ilca.org/i4a/pages/index.cfm?pageid=3337
919/861-5577

La Leche League
www.llli.org/WebUS.html
800/LALECHE (US), or 847/519-7730

Medela
www.medelabreastfeedingus.com/
800/TELL-YOU

United States Breastfeeding Committee
Directory of State/Territory/Tribal Breastfeeding Coalitions
http://www.usbreastfeeding.org/Coalitions/CoalitionsDirectory/tabid/74/Default.aspx

WIC (Special Supplemental Nutrition Program for Women, Infants, and Children)
Provides breastfeeding help to mothers and children enrolled in the WIC program
www.fns.usda.gov

Women's Health.gov: Breastfeeding
www.womenshealth.gov/breastfeeding/index.cfm

Children With Special Needs

Aaron's Tracheostomy Page
www.tracheostomy.com/

AboutFace International (support for facial birth defects)
www.aboutfaceinternational.org/index.php

American Academy for Cerebral Palsy and Developmental Medicine
www.aacpdm.org/patients/websites_of_interest.php

Children With Special Needs, continued

CHERUBS: The Association of Congenital Diaphragmatic Hernia Research, Awareness, and Support
www.cherubs-cdh.org

Cleft Palate Foundation
1/800-24CLEFT
www.cleftline.org

March of Dimes: Cleft Lip and Palate
http://www.marchofdimes.com/professionals/14332_1210.asp

National Dissemination Center for Children with Disabilities
www.nichcy.org/FamiliesAndCommunity/Pages/Default.aspx
800/695-0285

National Down Syndrome Society
www.ndss.org
800/221.4602

National Tay-Sachs & Allied Diseases Association
www.ntsad.org/
800/906-8723

New Visions (continuing education and therapy services to professionals and parents working with infants and children with feeding, swallowing, oral-motor, and pre-speech problems)
www.new-vis.com/index.htm

Spina Bifida Association
www.spinabifidaassociation.org/site/c.liKWL7PLLrF/b.2642297/k.5F7C/Spina_Bifida_
Association.htm

Support Group for Arthrogryposis Multiplex Congenita
www.amcsupport.org/

Support Organization for Trisomy 18, 13, and Related Disorders (SOFT)
www.trisomy.org

United Cerebral Palsy
www.ucp.org/

ECMO

ECMO Moms and Dads
www.medhelp.org/amshc/amshc341.htm.

Heart Disease

American Heart Association: Congenital Heart Disease
www.americanheart.org/presenter.jhtml?identifier=3058143

Congenital Heart Information Network
http://tchin.org

Cove Point Foundation: Congenital Heart Disease, Johns Hopkins University
www.pted.org/htms/list.php#1

The Mended Hearts, Inc
www.mendedhearts.org/
888/HEART99 (888/432-7899)

Hearing Impairment

Alexander Graham Bell Association for the Deaf and Hard of Hearing
www.agbell.org/DesktopDefault.aspx?linkid=1

Laurent Clerc National Deaf Education Center, Gallaudet University
http://clerccenter.gallaudet.edu/Clerc_Center/Information_and_Resources/Info_To_Go.
html/index.html

High-Risk Pregnancy and Birth

American College of Obstetricians and Gynecologists (ACOG)
www.acog.org/

Sidelines National High Risk Pregnancy Support Network
www.sidelines.org
888/447-4754 (888/HI-RISK4)

Loss of a Child

A Place to Remember (support materials and resources for those who have been touched by a crisis in pregnancy or the death of a baby)
www.aplacetoremember.com/aptrfront.html

Center for Loss in Multiple Birth (CLIMB, Inc.)
www.climb-support.org/

The Compassionate Friends, Inc.
www.compassionatefriends.org/
877/969-0010 or 630/990-0010

First Candle
www.sidsalliance.org/
800/221-7437

Resolve Through Sharing (catalog of resources)
www.bereavementprograms.com/catalog/

SHARE: Pregnancy & Infant Loss Support, Inc.
www.nationalshare.org/
800/821-6819

Twinless Twins Support Group, International (US)
www.twinlesstwins.org/
888/205-8962

Wright J. (2006). Back to Life: Your Personal Guidebook to Grief Recovery
www.recover-from-grief.com/heartbroken-from-grief.html

Medical Home

(Refers to the concept of parent-professional partnership for coordinated health care.)

AAP: Medical Home
http://aap.org/healthtopics/medicalhome.cfm

Medical Home Initiatives & Resources by State
www.medicalhomeinfo.org/states/index.html

Washington State Medical Home
www.medicalhome.org/families/

What is a Medical Home?
www.medicalhomeinfo.org/

Parenting

American Academy of Pediatrics Bright Futures
http://brightfutures.aap.org/Family_Resources.html

Canadian Parents: Canada's Parenting Community
www.canadianparents.com

Come Unity: Parenting Support for Your Unique Family
(articles, resource directories, expert interviews, and exclusive book reviews on
parenting, adoption, and children's special needs)
http://comeunity.com/

Family Voices (family-centered care for all children and youth with special health
care needs and/or disabilities)
www.familyvoices.org/info/about.php

Healthy Child Care America
www.healthychildcare.org/ResourcesFamilies.html

**Healthy Kids, Healthy Care: Parents as Partners in Promoting Healthy and Safe
Child Care**
www.healthykids.us/

Infant CPR Anytime (DVD helps family, care providers, and friends learn infant
CPR at home)
www.aap.org/family/infantcpranytime.htm

Juvenile Products Manufacturers Association
www.jpma.org/index2.cfm?section=BabySafety

National Lekotek Center (provides information about toys and play for children with
special needs)
www.lekotek.org/

Parents Helping Parents
www.php.com/
408/727-5775

The Father's Network
www.fathersnetwork.org/
425/653-4286

Preterm Babies

AAP Section on Perinatal Pediatrics
www.aap.org/sections/perinatal/families.html

Critical Elements of Care for Low Birth Weight Neonatal Intensive Care Graduates (and Extremely Low Birth Weight supplement)
www.medicalhome.org/diagnoses/lbw_cg_gc.cfm

March of Dimes: Premature Birth
www.marchofdimes.com/prematurity/index_about.asp

Meriter: Parenting Guide for Families of Premature Infants
www.meriter.com/living/preemie/index.htm

NICHD Neonatal Research Network
https://neonatal.rti.org/family/

Parents of Premature Babies, Inc.
www.preemie-l.org

Prematurity.org
http://prematurity.org/

Siblings

Kids Aid (sibling grief and loss)
www.kidsaid.com

Sibling Support Project
www.siblingsupport.org/

Smoking Cessation

1-800-QUIT-NOW
http://1800quitnow.cancer.gov

American Legacy Foundation: Become an EX
www.becomeanex.org

American Lung Association: Freedom From Smoking® Online
http://www.ffsonline.org/

Learn to Quit: Help and Support for Quitting Smoking
http://www.learntoquit.org/

National Institutes of Health (NIH): Smokefree.gov
www.smokefree.gov

Nicotine Anonymous
www.nicotine-anonymous.org

QuitNet
www.quitnet.com

State Tobacco Cessation Coverage (state-by-state resources for Medicaid, state employees, and private insurance coverage)
http://lungusa2.org/cessation2/

You Can Quit Smoking Consumer Guide
www.ahrq.gov/consumer/tobacco/quits.htm

Sudden Infant Death Syndrome (SIDS)

CJ Foundation for SIDS
www.cjsids.com

First Candle
www.sidsalliance.org/

Supplies

Children's Medical Ventures
www.childmed.com/

The Preemie Store and More
www.preemie.com/

Travel and Car Safety Seat Information

(see Appendix C for additional resources)

AAP Car Safety Seats: A Guide for Families 2009
www.aap.org/family/carseatguide.htm

Twins and Multiples

Mothers of Supertwins (MOST)
www.mostonline.org
631/859-1110

Multiple Births Canada/Naissances Multiples Canada (formerly POMBA)
www.multiplebirthscanada.org/english/index.php
705/429-0901 or toll-free in Canada 866/228-8824

National Organization of Mothers of Twins Clubs, Inc.
www.nomotc.org/

The Triplet Connection
www.tripletconnection.org/
435/851-1105

Twins & Multiples
http://multiples.about.com/

Visual Impairment

American Association for Pediatric Ophthalmology and Strabismus
www.aapos.org
415/561-8505

FamilyConnect (from American Foundation for the Blind)
www.familyconnect.org/parentsitehome.asp

National Eye Institute
www.nei.nih.gov
301/496-5248

Appendix E
Choking/CPR

CHOKING/CPR

LEARN AND PRACTICE CPR (CARDIOPULMONARY RESUSCITATION)

IF ALONE WITH A CHILD WHO IS CHOKING...
1. SHOUT FOR HELP.   2. START RESCUE EFFORTS.   3. CALL 911 OR YOUR LOCAL EMERGENCY NUMBER.

YOU SHOULD START FIRST AID FOR CHOKING IF...	*DO NOT* START FIRST AID FOR CHOKING IF...
• The child cannot breathe at all (the chest is not moving up and down). • The child cannot cough or talk, or looks blue. • The child is found unconscious. (Go to CPR.)	• The child can breathe, cry, or talk. • The child can cough, sputter, or move air at all. The child's normal reflexes are working to clear the airway.

FOR INFANTS YOUNGER THAN 1 YEAR

INFANT CHOKING

If the infant is choking and is unable to breathe, cough, cry, or speak, follow these steps. Have someone call 911, or if you are alone call 911 as soon as possible.

1 GIVE FIVE BACK SLAPS

ALTERNATING WITH

2 GIVE FIVE CHEST THRUSTS

Alternate back slaps and chest thrusts until the object is dislodged or the infant becomes unconscious. If the infant becomes unconscious, begin CPR.

INFANT CPR

To be used when the infant is unconscious or when breathing stops.

1 OPEN AIRWAY
- Open airway (tilt head, lift chin).
- Take 5 to 10 seconds to check if the child is breathing after the airway is opened. **Look** for up and down movement of the chest and abdomen. **Listen** for breath sounds at the nose and mouth. **Feel** for breath on your cheek. If opening the airway results in breathing, other than an occasional gasp, do not give breaths.
- If there is no breathing **look** for a foreign object in the mouth. **If you can see** an object in the infant's mouth, sweep it out carefully with your finger. Then attempt rescue breathing. **Do NOT** try a blind finger sweep if the object is not seen, because it could be pushed farther into the throat.

2 RESCUE BREATHING
- **Position** head and chin with both hands as shown— head gently tilted back, chin lifted.
- Take a normal breath (not a deep breath).
- **Seal** your mouth over the infant's mouth and nose.
- Give 2 breaths, each rescue breath over 1 second with a pause between breaths Each breath should make the chest rise.

If no rise or fall after the first breath, repeat steps 1 and 2. If still no rise or fall, continue with step 3 (below).

3 CHEST COMPRESSIONS
- **Place** 2 fingers of 1 hand on the breastbone just below the nipple line.
- **Compress** chest ⅓ to ½ the depth of the chest.
- **Alternate** 30 compressions with 2 breaths.
- **Compress** chest at rate of 100 times per minute.

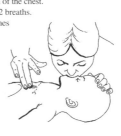

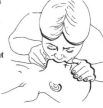

Be sure someone calls 911 as soon as possible. If you are alone, call 911 or your local emergency number after 5 cycles of breaths and chest compressions (about 2 minutes).

From: American Academy of Pediatrics. 3-in-1 First Aid, Choking, CPR Chart. Elk Grove Village, IL; American Academy of Pediatrics; 2006.

Bibliography

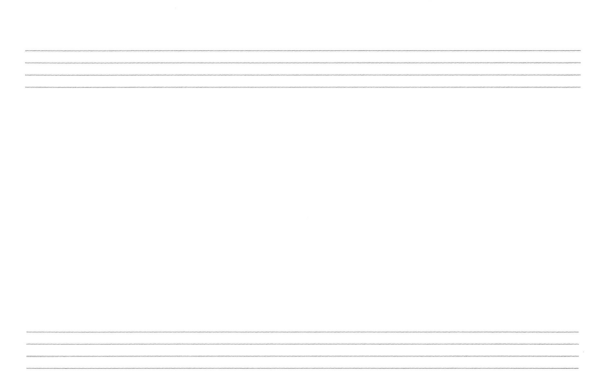

CHAPTER 1

American Academy of Pediatrics, American College of Obstetricians and Gynecologists. *Guidelines for Perinatal Care.* 6th ed. Elk Grove Village, IL: American Academy of Pediatrics; 2007

American Academy of Pediatrics, American Heart Association. *Textbook of Neonatal Resuscitation.* 5th ed. Elk Grove Village, IL: American Academy of Pediatrics; 2006

American Academy of Pediatrics Committee on Fetus and Newborn. Levels of neonatal care. *Pediatrics.* 2004;114:1341–1347

American College of Obstetricians and Gynecologists. Dystocia and augmentation of labor. *ACOG Practice Bull.* 2003;No. 49

American College of Obstetricians and Gynecologists. Induction of labor. *ACOG Practice Bull.* 1999;No. 10

American College of Obstetricians and Gynecologists. Intrapartum fetal heart rate monitoring. *ACOG Tech Bull.* 2005;No. 70

American College of Obstetricians and Gynecologists. Management of preterm labor. *ACOG Practice Bull.* 2003;No. 43

Freeman RK, Garite TJ, Nageotte MP. *Fetal Heart Rate Monitoring.* 3rd ed. Philadelphia, PA: Lippincott Williams & Wilkins; 2003

Garite TJ. Intrapartum fetal evaluation. In: Gabbe SG, Niebyl JR, Simpson JL, eds. *Obstetrics: Normal and Problem Pregnancies.* 5th ed. Philadelphia, PA: Churchill Livingstone Elsevier; 2007

Hawkins JL, Goetzl L, Chestnut DH. Obstetric anesthesia. In: Gabbe SG, Niebyl JR, Simpson JL, eds. *Obstetrics: Normal and Problem Pregnancies.* 5th ed. Philadelphia, PA: Churchill Livingstone Elsevier; 2007

Iams JD, Romero R. Preterm birth. In: Gabbe SG, Niebyl JR, Simpson JL, eds. *Obstetrics: Normal and Problem Pregnancies.* 5th ed. Philadelphia, PA: Churchill Livingstone Elsevier; 2007

Kilpatrick S, Garrison E. Normal labor and delivery. In: Gabbe SG, Niebyl JR, Simpson JL, eds. *Obstetrics: Normal and Problem Pregnancies.* 5th ed. Philadelphia, PA: Churchill Livingstone Elsevier; 2007

Landon MB. Cesarean delivery. In: Gabbe SG, Niebyl JR, Simpson JL, eds. *Obstetrics: Normal and Problem Pregnancies.* 5th ed. Philadelphia, PA: Churchill Livingstone Elsevier; 2007

Nielsen PE, Galan HL, Kilpatrick S, Garrison E. Operative vaginal delivery. In: Gabbe SG, Niebyl JR, Simpson JL, eds. *Obstetrics: Normal and Problem Pregnancies.* 5th ed. Philadelphia, PA: Churchill Livingstone Elsevier; 2007

CHAPTER 2
American Academy of Pediatrics, American College of Obstetricians and Gynecologists. *Guidelines for Perinatal Care.* 6th ed. Elk Grove Village, IL: American Academy of Pediatrics; 2007

American Academy of Pediatrics, American Heart Association. *Textbook of Neonatal Resuscitation.* 5th ed. Elk Grove Village, IL: American Academy of Pediatrics; 2006

American Academy of Pediatrics Section on Transport Medicine. *Handbook of Air and Ground Transport of Neonatal and Pediatric Patients.* 3rd ed. Elk Grove Village, IL: American Academy of Pediatrics; 2007:1–5

Gomella TL. *Neonatology Management, Procedures, On-Call Problems, Diseases, and Drugs.* 5th ed. New York, NY: McGraw-Hill Medical; 2003:48

Wood KS. Care of the sick or premature infant before transport. In: McInerny TK, Adam HM, Campbell DE, Kamat DM, Kelleher KJ, eds. *American Academy of Pediatrics Textbook of Pediatric Care.* Elk Grove Village, IL: American Academy of Pediatrics; 2009

CHAPTER 3
American Academy of Pediatrics Committee on Hospital Care. Family-centered care and the pediatrician's role. *Pediatrics.* 2003;112:691–696

Harris M, Little G. Family-centered care in the NICU. *Children's Hospitals Today.* Winter 2005

Institute for Family-Centered Care Web site. http://www.familycenteredcare.org/index.html

Institute for Healthcare Improvement. Patient-centered care. http://www.ihi.org/IHI/Topics/PatientCenteredCare/

Institute of Medicine Committee on Quality of Health Care in America. *Crossing the Quality Chasm: A New Health System for the 21st Century.* Washington, DC: National Academies Press; 2001

CHAPTER 4

Alhusen JL. A literature update on maternal-fetal attachment. *JOGNN.* 2008;37:315–328

Blackburn ST. *Maternal, Fetal & Neonatal Physiology: A Clinical Perspective.* Philadelphia, PA: WB Saunders; 2007

Cleveleand LM. Parenting in the neonatal intensive care unit. *JOGNN.* 2008;37:666–691

Lowman LB, Stone LL, Cole JG. Using developmental assessments in the NICU to empower families. *Neonatal Netw.* 2006;25:177–186

Thomas LM. The changing role of parents in neonatal care: a historical review. *Neonatal Netw.* 2008;27:91–99

CHAPTER 5

American Academy of Pediatrics, American College of Obstetricians and Gynecologists. *Guidelines for Perinatal Care.* 6th ed. Elk Grove Village, IL: American Academy of Pediatrics; 2007

American Academy of Pediatrics Section on Breastfeeding. Breastfeeding and the use of human milk. *Pediatrics.* 2005;115;496–506

American Dietetic Association, Dietitians of Canada. Position paper: dietary fatty acids *Am J Diet Assoc.* 2007;107:1599–1611

Askin D, Diehl-Jones WL. Improving on perfection: breast milk and breast-milk additives for preterm neonates. *Newborn Infant Nurs Rev.* 2005;5:10–18

Biancuzzo M. *Breastfeeding the Newborn: Clinical Strategies for Nurses.* 2nd ed. St Louis, MO: Mosby Inc; 2006

Brenna JT, Varamini B, Jenses RG, Diersen-schade DA, Boettcher JA, Arterburn LM. Docosahexaenoic and arachidonic acid concentrations in human breast milk worldwide. *Am J Clin Nutr.* 2007;85:1457–1464

Campbell DE. Care of the infant after transfer from neonatal intensive care. In: McInerny TK, Adam HM, Campbell DE, Kamat DM, Kelleher KJ, eds. *American Academy of Pediatrics Textbook of Pediatric Care.* Elk Grove Village, IL: American Academy of Pediatrics; 2009

Carlson SJ, Johnson K, Cress G, et al. Higher protein intake improves growth of VLBW infants fed fortified breast milk. *Pediatr Res.* 2004;45:278A

Collins CT, Ryan P, Crowther CA, et al. Effect of bottles, cups, and dummies on breastfeeding in preterm infants: a randomized controlled trial. *Br Med J.* 2004;329:193–198

DePasquale E, Giordano A, Donnenfeld AE. The genetics of ovarian cancer: molecular biology and clinical application. *Obstet Gynecol Surv.* 1998;53:248–256

Field CJ. The immunological components of human milk and their effect on immune development in infants. *J Nutr.* 2005;135:1–4

Fleith M, Clandinin MT. Dietary PUFA for preterm and term infants: review of clinical studies. *Crit Rev Food Sci Nutr.* 2005;45:205–229

Hanna N, Ahmed K, Anwar M, et al. Effect of storage on breast milk antioxidant activity. *Arch Dis Child Fetal Neonatal Ed.* 2004;89:F518–F520

International Society for the Study of Fatty Acids and Lipids. Polyunsaturated fatty acid recommendations. http://www.issfal.org.uk/pufa-recommendations.html

Isaacs CE. Human milk inactivates pathogens individually, additively and synergistically. *J Nutr.* 2005;135:1286–1288

Jim W-T, Shu C-H, Chio NC, et al. Transmission of cytomegalovirus from mothers to preterm infants by breast milk. *Pediatr Infect Dis J.* 2004;23:848-851

Jones E, King C. *Feeding and Nutrition in the Preterm Infant.* St Louis, MO: Churchill Livingstone; 2005

Jones F, Tully MR. *Best Practice for Expressing, Storing and Handling Human Milk in Hospitals, Homes and Child Care Settings.* Raleigh, NC: Human Milk Banking Association of North America; 2006

Karl DJ. Using principles of newborn behavioral state organization to facilitate breast-feeding. *MCN Am J Matern Child Nurs.* 2004;29:292–298

Kennedy K. Premature introduction of progestin-only contraceptive methods during lactation. *Contraceptive.* 1997;5:347–350

Kent JC, Ramsay DT, Doherty D, et al. Response of breasts to different stimulation patterns of an electric breast pump. *J Hum Lact.* 2003;19:179–186

Koletzko B, Cetin I, Brenna JT. Dietary fat intakes for pregnant and lactating women. *Br J Nutr.* 2007;98:873–877

Koletzko B, Lien E, Agostoni C, et al. The roles of long-chain polyunsaturated fatty acids in pregnancy, lactation and infancy: review of current knowledge and consensus recommendations. *J Perinat Med.* 2008;36:5–14

La Leche League International. *The Womanly Art of Breastfeeding.* 7th rev ed. Torgus J, Gotsch G, eds. New York, NY: Penguin Books; 2004

Lawrence RA, Lawrence RM. *Breastfeeding: A Guide for the Medical Profession.* 6th ed. St Louis, MO: Mosby; 2005

Merenstein GB, Gardner SL, eds. *Handbook of Neonatal Intensive Care.* 6th ed. St Louis, MO: Mosby; 2006

Mzuno K, Fujimaki K, Sawada M. Sucking behavior at breast during the early newborn period affects later breastfeeding rate and duration of breastfeeding. *Pediatr Int.* 2004;46:15–20

Newman J, Pitman T. *The Ultimate Breastfeeding Book of Answers: The Most Comprehensive Problem-Solving Guide to Breastfeeding From the Foremost Expert in North America.* New York, NY: Three Rivers Press; 2006

Ramsay DR, Kent JC, Owen RA, et al. Ultrasound imaging of milk ejection in the breast of lactating women. *Pediatrics.* 2003;113:361–367

Schleiss MR. Role of breast milk in acquisition of cytomegalovirus infection: recent advances. *Curr Opin Pediatr.* 2006;18:48–52

Sievers, Haase S, Oldings H-D, Scaub J. The impact of peripartum factors on the onset and duration of lactation. *Biol Neonate.* 2003;83:264–252

Sivin I. Contraceptives for lactating women: a comparative trial of a progesterone-releasing vaginal ring and the copper T380A IUD. *Contraception.* 1997;55:225–232

Vasan U, Meier P, Meier W, et al. Individualizing the lipid content of own mothers' milk: effect on weight gain for extremely low birth weight (ELBW) infants. *Pediatr Res.* 1998;43:270A

Walker M. *Breastfeeding Management for the Clinician: Using the Evidence.* Sudbury, MA: Jones and Bartlett Publishing; 2006

Wood S, Hildebrandt LA. Use of low-carbohydrate diets during lactation: implications for mothers and infants (report). *Top Clin Nutr.* 2004;19:286–296

Zeiger RS. Food allergen avoidance: the prevention of food allergy in infants and children. *Pediatrics.* 2003;11(suppl):1662–1671

Zhangm M, Xie X, Lee AH, Binns CW. Prolonged lactation reduces ovarian cancer risk in Chinese women. *Eur J Cancer Prev.* 2004;13:499–502

CHAPTER 6

Bakewell-Sachs S, Gennaro S. Parenting the post-NICU premature infant. *MCN: Am J Matern Child Nurs.* 2004;29:398–403

Browne JV, Talmi A. Family-based intervention to enhance infant-parent relationships in the neonatal intensive care unit. *J Pediatr Psychology.* 2005;30:667–677

Driscoll J. Psychosocial adaptation to pregnancy and postpartum. In: Simpson KR, Creehan PA, eds. *AWHONN Perinatal Nursing.* 3rd ed. Philadelphia, PA: Wolters & Kluwer/Lippincott, Williams & Wilkins; 2008:84–86

Dudek-Shriber L. Parent stress in the neonatal intensive care unit and the influence of parent and infant characteristics. *Am J Occup Ther.* 2004;58:509–520

Heermann JA, Wilson ME, Wilhelm PA. Mothers in the NICU: outsider to partner. *Pediatr Nurs.* 2005;31:176–200

Lusskin SI, Misri S. Postpartum blues and depression. Up To Date Online. http://www.UpToDateonline.com. Version 16.1. Accessed December 5, 2008

Maguire CM, Bruil J, Wit JM, Walther FJ. Reading preterm infants' behavioral cues: an intervention study with parents of premature infants born at 32 weeks. *Early Hum Dev.* 2007;83:419–424

CHAPTER 7

Centers for Medicare & Medicaid Services. Children's health insurance program. http://www.cms.hhs.gov/lowcosthealthinsfamchild/

Social Security Online: The Official Website of the US Social Security Administration. http://www.ssa.gov

Social Security Online: The Official Website of the US Social Security Administration. Supplemental security income (SSI). http:www.ssa.gov/pgm/links_ssi.htm

Statehealthfacts.org. Income Eligibility Levels for Children's Regular Medicaid and Children's SCHIP-funded Medicaid Expansions by Annual Incomes as a Percent of Federal Poverty Level (FPL), 2009. http://www.statehealthfacts.org/comparetable.jsp?ind=203&cat=4

US Department of Agriculture, Food and Nutrition Service. WIC Program. http://www.fns.usda.gov/wic/

US Department of Health and Human Services Office of Family Assistance Web site. http://www.acf.hhs.gov/programs/ofa/

US Department of Labor. The Family and Medical Leave Act of 1993. Information available at: www.dol.gov/esa/whd/fmla/.

Washington State Department of Health. *Finding Your Way in Managed Care: A Guide for Washington Families of Children with Special Health Care Needs.* Pages 43–46. http://www.doh.wa.gov/cfh/mch/documents/FYWayinEnglish.pdf

CHAPTER 8

Askin D. Newborn adaptation to extrauterine life. In: Simpson KR, Creehan PA, eds. *Perinatal Nursing.* 3rd ed. Philadelphia, PA: Wolters & Kluwer/Lippincott, Williams & Wilkins; 2008:527–545

Askin DF. Physical assessment of the newborn: part 2 of 2: inspection through palpation. *Nurs Womens Health.* 2007;11:304–313

Askin DF. Physical assessment of the newborn: part 1 of 2: preparation through auscultation. *Nurs Womens Health.* 2007;11:292–301

Broussard AB, Hurst HM. Antepartum-intrapartum complications. In: Verklan MT, Walden M, eds. *Core Curriculum for Neonatal Intensive Care Nursing.* 3rd ed. St Louis, MO: Saunders;2004:21–45

Efird MM, Hernandez JA. Birth injuries. In: Thureen PJ, Deacon J, Hernandez JA, Hall DM, eds. *Assessment and Care of the Well Newborn.* 2nd ed. St Louis, MO: Saunders; 2005:110–118

Furdon SA, Benjamin K. Physical assessment. In: Verklan MT, Walden M, eds. *Core Curriculum for Neonatal Intensive Care Nursing.* 3rd ed. St Louis, MO: Saunders; 2004:135–172

Gardner SL, Johnson JL. Initial nursery care. In: Merenstein GB, Gardner SL, eds. *Handbook of Neonatal Intensive Care.* 6th ed. St Louis, MO: Mosby Elsevier; 2006:79–121

Hernandez JA, Fashaw L, Evans R. Adaptation to extrauterine life and management during normal and abnormal transition. In: Thureen PJ, Deacon J, Hernandez JA, Hall DM, eds. *Assessment and Care of the Well Newborn.* 2nd ed. St Louis, MO: Saunders; 2005:83–109

Lee KG. Identifying the high-risk newborn and evaluating gestational age, prematurity, postmaturity, large-for-gestational-age, and small-for-gestational-age infants. In: Cloherty JP, Eichenwald EC, Stark AR, eds. *Manual of Neonatal Care.* 6th ed. Philadelphia, PA: Lippincott, Williams & Wilkins;2008:41–58

Lee-Parritz A, Cloherty JP. Diabetes mellitus. In: Cloherty JP, Eichenwald EC, Stark AR, eds. *Manual of Neonatal Care.* 6th ed. Philadelphia, PA: Lippincott, Williams & Wilkins; 2005:9–19

Lepley M, Gogoi RG. Prenatal environment: effect on neonatal outcome. In: Merenstein GB, Gardner SL, eds. *Handbook of Neonatal Intensive Care.* 6th ed. St Louis, MO: Mosby Elsevier; 2006:11–38

McElrath TF. Preeclampsia and related conditions. In: Cloherty JP, Eichenwald EC, Stark AR, eds. *Manual of Neonatal Care.* 6th ed. Philadelphia, PA: Lippincott, Williams & Wilkins; 2005:28–33

Nandyal RR. Update on group B streptococcal infections: perinatal and neonatal periods. *J Perinat Neonat Nurs.* 2008;22:230–237

Schrag S, Gorwitz R, Fultz-Butts K, Schuchat A. Prevention of perinatal group B streptococcal disease. Revised guidelines from CDC. *MMWR Recomm Rep.* 2002;51(RR-11):1–22

Thureen PJ, Davies JK, LeBel A, Hobbins JC. Maternal factors affecting the newborn. In: Thureen PJ, Deacon J, Hernandez JA, Hall DM, eds. *Assessment and Care of the Well Newborn.* 2nd ed. Philadelphia, PA: Saunders; 2005:3–26

Trotter CW. Gestational age assessment. In: Tappero EP, Honeyfield ME, eds. *Physical Assessment of the Newborn: A Comprehensive Approach to the Art of Physical Examination.* 3rd ed. Santa Rosa, CA: NICU Ink; 2003:21–40

Tumbaga PF, Philip AGS. Perinatal group B streptococcal infections and the new guidelines: an update. *NeoReviews.* 2006;7:e524–e530

Verklan MT. Adaptation to extrauterine life. In: Verklan MT, Walden M, eds. *Core Curriculum for Neonatal Intensive Care Nursing.* 3rd ed. St Louis, MO: Saunders; 2004:80–101

Working Group on High Blood Pressure in Pregnancy. Report of the National High Blood Pressure Working Group on High Blood Pressure in Pregnancy. *Am J Obstet Gynecol.* 2000;183:S1–S22

CHAPTER 9

Bancalari E, Claure N, Gonzalez A. Patent ductus arteriosus and respiratory outcome in premature infants. *Biol Neonate.* 2005;88:192–201

Baraldi E, Filippone M. Chronic lung disease after premature birth. *N Engl J Med.* 2007;357:1946–1955

Costeloe K, Hennessy E, Gibson AT, Marlow N, Wilkinson AR. The EPICure study: outcomes to discharge from hospital for infants born at the threshold of viability. *Pediatrics.* 2000;106:659–671

Early Treatment for Retinopathy of Prematurity Cooperative Group. Revised indications for the treatment of retinopathy of prematurity: results of the early treatment for retinopathy of prematurity randomized trial. *Arch Ophthalmol.* 2003;121:1684–1694

Eichenwald EC, Stark AR. Management and outcomes of very low birth weight. *N Engl J Med.* 2008;358:1700–1711

Fleck BW, McIntosh N. Retinopathy of prematurity: recent developments. *NeoReviews.* 2009;10:e20–e30

Henry MCW, Moss RL. Neonatal necrotizing enterocolits. *Semin Pediatr Surg.* 2008;17:98–109

Koivisto M, Marttila R, Kurkinen-Räty M, et al. Changing incidence and outcome of infants with respiratory distress syndrome in the 1990s: a population-based survey. *Acta Paediatr.* 2004;93:177–184

March of Dimes. Fact sheet: premature birth. http://www.marchofdimes.com/professionals/14332_1157.asp. Accessed January 2, 2009

Martin JA, Kung HC, Mathews TJ, et al. Annual summary of vital statistics: 2006. *Pediatrics.* 2008;121:788–801

Ohls RK. Transfusions in the preterm infant. *NeoReviews.* 2007;8:e377–e386

Schmidt B, Roberts RS, Davis P, et al. Caffeine therapy for apnea of prematurity. *N Engl J Med.* 2006;354:2112–2121

Spitzer AR, ed. *Intensive Care of the Fetus and Neonate.* 2nd ed. Philadelphia, PA: Elsevier, Inc.; 2005

Taeusch HW, Ballard RA, eds. *Avery's Diseases of the Newborn.* Philadelphia, PA: Elsevier Inc.; 2005

Volpe JJ. *Neurology of the Newborn.* 5th ed. Philadelphia, PA: WB Saunders; 2008

Walsh MC, Szefler S, Davis J, et al. Summary proceedings from the Bronchopulmonary Dysplasia Group. *Pediatrics.* 2006;117:S52–S56

Widness JA. Treatment and Prevention of Neonatal Anemia. *NeoReviews.* 2008;9:e526–e533

CHAPTER 10

American Heart Association. Common heart defects. http://www.americanheart.org/presenter.jhtml?identifier=158

Askin DF, ed. *Acute Respiratory Care of the Neonate.* 2nd ed. Santa Rosa, CA: NICU Ink; 1997

Cloherty JP, Eichenwald EC, Stark AR, eds. *Manual of Neonatal Care.* 6th ed. Philadelphia, PA: Lippincott, Williams & Wilkins; 2008

De Roo-Merritt L. Lasers in medicine: treatment of retinopathy of prematurity. *Neonatal Netw.* 2000;19:21–27

Gomella TL. *Neonatology: Management, Procedures, On-Call Problems, Diseases, and Drugs,* 5th ed. Norwalk, CT: Appleton & Lange; 2003

Kenner C, Lott JW. *Comprehensive Neonatal Nursing: An Interdisciplinary Approach.* 4th ed. Philadelphia, PA: WB Saunders; 2007

Merenstein GB, Gardner SL, eds. *Handbook of Neonatal Intensive Care.* 4th ed. St Louis, MO: Mosby; 2006

Taeusch HW, Ballard RA, Gleason CA, eds. *Avery's Diseases of the Newborn.* 8th ed. Philadelphia, PA: WB Saunders; 2005

Tappero E, Honeyfield ME, eds. *Physical Assessment of the Newborn: A Comprehensive Approach to the Art of Physical Examination.* 3rd ed. Santa Rosa, CA: NICU Ink; 2003

Zenk K, Sills JH, Koeppel RM. *Neonatal Medications & Nutrition: A Comprehensive Guide,* 3rd ed. Santa Rosa, California: NICU Ink; 2003

CHAPTER 11

American Academy of Pediatrics Committee on Fetus and Newborn, Committee on Drugs. Neonatal anesthesia. *Pediatrics.* 1987;80:446

American Academy of Pediatrics Committee on Fetus and Newborn, Section on Surgery, Section on Anesthesiology and Pain Medicine; Canadian Paediatric Society Fetus and Newborn Committee. Prevention and management of pain in the neonate: an update. *Pediatrics.* 2006;18:2231–2241

Anand KJS, Johnston C, Oberlander T, Taddio A, Lehr V, Waleg T. Analgesia and local anesthesia during invasive procedures in the neonate. *Clin Ther.* 2005;27:844–876

Berde C, Jaksic T, Lynn A, Maxwell L, Sorriano S, Tibboel D. Anesthesia and analgesia during and after surgery in neonates. *Clin Ther.* 2005;27:900–921

Berry F, Castro B. Neonatal anesthesia. In: Barash P, Cullen B, Stoelting R, eds. *Clinical Anesthesia.* 5th ed. Philadelphia, PA: Lippincott, Williams & Wilkins; 2006:1181–1204

Coleman M, Kolawole S., Smith C. Assessment and management of pain and distress in the neonate. *Adv Neonatal Care.* 2002;2:123–139

Fowler L, Gibbons S. A combined approach to pain management in the surgical neonate. *Newborn Infant Nurs Rev.* 2007;7:171–174

Gregory G. *Pediatric Anesthesia.* 4th ed. New York, NY: Churchill Livingston; 2002

Joint Commission. FAQs about the Universal Protocol for Preventing Wrong Site, Wrong Procedure, Wrong Person Surgery. Joint Commission Web site. 2008. http://www.jointcommission.org/JointCommission/Templates/GeneralInformation.aspx?NRMODE=Published&NRNODEGUID=%7b5D068A56-F2DE-475C-A2FD-997D4A477C5E%7d&NRORIGINALURL=%2fpatientsafety%2funiversalprotocol%2fup_faqs%2ehtm&NRCACHEHINT=Guest#4. Accessed December 2, 2008

Longobucco D, Ruth V. *Neonatal Surgical Procedures: A Guide for Care and Management.* Santa Rosa, CA: NICU Ink; 2007

Martin T, Stoner J. The neonate. In: Kirby R, Gravenstein N, Lobato E, Gravenstein J, eds. *Clinical Anesthesia Practice.* 2nd ed. Philadelphia, PA: Saunders; 2002

Venes D. *Taber's Cyclopedic Medical Dictionary Edition 19.* Philadelphia, PA: F.A. Davis Company; 2001

Welborn LG. Perioperative apnea in the preterm infant. *Anesthesiol Clin North Am.* 1991;9:885–897

Welborn LG, Hannallah RS, Fink R, Ruttimann UE, Hicks JM. High-dose caffeine suppresses postoperative apnea in former preterm infants. *Anesthesiology.* 1989;71:347–349

Welborn LG, Hannallah RS, Higgins T, Fink R, Luban N. Postoperative apnoea in former preterm infant: does anaemia increase the risk? *Can J Anaesth.* 1990;37:592

Welborn LG, Hannallah RS, Luban, NL, Fink R, Ruttimann UE. Anemia and postoperative apnea in former preterm infants. *Anesthesiology.* 1991;74:1003–1006

CHAPTER 12

Ballard RA, Hansen TN, Corbet A. Respiratory failure in the term infant. In: Taeusch HW, Ballard RA, Gleason CA, eds. *Avery's Diseases of the Newborn.* 8th ed. Philadelphia, PA: WB Saunders; 2005:705–722

Blackburn S. Assessment and management of the neurologic system. In: Kenner C, Lott J, eds. *Comprehensive Neonatal Nursing: A Physiologic Perspective.* 3rd ed. St Louis, MO: WB Saunders; 2003:647–649

Carlo WA, Martin RJ, Fanaroff AA. Assisted ventilation and complications of respiratory distress. In: Martin RJ, Fanaroff AA, Walsh MC, eds. *Neonatal-Perinatal Medicine: Disease of the Fetus and the Infant.* 8th ed. Philadelphia, PA: Mosby Elsevier; 2006:1108–1122

Clark RH, Kueser TJ, Walker MW, et al. Low-dose nitric oxide therapy for persistent pulmonary hypertension of the newborn. Clinical Inhaled Nitric Oxide Research Group. *N Engl J Med.* 2000;342:469

Clark RH, Huckaby JL, Kueser TJ, et al. Low dose nitric oxide therapy for PPHN: 1-year follow-up. *J Perinatol.* 2003;23:300

Davidson D, Barefield ES, Kattwinkel J, et al. Inhaled nitric oxide for the early treatment of persistent pulmonary hypertension of the term newborn: a randomized, double-masked, placebo-controlled, dose response, multicenter study. *Pediatrics.* 1998;101:325–334

Extracorporeal Life Support Organization. *Extracorporeal Life Support Registry Report, International Summary.* Ann Arbor, MI: Extracorporeal Life Support Organization; 2009

Extracorporeal Life Support Organization. *Neonatal ECMO Registry Report of the Extracorporeal Life Support Organization.* Ann Arbor, MI: Extracorporeal Life Support Organization; 2009

Fawer CL, Calame A. Ultrasound. In: Haddad J, Christmann D, Messer J, eds. *Imaging Techniques of the CNS of the Neonate.* New York, NY: Springer-Verlag; 1991:79–106

Faerber EN, Bulas DI, Cecil KM, Muzik O, Chugani HT. Imaging modalities. In: Slovis TL, ed. *Caffey's Pediatric Diagnostic Imaging.* 11th ed. Philadelphia, PA: Mosby Elsevier; 2008;623–643

Finer NN, Barrington KJ. Nitric oxide for respiratory failure in infants born at or near term. *Cochrane Database Syst Rev.* 2006;(4):CD000399

Floyer J. *An Essay to Restore the Dipping of Infants in Their Baptism; With a Dialogue Betwixt a Curate and a Practitioner, Concerning the Manner of Immersion.* London, UK: Holland; 1722

Frose AB, Bryon AC. Ventilation by high-frequency-oscillation—a preliminary report. In: Stern L, Salle B, Friis-Hanson B, eds. *Intensive Care of the Newborn.* New York, NY: Masson; 1981:271–273

Glass P, Wagner AE, Papero PH, et al. Neurodevelopmental status at age five years of neonates treated with extracorporeal membrane oxygenation. *J Pediatr.* 1995;127:447–457

Gluckman PD, Wyatt JS, Azzopardi D, et al. Selective head cooling with mild systemic hypothermia after neonatal encephalopathy: multicentre randomised trial. *Lancet* 2005;365:663–670

Gomella TL. Respiratory management. In: Gomella TL, ed. *Neonatology: Management, Procedures, On-Call Problems, Diseases, and Drugs.* 5th ed. New York, NY: Lange Medical; 2004:44–68

Gunn AJ, Hoehn T, Hansmann G, et al. Hypothermia: an evolving treatment for neonatal hypoxic ischemic encephalopathy. *Pediatrics.* 2008;121:648–649

Hagedorn MI, Gardner SL, Dickey LA, Abman SH. Respiratory diseases. In: Merenstein GB, Gardner S, eds. *Handbook of Neonatal Intensive Care.* 6th ed. St Louis, MO: Mosby Elsevier; 2006:595–698

Henderson-Smart DJ, Cools F, Bhuta T, Offringa M. Elective high frequency oscillatory ventilation versus conventional ventilation for acute pulmonary dysfunction in preterm infants. *Cochrane Database Syst Rev.* 2007;(3):CD000104

Jacobs S, Hunt R, Tarnow-Mordi WO, Inder T, Davis P. Cooling for newborns with hypoxic ischaemic encephalopathy. *Cochrane Database Syst Rev.* 2007;(4):CD003311

Kanto WP, Bunyapen C. Extracorporeal membrane oxygenation: controversies in selection of patients and management. *Clin Perinatol.* 1998;25:123–135

Keszler M. High-frequency ventilation: evidence-based practice and specific clinical indications. *NeoReviews.* 2006:7:e234–e249

Laptook AR. Brain cooling for neonatal encephalopathy: potential indications for use. In: Perlman JM, ed. *Neurology: Neonatology Questions and Controversies.* Philadelphia, PA: WB Saunders; 2008:66–78

Levene MI, de Vries L. Hypoxic-ischemic encephalopathy. In: Martin RJ, Fanaroff AA, Walsh MC, eds. *Neonatal-Perinatal Medicine: Disease of the Fetus and the Infant.* 8th ed. Philadelphia, PA: Mosby Elsevier, 2006:938–956

Lipkin P, Davidson D, Spivak I, et al. One-year neurodevelopmental and medical outcome of PPHN in term newborns treated with INO. *J Pediatr.* 2002;140:306

Mathur AM, Smith JR, Donze A. Hypothermia and hypoxic-ischemic encephalopathy: guideline development using the best evidence. *Neonatal Netw.* 2008;27:271–286

Menache CC, Huppi PS. Magnetic resonance imaging's role in the care of the infant at risk for brain injury. In: Perlman JM, ed. *Neurology: Neonatology Questions and Controversies.* Philadelphia, PA: WB Saunders; 2008:231–264

Mugford M, Elbourne D, Field D. Extracorporeal membrane oxygenation for severe respiratory failure in newborn infants. *Cochrane Database Syst Rev.* 2008;(3):CD001340

Page PL, Moe PC. Neourologic disorders. In: Merenstein GB, Gardner S, eds. *Handbook of Neonatal Intensive Care.* 6th ed. St Louis, MO: Mosby Elsevier, 2006:773–811

Rais-Bahrami K, Wagner AE, Coffman C, Glass P, Short, BL. Neurodevelopmental outcome in ECMO vs near-miss ECMO patients at 5 years of age. *Clin Pediatr.* 2000;39:145–152

Sahni R, Sanocks UM. Hypothermia for hypoxic-ischemic encephalopathy. *Clin Perinatol.* 2008;35:717–734

Sarnat HB, Sarnat MS. Neonatal encephalopathy following fetal distress: a clinical and electroencephalographic study. *Arch Neurol.* 1976;33:696-705

Schulzke SM, Rao S, Patole SK. A systematic review of cooling for neuroprotection in neonates with hypoxic ischemic encephalopathy—are we there yet? *BMC Pediatr.* 2007;7:1–10

Shah PS, Ohlsson A, Perlman M. Hypothermia to treat neonatal hypoxic ischemic encephalopathy: systematic review. *Arch Pediatr Adolesc Med.* 2007;161:951–958

Shankaran S, Laptook AR, Ehrenkranz RA, et al. Whole body hypothermia for neonates with hypoxic-ischemic encephalopathy. *N Engl J Med.* 2005;353:1574–1584

Schwartz JE. New technologies applied to the management of the respiratory system. In: Kenner C, Lott J, eds. *Comprehensive Neonatal Nursing: A Physiologic Perspective.* 3rd ed. St Louis, MO: WB Saunders; 2002:363–375

Steinhorn RH, Kinsella JP. Use of inhaled nitric oxide in the preterm infant. *NeoReviews.* 2007;8:e247–e253

Stork EK. Therapy for cardiorespiratory failure. In: Martin RJ, Fanaroff AA, Walsh MC, eds. *Neonatal-Perinatal Medicine: Disease of the Fetus and the Infant.* 8th ed. Philadelphia, PA: Mosby Elsevier; 2006:1168–1180

Strain JD, Jenkins JC. Diagnostic imaging in the neonate. In: Merenstein GB, Gardner S, eds. *Handbook of Neonatal Intensive Care.* 6th ed. St Louis, MO: Mosby Elsevier; 2006: 157–174

Theorell C, Montrowl S. Diagnostic processes. In: Kenner C, Lott J, eds. *Comprehensive Neonatal Nursing: A Physiologic Perspective.* 3rd ed. St Louis, MO: WB Saunders, 2003; 810–831

Volpe JJ. Hypoxic-ischemic encephalopathy: clinical aspects. In: Volpe J, ed. *Neurology of the Newborn.* 5th ed. Philadelphia, PA: 2008:400–461

Vancher YE, Dudell GG, Bejar R, Gist K. Predictors of early childhood outcome in candidates for extracorporeal membrane oxygenation. *J Pediatr.* 1996;128:109–117

CHAPTER 13

American Academy of Pediatrics Committee on Hospital Care, Section on Surgery. Pediatric organ donation and transplantation. *Pediatrics.* 2002;109:982–984

Bailey NA, Lay P, Loma Linda University Infant Heart Transplant Group. New horizons: infant cardiac transplantation. *Heart Lung.* 1989;18:172–178

Callister LC. Perinatal loss: a family perspective. *J Perinat Neonatal Nurs.* 2006;20:227–234

Gold KJ, Dalton VK, Schwenk TL. Hospital care for parents after perinatal death. *Obstet Gynecol.* 2007;109:1156–1166

Kafrawy U, Stewart D. An evaluation of brainstem death documentation: the importance of full documentation. *Pediatr Anesth.* 2004;14:584–588

Kobler K, Limbo R, Kavanaugh K. Meaningful moments. MCN *Am J Matern Child Nurs.* 2007;32:288–295

Kubler-Ross E, Kessler D. *On Grief and Grieving: Finding the Meaning of Grief Through the Five Stages of Loss.* New York, NY: Simon & Schuster; 2005

Lamb EH. The impact of previous perinatal loss on subsequent pregnancy and parenting. *J Perinat Educ.* 2002;11:33–40

Levetown M, American Academy of Pediatrics Committee on Bioethics. Communicating with children and families: from everyday interactions to skill in conveying distressing information. *Pediatrics.* 2008;121; e1441-e1460. Accessed at http://www.pediatrics.org/cgi/content/full/121/5/e1441

Limbo RK, Wheeler SR. *When a Baby Dies: A Handbook for Healing and Helping.* La Crosse, WI: RTS Bereavement Services; 1986:14, 56, 59, 74

Mehren E. *Born Too Soon.* New York, NY: Doubleday; 1991

Mellichamp P. End-of-life care for infants. *Home Health Care Nurs.* 2007;25:41–44

Merenstein GB, Gardner SL. *Handbook of Neonatal Intensive Care.* 6th ed. St Louis, MO: Mosby-Elsevier; 2006

Moskop JC, Saldanha RL. The Baby Doe rule: still a threat. *Hastings Center Report.* 1986;16:8–14

Sanderson HM. Loss and bereavement. In: Potts NL, Mandleco BL, eds. *Pediatric Nursing: Caring for Children and Their Families.* Clifton Park, NY: Thomson Delmar Learning; 2007:565–584

Scully T, Scully C. *Playing God: The New World of Medical Choices.* New York, NY: Simon & Schuster; 1987:121–151, 194–229

Sornaienchi JM. Chronic sorrow: one mother's experience with two children with lissencephaly. *J Pediatr Health Care.* 2003;17:290–294

Stinson R, Stinson P. *The Long Dying of Baby Andrew.* Boston, MA: Little, Brown; 1983

Sumer LH, Kavanaugh K, Moro T. Extending palliative care into pregnancy and the immediate newborn period: state of the practice of perinatal palliative care. *J Perinat Neonatal Nurs.* 2006;20:113–116

Wright J. *Back to Life: Your Personal Guidebook to Grief Recovery.* http://www.recover-from-grief.com/heartbroken-from-grief.html

CHAPTER 14
Brodsky D, Ouellette MA. *Primary Care of the Premature Infant.* St Louis, MO: WB Saunders; 2008

Campbell DE. Care of the infant after transfer from neonatal intensive care. In: McInerny TK, Adam HM, Campbell DE, Kamat DM, Kelleher KJ, eds. *American Academy of Pediatrics Textbook of Pediatric Care.* Elk Grove Village, IL: American Academy of Pediatrics; 2009

Jana LA, Shu J. *Heading Home With Your Newborn: From Birth to Reality.* Elk Grove Village, IL: American Academy of Pediatrics; 2005

Kenner C, Ellerbee S. Transition to home. In: Kenner C, Lott JW, eds. *Comprehensive Neonatal Care.* 4th ed. St Louis, MO: WB Saunders Elsevier; 2007

Ludwig SM, Waitzman KA. Changing feeding documentation to reflect infant-driven feeding practice. *Newborn Infant Nurs Rev.* 2007;7:155–160

McClure VS. *Infant Massage: A Handbook for Loving Parents*. 3rd ed. New York, NY: Bantam Books; 2000

Verklan MT, Walden M, eds. *Core Curriculum for Neonatal Intensive Care Nursing*. 3rd ed. St Louis, MO: WB Saunders Elsevier; 2004

CHAPTER 15

American Academy of Pediatrics. Recommended immunization schedule for persons aged 0-6 years. In: *Patient Education Online: Health Care Advice for Children, Teens, and Parents*. http://patiented.aap.org/.

American Academy of Pediatrics Section on Ophthalmology, American Academy of Ophthalmology, American Association for Pediatric Ophthalmology and Strabismus. Screening examination of premature infants for retinopathy of prematurity [published erratum appears in *Pediatrics*. 2006;118:1324]. *Pediatrics*. 2006;117:572–576

American Academy of Pediatrics Committee on Fetus and Newborn. Hospital discharge of the high-risk infant. *Pediatrics*. 2008;122:1119–1126

Campbell DE. Care of the infant after transfer from neonatal intensive care. In: McInerny TK, Adam HM, Campbell DE, Kamat DM, Kelleher KJ, eds. *American Academy of Pediatrics Textbook of Pediatric Care*. Elk Grove Village, IL: American Academy of Pediatrics; 2009

Cochran WD, Lee KG. Assessment of the newborn. In: Cloherty JP, Eichenwald EC, Stark AR, eds. *Manual of Neonatal Care*. 5th ed. Philadelphia, PA: Lippincott, Williams & Wilkins; 2004:35

Fraser Askin D. Chest and Lungs Assessment. In: Tappero EP, Honeyfield ME, eds. *Physical Assessment of the Newborn: A Comprehensive Approach to the Art of Physical Examination*. 3rd ed. Santa Rosa, CA: NICU Ink; 2003:69

Gracey K, Hummel P, Cronin J. Choosing a home care provider. *Adv Neonatal Care*. 2004;4:365–366

Jana LA, Shu J. *Heading Home With Your Newborn: From Birth to Reality*. Elk Grove Village, IL: American Academy of Pediatrics; 2005

Long CM, Campbell DE. Discharge planning for the high-risk newborn requiring intensive care. In: McInerny TK, Adam HM, Campbell DE, Kamat DM, Kelleher KJ, eds. *American Academy of Pediatrics Textbook of Pediatric Care*. Elk Grove Village, IL: American Academy of Pediatrics; 2009

New England SERVE. *The Medical Home Partnership: Building a Home Base for Your Child with Special Health Care Needs.* 2nd ed. http://www.neserve.org/neserve/pdf/NES%20Publications/Medical_Home_Tips_for_Families_2ndEd.pdf. Accessed December 15, 2008

Washington State Department of Health. *Does Your Child Have a Medical Home?* http://www.medicalhome.org/leadership/brochures.cfm. Accessed December 15, 2008

CHAPTER 16

Care of the Percutaneous Endoscopic Gastrostomy (PEG) and the Button Replacement Gastrostomy. Billerica, MA: CR Bard; 1987:3–12

Ahmann E. *Home Care for the High Risk Infant.* Rockville, MD: Aspen; 2007

Als H. Toward a synactive theory of development: promise for the assessment and support of infant individuality. *Infant Ment Health J.* 1982;3:229–243

American Academy of Pediatrics. The first month. In: Shelov SP, Hannemann RE, eds. *Caring for Your Baby and Young Child—Birth to Age 5—The Complete and Authoritative Guide.* 4th ed. New York, NY: Bantam; 2004

American Academy of Pediatrics. Bottle feeding tips [audiotape]. In: *Patient Education Online: Health Care Advice for Children, Teens, and Parents.* http://patiented.aap.org/

American Academy of Pediatrics. Crying and your baby: how to calm a fussy or colicky baby. In: *Patient Education Online: Health Care Advice for Children, Teens, and Parents.* http://patiented.aap.org/

American Academy of Pediatrics. Dangers of secondhand smoke. In: *Patient Education Online: Health Care Advice for Children, Teens, and Parents.* http://patiented.aap.org/

American Academy of Pediatrics. Fever and your child. In: *Patient Education Online: Health Care Advice for Children, Teens, and Parents.* http://patiented.aap.org/

American Academy of Pediatrics. A guide to your child's medicines. In: *Patient Education Online: Health Care Advice for Children, Teens, and Parents.* http://patiented.aap.org/

American Academy of Pediatrics. How to take your child's temperature. In: *Patient Education Online: Health Care Advice for Children, Teens, and Parents.* http://patiented.aap.org/

American Academy of Pediatrics. Immunizations: what you need to know. In: *Patient Education Online: Health Care Advice for Children, Teens, and Parents.* http://patiented.aap.org/

American Academy of Pediatrics. SIDS: important information for parents. In: *Patient Education Online: Health Care Advice for Children, Teens and Parents.* http//patiented.aap.org

American Academy of Pediatrics. TIPP—The Injury Prevention Program 6 to 12 months: safety for your child. In: *Patient Education Online: Health Care Advice for Children, Teens, and Parents.* http://patiented.aap.org/

American Academy of Pediatrics Committee on Fetus and Newborn. Policy statement: apnea, sudden infant death syndrome, and home monitoring. *Pediatrics.* 2003;111:914–917

American Academy of Pediatrics Task Force on Infant Positioning and SIDS. Positioning and SIDS [published erratum appears in *Pediatrics.* 1992;90: 264]. *Pediatrics.* 1992;89:1120–1126

American Academy of Pediatrics Task Force on Sudden Infant Death Syndrome. Policy statement: the changing concept of sudden infant death syndrome: diagnostic coding shifts, controversies regarding the sleeping environment, and new variables to consider in reducing risk. *Pediatrics.* 2005;116:1245–1255

American Heart Association. *Instructor's Manual for Pediatric Basic Life Support.* Dallas, TX: American Heart Association; 2006

American Heart Association. *Instructor Manual for Pediatric First Aid.* Dallas, TX: American Heart Association; 2006

AWHONN Practice Resource. *Preparation for Home Care of Technology-Dependent Infants.* Washington, DC: Association of Women's Health, Obstetric, and Neonatal Nurses; 1993:2–8

Bakewell-Sachs S, Blackburn S. March of Dimes nursing module. In: Wieczork RR, ed. *Discharge and Follow-Up of the High-Risk Preterm Infant.* White Plains, NY: March of Dimes; 2001:19–93

Bernbaum JC, Campbell DE, Imaizumi SO. Follow-up care of the graduate from the neonatal intensive care unit. In: McInerny TK, Adam HM, Campbell DE, Kamat DM, Kelleher KJ, eds. *American Academy of Pediatrics Textbook of Pediatric Care.* Elk Grove Village, IL: American Academy of Pediatrics; 2009:867–882

Bound JP, Voulvoulis N. Household disposal of pharmaceuticals as a pathway for aquatic contamination in the United Kingdom. *Environ Health Perspect.* 2005;113:1705–1711

Brazelton TB. Touchpoints: *Your Child's Emotional and Behavioral Development, Birth to 3—The Essential Reference for the Early Years.* Reading, MA: Addison-Wesley; 1992:60–64, 92–94, 231–238

Buzz-Kelly L, Gordin P. Teaching CPR to parents of children with tracheostomies. *MCN Am J Matern Child Nurs.* 1993;18:158–163

Consumer Product Safety Commission. Baby safety checklist. CPSC document #206. http://www.cpsc.gov/cpscpub/pubs/206.html

Consumer Product Safety Commission. Locked up poisons: prevent tragedy. CPSC document #382. http://www.cpsc.gov/cpscpub/pubs/382.html

Davidson Ward SL, Keens TG. Ventilator management at home. In: Ballard RA, ed. *Pediatric Care of the ICN Graduate.* Philadelphia, PA: WB Saunders, 1988:166–176

Eisenberg A, Murkoff HE, Hathaway SE. *What to Expect the First Year.* New York, NY: Workman; 2003

Finston P. *Parenting Plus: Raising Children with Special Health Needs.* New York, NY: Dutton; 1990:63

Fitzgerald K. SIDS Global Strategy Task Force: SIDS International. http://www.sidsinternational.org/

Gennaro S, Bakewell-Sachs S. Discharge planning and home care for low-birth-weight infants. *NAACOGS Clin Issu.* 1991;3:129–145

Gorski PA. Fostering family development after preterm hospitalization. In: Ballard RA, ed. *Pediatric Care of the ICN Graduate.* Philadelphia, PA: WB Saunders, 1988:27–32

Howell LJ. Home ostomy care. In: Ballard RA, ed. *Pediatric Care of the ICN Graduate.* Philadelphia, PA: WB Saunders; 1988:306–316

Huggins K. *The Nursing Mother's Companion.* Rev ed. Boston, MA: The Harvard Common Press; 2005

Jonville-Bera AP, Autret-Leca E, Barbeillon F, Paris-Llado J. The French Reference Centers for SIDS: sudden unexpected death in infants under 3 months of age and vaccination status—a case-control study. *Br J Clin Pharmacol.* 2001;51:271–276

Kenner C, Bagwell GA. Assessment and management of the transition to home. In: Kenner C, Brueggemeyer A, Gunderson LP, eds. *Comprehensive Neonatal Nursing: A Physiologic Perspective.* Philadelphia, PA: WB Saunders; 1991:1134–1147

Linden DW, Paroli ET, Doron MW. *Preemies: The Essential Guide for Parents of Premature Babies.* New York, NY: March of Dimes NICU Family Support; 2000

Long CM, Campbell DE. Discharge planning for the high-risk newborn requiring intensive care. In: McInerny TK, Adam HM, Campbell DE, Kamat DM, Kelleher KJ, eds. *American Academy of Pediatrics Textbook of Pediatric Care.* Elk Grove Village, IL: American Academy of Pediatrics; 2009

MacIntyre CR, Leask J. Immunization myths and realities: responding to arguments against immunization. *J Pediatr Child Health.* 2003;39:487–491

Martin JA, Kung H-C, Matthews TJ, et al. Annual summary of vital statistics. *Pediatrics.* 2008;121:788–801

Meier PP, Mangurten HH. Breastfeeding the pre-term infant. In: Riordan J, Averbach KG, eds. *Breastfeeding and Human Lactation.* 2nd ed. Boston, MA: Jones & Bartlett; 1999

Parker L, Richardson C. *Ochsner NICU Babybook: Parent Edition.* New Orleans, LA: Alton Ochsner Medical Foundation; 1990, 2008 (revised)

Platzker ACG. Chronic lung disease in infancy. In: Ballard RA, ed. *Pediatric Care of the ICN Graduate.* Philadelphia, PA: WB Saunders; 1988:129–156

Platzker ACG, Lew CD, Cohen SR, et al. Home care of infants with chronic lung disease. In: Ballard RA, ed. *Pediatric Care of the ICN Graduate.* Philadelphia, PA: WB Saunders; 1988:289–294

Sears W, Sears M, Sears R, Sears J. *The Baby Book: Everything You Need to Know about Your Baby—From Birth to Age Two.* Boston, MA: Little, Brown; 2003

Silvers LE, Varricchio FE, Ellenberg SS, Krueger CL, Wise RP, Salive ME. Pediatric deaths reported after vaccination: the utility of information obtained from parents. *Am J Prev Med.* 2002;22:170–176

Smith GCS, White IR. Predicting the risk for sudden infant death syndrome from obstetric characteristics: a retrospective cohort study of 505,011 live births. *Pediatrics.* 2006;117:60–66

TeKolste K, Bragg J, Wendel S, eds. Extremely low birth weight NICU. Supplement to: *Critical Elements of Care: Low Birth Weight Neonatal Intensive Care Unit Graduate (CEC_LBW).* Seattle, WA: Washington State Department of Health, Children with Special Health Care Needs; 2004:1–25. http://www.medicalhome.org

Tomasheck KM, Wallman C, American Academy of Pediatrics Committee on Fetus and Newborn. Cobedding twins and higher order multiples in a hospital setting. *Pediatrics.* 2007;120:1359–1366

University of California San Francisco Center for Consumer Self Care Publication. *Don't Flush Your Medicines Down the Toilet!* San Francisco, CA: UCSF School of Pharmacy; 2008

Wake M, Morton-Allen E, Poulakis Z, Hiscock H, Gallagher S. Prevalence, stability, and outcomes of cry-fuss and sleep problems in the first 2 years of life: prospective community-based study. *Pediatrics.* 2006;117:836–842

Winickoff JP, Friebely J, Tanski SE, et al. Beliefs about the health effects of "thirdhand" smoke and home smoking bans. *Pediatrics.* 2009;123:e74–e79

Washington State Consensus Project. *Critical Elements of Care: Low Birth Weight Neonatal Intensive Care Unit Graduate.* Seattle, WA: Washington State Department of Health, Children with Special Health Care Needs; 2005:1–49. http://www.medicalhome.org/4Download/cec/CEC.pdf

CHAPTER 17

Ahmann E. *Homecare for the High Risk Infant.* Rockville, MD: Aspen; 2007

American Academy of Pediatrics Council on Children with Disabilities. Policy statement: provision of educationally related services for children and adolescents with chronic diseases and disabling conditions. *Pediatrics.* 2007;119:1218–1223

Ancol PY, Livinec F, Larroque B, et al. Cerebral palsy among very preterm children in relation to gestational age and neonatal ultrasound abnormalities: the EPIPAGE Cohort Study. *Pediatrics.* 2006;117:828–835

Bayley N. *Bayley Scales of Infant and Toddler Development Manual.* 3rd ed. San Antonio, TX: Psychological Corp, Harcourt Assessment, Inc; 2006

Belcher HME. Developmental screening. In: Capute AJ, Accardo PJ, eds. *Developmental Disabilities in Infancy and Childhood.* Baltimore, MD: Paul H. Brookes; 1991:113–131

Bernbaum JC, Campbell DE, Imaizumi SO. Follow-up care of the graduate from the neonatal intensive care unit. In: McInerny TK, Adam HM, Campbell DE, Kamat DM, Kelleher KJ, eds. *American Academy of Pediatrics Textbook of Pediatric Care.* Elk Grove Village, IL: American Academy of Pediatrics; 2009:867–882

Bakewell-Sachs S, Blackburn S. March of Dimes nursing module. In: Wieczork RR, ed. *Discharge and Follow-Up of the High-Risk Preterm Infant.* White Plains, NY: March of Dimes; 2001:19–93

Campbell DE, Imaizumi SO, Bernbaum, JC. 2009. Health and developmental outcomes of infants requiring neonatal intensive care. In: McInerny TK, Adam HM, Campbell DE, Kamat DM, Kelleher KJ, eds. *American Academy of Pediatrics Textbook of Pediatric Care.* Elk Grove Village, IL: American Academy of Pediatrics; 852–866

Fily A, Pierrat V, Delporte V, Breart G, Truffert P, EPIPAGE Nord-Pas-de-Calais Study Group. Factors associated with neurodevelopmental outcome at 2 years after very preterm birth: the population-based Nord-Pas-de-Calais EPIPAGE Cohort. *Pediatrics.* 2006;117:357–366

Finston P. *Parenting Plus: Raising Children with Special Health Needs.* New York, NY: Dutton; 1990:193–200

Frankenburg WK, Dobbs J, Archer P, et al. *Denver II Screening Manual.* Denver, CO: Denver Developmental Materials; 1990:1–48

Gennaro S, Bakewell-Sachs S. Discharge planning and home care for low-birth weight infants. *NAACOGS Clin Issu.* 1991;3:129–145

Gorski PA. Fostering family development after preterm hospitalization. In: Ballard RA, ed. *Pediatric Care of the ICN Graduate.* Philadelphia, PA: WB Saunders; 1988:27–32

Green M, Solnit A. Reactions to the threatened loss of a child: a vulnerable child syndrome. *Pediatrics.* 1964;34:58–66

Hack M, Wilson-Costello D, Friedman H, et al. Neurodevelopment and predictors of outcomes of children with birth weights of less than 1000 g: 1992–1995. *Arch Pediatr Adolesc Med.* 2000;154:725–731

Hanson MJ, VandenBerg KA. *Homecoming for Babies After the Intensive Care Nursery: A Guide for Parents in Supporting Their Baby's Early Development.* Austin, TX: Pro-Ed; 1993:19–25

Kidsource Online. What is early intervention? http://www.kidsource.com/kidsource/content/early.intervention.html

Leonard CH. Developmental and behavioral assessment. In: Ballard RA, ed. *Pediatric Care of the ICN Graduate.* Philadelphia, PA: WB Saunders; 1988:94–110

Linden DW, Paroli ET, Doron, MW. *Preemies: The Essential Guide for Parents of Premature Babies.* New York, NY: March of Dimes NICU Family Support: 2000:33–37, 394–480

Long CM, Campbell DE. Discharge planning for the high-risk newborn requiring intensive care. In: McInerny TK, Adam HM, Campbell DE, Kamat DM, Kelleher KJ, eds. *American Academy of Pediatrics Textbook of Pediatric Care.* Elk Grove Village, IL: American Academy of Pediatrics; 2009:709–766

Marlow N, Hennessy EM, Bracewell MA, Wolke D, EPICure Study Group. Motor and executive function at 6 years of age after extremely preterm birth. *Pediatrics.* 2007;120:793–804

Martin JA, Kung H-C, Matthews TJ, et al. Annual summary of vital statistics. *Pediatrics* 2008;121:788–801

Merialdi M, Murray J. The changing face of preterm birth. *Pediatrics* 2007;120:1133–1134

New York State Department of Health. The early intervention program: a parents guide. http://www.,health.state.ny/us/community/infants_children/early_intervention/parents_guide.html

Pacer Center ACTion Sheet: PHP-c158. Preparing for transition from early intervention to an individualized education program. http://www.pacer.org.

Parker L, Richardson C. *Ochsner NICU Babybook*. New Orleans, LA: Alton Ochsner Medical Foundation; 1990 (revised 2008)

Pearson SR, Boyce WT. Vulnerable child syndrome, *Pediatr Rev.* 2004;25:345–34

Seidl Z, Sussova J, Obenberger J, et al. Magnetic resonance imaging in diplegic form of cerebral palsy. *Brain Dev.* 2001;23:46–49

Sumner G, Spietz A, eds. *NCAST Caregiver/Parent-Child Interaction Teaching Manual.* Seattle, WA: NCAST Publications, University of Washington, School of Nursing; 1994:3

TeKolste K, Bragg J, Wendel S. eds. Extremely low birth weight. NICU supplement to: *Critical Elements of Care for the Low Birth Weight Neonatal Intensive Care Graduate (CEC_LBW).* Seattle, WA: Washington State Department of Health, Children with Special Health Care Needs; 2004:1–25. http://www.medicalhome.org

Tommiska V, Heinonen K, Lehtonen L, et al. No improvement in outcome of nationwide extremely low birth weight infant populations between 1996–1997 and 1999–2000. *Pediatrics.* 2007;119:29–36

Vohr BR, Wright LL, Dusick AM, et al. Neurodevelopmental and functional outcomes of extremely low birth weight infants in the National Institute of Child Health and Human Development Neonatal Research Network, 1993–1994. *Pediatrics.* 2000;105:1216–1226

Washington State Consensus Project. *Critical Elements of Care: Low Birth Weight Neonatal Intensive Care Unit Graduate.* Seattle, WA: Washington State Department of Health, Children with Special Health Care Needs; 2005:1–49. http://www.medicalhome.org/4Download/cec/CEC.pdf

Wilson-Costello D, Friedman H, Minich N, et al. Improved neurodevelopmental outcomes for extremely low birth weight infants in 2000–2002. *Pediatrics.* 2007;119:37–45

Wood NS, Marlow N, Costeloe K, Gibson AT, Wilkinson AR. Neurologic and developmental disability after extremely preterm birth. EPICure study group. *N Engl J Med.* 2000;343:378–384

Wright PWD. IDEA 2004 regulations subpart A: general; purposes and applicability. http://www.wrightslaw.1com/idea/law.html

Yeargin-Allsopp M, VanNaarden Braun K, Doernberg NS, Benedict RE, Kirby RS, Durkin MS. Prevalence of cerebral palsy in 8-year-old children in three areas of the United States in 2002: a multisite collaboration. *Pediatrics.* 2008;121:547–554

Glossary

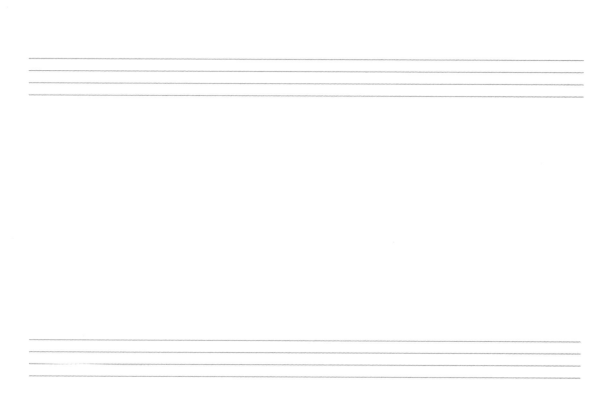

A

ABG: See **Blood gas, arterial.**

Account manager: An individual, employed by the hospital treating your baby, who is assigned to handle the financial details of your baby's case.

Acetaminophen: Medication for relief of pain and lowering of body temperature that does not contain aspirin. Tylenol and Tempra are 2 of the brand names for acetaminophen.

Acrocyanosis: A bluish color to the skin of the hands and feet, caused by decreased circulation (especially if the infant's hands or feet are cool). A normal occurrence in newborns.

Acquired immune deficiency syndrome: See **AIDS.**

Acuity, visual: Sharpness of sight.

Acute care: Care given in an emergency or life-threatening situation.

Admitting privileges: Authorization (or authority) of a medical provider to have patients cared for at a given hospital.

ADN: Associate degree in nursing. A 2-year community college nursing training program. Denotes educational level, not professional nursing licensure.

Advanced registered nurse practitioner: See **ARNP.**

Adverse event: Injury caused by medical management; not a result of baby's underlying problems.

Advocate: Someone who speaks for and actively promotes another's best interests.

AIDS: Acquired immune deficiency syndrome. Caused by infection with the human immunodeficiency virus (HIV), which impairs the body's immune response. Increases the body's susceptibility to one or more secondary (opportunistic) infections that characterize the syndrome.

Air leak, pulmonary: Caused when air tears one or more breathing sacs (alveoli) in the lungs and leaks into spaces around the lung tissue.

Airway: The route by which air passes from the nose or mouth to the lungs; the breathing passages. Also, a tube or oral appliance used to provide a route for air to the lungs.

Albumin: The protein portion of the blood serum. Important for maintenance of blood volume.

Alveoli: Small air sacs in the lung.

Amino acid: The protein component essential to body cells.

Amniotic fluid: Liquid that surrounds the fetus inside the mother's uterus.

Amniotic membrane: The sac that surrounds the fetus inside the mother's uterus. Breaks before or during labor, allowing the amniotic fluid inside to escape (often referred to as when "the mother's water breaks").

Amniotomy: See **Artificial rupture of membranes.**

Analgesia: Pain medication that relieves or decreases awareness of pain. Analgesia does not cause unconsciousness or loss of sensation (numbness).

Anemia: A condition marked by lower-than-normal hemoglobin and hematocrit levels in the blood.

Anesthesia: A medication that reduces or eliminates the sensation of pain or that produces loss of consciousness and, as a result, inability to feel pain.

Anesthesia, epidural: A type of regional anesthesia used during labor or cesarean birth to make a patient unable to feel pain from the navel to the midthigh; body coverage can be extended, depending on the patient's anesthesia needs. An epidural block is injected through a catheter into the space outside the covering of the spinal cord.

Anesthesia, general: A drug given through an intravenous (IV) line and/or through inhalation. Produces unconsciousness and, as a result, blocks any sensation of pain.

Anesthesia, local: A type of nerve block that makes a patient unable to feel pain in a small specific area of the body. Does not cause loss of consciousness.

Anesthesia, regional: A type of nerve block that makes a patient unable to feel pain in a specifically targeted area of the body. Does not cause unconsciousness. Epidural block and spinal anesthesia are examples of regional anesthesia.

Anesthesia, topical: Medication applied to the skin that causes numbness. Used for minor surgical procedures.

Anesthesiologist: A physician with specialized training in giving medications that reduce or abolish pain and/or cause unconsciousness.

Ankyloglossia: A physical characteristic in which a shorter than normal connection exists between the tongue and the floor of the mouth and interferes with free protrusion of the tongue. Commonly called *tongue-tied*.

Anomaly, congenital: A defect existing at birth; an external or internal abnormality of an organ or structure. Commonly called a *birth defect*. See also **Malformation, congenital.**

Anterior: Located in the front or forward section of a body part or organ.

Antibiotic: A drug that kills bacteria or reduces their growth. Used to treat infection.

Antibiotic ointment: Medication applied to the skin surface to fight infectious bacteria.

Antibody: A disease-fighting substance in the blood; antibodies attack foreign substances in the body.

Anticonvulsant: Medication that prevents, controls, or relieves involuntary muscle contractions (seizures).

Aorta: A large, branched artery that carries blood from the heart to the main arteries of the body.

Aortic arch: The part of the aortic artery that extends upward over the heart, through which blood passes as it flows to the body.

Aortic stenosis: A narrowing of the valve between the left ventricle of the heart and the aorta; reduces blood flow to the body. Can result from a birth defect.

Apgar score: The numerical result of a newborn assessment generally done at 1 minute and again at 5 minutes after birth; assesses heart rate, breathing, color, tone, and reflexes. A maximum of 2 points for each sign is given. A 10, the highest score, indicates an infant in excellent condition; lower scores indicate less responsiveness (or for preterm infants, less ability to respond due to immaturity). Apgar scoring may be continued every 5 minutes for up to 20 minutes or until 2 successive scores are more than 7.

Apnea: Pause in breathing (by strict definition, a pause of 20 seconds or longer), or pause of any length accompanied by bradycardia and oxygen desaturation.

Apnea monitor: A mechanical device that is usually set to alarm if apnea occurs and/or if the heart rate slows or speeds up abnormally. This term usually refers to the monitor used by selected babies who require monitoring at home after discharge.

Apneic: A term to describe a baby experiencing apnea.

Appropriate for gestational age (AGA): A newborn whose weight (and possibly length and head circumference) falls between the 10th and 90th percentiles on a standard intrauterine growth chart; indicates appropriate growth for the length of time the baby was in the uterus. An AGA baby can be preterm, term, or post-term.

Areola: The brownish or pink circular area around the nipple of the breast.

ARNP: Advanced registered nurse practitioner. A legal term for professional licensure; may be used by a neonatal nurse practitioner. In some states, denoted by *APRN*.

Arrhythmia: A change in the regularity of the heartbeat.

Arterial line: A tube inserted into a major artery; used for administration of fluids and/or medications and sometimes for monitoring blood pressure. Some types can be used to withdraw blood for laboratory work.

Arterioles: A small branch of an artery, leading into many small vessels.

Artificial rupture of membranes (AROM): A procedure in which the physician or midwife "breaks" the bag of waters surrounding the fetus; used to augment labor. Also called an *amniotomy*.

Asphyxia: The result of insufficient oxygen reaching the body cells. The term denotes progressive hypoxia and an accumulation of carbon dioxide and acid waste products in the blood. If left uncorrected, asphyxia can result in permanent brain and organ damage or in death.

Aspirate/Aspiration: Breathing of a substance other than air (for example, stomach contents, meconium, or milk) into the trachea or lungs. Also, the removal of fluids from the body by suctioning.

Assessment: An evaluation of a baby's general condition and one method to determine anything that differs from the baby's usual status. Nursing and medical actions are based on continuous assessment of the baby's condition.

Associate Degree in Nursing: See **ADN.**

Asthma: A condition in which breathing (especially exhalation) is difficult and often accompanied by wheezing and tightness in the chest.

Asymmetry: A lack of balance, equality, or sameness on opposite sides of a dividing line (such as the left and right sides of the body); affects corresponding parts differently.

Atelectasis: The collapse of groups of alveoli (air sacs) in the lungs.

Atresia: A birth defect in which a passage (such as a valve, a vein, or an artery) is completely blocked or is absent.

Atretic: Having to do with an atresia.

Atrial: Having to do with the atrium (1 of the 2 upper chambers of the heart).

Atrial septal defect (ASD): A birth defect in which a hole is present in the wall (septum) between the 2 upper chambers (atria) of the heart.

Atrium: One of the 2 upper chambers of the heart (plural: atria).

Attending physician: The physician who oversees your baby's treatment; may or may not perform all procedures.

Audiologist: A physician who specializes in diagnosing and treating hearing difficulties.

Audiology screening: A hearing test.

Auditory: Having to do with hearing.

Augmentation, labor: A method used to promote more effective uterine contractions when labor has already begun or contractions have stopped.

Autopsy: An examination by a pathologist of a body after death to determine the cause.

Aversion, oral: A negative association with or response to anything placed in or near the mouth.

Axillary: Having to do with the armpit.

Axillary temperature: A body temperature taken by placing a thermometer snugly between the skin of the chest and the inner upper arm.

B

Bachelor of science in nursing: See **BSN.**

Back transport: The return of a baby from the hospital of current treatment to the hospital where the pregnant woman or newborn was originally admitted and previously treated or to a local hospital for further care when the problems that required transport have resolved. Also called *return transport.*

Bacteria: Single-cell microorganisms that can cause infection in humans; can also be protective or helpful, however.

Bagging: Gently pumping "breaths" into the lungs using a resuscitation bag and a face mask or endotracheal tube. Also called *hand-bagging.* See also **Bag-mask ventilation.**

Bag-mask ventilation: A method used to "breathe" for a baby; the face mask is placed firmly over the nose and mouth of the baby, and air or an air/oxygen mix is puffed into the baby's lungs. This method of positive pressure ventilation is also called *bagging the baby.*

Balloon atrial septostomy: A procedure used during heart catheterization to enlarge the hole in the wall between the 2 upper chambers of the heart.

Balloon valvuloplasty: A procedure used to enlarge a constricted heart valve. A balloon is fed into the heart inside a catheter and then inflated inside the valve.

Barrier property: The protective function of the skin; insulates and protects from infection.

Behavioral disorganization: Unpredictable activity patterns. Usually refers to the preterm infant's inability to organize endogenous rhythms, physiologic functions, and behavior to respond appropriately to the environment.

Bile: Green-colored liquid secreted by the liver and stored in the gallbladder. Intermittently ejected into the duodenum (upper portion of the small intestine).

Bilirubin ("bili"): The substance released when the body breaks down red blood cells; converted by the liver and disposed of mainly in the stool. Buildup of bilirubin in the blood may cause jaundice (yellow color to skin).

Birth defect: See **Anomaly, congenital.**

Bleed, a: Medical jargon for an intracranial or intraventricular hemorrhage.

Bleeding time: A laboratory test in which the time required for a sample of blood to clot is measured for the purpose of assessing normal blood clotting functions.

Blood culture: A laboratory test in which blood is microscopically monitored to see if harmful microorganisms grow. The purpose is to determine the presence and type of infectious agent.

Blood gas, arterial (ABG): A laboratory test performed on blood taken from an artery to determine levels of oxygen, carbon dioxide, and acid. The oxygen level of an ABG is more reliable than the oxygen level from veins or capillaries in helping to evaluate the baby's respiratory status.

Blood gas, capillary (CBG): A laboratory test performed on blood taken from a capillary (generally by pricking the baby's heel) to determine levels of oxygen, carbon dioxide, and acid. An important test for evaluating a baby's respiratory status.

Blood gas, venous (VBG): A laboratory test performed on blood taken from a vein to determine levels of oxygen, carbon dioxide, and acid. An important test for evaluating a baby's respiratory status.

Blood glucose: The concentration of glucose (sugar) in the blood.

Blue: A term denoting poor tissue oxygenation. See also **Color** and **Cyanosis.**

Board certified: A term for a health care provider who has taken and passed a standardized examination specific to a given specialty. Not required for state licensure; denotes professional excellence in the specialty.

Bolus: A volume of fluid given all at once, instead of over a long period.

Booster: A dose of vaccine given sometime after the original vaccine is given to maintain or increase the effectiveness of an immunization.

Boundaries: Physical things (such as blankets, special buntings, or a hand) used to encircle or contain a baby or to create a sort of nest and to help the baby bring and keep the arms and legs close to the body; provide a feeling of security and promote behavioral organization.

Bradycardia: A significant slowing of the heart rate below the individual's normal rate. Generally, bradycardia for a newborn may be defined as a heart rate of less than 100 beats per minute. May accompany apnea and/or cyanosis, or occur independently.

Brain stem: One of 3 primary divisions of the brain; the stalk of the brain. All nerve fibers relaying signals between the spinal cord and the higher brain centers pass through the brain stem.

Breast pump: A mechanical device used to remove milk from the breasts.

Breathing, periodic: A cyclic pattern of brief (about 5- to 10-second) pauses in breathing, without any change in heart rate or skin color. A common pattern in preterm infants; also seen in some healthy term infants in the first few days of life.

Breech presentation: The birth position in which a baby's buttocks or feet approach the opening to the birth canal before the head.

Bronchioles: Small airways in the lungs; a subdivision of the bronchial tree.

Bronchitis: Inflammation or infection of the tubes leading to the lungs (the bronchial tubes).

Bronchopulmonary dysplasia (BPD): A chronic lung disease primarily affecting premature infants less than 32 weeks' gestation who have required oxygen therapy for at least 4 weeks and continue to require supplemental oxygen at 36 weeks' corrected gestational age.

Bronchospasm: A contraction of the smooth muscle and a narrowing of the large air passages that lead to the lungs. Seen in asthma and bronchopulmonary dysplasia.

Brown adipose tissue (BAT): A special kind of fat around the shoulders, the base of the neck, the breast bone, and some organs in newborns. Newborns use BAT to produce heat because it breaks down more easily and makes heat more quickly than white fat does. Preterm babies have only small amounts.

BSN: Bachelor of science in nursing. A 4-year college nursing training program. Denotes educational level, not professional licensure.

Bulb syringe: A tool used to apply suction by hand to remove secretions from the nose and the mouth of an infant.

Button gastrostomy: A modification of a gastrostomy with a valve on the abdominal wall. Usually done when an infant with long-term feeding problems reaches about 10 pounds. Permits removal of the gastrostomy tube after each feeding; the flap closes the "button" and prevents feeding loss.

C

C-section: See **Cesarean section.**

Caffeine: A medication that stimulates the central nervous system; can be given to infants to reduce occurrences of apnea of prematurity.

Calorie: A measure of the energy value of food.

Cannula, nasal: A soft plastic tubing that wraps around a baby's face and has openings under the baby's nose. Used to deliver oxygen.

Cannulation: A surgical procedure performed to place catheters into the body, as in extracorporeal membrane oxygenation (ECMO) therapy.

Capillaries: Extremely tiny blood vessels that form networks in most tissues, supply cells with oxygen and nutrients, and remove wastes.

Car safety seat trial: Recommended prior to discharge home for babies born premature or discharged with cardiac, respiratory, neurologic, or musculoskeletal problems. Baby is placed in car safety seat while heart rate, breathing, and oxygen saturation are monitored to determine if baby can tolerate upright position in car safety seat; also determines safety of upright position in infant carrier, baby seat, or swing.

Carbon dioxide (CO_2): A waste product of energy production in the body. Removed from the blood as it passes through the lungs and is exhaled.

Cardiac: Having to do with the heart.

Cardiac output: The amount of blood that the heart pumps out in a given period.

Cardiologist: A physician who specializes in diagnosing and treating problems associated with the heart.

Cardiopulmonary resuscitation (CPR): A technique for reviving someone whose breathing has stopped (or has slowed greatly) or whose heart is not beating (or is beating very slowly). Cardiopulmonary resuscitation involves artificial respirations and cardiac compressions.

Cardiorespiratory monitor: An electronic device attached to babies in NICUs to monitor heart rate and rate of breathing; sounds an alarm if either falls below or exceeds a desirable level.

Cardiorespiratory system: The body system made up of the heart, blood vessels, and lungs.

Cardiovascular: Having to do with the heart and blood vessels.

Care conference: A scheduled meeting at which members of a baby's health care team update parents on baby's health status, changes in the care plan, and expectations for improvement; questions are answered; parental involvement in care is desirable.

Care map: See **Clinical pathway.**

Care plan: An individualized outline that guides medical and nursing activities for a baby; revised as the baby's condition changes. Helps provide consistent methods of caregiving to meet the individual needs of the baby.

Carotid arteries: Large arteries in the neck that carry oxygenated blood from the heart to the brain. Internal and external carotid arteries are located on each side of the neck.

Case manager: A patient advocate who coordinates formal and informal health services during hospitalization and ensures orderly progress toward hospital discharge.

Catastrophic illness: In reference to health care coverage, a major illness involving a lengthy hospital stay (usually) and high medical bills. If an insurance carrier provides catastrophic coverage, it pays 100% of the bills above a stated dollar amount of costs.

Catheter: A thin, flexible tube through which fluids are given to or removed from the body.

Catheter, umbilical arterial (UAC): A thin, flexible tube inserted into 1 of the 2 arteries (blood vessels) in the umbilical cord of a newborn. Can be used to provide fluids and medications, to remove blood for testing, and to monitor blood pressure. Also called an *umbi line*.

Catheter, umbilical venous (UVC): A thin, flexible tube inserted into a vein in the umbilical cord of a newborn to facilitate administration of medications and/or fluids into the baby's bloodstream, especially used for birth resuscitation.

Catheterization: A procedure in which a thin, flexible tube (a catheter) is inserted into the body. In cardiac catheterization, the tube is fed (slowly advanced) into arteries or veins of the arms or legs and into the heart and may contain an inflatable balloon to enlarge or open a constricted heart passage.

CBG: See **Blood gas, capillary.**

Central nervous system (CNS): The body system made up of the brain and spinal cord.

Cephalhematoma: A localized swelling on the head of a newborn caused by a collection of blood between one of the skull bones and its membranous covering.

Cerebellum: The rounded portion of the hindbrain. Serves to coordinate movement, posture, and balance.

Cerebral: Having to do with the brain.

Cerebral cortex: The outer layer (and nerve center) of the brain.

Cerebral palsy (CP): Abnormality of tone or coordination of body movement. Risk factors for development of CP include lack of blood flow or oxygen to the brain, prematurity, severe brain hemorrhage, infection, or periventricular leukomalacia. The cause of CP is often unknown.

Cerebrospinal fluid: Fluid surrounding the brain and spinal cord. Acts as a cushion for those organs.

Certified registered nurse anesthetist: See **CRNA.**

Cervix: The narrow passage at the end of the uterus closest to the vagina (birth canal). The passage dilates (expands) as labor progresses.

Cesarean section: A surgical procedure in which an incision is made through the abdomen into the uterus to deliver the baby. Also called a *C-section*.

Chorioamnionitis: An infection of the membranes that contain the amniotic fluid in the uterus.

Chromosome: One of 46 threadlike structures (23 coming from the mother and 23 from the father) that make up the center of each cell in the human body. Chromosomes carry genetic information in the form of genes.

Chromosome defect: See **Genetic defect.**

Chronic: Lasting for a long time; long term.

Chronic-care facility: See **Long-term care facility.**

Chronic sorrow: An ongoing, unresolved feeling of sadness (sometimes intense; other times barely recognizable) in response to a negative situation that cannot be made right or resolved.

Chronic stress: Ongoing, long-term stress, often resulting from an unresolvable situation.

Circulatory system: The body system made up of the vessels through which blood and other fluids move.

Circumcision: The surgical procedure in which the foreskin covering the tip of the penis is removed.

Cleft lip: A birth defect marked by internal and external malformations of the mouth and nose areas. Usually involves an opening or slit from the upper lip to one or both nostrils. Sometimes accompanied by cleft palate.

Cleft palate: A birth defect marked by an opening in the roof of the mouth connecting the oral and nasal cavities. Sometimes accompanied by cleft lip.

Clinical nurse specialist: See **CNS.**

Clinical pathway: The normal, expected pattern or progression of a disease or a developmental sequence over a specific period in most patients; not specific to an individual patient. Also called a *care map* or a *critical pathway.*

CNS: Clinical nurse specialist. A registered nurse with a master's degree who provides clinical expertise and information to the nursing staff; may be involved in teaching, research, consultation, and program development, as well as in patient care. Also an abbreviation for central nervous system.

Coarctation of the aorta: A birth defect in which the main artery from the heart to the body (the aorta) is constricted, obstructing blood flow to the body.

Cold stress: Physiologic responses to a lower than normal body temperature such as increased metabolism and increased oxygen consumption; cold stress can lead to weight loss or failure to gain weight and respiratory distress.

Color: In reference to a baby, the look of the skin denoting general health, especially oxygenation. Normal color of the mucous membranes (inner lips, tongue, and gums) is a healthy pink, regardless of ethnicity. A pale, dusky (bluish pink), or blue color of the mucous membranes or a yellowish skin color may indicate medical problems.

Colostomy: A surgical opening made in the abdominal wall so that part of the large intestine can be attached to the abdominal wall surface; stool then drains from the bowel into a collecting bag or pouch placed over the opening. Often performed after surgical removal of part of the intestine because of disease (most commonly necrotizing enterocolitis) or malformation.

Colostrum: The thick clear or yellowish secretion produced by the breasts of pregnant women beginning about week 16 of pregnancy; changes to a thinner, whiter substance called *mature milk* within a few days after the birth of a baby. Colostrum is rich in protein and immune factors.

Community hospital: A local hospital. Usually has an obstetrics and newborn area equipped to care for healthy mothers and newborn babies, to evaluate and stabilize patients for transport and, in some cases, to care for mildly ill and convalescing mothers and babies. See also **Level I nursery** and **Level II nursery.**

Complete blood count (CBC): A laboratory test that measures the cellular components—red blood cells (RBCs), white blood cells (WBCs), and platelets—in the blood. Often done as one of a series of tests to detect infection.

Compliance: When referring to the lung, the degree of flexibility.

Complication: An unwelcome by not unexpected setback or physical difficulty related to (and resulting from) a medical condition, disease, or problem or to the treatment for that problem.

Compression, chest: Application of pressure to the chest, squeezing the heart between the breastbone and the spine to artificially pump the heart.

Computed tomography (CT) scan: A diagnostic imaging technique that uses a narrow beam of radiation (x-ray) rotated around the body and a computer to construct 2-dimensional cross-sectional pictures of internal body structures. Among other uses, aids in diagnosis of bleeding or excess fluid in the brain.

Conditioned response: A learned action that occurs uncontrollably in reaction to a specific stimulus.

Congenital: Existing at birth.

Congenital diaphragmatic hernia (CDH): A life-threatening birth defect caused by the fetal bowel pushing up into the chest cavity through an abnormal hole in the muscle (the diaphragm) separating the chest from the abdomen.

Congenital heart defect: A malformation of the heart or of the blood vessels near it that exists at birth. Caused by abnormal development of the organ or vessels during gestation. Can be minor or life-threatening.

Congestive heart failure (CHF): A condition in which the heart has trouble meeting the body's energy needs. Not a disease itself, but the result of an underlying condition such as a congenital heart defect, severe anemia, or a patent ductus arteriosus.

Consent: Written permission granted for a specific medical procedure, often a surgery. "Giving informed consent" means that you understand what you are agreeing to and that all of your questions have been answered.

Constrict: To narrow or compress.

Containment, body: The encircling or nesting of a baby in the hospital using boundaries (rolled blankets, special buntings, or a hand) to help the baby bring and keep the arms and legs close to the body. Provides a feeling of security and promotes behavioral organization. See also **Nest.**

Continuity, patient: For a health care provider (especially a nurse), a system that promotes familiarity with patients through consistency in patient care assignments.

Continuous positive airway pressure (CPAP): Air or an air-oxygen mixture mechanically pushed into a baby's lungs to keep the air sacs open after the baby takes a breath, reducing the effort the baby must make to breathe; commonly delivered through short tubes placed in the nose (nasal CPAP) or through an endotracheal (ET) tube.

Contracture: A tightness or stiffness (resistance to stretching) of a muscle or joint.

Contraindication: A reason a patient may not receive a medication or a treatment.

Contrast enhancement: A dye or some other material injected into the body to produce a difference between the appearance of 2 types of body structures on the images produced by radiography (conventional x-ray or CT scan).

Coping mechanism: A way or ways in which individuals deal with difficult situations and the stress they produce. Also called a *coping strategy.*

Corrected age: The number of weeks or months since a baby's birth, minus the number of weeks or months the baby was born before the due date. An important consideration when assessing the developmental level of the preterm infant. Example: a baby born at 32 weeks' gestation who is now 12 weeks old has a corrected age of 4 weeks old (12 weeks old minus 8 weeks premature = 4 weeks old corrected age).

Cot death: See **Sudden infant death syndrome.**

CPAP: See **Continuous positive airway pressure.**

CPR: See **Cardiopulmonary resuscitation.**

Crib death: See **Sudden infant death syndrome.**

Critical pathway: See **Clinical pathway.**

CRNA: Certified registered nurse anesthetist. A registered nurse with advanced practice education who, under the supervision of and in collaboration with an anesthesiologist, is qualified to give medications that reduce or abolish pain and/or cause unconsciousness.

CT scan: See **Computed tomography scan.**

Cue: An action or behavior that can indicate a baby's readiness for and reaction to stimulation; one means of infant communication.

Culture: A laboratory test in which blood or another body fluid is placed in nutritive substance to see if microorganisms grow. The purpose of a culture is to determine presence and type of infection.

Cyanosis: A condition in which the skin and mucous membranes have a bluish color, caused by lack of oxygen in the tissues.

Cyanosis, central: A condition in which the skin over the entire body and of the mucous membranes has a bluish color, caused by lack of oxygen in the tissues. Also called *central cyanosis.*

Cyanosis, circumoral: A condition in which the skin around the mouth has a bluish color, caused by lack of oxygen to the cells.

Cyanotic defect: A heart defect that causes blood going to the body to contain a lower than normal amount of oxygen.

Cyst: A membrane-covered sac (often filled with liquid or a semisolid material) that develops abnormally in a body cavity or structure.

D

Decannulation: The removal of a tube, such as a catheter used in extracorporeal membrane oxygenation therapy or a tracheostomy tube.

Deductible: In reference to health care coverage, the amount you must pay before the insurance carrier begins to cover the bills.

Defense mechanism: One of the factors in the human body that protect it from infection.

Dehydrate: To lose body fluids or water.

Dehydration: The loss of water or fluids from the body.

Dependence, drug: The state of having grown accustomed to a drug's effects. Characterized by withdrawal symptoms experienced when the drug is stopped.

Depression: A mental and emotional state marked by fatigue, sadness, reduced activity, difficulty thinking, changes in eating and sleeping patterns, feelings of hopelessness, and sometimes thoughts of suicide.

Desaturation, oxygen: Too little oxygen bound to hemoglobin molecules in the bloodstream; causes lack of oxygen in the tissues.

Developmental delay: A slowness in mastering motor coordination skills (such as lifting the head, rolling over, or sitting), behavioral skills (such as self-calming or controlling anger), and living skills (such as learning simple tasks or mastering more complex schoolwork).

Developmental milestone: One of the many important basic skills an average baby masters at a specific age—for example, sitting with support by 6 months of age.

Developmental outcome: A baby's ability, as he or she grows, to master physical, behavioral, and emotional skills of living.

Developmental specialist: A health care provider who has special training in diagnosing and treating delays in a child's mastery of motor coordination and behavioral and learning skills.

Diagnosis: A conclusion about the cause of a medical problem.

Diagnostic imaging: Producing "pictures" of the inside of the body without opening it up, to identify the cause(s) and to help in the treatment of medical problems. Types of diagnostic imaging include the computed tomography (CT) scan, ultrasound, and magnetic resonance imaging (MRI).

Diagnostic testing: Laboratory and other tests (such as imaging techniques that produce "pictures" of the inside of the body) performed to help medical caregivers determine what is wrong with a patient.

Diaphragm: The dome-shaped muscle just below the lungs and above the stomach that separates the chest cavity from the abdominal cavity. Plays an important role in breathing.

Diaphragmatic hernia: See **Congenital Diaphragmatic Hernia**

Diarrhea: Frequent watery or liquid stools (feces); often foul smelling.

Dilate: To enlarge, stretch, or widen.

Diploma program: A 2- or 3-year hospital training program for nursing. Denotes educational preparation, not nursing licensure.

Disability: A physical or mental abnormality or restriction.

Discharge coordinator: See **Discharge planner.**

Discharge planner: A nurse or other trained individual on the hospital's staff who makes all arrangements for a baby's release from the hospital and for any special care the baby may need after discharge. Also called a *discharge coordinator.*

Discharge planning: The process carried out by trained hospital staff to ensure that all designated medical care activities, tests, and parent teaching are completed before a baby's release from the hospital and that arrangements are made for any needed follow-up or special care.

Discharge summary: A written report of a baby's prenatal history and events of labor, birth, and hospitalization.

Disseminated intravascular coagulation (DIC): Bleeding at more than one location in the body because of toxins in the bloodstream released by infectious microorganisms.

Distention: An enlargement or swelling, especially caused by pressure from the inside.

Diuretic: A medication that removes excess fluid from the body by increasing urine production.

Do not resuscitate (DNR) order: A medical order written when a terminally ill or severely disabled patient is to be permitted to die peacefully; the DNR order ensures no vigorous lifesaving measures will be taken.

Doppler ultrasound: An enhancement to a regular ultrasound scan. Detects blood flow disturbances caused by abnormalities in internal body structure. Used for an echocardiogram.

Down syndrome: A birth defect characterized by specific physical features and caused by an extra 21st chromosome. Also called *trisomy 21.*

DTaP: Diphtheria-tetanus-pertussis vaccine.

Ductus arteriosus: A short vessel connecting the pulmonary artery with the aorta in the fetus. Before birth, sends most of the blood directly from the right ventricle of the heart to the aorta, bypassing the lungs; normally closes shortly after birth.

Duodenal atresia: A birth defect marked by a blockage in the upper portion (duodenum) of the small bowel.

Durable medical equipment (DME): Medical equipment prescribed for home use (such as oxygen or suction machine); the DME company's staff trains users in its operation and maintenance, and deals with equipment problems.

Dusky: A descriptive term for the bluish-pink color of skin and mucous membranes of babies who are cyanotic (whose cells lack oxygen).

Dynamics: The ways in which individuals interact; includes such aspects as who leads and who follows and whether members share thoughts and feelings openly.

E

Early intervention program: A public program designed to prevent developmental delays in at-risk children and to aid children already showing delays.

ECG: See **Electrocardiogram.**

Echocardiogram: An ultrasound of the heart.

Echocardiography: A diagnostic imaging technique in which an ultrasound of the heart is made.

Eclampsia: A term used to denote neurologic involvement that results in a seizure as a result of gestational hypertension. A woman with this condition is said to be eclamptic.

ECMO: See **Extracorporeal membrane oxygenation.**

ECMO specialist: A trained medical caregiver (usually a specially trained nurse or respiratory therapist) who monitors and maintains an ECMO circuit at all times while it is operating.

Edema: An accumulation of excess fluid in body tissues, generally causing swelling.

EEG: See **Electroencephalogram.**

EFM: See **Electronic fetal monitoring.**

EKG: See **Electrocardiogram.**

Electrocardiogram (ECG or EKG): A diagnostic test that records the electrical activity of the heart and helps caregivers determine how well it is functioning.

Electrode: See **Lead.**

Electroencephalogram (EEG): A diagnostic test that records the electrical impulses of the brain; helps caregivers determine how well it is functioning.

Electrolytes ("lytes"): Basic body chemicals in the blood; essential for proper cell functioning. Include sodium (Na), potassium (K), chloride (Cl), calcium (Ca), and magnesium (Mg). Also, a laboratory test that measures the balance of these elements in the blood.

Electronic fetal monitor (EFM): An electronic device, often used during labor, to track fetal heart rate and monitor maternal uterine contractions. EFM is one tool for assessing how well the mother and baby are progressing through labor and birth.

Embolus, air: A bubble of air obstructing blood flow through a blood vessel (plural: emboli).

Endothelial-derived relaxing factor (EDRF): A natural substance released by the body that helps relax and therefore open the arterioles (blood vessels near the breathing sacs in the lungs) after birth. Nitric oxide is an EDRF.

Endotracheal (ET) tube: A tube placed into the windpipe (trachea) through the nose or mouth to assist babies with breathing difficulties. Insertion of the tube is called *intubation;* removal, *extubation.* A baby with an ET tube is assisted with continuous positive airway pressure (CPAP) or a ventilator.

Engorgement, postpartum: A condition caused by increased blood flow and overfilling of the woman's breasts with milk, often 2 to 3 days after delivery. Breasts become hard, painful, and warm; the skin covering them may feel tight; and swelling may extend into the armpits.

Enterohepatic shunt: A mechanism by which bilirubin (that has been processed by the liver [hepatic]) is unprocessed in the intestine (entero). In the first week of life, there is a high concentration of the enzyme that initiates this conversion.

Enzyme: A complex protein produced by body cells. Makes possible certain necessary chemical reactions in the body.

Episiotomy: A surgical incision to enlarge a woman's vaginal opening shortly before the birth of a baby.

Erythropoietin: A hormone that controls red blood cell production.

Esophageal atresia: A birth defect marked by blockage or malformation of the esophagus (food pipe).

Esophagus: The passage from the mouth to the stomach.

Estrogen: A hormone produced mainly by the ovaries; controls female sexual development.

Ethics: An area of study that involves moral principles or practice.

ET tube: See **Endotracheal tube.**

Exogenous: Not produced by the body.

Expiration, active: The mechanical pulling of gas out of the lung during the exhalation part of a breath; used in high-frequency oscillatory ventilation.

Expiration, passive: An exhalation portion of a breath that is allowed to occur naturally through relaxation (automatic recoil) of the breathing muscles of the chest wall and diaphragm; used in conventional ventilation, high-frequency positive-pressure ventilation, high-frequency jet ventilation, and unassisted breathing.

Extracorporeal membrane oxygenation (ECMO): A mechanical technique for supporting both the heart and lung functions of critically ill term or late preterm babies with severe lung failure; used when the baby does not respond to conventional ventilation and/or medication therapy. Equipment is a modified version of the heart-lung bypass machine used during open-heart surgery.

Extrauterine: Outside the uterus.

ELBW: Extremely low birth weight. Any baby weighing less than 2 pounds, 4 ounces (1,000 grams) at birth, regardless of gestational age.

Extubate: To remove an endotracheal (ET) tube.

Eye patches: Soft coverings placed over a baby's eyes during phototherapy treatment to prevent possible injury to the eyes from bright light.

F

Feeding on demand: Letting the baby decide when and how much to eat.

Feeding pump: A device attached to a feeding tube and used to feed babies who cannot handle large amounts of food at one time. Meters a tiny amount of breast milk or formula into the feeding tube and allows for continuous tube feeding.

Feeding tube: A narrow, flexible tube inserted through the infant's nose (nasogastric) or mouth (orogastric) and on into the stomach to provide a route for breast milk or formula. Also called a *gavage tube.*

Fellow, neonatal: In a teaching hospital, a physician who has completed medical school and pediatric residency and is training to become a neonatologist.

Fetal: Having to do with an unborn baby (a fetus).

Fetal circulation: The movement of blood through a fetus's body before birth, specifically through the fetal heart and lungs. Much of the blood bypasses the fetus's lungs because of 2 open fetal shunts: the foramen ovale and the ductus arteriosus.

Fetus: An unborn baby of at least 8 weeks' gestation.

Fever: In an infant, a body temperature higher than 100.4°F (38°C) rectally.

Fever strip: A temperature-sensitive material applied to the forehead to estimate skin temperature.

Fiberoptic blanket: A flat, flexible wrapping covered with fiberoptic lights and used for phototherapy treatment; a baby can lie on it, or the blanket can be wrapped around the baby's torso to provide phototherapy treatment.

Finger feeding: An alternative technique for feeding a breastfeeding baby; caregiver places a clean, gloved finger in the baby's mouth with a feeding tube filled with milk beside it. When the baby sucks on the finger, milk is drawn from the feeding tube.

Fistula: An abnormal passage or connection between 2 parts of the body.

Flaring, nasal: A condition that accompanies respiratory distress in an infant; the nostrils open widely during each inspiration in order to take in as much air as possible with each breath.

Flex: To bend, especially at a joint.

Fontanel: The soft spot on the top of a baby's head; a normal opening between the bones of the skull of a fetus or young infant where skull development is incomplete.

Foramen ovale: An opening in the wall between the 2 upper chambers (atria) of the fetal heart; normally closes at birth.

Forceps: Curved metal tongs used by medical personnel to help deliver a baby's head during the final stages of birth.

Foremilk: Breast milk produced at the beginning of a feeding; lower in fat and calories than the milk produced toward the end of the feeding (hindmilk).

Foster care: Care given to a child (usually for a temporary period) by one or more individuals who are not related to the child by blood or under law; foster care providers generally must follow government regulations and usually receive some financial compensation for their services.

Frenulum: Fold of mucous membrane under the tongue; a short frenulum refers to a shorter than normal band of tissue that anchors the tongue to the bottom of the mouth.

Free flow oxygen: Stream of oxygen/air mixture directed toward the nose and mouth of a baby who is breathing but requires supplemental oxygen.

Fundoplication: Surgical treatment for gastroesophageal reflux. Tightens the connection between the esophagus (food pipe) and the stomach; prevents food from moving back up into the baby's esophagus.

Fungus: A microorganism that can cause infection; yeast *(Candida)* is a common fungus.

G

Gas exchange: In the lungs, addition of oxygen to the blood with removal of carbon dioxide.

Gastroenteritis: An inflammation in the bowel, usually due to infection.

Gastroesophageal reflux (GER): Condition that occurs when the opening to the entrance of the stomach allows food to move back up into the esophagus. Most preterm babies outgrow GER; however, some require medication or surgery (fundoplication).

Gastrointestinal: Having to do with the stomach and intestines.

Gastrointestinal (GI) system: The body system made up of the stomach and intestines.

Gastrointestinal (GI) tract: The stomach and intestines. Also called the *gut.*

Gastroschisis: A birth defect in which abdominal organs push outside the baby's body through an opening in the wall of the abdomen usually just to the right of the umbilical cord.

Gastrostomy: A surgical opening in the abdominal wall through which part of the stomach can be attached to the abdominal skin; a feeding tube can be inserted into the opening. Usually used only in babies expected to have long-term feeding problems.

Gastrostomy (GT) tube: A feeding tube inserted into a surgically created opening in the abdominal wall to which a portion of the stomach is attached (a gastrostomy). During feeding, a measured amount of breast milk or formula flows through the tube by gravity into the baby's stomach.

Gavage feeding: Feeding a baby through a tube inserted through the mouth (orogastric) or nose (nasogastric) into the stomach (or occasionally, the intestine). Also called *tube feeding.*

Gavage tube: See **Feeding tube.**

GBS pneumonia: A type of pneumonia in babies caused by group B beta-hemolytic streptococcus (GBS).

Gene: A unit of heredity. Found in the chromosomes in each cell of the body. Determines certain traits and physical characteristics (such as eye color) of a baby.

Generic: General. In reference to a drug, one that is not proprietary—that is, is not manufactured or controlled by a single company and does not have a trademarked (brand) name. For example, acetaminophen is a generic drug; Tylenol is a brand name for an acetaminophen-containing medication.

Genetic: Having to do with the genes; something one is born with or inherits.

Genetic defect: An abnormality caused by improper development of the chromosome pairs when the egg is fertilized. Also called a *chromosome defect.*

Gestation: The time required for a fertilized egg cell to develop into a baby ready for birth. Human gestation averages 266 days (or 280 days from the first day of the last menstrual period).

Gestational age: The number of completed weeks that have elapsed between the first day of the last menstrual period (not the presumed time of conception) and the date of birth.

Gestational hypertension: A multiorgan disease process during pregnancy involving high blood pressure as an important symptom; onset is usually after 20 weeks' gestation. Renal, neurologic, liver, and hematologic involvement are possible during the course of the disease. Previously called *pregnancy-induced hypertension (PIH).*

Glucose: A simple sugar used by the body for energy.

Glucose polymers: Additives for breast milk or formula that provide sugars in a form that immature newborns can digest and absorb easily.

Glycogen: A form of glucose (sugar) that a fetus stores for use during the energy-consuming process of birth and transition to extrauterine life.

Group B beta-hemolytic streptococcus: See **Streptococcus, group B beta-hemolytic.** See also **GBS pneumonia.**

Growth factor: A substance that promotes growth, especially of the cells of the body.

Grunting: The audible sound made by an infant at exhalation that indicates a breathing problem. A compensatory mechanism that prevents the small air sacs of the lungs from completely deflating after every breath.

Gut: See **Gastrointestinal tract.**

H

Hand-bagging: See **Bagging.**

Heart murmur: A characteristic swishing sound made as blood flows through the heart. Many heart murmurs are not associated with problems.

Heelstick: A prick of a baby's heel to obtain a small amount of capillary blood for testing.

Hematocrit ("crit"): The percentage of red blood cells in the blood. Also, a laboratory test that measures the percentage; results help show a baby's ability to supply oxygen to the body tissues.

Hematologic system: The body system made up of the blood and its components: plasma (the liquid portion), red blood cells, white blood cells, and platelets (the cellular portion).

Hemoglobin (Hgb): The substance in red blood cells that carries oxygen to body cells. Also, a laboratory test that measures the amount of this substance in the cells.

Hemolysis: Destruction of red blood cells.

Hemorrhage: Heavy or uncontrollable bleeding.

Hemorrhage, postpartum: The loss of more than 500 milliliters of blood by a mother following the birth of a baby.

Heparin: A substance that keeps blood from clotting.

Heparin lock: A cap applied to the end of the insertion site of an intravenous (IV) line so that the long tubing can be disconnected and reconnected as needed while keeping the IV patent (open and unclotted); lets the patient move more freely between administration of medication and fluids. Also called a *heparin well.*

Heparin well: See **Heparin lock.**

Hepatitis: A disease that causes inflammation of the liver; different types (A, B, and so on) are caused by different viruses and are transmitted by different means (water, fecal contamination, or blood and blood products).

Hernia: A protrusion of part of an internal organ through a tissue that normally contains it.

Herpes: An inflammatory disease of the skin or mucous membranes caused by a virus that reproduces in the nuclei of body cells.

Herpes simplex virus: A microorganism that reproduces in the nuclei of body cells and causes herpes.

HFV: High-frequency ventilation; type of mechanical breathing assistance that delivers very small breaths at extremely rapid rates.

Hindmilk: Breast milk produced at the end of a feeding; higher in fat and calories than the first milk produced (the foremilk).

Hirschsprung disease: A congenital problem in which the rectum and sometimes the lower colon have failed to develop a normal nerve network. Contents of the bowel accumulate and distend the upper colon. Treatment requires surgery.

HIV: Human immunodeficiency virus, the virus that causes acquired immune deficiency syndrome (AIDS).

Home care: Care for a sick or disabled individual in the individual's home instead of at a hospital or care facility.

Home health agency: A health care organization that provides skilled nursing and/or rehabilitation services in the home or place of residence.

Home visit: A visit to your home by a nurse or trained home health care provider after your baby's discharge to assess your baby's well-being and progress, review care procedures, and answer your questions.

Hood: See **Oxygen hood.**

Hormone: A substance produced by body cells; circulates in body fluids and stimulates the activity of other body cells.

Hospice: Care services from a team of professionals that help ensure a comfortable and peaceful death.

Hospitalist, pediatric: A physician who has completed a pediatric residency and has developed specific skills and interest in caring for infants and children who require in-patient hospital care. Some hospitalists choose to spend part or all of their time working in a NICU.

Human immunodeficiency virus: See **HIV.**

Humidifier: A mechanical device that adds moisture to the air.

Hyaline membrane disease (HMD): See **Respiratory distress syndrome.**

Hydrocephalus: Literally "water on the brain"; backup of cerebrospinal fluid in the ventricles (chambers) of the brain, producing pressure that causes head enlargement and can damage brain tissue. Spina bifida and intraventricular hemorrhage are conditions associated with hydrocephalus.

Hyperactivity: Greater than normal movement or activity.

Hyperbilirubinemia: A higher than normal level or faster than normal rise in the level of bilirubin in the blood.

Hyperglycemia: A higher than normal level of glucose (sugar) in the blood.

Hypertension: High blood pressure.

Hyperventilation: Faster than normal breathing at rest.

Hypervigilance: A constant high level of worrying and watching.

Hypocalcemia: A lower-than-normal level of calcium in the blood.

Hypoglycemia: A lower than normal blood sugar level.

Hypoplastic left heart syndrome (HLHS): A congenital heart defect that is fatal without treatment. Includes a small aorta, heart valve narrowing or absence, and a small left atrium and ventricle. Previously treated only somewhat successfully through a series of surgeries, but improved surgical techniques and heart transplants have increased the survival rate.

Hypotension: A lower than normal blood pressure.

Hypothermia: A lower than normal body temperature. In infants, can lead to breathing problems, low blood sugar, and weight loss.

Hypovolemia: A lower than normal blood volume (amount circulating in the body).

Hypoxia: Insufficient oxygen in the tissues.

Hypoxic-ischemic encephalopathy (HIE): A common cause of brain damage in the newborn that occurs when blood flow to the placenta is inadequate, resulting in a newborn who does not begin to breathe and circulate oxygenated blood at birth. HIE is caused by hypoxia (lack of oxygen in the blood) and ischemia (reduced blood flow to the brain). These events lead to asphyxia and brain dysfunction (encephalopathy).

I

I & O: Intake and output. A method of measuring and recording all fluids that go into and come out of the baby's body to ensure correct fluid balance.

Idiopathic: A term for a condition for which no cause can be identified.

Ileostomy: A surgical opening in the abdominal wall made so that part of the small intestine can be attached to the abdominal wall surface. Stool then drains from the bowel into a collecting bag or pouch placed over the opening. Often performed after surgical removal of part of the intestine because of disease or malformation.

Immaturity: A state of incomplete growth or development.

Immune: Having resistance, antibodies, or lack of susceptibility to something—generally, to infectious agents such as bacteria or viruses.

Immunization: A vaccination given to eliminate or reduce a person's likelihood of getting a specific disease.

Immunoglobulin: A protein molecule that acts as an antibody, a disease-fighting substance in the blood. Some types of immunoglobulins can cross the placenta from mother to fetus during the final 3 months of pregnancy. Breast milk also contains immunoglobulins. Some types of immunoglobulins can be given to high-risk infants through an intravenous line as a preventive measure.

Imperforate anus: A birth defect in which the anal canal and/or opening is absent. Also called *anal atresia.*

Incarcerated hernia: A hernia in which the protruding body organ becomes trapped in the space it has invaded.

Incision: The cut made into tissue with a scalpel for a surgical procedure.

Incubator: A transparent, boxlike enclosure in which sick or preterm babies are placed. Allows control of the temperature around the baby and provides limited protection of the baby from infectious agents. See also **Isolette.**

Individualized family service plan (IFSP): An outline for action prepared by a team of professionals participating in a state-sponsored early intervention program who have assessed a developmentally delayed baby's needs, along with those of the family.

Induction, labor: Refers to deliberate initiation of uterine contractions with medication before labor begins on its own. Used only when medically indicated.

Infant of a diabetic mother (IDM): A baby, often preterm and large for gestational age, born to a diabetic mother.

Infection: An invasion of body cells and/or tissues by harmful microorganisms (bacteria, viruses, fungi, or protozoa) that generally multiply once established. Also, the body's response to the invasion.

Infection, acquired: Infection passed to a baby after birth; results from exposure to infectious agent while in the health care (hospital) setting. Also called *nosocomial infection.*

Infection, congenital: See **Infection, intrauterine.**

Infection, intrauterine: Infection contracted by a fetus across the placenta (vertical transmission). Also called a *congenital infection.* For types, see **TORCH.**

Infection, perinatal: Infection passed to the fetus through the birth canal prior to birth (especially if the amniotic membranes are ruptured) or contracted by the baby as he or she passes through the birth canal.

Infiltrated IV: An intravenous (IV) line that has become obstructed or dislodged from the vein, causing IV fluid to leak out of the vein and into the surrounding tissue.

Infusion, IV: Continuous instillation of a solution into a vein. Usually metered by a pump.

Inguinal hernia: A protrusion of part of the intestine into the scrotum through a gap in the muscle wall. In females, part of the intestine can slide into the groin. Inguinal hernia is more common in males.

Inhalatory: A term used to describe something (usually a medication) taken by breathing it in.

Insulin: A hormone produced by the pancreas. Helps move glucose from the blood into the cells.

Insurance case manager: An individual employed by your insurance carrier and assigned to handle the financial aspects of your baby's case.

Intensive care nursery: See **Level III nursery.**

Intermediate care: The level of care for sick and convalescing babies who do not require intensive care but do require medical and nursing supervision and caregiving; the form of care focused on preparing recovering babies for hospital discharge.

Intervention: A medical or nursing action or procedure.

Intracranial hemorrhage: A bleeding in or around the brain. Also called a *bleed.*

Intramuscular (IM): A term for a medication route into the muscle by needle. In lay terms, a "shot" is administration of an intramuscular medication.

Intraparenchymal: Within the functional tissue of an organ.

Intravenous (IV) catheter/line: A thin tube inserted into a vein by means of a needle (the needle is removed after the catheter is in the vein). Supplies medications, fluids, or nutrients directly into the bloodstream. Also called a *peripheral line.*

Intraventricular hemorrhage (IVH): Usually, bleeding in the brain tissue that may extend into the chambers (ventricles) of the brain. A type of intracranial hemorrhage. Severity is indicated by number, ranging from Grade 1 (least severe) to Grade 4 (ventricular enlargement and bleeding into surrounding brain tissue). Also called a *bleed.*

Intubation: Insertion of an endotracheal (ET) tube.

Invasive: A term that describes a diagnostic or treatment procedure involving cutting into the skin or inserting something (an instrument or device; a foreign substance) into the body.

Inverted nipples: Nipples that do not protrude from the areola of the breast, but are recessed (sunken) into the breast.

IQ: The abbreviation for "intelligence quotient." A person's IQ score is the result of a standardized test that expresses an individual's intellectual ability relative to the rest of the population. The best known for children are the Wechsler Intelligence Scale for Children (WISC) and the Stanford-Binet Intelligence Scale.

Isolette: A trade name for an incubator. Often used as a common term for an incubator.

IV: See **Intravenous catheter/line.**

J

Jaundice, pathologic: Jaundice (buildup of bilirubin in the fatty tissues that results in yellow skin color) that occurs within the first 24 hours of life; or visible persistent jaundice after 1 week of age in term infants (2 weeks in preterm infants); or bilirubin values that exceed defined norms. Usually a result of increased production of bilirubin caused by hemolysis, as in Rh or blood type incompatibility.

Jaundice, physiologic: A condition in which the skin color in newborns is yellowish because of a buildup of bilirubin in the fatty tissues. A common condition caused by immature liver function.

K

Kangaroo care: The practice of holding a NICU infant skin to skin against a parent's chest (often between the mother's breasts) to provide close human contact between parent and baby and to facilitate parent-infant attachment. Additional benefits usually include stable vital signs, more time in sleep and quiet alert states, increased weight gain, and improved feeding.

Kernicterus: A rare complication of hyperbilirubinemia. Occurs with very high levels of bilirubin, when bilirubin passes into the brain. Can cause permanent brain damage.

Kidney: A bean-shaped body organ that disposes of the waste products of metabolism as urine. Humans have 2 kidneys, one on either side of the spine.

L

Lactation: Milk production in the breasts of a woman. Also, broadly, breastfeeding.

Lactation consultant/specialist: A nurse or other health care provider with special training and expertise related to breastfeeding. A nurse lactation specialist with advanced education is most often used to manage the complex problems of breastfeeding mothers and babies in the NICU and in the community after hospital discharge; a layperson may be used in the community to offer support and education to breastfeeding mothers of healthy babies.

Lanugo: The soft, downy hair covering a preterm infant. Most evident on the upper back and shoulders. Disappears with maturation.

Large for gestational age (LGA): A term for a newborn whose weight (and possibly length and head circumference) falls above the 90th percentile on a standard intrauterine growth chart; indicates a larger than expected baby for the length of time the baby was in the uterus. An LGA baby can be preterm, term, or post-term.

Laryngeal mask: An inflatable airway device that slides into the infant's throat, forms a seal over the esophagus, and holds open the trachea during assisted breathing.

Laser therapy: A treatment that uses high energy concentrated in the form of a beam of light to destroy problem tissue.

Late preterm infant: Term used to describe a baby born at 34 to 36 weeks' gestation.

Lead: An adhesive patch placed on a baby's chest or abdomen that connects the baby to the cardiorespiratory monitor. Also called an *electrode*.

Learning disability: A disorder that interferes with one's learning processes.

Lesion: Any break in normal tissue or change in the structure of an organ because of disease or injury.

Let-down reflex: Contractions (caused by the hormone oxytocin) that squeeze a mother's breast milk into the holding reservoirs just behind the nipples. May be experienced as a gripping sensation or as "pins and needles" in the breasts. Milk may drip from the nipples as the milk "lets down." Also called a *milk-ejection reflex*.

Lethargy: Lack of energy; sluggishness.

Level I nursery: A hospital classification of perinatal care indicating obstetric and neonatal units equipped to manage healthy mothers and babies and to stabilize and initiate transport of ill and/or complex mothers and newborns.

Level II nursery: A hospital classification of perinatal care indicating obstetric and neonatal units equipped to care for selected complicated pregnancies and neonatal problems and for infants convalescing after a stay in a Level III nursery.

Level III nursery: Identifies an obstetric unit/nursery, generally in a regional medical center and often affiliated with a university, equipped to diagnose and treat all perinatal problems; provides intensive care for infants requiring technological support or surgery. Also called a *neonatal intensive care unit* or an *intensive care nursery*.

Licensed practical nurse (LPN): A designation of state licensure; a nurse who provides basic bedside care under the supervision of an RN. Also called a *licensed vocational nurse (LVN)*.

Licensed vocational nurse (LVN): See **Licensed practical nurse.**

Long-term care facility: A facility that cares for patients with poor prognosis, severe physical or mental disabilities, or with fatal conditions. Also called a *chronic care facility*.

Low birth weight (LBW) infant: Any infant who weighs less than 2,500 grams (5 pounds, 8 ounces) at birth, regardless of gestational age.

LPN: See **Licensed practical nurse.**

Lumbar puncture: Insertion of a needle into the lower back, through the membranous space covering the brain and spinal cord to withdraw spinal fluid; procedure is used in diagnosis and treatment. Also called a *spinal tap*.

LVN: Licensed vocational nurse. See **Licensed practical nurse.**

Lymphocyte: A type of white blood cell that fights invading microorganisms.

M

Magnetic resonance imaging (MRI): A diagnostic imaging technique involving interaction between a magnetic field and the atoms in the body; does not use radiation. Produces better images of soft tissue than does CT scanning or ultrasound, and dense bone and fatty tissue do not interfere with the image (as they can in ultrasound).

Magnetic resonance spectroscopy (MRS): Used with MRI to formulate a plan of care, especially for babies with hypoxic-ischemic encephalopathy (HIE). MRS produces a graph representing the chemical composition of a region of tissue; improves diagnostic capabilities and helps predict future neurologic outcome.

Malformation, congenital: An anatomic abnormality (external or internal) present in a baby at birth.

Master's degree in social work: See **MSW.**

Mastitis: Bacterial infection of the breast that shows itself as a hot, red, tender area on the breast and is usually accompanied by fever, chills, and flulike symptoms.

Maternal transport: The physical moving of a pregnant woman (by ground or air) from one medical facility to another for special care or delivery of a newborn expected to require neonatal intensive care.

Mature milk: Thin, whitish breast milk produced by a mother a few days after the birth of her baby. Follows production of colostrum.

Mean arterial pressure (MAP): One aspect of the blood pressure. Often monitored by a transducer connected to an umbilical arterial catheter.

Mechanical ventilation: Use of a machine (called a *respirator* or *ventilator)* to supply a number of breaths per minute and a mixture of air, oxygen, and pressure with each breath. The machine is connected to an endotracheal tube or a tracheostomy tube.

Meconium: Dark green to blackish material present in the large intestine of the fetus before birth. Usually passed during the first few days of life.

Meconium aspiration: "Breathing" into the trachea or lungs of meconium (a stool-like material that a fetus may excrete from its intestine into the amniotic fluid) by a fetus before or in the first moments after birth. Can cause breathing difficulties.

Meconium aspiration syndrome (MAS): Severe breathing problems after birth caused by meconium "breathed" into the airways while a baby is in the uterus or in the first moments after birth.

Medical home: A concept of care that means families and care providers work together to coordinate all of a child's care; a "home base" for health care focused on all needs of the child.

Medium-chain triglyceride (MCT) oil: An additive for breast milk or formula that contains fats that can be digested and absorbed by immature newborns who are not yet producing certain enzymes and bile salts.

Memory cell: An infection-fighting blood cell that, after once contacting a specific microorganism, remembers the microorganism and immediately begins to destroy it if it appears again.

Meningitis: Inflammation of the membranes lining the brain and spinal column; usually caused by a bacterium or a virus.

Metabolic: Having to do with metabolism.

Metabolic activity: Chemical reactions in which the body changes the nutrients in food into substances it needs to function or to build cells and tissues.

Metabolism: All the processes carried out by and chemical reactions that occur in the cells of the body as energy is produced and used.

Metoclopramide hydrochloride: A drug that may increase milk supply in lactating women.

Micrognathia: A birth defect marked by an abnormally small jaw.

Milk ejection reflex: See **Let-down reflex.**

Motor development: The learning of skills having to do with muscle movement and coordination.

Mottled: A marbled or blotched appearance; a term used to describe skin color.

MSW: Master's degree in social work. A social worker with a postgraduate degree with focus on support of hospital patients and families with socioeconomic and psychosocial problems. See also **Social worker.**

Multidisciplinary: Having many different areas of expertise or specialization; in a hospital setting, may refer to medicine, nursing, social work, respiratory care, etc.

Murmur: A characteristic swishing sound made by blood flowing through the heart. Many heart murmurs are not associated with problems.

Myelomeningocele: See **Spina bifida.**

N

Narcotic: A medication that relieves pain and dulls the senses—for example, morphine.

Nasal cannula: See **Cannula, nasal.**

Nasogastric (NG) tube: A feeding tube inserted through a baby's nostril into the esophagus (food pipe) and on to the stomach. Formula or breast milk flows through the tube into the baby's stomach. An NG tube is usually left in place for a number of feedings after insertion.

Nebulizer: A device for giving medication that must be breathed into the airway; administers a liquid in the form of a fine spray. A type of inhaler, a "puffer."

Necrotizing enterocolitis (NEC): A serious inflammatory bowel disease, most common in preterm babies.

Neonatal: Having to do with a newborn baby, from birth to 28 days of age.

Neonatal intensive care: Special care provided, usually at a regional medical center, to newborns with major health problems.

Neonatal intensive care unit (NICU): A nursery, usually located in a regional medical facility, equipped to treat newborns who have serious health problems; staffed with neonatologists, anesthesiologists, surgeons, and nurses with special training and experience in the care of sick newborns. See **Level III nursery.**

Neonatal nurse: A registered nurse with special training in the care of newborn babies.

Neonatal nurse practitioner: See **NNP.**

Neonatal physician assistant: See **NPA.**

Neonatal team: A group of health care professionals who care for a newborn baby in a hospital setting.

Neonatal transport: The moving of a newborn who requires special care or surgery from one hospital (often a community facility) to another (usually a Level III nursery).

Neonatologist: A physician who specializes in care and development, diagnosis, and treatment of ill newborn babies; has 3 years of training beyond that required for general pediatricians.

Neonatology: A branch of medicine that deals with the diagnosis, care, and treatment of disorders of newborn babies.

Nerve block: A type of anesthesia that makes the patient unable to feel pain—"blocks" the sensation—either locally (in a limited area of the body) or regionally (over a larger area of the body). See also **Anesthesia, local; Anesthesia, regional.**

Nerves: Bandlike tissues that transmit impulses from the brain or spinal cord to motor and sensory nerves in a particular body region.

Nervous system: The body system designed to carry information to and from all parts of the body in the form of nerve impulses; made up of the brain and spinal cord (central nervous system) and the remaining nerves and ganglia outside the brain and spinal cord (peripheral nervous system).

Nest: To surround a hospitalized baby with rolled blankets or other things (even the hands) that act as boundaries. Promotes behavioral organization and a feeling of security. See also **Containment, body.**

Neurochemical: Having to do with the chemistry of the nervous system.

Neurologist: A physician who specializes in the structure, function, diagnosis, and treatment of nervous system disorders.

Neuromuscular: Having to do with both the nerves and the muscles.

Neuron: A nerve cell specialized to transmit electrical nerve impulses and to carry information from one part of the body to another.

NICU: See **Neonatal intensive care unit; Level III nursery.**

Nitric oxide (NO) therapy: Therapy commonly used for treatment of persistent pulmonary hypertension of the newborn (PPHN), a serious condition in infants that causes high blood pressure in the arteries supplying blood to the lungs. When breathed into the lungs, NO relaxes the walls of the blood vessels near the breathing sacs, opening or enlarging those vessels and improving oxygen and carbon dioxide exchange.

NNP: Neonatal nurse practitioner. A registered nurse who has advanced education (usually a master's degree) in the care and treatment of newborns and their families. Working in collaboration with a neonatologist or attending physician, the NNP is an expert in neonatal resuscitation; examines, diagnoses, and designs a care plan for your baby; and serves as an education resource for all members of the NICU team. The NNP may also perform procedures such as intubation, central line placement, chest tube insertion, and lumbar puncture.

Nonnutritive sucking: Sucking on a pacifier or a finger (the baby's own finger or a caregiver's). Aids motor skill development. May enhance digestion and absorption of food and improve weight gain and oxygenation. Does not supply nutrition.

Nonpharmacologic: Without the use of drugs or medications.

Nonspecific sign: A change in body function that may be caused by any one of many disorders or illnesses.

NPA: Neonatal physician assistant. A physician assistant who has completed education and training in the care and treatment of infants and their families. The NPA works under the supervision of a neonatologist or attending physician. An NPA performs delivery room resuscitation and has been trained to assess, diagnose, and design a care plan for your baby. The NPA may also perform procedures such as intubation, central line placement, chest tube insertion, and lumbar puncture and may serve as an education resource for members of the NICU team.

NPO: Abbreviation of the Latin for a medical order meaning "nothing by mouth"; indicates that a patient should be given neither food nor fluids orally.

Nursery monitor: A listening device (transmitter) placed in a baby's room to allow caregivers in another room to hear (through the receiver) any equipment alarms or sounds the baby makes. The device is not attached to the baby and is not considered medical equipment.

Nursing supplementer: A device consisting of a bag or bottle to hold breast milk or formula and a tube that is taped beside a woman's nipple. Provides extra milk or supplemental nutrients to a nursing baby during the breastfeeding session.

Nutrients: Proteins, carbohydrates, fats, vitamins, and minerals that humans need for life.

O

Obstetrician: A physician trained to meet the special health care needs of women during pregnancy, labor, delivery, and the postpartum period.

Occupational therapist: A specially trained health care provider who uses structured activity to promote recovery or rehabilitation. In infants, may focus on developmental and behavioral tasks (such as feeding or positioning).

Oligohydramnios: A condition in which less amniotic fluid than normal surrounds the unborn baby in the uterus.

Omphalocele: A birth defect in which some or all of the intestine (or another abdominal organ) pushes out through the abdominal wall at the base of the umbilical cord.

Ophthalmologist: A physician who specializes in diagnosing and treating problems of the eye.

Opiate: A drug made from opium. Relieves pain; calms; and produces restfulness, lack of action, and often sleep. Sometimes used to refer to any narcotic.

Optic nerve: A nerve that controls sharpness of vision and ability to focus on and follow objects.

OR: Operating room.

Oral: Having to do with the mouth.

Oral feeding: Feeding a baby breast milk or formula; methods include, among others, gavage, bottle, and breast.

Oral-motor development: Having to do with the mouth and with movement. Ability to coordinate movements involving the muscles and nerves of the mouth—for example, the sucking movements used in feeding.

Organ: A body structure that performs a specific function. The heart, lungs, kidneys, liver, and brain are all organs.

Orogastric (OG) tube: A feeding tube inserted through a baby's mouth into the esophagus (food pipe) and on to the stomach. Formula or breast milk flows through the tube into the baby's stomach. Usually inserted at each feeding and removed afterward.

Orthopedic: Having to do with correction of problems in the bones and joints.

Orthopedist: A physician with specialized training in preventing, diagnosing, and treating problems with the bones (skeleton) and connective tissues.

Ostomy: A surgical opening into an organ or body part. See also **Colostomy, Gastrostomy, Ileostomy, Tracheostomy.**

Otolaryngologist: A physician with specialized training in diagnosing and treating problems of the ear, nose, and throat.

Ototoxic: A term for a medication with side effects that can cause hearing loss.

Outpatient clinic: A medical facility, staffed by a team of health care providers, at which individuals with medical problems are examined and treated without staying overnight.

Oxygen (O_2): A substance contained in air necessary for proper functioning of body cells. Absorbed into the blood from air breathed into the lungs (called *oxygenation*).

Oxygen, free-flow: A stream of air/oxygen mixture that flows from a tube placed near a baby's nose and mouth to provide a breathing baby with supplemental oxygen.

Oxygen, supplemental: An air/oxygen mixture provided to an infant who, because of prematurity or illness, requires a higher concentration of oxygen than the 21% found in room air.

Oxygenation: The level of oxygen in the blood. Also, supplying oxygen to the blood.

Oxygen hood: A clear plastic box or hood placed over a baby's head to hold supplemental oxygen. Also called an *oxyhood* or a *hood*.

Oxygen saturation monitor: See **Pulse oximeter.**

Oxygen tent: A plastic apparatus placed around a baby's upper body to contain supplemental oxygen.

Oxyhood: See **Oxygen hood.**

Oxytocin: A hormone that causes contractions (of the uterus during labor and of the muscles surrounding the milk glands in women who have just given birth). Produces the let-down (or milk-ejection) reflex.

P

Pacifier: A nipple-shaped device on which a baby can suck; provides no nutrition.

Palate: The roof of the mouth.

Pale: A term denoting a deficiency of skin color, usually caused by reduced blood flow through the skin.

Palliative care: A term for a service that provides relief from a condition but does not cure it. Includes pain management if needed, social support, and access to resources.

Paramedic: A specially trained medical technician who provides emergency services before or during transport to a hospital.

Patent: Open.

Patent ductus arteriosus (PDA): A ductus arteriosus that has not closed shortly after birth as it normally would. See also **Ductus arteriosus.**

Pathologist: A physician with specialized training in interpreting and identifying changes in the body caused by disease.

Pediatric developmentalist: A health care provider specially trained to evaluate and treat babies who are at risk or have problems mastering developmental skills, commonly because of preterm birth or a long hospital stay.

Pediatric neurologist: A physician who specializes in the structure, function, diagnosis, and treatment of nervous system disorders in babies and children.

Pediatric nurse: A registered nurse with special training in the care of children from birth to age 18 (sometimes up to age 21).

Pediatrician: A physician specially trained to diagnose and treat children from birth to age 18.

Percutaneous endoscopic gastrostomy (PEG) tube: A type of gastrostomy tube that can be inserted with an endoscope (a floppy tube with a light on the end). The endoscope guides placement of the tube as it is passed through the mouth, into the stomach, and out through a small hole made through the skin of the abdomen.

Perforate: To tear or rupture.

Perfusion: The passage of fluid through a tissue; especially refers to blood passing through the lungs to pick up oxygen.

Perinatal: The period before and after birth; a broad definition is from week 20 of pregnancy until 1 month after birth.

Perinatal center: The maternal-fetal-neonatal components of a regional medical center.

Perinatologist: A physician specially trained in diagnosing and treating problems of the pregnant woman and the fetus during pregnancy, labor, delivery, and postpartum.

Peripheral line: See **Intravenous (IV) catheter/line.**

Peritonitis: An infection of the abdominal cavity.

Periventricular leukomalacia (PVL): Damaged brain tissue resulting in brain cysts, usually as a result of brain hemorrhage.

Permeability, skin: In newborns, refers to the ability of the skin to absorb substances such as applied lotions and oils and to the skin's susceptibility to water loss and heat loss. Has to do with the ability of liquids or gases to pass through (penetrate) tiny openings in the skin.

Persistent pulmonary hypertension of the newborn (PPHN): A serious condition in which high blood pressure (hypertension) in the arteries supplying blood to the lungs forces blood away from the lungs, decreasing the amount of oxygen in the blood going to the body.

Phototherapy: Light treatment for hyperbilirubinemia. Light waves break down indirect bilirubin so that the baby's system can eliminate it in urine.

Physical therapist: A specially trained health care provider who uses physical and mechanical methods (such as exercise; electric current treatment; massage; and water, light, and heat treatments) to promote recovery or rehabilitation. Also known as a *physiotherapist.*

Physiologic: Having to do with normal body processes.

Placenta: An organ inside the uterus that attaches the developing baby to the wall of the uterus. Provides the fetus with nutrients, eliminates wastes, and exchanges respiratory gases. Commonly called the *afterbirth* because it is expelled after the birth of the baby.

Placenta previa: A placenta that is positioned low in the uterus and partly or completely covers the opening of the uterus. Potentially dangerous to mother and baby because of a risk of bleeding before or during delivery.

Placental abruption: Separation of the placenta from the uterine wall before delivery of a baby. Causes bleeding that can be life-threatening for both the unborn baby and the mother.

Platelet: A component of the blood involved in clotting. Also called a *thrombocyte*.

Pneumocardiogram (PCG): A test that may help determine the cause of apnea and bradycardia. Philosophies vary regarding use, and not all NICUs use them. Interpretation varies regionally. Test equipment is similar to the cardiorespiratory monitor but has channels to record heart rate, respirations, air flow through the nose, and oxygen saturation. Also called a *sleep study* or a *pneumogram*.

Pneumomediastinum: Leakage of air into the space in the center of the chest containing the heart and major blood vessels.

Pneumonia: Inflammation or infection of the lungs.

Pneumopericardium: Collection of air in the sac around the heart; life-threatening.

Pneumothorax: Air trapped between the lung and the chest wall. Also called a *pulmonary air leak*.

Polyhydramnios: A condition in which more amniotic fluid than normal is present in the mother's uterus during pregnancy. Sometimes a sign of a fetal anomaly.

Postnatal: Taking place after birth.

Postoperative: The period after surgery.

Postpartum: Taking place after delivery of a baby.

Precipitous birth: An unusually fast vaginal delivery; by strict definition, a labor and birth that takes 3 hours or less.

Preeclampsia: A term used to denote renal involvement caused by gestational hypertension. A woman with this condition is said to be preeclamptic.

Preemie: A preterm or premature baby, or used to describe something used by a preterm baby.

Preemie nipple: A small, soft, pliable nipple designed for bottle-feeding a baby with a weak or immature suck. Provides more formula with less sucking effort.

Premature: A term for a baby born before week 38 of gestation. Also called *preterm*.

Premature rupture of membranes (PROM): Term used when the amniotic sac breaks ("water breaks") prior to the onset of labor. If the amniotic sac breaks prior to the onset of labor contractions and before the 38th week of gestation, the condition is called *preterm premature rupture of membranes*.

Prematurity: The condition of being born early, before week 38 of gestation.

Prenatal: Having to do with the period before birth.

Preterm: See **Premature.**

Primary nurse: A nurse who works with a baby and his/her family throughout the hospitalization to coordinate care and teach and support the family.

Progesterone: The hormone that stimulates growth of the endometrium (lining of the uterus); needed for growth of a fertilized egg.

Prognosis: The outlook or forecast for a baby's recovery or future condition.

Prolactin: A hormone that causes the milk glands to begin secreting milk in the breasts of a woman who has just given birth. Released by the body whenever the nipples of a postpartum woman are stimulated.

Prolonged rupture of membranes: Term used when 12 to 24 hours or more pass after the amniotic sac breaks without delivery of the newborn. Because the amniotic sac provides a barrier to infection, the infant can be at risk for infection if labor and delivery do not occur for a prolonged period after the membranes rupture.

Prone: Lying on the stomach.

Prophylactic treatment: Treatment designed to prevent something from developing or occurring.

Protocol: A standard plan or standard instructions for a specific situation.

Psychologist: A care provider (not a physician) who specializes in diagnosing and treating mental and behavioral problems.

Public Law (PL) 94-142: Education for All Handicapped Children Act. A 1975 federal law requiring special education programs for all disabled children from 6 to 21 years of age.

Public Law (PL) 99-457, part H: Education of the Handicapped Amendments. A 1986 federal law providing early intervention programs for disabled or at-risk babies (from birth to age 2) and offering incentives for states to expand services for disabled children between ages 3 and 5.

Pulmonary: Having to do with the lungs.

Pulmonary atresia: A cyanotic heart defect in which the valve that allows blood to flow from the right ventricle of the heart to the lungs (the pulmonary valve) is absent.

Pulmonary edema: Leakage of fluid into the tissues of the lungs.

Pulmonary hypoplasia: A term describing limited lung development, resulting in inadequate blood flow to the lungs. May be a consequence of congenital diaphragmatic hernia, abnormal kidney development, inadequate amniotic fluid, or other problems that cause inadequate fetal breathing movement.

Pulmonary interstitial emphysema (PIE): Leakage of air from torn breathing sacs (alveoli) in the lungs into spaces around the lung tissue.

Pulmonary stenosis: A birth defect in which the valve that allows blood to flow from the heart to the lungs is narrowed, reducing blood flow through the pulmonary artery to the lungs. May be isolated or combined with other heart defects.

Pulmonary valve: A heart valve that opens to allow blood to flow from the right ventricle through the pulmonary artery and to the lungs.

Pulmonologist: A physician who specializes in the structure and function of the lungs and diagnosis and treatment of breathing difficulties and problems of the lungs.

Pulse: A measurement of the rate at which the heart is beating; the heart rate.

Pulse oximeter: A device that wraps around the hand or foot of an infant and uses a light sensor to determine the amount of oxygen bound to the hemoglobin molecules in the blood. A general indicator of a baby's oxygenation. Also called an *oxygen saturation monitor*.

R

R-1: A resident in the first year of a physician training program. Formerly called an *intern*.

R-2: A resident in the second year of a physician training program.

R-3: A resident in the third year of a physician training program.

Radiant warmer: An open mattress, usually on a mobile cart, with a heat source above it. Used to stabilize and warm a baby immediately after delivery, for easy access to the baby during caregiving in the NICU, and in other situations (during in-hospital transport and during surgery, for example). The baby is said to be "on a warmer."

Radiation: A type of energy involved in x-rays. Large amounts can damage body tissues and cells.

Radiology: The branch of medicine that performs and interprets radiographic (x-ray) and ultrasound procedures.

Recovery: A restoration period when a patient is to regain health or strength.

Rectal: Having to do with the rectum, the lower part of the intestine just inside the anus.

Rectal temperature: The body temperature taken by inserting a blunt-end thermometer into the lower part of the intestine just inside the anus (the rectum).

Rectal thermometer: A device inserted into the rectum to measure body temperature.

Rectum: The lower part of the intestine just inside the anus.

Red blood cell (RBC): A part of the blood that contains hemoglobin, which carries oxygen to the tissues of the body.

Referral: A recommendation for a care provider.

Reflexes, feeding: Unconscious, automatic responses of the nerves to certain kinds of stimuli. Includes gagging, sucking, swallowing, and rooting reflexes.

Reflux, gastroesophageal: The backward flow of stomach contents into the esophagus (food pipe); in infants, may trigger apnea and/or bradycardia.

Regional medical center: A hospital facility, often associated with a university, staffed with medical specialists. Provides patient care, research, and regional education and consultation. Also called a *tertiary care center*.

Registered nurse: See **RN.**

Regressive behavior: A return to past ways of acting, often to less mature approaches. May be seen in children under stress or who want attention—for example, bed-wetting may be regressive behavior in a toilet-trained preschooler.

Rehabilitation facility: See **Transitional care facility.**

Renal: Having to do with the kidneys.

Rescue therapy: Treatment given for an existing medical problem (as opposed to prophylactic therapy, which is given to treat an anticipated problem). For example, surfactant replacement therapy can be given as a prophylactic therapy (immediately following delivery) or as rescue therapy (after respiratory distress syndrome is diagnosed).

Resident: A physician who has graduated from medical school and has progressed to the first year of a residency program (a hospital-based program of specialized training). A physician in his second year of training (R-2) or third year of training (R-3) usually instructs R-1s and works with senior residents and/or attending physicians. Many residents in NICUs are enrolled in pediatric residencies.

Residual: Food remaining in the stomach from the previous feeding at the time of the next feeding. Large residuals indicate feeding intolerance.

Respirations: Breaths.

Respirator: See **Ventilator.**

Respiratory: Having to do with breathing.

Respiratory care practitioner: A health care provider who specializes in treating problems of the respiratory (breathing) system.

Respiratory depression: A reduction in or lack of breathing effort.

Respiratory distress syndrome (RDS): A condition that affects the lungs of preterm newborns, making it difficult for them to breathe. Caused by a lack of surfactant. Sometimes called *hyaline membrane disease.*

Respiratory syncytial virus (RSV): A virus that commonly causes infections of the upper and lower respiratory tract; the major cause of bronchiolitis and pneumonia in young children.

Respiratory therapist (RT): See **Respiratory care practitioner.**

Respite care: The assumption of total care for an ill or disabled individual by an outside facility or individual for a short time to permit the regular caregiver(s) to rest, relax, and re-energize.

Resuscitate/resuscitation: To restore breathing and/or heart and circulatory function when either or both are functioning insufficiently to support life.

Reticulocyte ("retic") count: A laboratory test that shows how many red blood cells the body is producing. A reticulocyte is an immature red blood cell.

Retina: The light-sensitive lining of the interior of an eye. Receives visual images.

Retinopathy of prematurity (ROP): A disease affecting the retina of a preterm baby's eye. Involves rapid, irregular growth of blood vessels that can lead to bleeding and scarring of the retina. Can cause retinal detachment and blindness if severe.

Retraction: The drawing in of the chest wall with each breath. Most visible at the breast-bone, between the ribs, and above the collarbone. Generally indicates difficulty breathing.

Return transport: See **Back transport.**

Risk factor: Something (usually some characteristic or physical condition) that makes it more likely that a baby will experience problems.

RN: Registered nurse. A designation of state licensure. A person can prepare for state licensure as an RN by graduating from a diploma program (hospital training), a 2-year college (associate degree) program, or a 4-year university program (bachelor's degree).

Robin sequence: Birth defects involving the skull and face: micrognathia (abnormally small jaw) in association with cleft palate and glossoptosis (displacement of the tongue). Causes breathing difficulty because of a blocked upper airway.

Rooming-in: Staying overnight at the hospital with your baby shortly before discharge; a "trial run" when parents care for their baby independently and use nursing staff only if necessary.

Rooting reflex: A baby's response to stroking of the face: head turns in the direction of the stroking and mouth opens.

Rotation, physician: For residents, the changing of assignment from one patient care specialty area to another; often takes place about once a month. Attending physicians, fellows, and interns may also rotate.

Rounds: Daily patient visits during which members of the health care team discuss and review each patient's condition and medical plan. In some NICUs, parents participate in rounds for their baby.

S

Saline, normal: A liquid solution containing 0.9% sodium chloride; used to dilute some drugs for injection; also used to flush fluid through an IV line and ensure patency. Normal saline can also be used to increase plasma volume and thereby increase blood pressure.

Saturation, oxygen: The degree to which oxygen is bound to hemoglobin (a substance in red blood cells). Expressed as a percentage. Pulse oximetry is used to monitor oxygen saturation.

Screening test: A structured examination or review by a health care professional to identify potential or existing physical, mental, behavioral, or emotional problems.

Scrotum: In males, the pouch between the legs that contains the testes.

Secretion: A substance (such as mucus) produced by a gland and released to an external or internal body surface.

Sedate: To medicate to calm excitement or agitation.

Seizure: Abnormal brain electrical activity often accompanied by involuntary muscle contraction and relaxation (spasms).

Self-comforting: A term for a behavioral skill in which a baby takes actions (brings the hands to the mouth; sucks on a finger, a fist, or a pacifier; or clasps the hands together) to make himself or herself feel better. Facilitates behavioral organization.

Sensory system: The body system made up of the organs used to see, hear, feel, taste, and touch.

Separation anxiety: Concern or anxiousness about what will happen when one leaves a familiar environment or familiar people for an unknown situation.

Sepsis: The presence of harmful microorganisms in the blood and their effects on the body; a general infection.

Sepsis workup: The collection and laboratory culture (growth) of blood, urine, and/or spinal fluid samples to determine whether microorganisms are present in them. Used to identify the presence of infection.

Septal defect: A birth defect marked by a hole in the wall (the septum) separating the left and right sides of the heart. May be atrial or ventricular.

Septicemia: An infection in the blood.

Sequela: A consequence that results from a preceding disease. For example, visual impairment is a potential sequela of retinopathy of prematurity.

Servomechanism/servocontrol: A thermostat mechanism for regulating the body temperature of an infant on a radiant warmer or in an incubator. A skin temperature probe senses the infant's skin temperature and decreases or increases the heat source when the skin temperature is above or below a preset level.

Sexually transmitted infection (STI): An infection passed from one person to another during sexual activity.

Shock: An unstable condition marked by circulatory collapse: inadequate blood flow, insufficient oxygen to the tissues, and inadequate removal of waste products from them. Can occur in the presence of sepsis, acute blood loss, heart problems, or allergic reaction.

Short bowel syndrome: Having only a small length of healthy bowel (potential sequela of a disease like necrotizing enterocolitis); limits the bowel's ability to absorb nutrients and water from the stool. Also called *short gut.*

Short gut: See **Short bowel syndrome.**

Shunt: A thin tube used to drain fluid from one area of the body to another. Also, an abnormal connection between 2 areas of the body (as in a patent ductus arteriosus in a newborn).

Shunt, left-to-right: In newborns, a blood circulation pattern in which some of the blood leaving the heart flows back from the aorta into the lungs through a patent ductus arteriosus. Generally seen in a baby recovering from respiratory distress syndrome. The overabundance of blood entering the lungs can lead to signs and symptoms of a patent ductus arteriosus (for example, worsening respiratory problems).

Shunt, right-to-left: In newborns, a blood circulation pattern in which some of the blood entering the heart is directed away from the blood vessels in the lungs, which are narrowed by the effects of respiratory distress syndrome or pulmonary hypertension, causing oxygen-poor blood to be sent to the body.

Sibling: A brother or sister.

Side effect: A secondary effect of a medication or drug; can be undesirable.

SIDS: See **Sudden infant death syndrome.**

Sleep study: See **Pneumocardiogram.**

Small for gestational age (SGA): Term for a newborn whose weight (and possibly length and head circumference) falls below the 10th percentile on a standard intrauterine growth chart; indicates small size for the length of time the baby was in the uterus. An SGA baby can be preterm, term, or post-term.

Social worker: An individual on the hospital staff who has training (and usually a master's degree) in helping patients and their families cope with stress, deal with financial concerns related to the hospitalization, use hospital and community resources, and prepare for discharge.

Socioeconomic status: In combination, the social and financial factors that determine a person's position in society relative to others.

Sonographer: A medical technician who performs ultrasounds.

Spastic diplegia: Stiffness and awkward movement of the limbs; a form of cerebral palsy.

Special care nursery: A unit in a hospital that has staff trained to care for any baby requiring more than routine, well-born care. In some hospitals, the term may denote a unit for babies requiring intermediate or convalescent care.

Special needs infant: A baby who requires technological support or medications to live or who requires special intervention and attention to develop and grow normally.

Spina bifida: A birth defect in which the spinal column does not close completely and the covering of the spinal cord pushes out through the gap between the vertebrae, forming an external sac. Myelomeningocele is one type.

Spinal tap: See **Lumbar puncture.**

State, behavioral: Level of awareness. Babies experience these 6 states: deep sleep, light sleep, drowsy, quiet alert, active alert, and crying.

Stenosis: A birth defect in which a passage (such as a valve, a vein, or an artery) is narrowed. Flow through the passage is limited.

Stenotic: Having to do with a stenosis.

Stenotic lesion: An abnormal narrowing of a blood vessel or valve.

Step-down unit: A hospital nursery for recuperating babies that provides less intensive care than that given in a NICU; may be called an *intermediate care unit (ICU),* a *Level II unit,* or a *special care unit.*

Steroid: A drug given in the NICU to reduce inflammation and raise blood pressure.

STI: See **Sexually transmitted infection.**

Stimulation, oral: Sensory input (either positive or negative) to the area in and around the baby's mouth.

Stimulation, tactile: Gentle alerting of a baby by touching, stroking, rubbing, or flicking a body surface such as the soles of the feet. Used in this way to encourage breathing in an apneic infant.

Stimulus: Something that excites, alerts, or promotes activity (plural: stimuli).

Stoma: The artificial opening of a hollow organ. For a colostomy, the stoma is on the abdomen. For a tracheostomy, the stoma is on the neck.

Stool: Feces; the result of a bowel movement.

Streptococcus, Group B beta-hemolytic: A type of bacteria sometimes found in the vagina and rectum; usually harmless for a pregnant woman; however, can cause pneumonia and meningitis in an exposed newborn. Newborn risk is reduced through maternal screening at 36–37 weeks of pregnancy; GBS+ women are treated with intravenous (IV) antibiotics during labor.

Stress: The body's response to disturbances in the environment (including emotional concerns), to pain, and often to infection. Signs include changes in heart rate, breathing patterns, blood pressure, and oxygen consumption. Also called *physiologic stress.*

Stress, environmental: Irritation caused by disturbance from light, sound, and temperature in the area around (environment of) a baby. Can produce physical (physiologic) changes in heart rate, breathing patterns, blood pressure, and/or oxygen consumption.

Stressor: Something that causes stress.

Subarachnoid: Located below the innermost membrane covering the brain.

Subdural: Located below the outermost membrane covering the brain.

Subependymal: Located beneath the lining of the brain chambers (the ventricles).

Subglottic stenosis: A narrowing of the trachea (windpipe); may be caused by prolonged mechanical ventilation or repeated intubations.

Substance abuse: Misuse or excessive use of a legal or illegal drug or a substance containing a drug.

Suction: Mechanical removal (drawing out) of air or fluid from the body.

Sudden infant death syndrome (SIDS): The sudden death of an infant younger than 1 year that remains unexplained after a thorough case investigation, including performance of a complete autopsy, examination of the death scene, and review of the clinical history. Also called *crib death* or *cot death.*

Suffocation: An inability to breathe, as with drowning or smothering; can cause unconsciousness or death.

Support group: A group of individuals who meet to share a common concern or focus. Intended to promote sharing of information, feelings, and concerns.

Surfactant: A soap-like substance (made up mainly of fat) produced by lung cells. Coats inner surfaces of airways and air sacs in the lungs to keep those passages open between breaths. Absent or lacking in babies born preterm (production begins at about 24 weeks' gestation but is not well developed until 36 weeks). Also, a manufactured substitute (exogenous surfactant) used to treat respiratory distress syndrome in preterm infants.

Surfactant replacement therapy: A treatment in which a preterm infant with expected or confirmed respiratory distress syndrome is given a natural or artificial substance (called an *exogenous surfactant)* through a tube placed in the windpipe (trachea) to replace the natural surfactant the baby lacks because of early birth.

Suture: The material used to sew up a surgical wound or close an incision. Can also refer to the thin line of connective tissue between 2 bones, as in "cranial suture."

Syndrome: A pattern of signs and/or symptoms occurring together that form a clinical picture indicative of a specific disorder.

Syringe: A device for injecting fluids into or withdrawing them from the body or for washing out a body cavity.

System, body: The series of interdependent body parts (organs, vessels, muscles, nerves, and so on) that work together to accomplish something; the heart and the blood vessels, for example, make up the cardiovascular system, through which blood moves to every part of the body.

Systemic: Having to do with or affecting the whole body.

T

Tachycardia: A faster than normal heart rate.

Tachycardic: A term for a baby whose heart rate is faster than normal.

Tachypnea: A faster than normal breathing rate.

Tachypneic: A term for a baby who is breathing faster than normal.

Teaching hospital: A hospital associated with a university; offers programs designed to accommodate learning needs of students in health care–related fields of study.

Technician: A trained hospital staff member who performs a specific function, often related to a diagnostic procedure.

Technology: An application of knowledge to achieve a desired outcome. In the NICU, technology includes state-of-the-art equipment and therapy used to treat infants.

Technology dependent: Needing mechanical equipment to survive.

Teratogen: An environmental agent (such as a drug, chemical, or toxin) that can cause birth defects if the fetus is exposed to it during development, especially during the first 3 months.

Term: A word for a baby born between the beginning of week 38 and the end of week 42 of gestation.

Tertiary care center: See **Regional medical center.**

Test weight: Method used in some NICUs to assess the infant's intake of breast milk after breastfeeding. Baby is weighed on an electronic scale (clothed and diapered) before and after feeding. Increase in grams equals intake in milliliters of breast milk.

Tetralogy of Fallot: A cyanotic heart defect involving 4 abnormalities of the heart and its vessels: a ventricular septal defect (VSD), pulmonary stenosis, an overly muscular right ventricle, and positioning of the aorta over the VSD.

Theophylline: A medication that stimulates the central nervous system. Given to reduce occurrences of apnea in selected babies.

Therapeutic hypothermia: Method of head cooling or body cooling used to treat newborns with hypoxic-ischemic encephalopathy (HIE) in an effort to protect the brain from long-term damage.

Thermal stress: Undesirable changes in the body's vital signs caused by high or low environmental temperatures.

Thirdhand smoke: contamination from tobacco products that remains after the item is extinguished; for example, thirdhand smoke is found on clothing of a smoker or furniture or car where smoker uses tobacco. Infants and children risk exposure to neurotoxic chemicals when they breathe, touch, or mouth smoke-contaminated surfaces.

Thoracic: Having to do with the chest.

Thrombocyte: See **Platelet.**

Thrombocytopenia: A term for a low platelet count.

Thrush: A yeast (fungal) infection common in babies who have been on antibiotics; appears as a patchy white coating on the tongue and gums or as a persistent, pebbly diaper rash.

Tidal volume: The amount of air breathed in (inhaled) and breathed out (exhaled) with one normal breath.

Time-out: A method used to calm an infant and facilitate behavioral organization; involves decreasing sound, light, and movement for a time.

Titrate: To adjust the dose of a drug to use the smallest amount that will produce a desired effect.

Tocotransducer ("toco"): The component of external electronic fetal monitoring that senses pressure changes on the pregnant woman's abdomen. Used to monitor frequency and duration of uterine contractions.

Tolerance: In reference to a drug, the need over time for an increasingly higher dose to achieve the same effect.

Tolerate: In reference to a baby receiving breast milk or formula, to retain, digest, and absorb the feeding.

Tongue-tied: See **Ankyloglossia.**

Topical: Applied to a limited surface area of the skin and affecting only that area.

Topical anesthetic: A preparation applied to the skin surface to numb it, temporarily blocking feeling in the area to which it is applied.

TORCH: A term that stands for the names of intrauterine, or congenital, infections that can cross the placenta to the fetus: toxoplasmosis, other viruses, rubella virus, cytomegalovirus, and herpes simplex virus.

Total anomalous pulmonary venous connection or return (TAPVR): A cyanotic heart defect in which the veins that return oxygenated blood from the lungs to the heart are not connected to the left atrium as they should be, but instead the blood drains through abnormal connections to the right atrium, mixes with unoxygenated blood, and passes through an atrial septal defect into the left atrium and out to the body.

Total parenteral nutrition (TPN): The provision of essential nutrients (proteins, fats, sugar, vitamins, and minerals) and water through an intravenous line to replace or supplement a baby's intake by mouth.

Trach (pronounced "trake"): See **Tracheostomy.**

Trachea: The windpipe.

Tracheoesophageal (T-E) fistula: A birth defect marked by an abnormal connection between the trachea (windpipe) and the esophagus (food pipe).

Tracheomalacia: A condition in which the airway is soft and collapses during breathing.

Tracheostomy: A surgical opening through the neck and into the windpipe (trachea) through which a breathing tube is inserted.

Tracheostomy tube: A breathing tube inserted into the windpipe (trachea) through a surgical opening in the neck.

Transcutaneous monitor (TCM): A device placed on the skin that, when calibrated with a laboratory test called a *blood gas,* approximates the oxygen and carbon dioxide levels in the blood.

Transducer: A device that converts energy from one form to another.

Transfusion: The giving of fluid, such as whole blood or a blood component (such as red blood cells, to treat anemia), directly into the bloodstream through a catheter.

Transfusion, exchange: A method for replacing (exchanging) a portion of the blood volume through repeated removal of small amounts of blood and replacement with equal amounts of donor blood. Done to reduce the concentration of undesirable elements in the blood, such as excess bilirubin.

Transient tachypnea of the newborn (TTN): A respiratory condition caused by delay in the body's absorption after birth of the fluid that fills the fetal lungs.

Transillumination: An assessment/diagnostic technique that involves shining a bright light through body tissues.

Transitional care: The level of medical care that falls between what is provided in a hospital and what can be provided in the home.

Transitional care facility: A facility that provides care that falls between what is provided in a hospital and what can be provided in the home. The goal is independent caregiving and discharge home. Also called a *rehabilitation hospital.*

Transposition of the great arteries: A cyanotic heart defect in which the pulmonary artery (which normally carries unoxygenated blood to the lungs) and the aorta (which carries oxygenated blood to the body) are reversed, resulting in oxygen-poor blood being sent to the body.

Transpyloric feeding: Feeding through a tube that descends beyond the stomach and is placed in the upper intestine.

Tricuspid atresia: A cyanotic heart defect in which the valve that allows blood to flow from the right atrium of the heart to the right ventricle (the tricuspid valve) is absent.

Trisomy 21: See **Down syndrome.**

Trophic feeds: Tiny amounts of milk, preferably breast milk, given as first feedings to prepare a very premature baby's immature intestines for digesting nutrition. Also called *minimal enteral nutrition (MEN)* or *gut priming.*

Truncus arteriosus: A complex heart defect in which only one artery (a combination of the aorta and the pulmonary artery) leaves the heart.

Tube feeding: See **Gavage feeding.**

Tuberculosis: A communicable disease affecting the lungs. Caused by a bacterium.

Tympanic thermometer: A device that measures body temperature through a probe inserted a short distance into the ear.

U

UAC: See **Catheter, umbilical arterial.**

Ultrasonography: A diagnostic imaging technique that uses reflections of high-frequency sound waves (called *echoes)* to make 2-dimensional images of internal body structures, tissues, and blood flow; often used to scan the brain. Does not involve radiation. Often can be done at the baby's bedside.

Umbilical cord: A cord connecting the fetus with the placenta. Contains 2 arteries and 1 vein. Is clamped and cut at birth. The location at which it attaches to the infant becomes the navel (belly button).

Umbilical hernia: A skin-covered protrusion of part of the intestine through a weakness in the abdominal wall at the navel (the umbilicus).

Umbilicus: The navel or belly button.

Uterus: In a woman, the organ that surrounds and protects the unborn baby (fetus) during development and until birth; the womb.

UVC: See **Catheter, umbilical venous.**

V

Vaccine: A killed or less-powerful version of a bacterium or a virus given to stimulate the development of antibodies (blood protein that attacks any foreign substance) and thus give immunity (resistance to infection) to disease.

Vacuum extraction: A method of birth assistance in which a suction cup is applied to the top of the unborn baby's head in the final pushing stage of labor; working with uterine contractions, the physician applies gentle traction to assist with delivery of the baby's head.

Validate: To ensure that someone understands what has been said, perhaps by asking the person to repeat the information in his or her own words.

Vasoconstriction: The narrowing, tightening, or partial closure of blood vessels, reducing blood flow through them and producing more resistance to flow.

Vasodilate: To widen or open blood vessels. Produces less resistance to flow.

Vasodilator: A drug that widens or opens blood vessels, reducing resistance to flow.

Vasopressor: Medication used to increase blood pressure, increase strength of cardiac contractions, and increase heart rate. Dobutamine and dopamine are vasopressors. Sometimes called *pressors*.

Venoarterial (VA) bypass: A technique used to start extracorporeal membrane oxygenation therapy. Involves inserting parallel catheters into the right side of the neck. One, placed in a vein, is threaded into the upper right chamber of the heart; the other, placed in the carotid artery, is threaded to the aortic arch. Insertion of the catheters is called *cannulation*.

Venoarterial extracorporeal membrane oxygenation (VA ECMO) therapy: A therapy used to treat babies who have both lung and heart function or blood pressure problems; requires insertion of 2 catheters, one in a vein and the other in an artery. Blood is drained from the upper right chamber of the infant's heart by gravity through the catheter in the vein, carbon dioxide is removed, oxygen is added, and the blood is then warmed and pumped back to the aortic arch and into the baby's body through the catheter in the artery. The ECMO equipment circuit includes a membrane oxygenator (artificial lung) and a pump. See also **Extracorporeal membrane oxygenation.**

Venovenous (VV) bypass: A technique used to start extracorporeal membrane oxygenation therapy; involves inserting a double lumen catheter into a large vein in the right side of the neck and threading it into the upper right chamber of the heart. Insertion of the catheter is called *cannulation*.

Venovenous extracorporeal membrane oxygenation (VV ECMO) therapy: A therapy used to treat babies who have lung problems but whose heart function and blood pressure are normal; requires insertion of a split catheter into a vein in the neck. Blood is drained from the upper right chamber of the heart by gravity through one side of the tube, carbon dioxide is removed, oxygen is added, and the blood is then warmed and pumped back into the baby's heart through the other side of the catheter. The ECMO equipment circuit includes a membrane oxygenator (artificial lung) and a pump. See also **Extracorporeal membrane oxygenation.**

Ventilation: Mechanical breathing assistance; passage of air in and out of the airways.

Ventilator: A mechanical device that assists breathing and supplies an air/oxygen mixture under pressure. Used with an endotracheal tube or tracheostomy tube. Also called a *respirator*.

Ventricle: A small chamber; one of the central chambers in the brain or 1 of the 2 lower chambers of the heart.

Ventricular septal defect (VSD): A birth defect marked by a hole in the wall (septum) between the 2 lower chambers (ventricles) of the heart.

Vernix caseosa: Greasy white or yellow, cheeselike material from fetal oil glands; made up of skin cells and fine hairs that cover the skin of the fetus. Protects the fetal skin from abrasions, chapping, and hardening before birth.

Very low birth weight (VLBW) infant: Any infant who weighs less than 1,500 grams (3 pounds, 5 ounces) at birth, regardless of gestational age.

Virus: An infectious microorganism that can live and multiply in the cells of the body.

Visual: Having to do with sight.

Vital signs: Body temperature, pulse (heart) rate, and rate of respirations (breathing) and, if clinically indicated, blood pressure.

Vulnerable child syndrome: A tendency to continue to see a child who was once sick or physically disabled as still sickly or very susceptible to disease or injury despite normal findings on physical examination.

W

Warmer: See **Radiant warmer.**

Wean: To gradually stop one method of doing something and accustom the baby to another method; commonly used in reference to removal of a baby from technological support, such as weaning from the ventilator to independent breathing. To slowly decrease the use of an intervention, such as a medication.

White blood cell (WBC): The part of the blood that plays a role in defending against infection.

X

X-ray: An electromagnetic wave that produces an image of internal body parts. Used in diagnosis.

Y

Yeast infection: Infection with a fungus such as *Candida.* An oral yeast infection, called *thrush,* is common in babies who have been treated with antibiotics. Babies may get this type of infection in their mouths; nursing mothers may get it on their nipples. A systemic yeast infection (in the blood) can be life-threatening for NICU babies.

Index

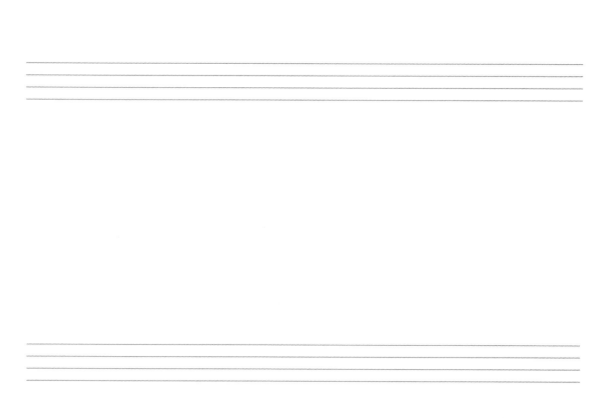